East Coast Fever

The Disease, its Impact and Control

East Coast Fever

The Disease, its Impact and Control

Edited by

W. Ivan Morrison PhD, BVMS, FRC Path

and

Philip Toye PhD, BVSc, Dip. Immunology

CABI

CABI is a trading name of CAB International

CABI
Nosworthy Way
Wallingford
Oxfordshire OX10 8DE
UK

Tel: +44 (0)1491 832111
E-mail: info@cabi.org
Website: www.cabi.org

CABI
200 Portland Street
Boston
MA 02114
USA

T: +1 (617)682-9015
E-mail: cabi-nao@cabi.org

A catalogue record for this book is available from the British Library, London, UK.

ISBN-13: 9781800626300 (hardback)
9781800626317 (ePDF)
9781800626324 (ePub)

DOI: 10.1079/9781800626324.0000

Commissioning Editor: Alex Lainsbury
Editorial Assistant: Theresa Regueira
Production Editor: Rosie Hayden

Typeset by Exeter Premedia Services Pvt Ltd, Chennai, India
Printed and bound in the UK by CPI Group (UK) Ltd, Croydon, CR0 4YY

Contents

Preface

The tick-borne protozoan parasite *Theileria parva* causes an acute, often fatal disease of cattle in Africa known as East Coast fever (ECF). The parasite is found only in Africa and is believed to have evolved in the African buffalo (*Syncerus caffer*), which is fully susceptible to infection but does not suffer disease. The presence of the parasite throughout a large part of eastern and southern Africa is dictated by the distribution of the main tick vector, *Rhipicephalus appendiculatus*. All buffalo residing in tick-infested areas, as well as cattle that have recovered from infection, harbour low-level, persistent infections with *T. parva*.

ECF is one of the most devastating diseases of cattle on the African continent. The acute and frequently fatal nature of the disease, the presence of the buffalo reservoir and the widespread distribution of the parasite and tick vector present major challenges to achieving effective control of ECF. Despite intensive research efforts over the past century, control still relies largely on frequent application of acaricide to reduce tick infestation. Consequently, the disease imposes a major financial burden on livestock producers, particularly smallholder, resource-poor farmers, whose livelihood is heavily dependent on cattle. Although some indigenous populations of cattle are able to survive in ECF-endemic areas, they are of relatively low productivity. Genetic improvement through interbreeding with more productive European taurine breeds is thwarted by the high susceptibility of these breeds to ECF.

Cattle are the most numerous domestic ruminant species in Africa and the most important source of animal products for human food consumption. They will continue to be a vital source of human dietary protein for the foreseeable future. However, given the impact of livestock on the global carbon footprint, there will be increasing pressure to improve the efficiency of generating cattle products. As ECF is one of the most important diseases that constrain productivity, more efficient and sustainable methods to control the disease are urgently needed.

In addition to its economic importance, *T. parva* is of significant comparative biological interest. It is a member of the apicomplexan group of parasites, which includes other important human and animal pathogens, most notably those causing human malaria. These pathogens each have distinct, complex life cycles, but much can be gained by recognition of common features in their host–parasite relationships and immunobiology. The capacity of *T. parva* and several other *Theileria* species to transform their host leucocytes into a proliferative, cancer-like state is unique among eukaryotic pathogens. The ability to cultivate these parasitized cells as continuously growing cell lines and to reverse their transformed state by removal of the parasite presents an attractive model for studying mammalian cell transformation, which has attracted the interest of cancer biologists.

The origins of this book arose from our discussions of the current state of knowledge of *T. parva* and the viability and sustainability of efforts to control ECF. As we neared retirement from several decades of active research on *T. parva* and stepped back from our respective areas of interest, we concluded that there was a need to assemble current information on the disease. The most recent book dedicated to theileriosis was published over 30 years ago and was focused largely on the epidemiology of the disease. This volume aims to provide a broad account of the available knowledge of the parasite and the disease, including current and potential measures aimed at its control. To this end, we have been fortunate to attract research leaders in different disciplines to contribute chapters to the book. Since there is a wealth of information on ECF in historical literature, which is not easily accessible by today's researchers, we have encouraged authors to include such information where relevant. In the final chapter of the book, we have attempted to identify gaps in the knowledge of ECF that we believe need to be addressed in future research, focusing particularly on aspects that will underpin development of new control measures to mitigate the effects of this important disease.

W.I. Morrison
P.G. Toye

Foreword

Graduating from the University of Queensland School of Veterinary Science in 1962, I spent a decade employed as a veterinary diagnostic pathologist and experimental pathologist/neuropathologist at the Queensland Department of Primary Industries Animal Research Institute (ARI), Brisbane, then at the Moredun Research Institute, Edinburgh. A 'side job' at the ARI was to be on the weekend veterinarian roster for monitoring the clinical status of stud cattle injected with blood containing vaccine strains of *Babesia bovis* and *B. bigemina* (grown up in splenectomized calves). Elevated body temperature was a primary indicator for drug treatment to reduce parasite load and protect these 'valuable vaccinees'. At that time, a similar 'infection and treatment' vaccination regime was being developed in Africa for *Theileria parva*, the cause of East Coast fever (ECF) and the subject of this book. LL (Bill) Callow, who ran the Queensland *Babesia* vaccine programme, served as a Board member of the International Laboratory for Research on Animal Diseases (ILRAD) in Nairobi. Much later in my career, I was to follow Bill in serving as a Board member of ILRAD (now the International Livestock Research Institute, ILRI), where a lot of great research has been done on ECF and the bovine immune system. More of that later.

These tick-borne apicomplexan parasites, along with the mosquito-transmitted *Plasmodia* that cause malaria in a variety of species (including us), all multiply both in their arthropod vector and in one or other warm-blooded (homeothermic) vertebrate hosts. Replicating in the salivary gland of a 'vector' tick or mosquito, the process of taking a blood meal results in the sporozoite stage of the parasite entering the vertebrate host. Sometimes the infection can be essentially asymptomatic, as is the case for *T. parva* in African buffalo that are regarded as a 'reservoir' host, with the same parasite causing severe disease in domestic cattle. Diagnostically, all these parasites are detected by optical microscopy as 'piroplasms' in the cytoplasm of infected red blood cells (RBCs), which in turn transmit the pathogen back to any uninfected, feeding arthropod. While parasitism by the *Babesia* species is restricted to RBCs, the incoming *Theileria* and *Plasmodia* sporozoites differentiate to an asexual replicative/segmentation phase (schizogony) in nucleated cells that leads, in turn, to the piroplasm–RBC relationship. For the *Plasmodia*, the schizogony phase occurs in the liver, while for *Theileria*, that happens in a spectrum of white blood cells (WBCs).

Therein lies the unique biological fascination of *T. parva*, with the parasitized WBCs showing an essentially transformed phenotype and, as a consequence, causing lymphomatosis in infected cattle. For the laboratory scientist, the schizont-bearing WBCs can easily be grown out and continue to replicate in cell culture. Unlike in cancer, this apparently 'transformed' phenotype depends on the continued presence of the parasite. Drug-treat the cultured lymphocytes to eliminate the schizonts and they stop dividing and die.

If ECF were a human disease, it might well have been of considerable interest for cancer researchers. But, as a specifically veterinary problem, ECF and *T. parva* have not been obvious targets for biomedical research funding, and I expect that few oncology-focused investigators are even aware of the disease. That's one reason that the current book is of particular value: it represents a 'one-stop reading shop' for any researcher who suddenly becomes aware of this fascinating pathogenesis. Otherwise, for protozoologists, especially malariologists who may be marginally aware of ECF, this is a useful summary.

Growing up in Queensland where bovine babesiosis is a major economic problem, I had thought that – as an altruistic young veterinary student who was aiming for a research career focused on ameliorating the diseases of food-producing animals – I might go down the parasitology road. The University of Queensland Veterinary School was at that time home to an outstanding Parasitology department led by the eminent parasitologist J.F.A. Sprent. In a short course that he gave on parasitism, John Sprent incorporated the insights of Australian virologist/immunologist F.M. Burnet, a conceptually driven researcher who shared the 1960 Nobel Prize for Medicine with experimentalist P.B. Medawar for his thoughts on immunological tolerance. I was fascinated by John's little venture into parasitism, but totally turned off by the complexity of parasite life cycles, his own professional interest. Viruses looked to be a simpler way to go!

As a consequence, following an early foray into bacteriology studying leptospirosis in cattle, my own research career has focused on dissecting the intricacies of viral pathogenesis and immunity. After 5 years at the Moredun Research Institute, I was in the process of negotiating a senior job at the CSIRO (Commonwealth Scientific and Industrial Research Organisation) Division of Animal Health in Melbourne, when I heard a lecture by cancer immunologist Mel Greaves that convinced me I needed to develop a better understanding of the then emerging field of cell-mediated immunity. That led to my taking what I thought would be a 2-year break from the veterinary world to learn basic immunology in Canberra at the Australian National University John Curtin School of Medical Research, where R.V. Blanden and C.A. Mims had published intriguing findings on T cell responses to the ectromelia (mouse pox) and murine lymphocytic choriomeningitis (LCM) viruses. Mims left for the UK just as I arrived and I 'inherited' his technician and the LCM model he'd been studying. Then, working with a young Swiss MD, Rolf Zinkernagel (from 1973 to 1975), we made the chance discovery, then developed a theory of immunological surveillance that led to our being awarded the 1996 Nobel Prize for Medicine for 'illuminating the nature of the cellular immune defence'. Key initial findings published in 1974 in *Nature* led to our immediate prominence in immunology, and I spent the rest of my career working in biomedical research institutes, medical schools in research universities and in a paediatric research hospital.

Through that first 20+ years after our big discovery, my only close contact with the veterinary world was to serve as a Board member, then Chair of the Scientific Committee, for ILRAD. I was ideal for this as, with a veterinary training and good credentials as a disease-focused immunologist funded to do basic biomedical research, I had absolutely no conflict of interest for any research group that was dedicated to developing novel vaccination strategies for ECF or bovine trypanosomiasis. As I recall the story, the establishment of ILRAD resulted from the input of leading immunologists serving on WHO committees who evidently thought that, while the parasitologists and practical veterinarians who were the intellectual curators of the ECF and Trypanosome worlds were no doubt 'solid (if not stolid) chaps', adding the brilliant insights of the basic immunology community would rapidly move the field forward and lead to elegant solutions. By then, I'd been engaging with virus diseases for 20 years and was, to put it mildly, somewhat sceptical. Immunologists were arguing we'd be close to an affordable vaccine for human malaria within 5–10 years. As summarized in this book for *T. parva*, the vaccine field for apicomplexan parasites has moved forward, but production of effective and affordable vaccines has proved difficult to achieve. Malaria has continued to be a major global human health problem, exacerbated by the evolution of strains resistant to preventive/therapeutic drugs. Control has continued to rely largely on control of the mosquito vector. However, in the past few years, vaccines targeting the sporozoite stage of *P. falciparum*, which provide significant but incomplete protection against the disease, have been approved for use in humans.

Yet, while the underlying premise for establishing ILRAD may have been a bit naïve, it was a brilliant initiative, and we can only be thankful to all those who were involved in setting it up under the broad aegis of the World Bank, the Consultative Group for International Agricultural Research (CGIAR) and its Technical Advisory Committee (the TAC). Through my time on the Board, the TAC had a kind of papal authority in any discussion of CGIAR strategies and science! For once, with ILRAD, the study of two economically and socially important veterinary diseases was properly funded, and researchers were encouraged to engage with the latest ideas, instrumentation and technology. And, from a personal aspect, one of the great pleasures for me during weeks spent in Nairobi was getting to know African students, researchers and Board colleagues.

There can be a strange myth in the approach to veterinary diseases based on the premise that, as the problem involves animals, it's in some way simpler (and cheaper) to research than a comparable challenge in us. In fact, ECF is no easier to solve than malaria, though the $ amounts allocated are infinitely smaller. And it is a major human problem. As I recall, perhaps incorrectly, there's a Maasai saying: 'When the cattle die, the people die also.' In fact, that echoes a theme expressed in the Norse sagas. Under the donor country/AID model used by the World Bank and the CGIAR to fund ILRAD, the Scandinavian nations were among the very top donors! Overall, that generous international support from the more prosperous nations has fallen off, with the worst blow being the recent, precipitous decision to effectively shut down the USAID agency.

As you can read in this multi-author volume, the ILRAD researchers who studied *T. parva* – including a cohort who trained there, then seeded out to staff veterinary schools particularly in Britain and in Western Europe – generated (with others working on Western campuses) a new molecular understanding of ECF and, at the same time, developed key reagents and strategies for defining the bovine immune system. Even more brilliantly, ILRAD nurtured a group of young African molecular biologists and immunologists who, with others who trained as expatriates, have greatly advanced the practice of science in Africa. During my later, 9-year involvement with the International Union of Immunological Societies, as President-elect, President and Past President, the veterinary committee was generally dominated by former ILRAD scientists.

The complex scientific story outlined in this book is both intriguing and, at the same time I suspect, largely unknown outside the protozoal disease research community. These researchers aren't driven by any search for fame and great fortune, but by the desire to understand then solve a problem that is both intellectually fascinating and impacts on human well-being. Especially in Africa and parts of Asia, animal agriculture remains massively important for food supply and to sustain the livelihoods of rural communities and alleviate poverty.

This unique book should ideally be available in any comprehensive veterinary or biomedical library. It exemplifies the reality that 'comparative medicine and pathology', as they were once called, continue to offer important lessons for the study of infectious disease. Going way back, the second ever Nobel Prize for Medicine (in 1902) was awarded to Ronald Ross for his work on malaria. His illuminating experimental studies were done in birds using Plasmodium species that, while they do not infect people, cause a disease that has many features in common with human malaria.

A very recent example comes from the COVID-19 pandemic. Many of us, at least initially, underestimated both the complexity of the disease and the (to date) impossibility of developing a 'sterilizing' vaccine. That might have been avoided if the relevant scientific community had been more aware of the long history of attempts to control/prevent comparable coronavirus infections in cats, pigs, chickens and cattle. Perhaps there could have been more effort directed early on at developing small-molecule anti-viral therapeutics that, like the analogous drugs developed to control human influenza, might well work against all coronavirus infections, in any species.

Reflecting on the complexity of infectious diseases where at least two genomes (that of the host and the parasite) interact, we must surely be conscious of an underlying reality: we are 'instructed by nature'. That's even more so with these apicomplexan parasites, where we have the additional complication of the arthropod vector. At every level, the *T. parva*/ECF story both challenges and illuminates.

Peter C. Doherty, Nobel Laureate in Physiology or Medicine, 1996
University of Melbourne Medical School at the Doherty Institute,
792 Elizabeth St, Victoria 3000, Australia

About the Editors

W. Ivan Morrison PhD, BVMS, FRC Path
Emeritus Professor of Veterinary Immunology, The Roslin Institute, Royal (Dick) School of Veterinary Studies, University of Edinburgh

W. Ivan Morrison graduated in veterinary medicine from the University of Glasgow in 1972 and completed a PhD at the same University in 1975. He then joined the newly established International Laboratory for Research on Animal Diseases (ILRAD) in Nairobi, eventually heading the Institute's *Theileria* research programme. Returning to the UK in 1990, he joined the BBSRC Institute for Animal Health, before moving to the University of Edinburgh in 2002. His research has focused on studying the immunology and pathogenesis of infectious diseases of cattle, with a major emphasis on *Theileria parva*. His work on immune responses to *T. parva* demonstrated that immunity is mediated by T cell responses and specifically identified the importance of CD8 T cells both in providing protection and in determining the strain specificity of immunity. This work laid the foundation for subsequent research on subunit vaccine development for this parasite.

Philip Toye, PhD (Adelaide), BVSc (Queensland), Dip. Immunology (Monash)
Recently retired Principal Scientist, International Livestock Research Institute, Nairobi, Kenya

Philip Toye graduated as a bachelor of veterinary science from the University of Queensland. He completed a PhD in immunoparasitology from the University of Adelaide, which was followed by a postdoctoral appointment to the Harvard Medical School and Harvard School of Public Health, Boston. His research background is in the immunology and molecular biology of infectious diseases. He has spent over 20 years undertaking research on East Coast fever at ILRAD and its successor institute ILRI in Nairobi. This work initially entailed the identification of vaccine and diagnostic antigens and the characterization of the Muguga cocktail vaccine stabilates. He managed the 2007 production of the Muguga cocktail at commercial scale at ILRI and was involved in its registration and initial distribution. More recently, he led the team which discovered a paternal line of indigenous cattle resistant to ECF, leading to a collaboration with the Roslin Institute, University of Edinburgh, and the identification of a region of the bovine genome strongly associated with resistance.
He has also conducted research on contagious bovine pleuropneumonia, porcine cysticercosis and peste des petits ruminants, and was a co-leader of a large epidemiological study that documented the infectious diseases of a cohort of 548 indigenous calves in western Kenya during the first 12 months of life.

Acknowledgements

The editors wish to thank all the contributors for the considerable amount of time and effort that they so willingly devoted to the book.

The editors are also deeply grateful to Sheila Morrison and Vanessa Toye for their steadfast support and patience throughout the preparation of this book.

Contributors

Richard P. Bishop, Department of Veterinary Microbiology and Pathology, Washington State University, Pullman, USA. bishop5030@gmail.com

Gemma Chaters, Lancaster Medical School, University of Lancaster, Lancaster, UK. g.chaters@lancaster.ac.uk

Timothy Connelley, Roslin Institute, University of Edinburgh, Edinburgh, UK. timothy.connelley@roslin.ed.ac.uk

Jorge Del-Pozo, Roslin Institute, University of Edinburgh, Edinburgh, UK. Jorge.Del.Pozo@ed.ac.uk

Olivier Hanotte, International Livestock Research Institute, Addis Ababa, Ethiopia. o.hanotte@cgiar.org

Boitumelo B. Maboko, Epidemiology, Parasites and Vectors, Agricultural Research Council-Onderstepoort Veterinary Research, Onderstepoort, South Africa. BPule@arc.agric.za

Maxime Madder, Clinglobal, Tamarin, Mauritius. Maxime.Madder@clinglobal.com

Ben J. Mans, Epidemiology, Parasites and Vectors, Agricultural Research Council-Onderstepoort Veterinary Research, Onderstepoort, South Africa. MansB@arc.agric.za

Nick McHardy (now deceased)

Liam J. Morrison, Roslin Institute, University of Edinburgh, Edinburgh, UK. Liam.Morrison@roslin.ed.ac.uk

Andrew Peters, Arpexas (Scotland) Ltd, Edinburgh, UK. andrewrpeters@outlook.com

Ronel Pienaar, Epidemiology, Parasites and Vectors, Agricultural Research Council-Onderstepoort Veterinary Research, Onderstepoort. VolschenkR@arc.agric.za

Ashley Flynn Railey, Oklahoma State University, Oklahoma, USA. arailey@iu.edu

Jonathan Rushton, Roslin Institute, University of Edinburgh, Edinburgh, UK. jrushton@ed.ac.uk

Brian Shiels, College of Medical, Veterinary and Life Sciences, University of Glasgow, Glasgow, UK. Brian.Shiels@glasgow.ac.uk

Joana C. Silva, School of Medicine, The University of Maryland, Baltimore, USA. jcsilva@som.umaryland.edu

Kerry Woods, Institute of Animal Pathology, Vetsuisse Faculty, University of Bern, Bern, Switzerland. kerry.woods@unibe.ch

1 A Brief History of the Discovery of *Theileria parva* and Subsequent Research Revealing its Epidemiology and Capacity to Cause Disease

W. Ivan Morrison*
Roslin Institute, University of Edinburgh, Edinburgh, UK

1.1 Introduction

Unravelling the infectious nature of diseases was a relatively recent historical advance. Although the clinical features of many important human infectious diseases had been recognized by the ancient Greeks, the nature of the causative agents was only revealed within the past 150 years. Prior to that, diseases were widely considered to be due to interaction between individuals and their environment, including weather and geographical features – a concept known as the 'atmospheric-miasmic theory' of disease (Magner, 2009). A notable example was malaria, so named by the Romans (*mal aria* = bad air), who believed that it was caused by foul vapours emanating from stagnant waters in swampy areas where the disease was prevalent (Cunha and Cunha, 2008). The first proposal of the contagious nature of disease came in 1547 from an Italian physician, Girolamo Fracastoro, based on his studies of syphilis. However, his ideas received little attention and it was not until the latter half of the 19th century, when the studies of Louis Pasteur and Robert Koch established the '*germ theory of disease*', that the infectious nature of disease was gradually accepted. It was during this period that the modern disciplines of medical/veterinary microbiology and infectious disease medicine were established and led to a period of active research aimed at determining the causes of human and animal diseases. Much of the work on bacterial and protozoal diseases was made possible by the earlier invention of the microscope by Antonie van Leeuwenhoek in the 18th century, which for the first time permitted visualization of microorganisms. Among his early observations, van Leeuwenhoek described organisms resembling protozoa, which he referred to as 'animalcules', in samples of stagnant water. However, the first discoveries of pathogenic protozoa were not made until the closing stages of the 19th century (reviewed for human diseases by Cox, 2002). These early discoveries included several of the most important protozoal pathogens of man and animals, subsequently classified in the phylum *Apicomplexa*, which includes *Theileria* species. In 1880, a French scientist, Alphonse Laveran, identified *Plasmodium* parasites in patients with malaria (Laveran, 1880), and subsequently, Douglas Ross, a British scientist working in India, demonstrated that malaria is transmitted by mosquitos (Ross, 1898, 1923). *Babesia* parasites were identified as the cause of disease in cattle by

*Corresponding author: Ivan.Morrison@ed.ac.uk

 East Coast Fever: The Disease, its Impact and Control (eds W.I. Morrison and P. Toye)
DOI: 10.1079/9781800626324.0001

a Romanian scientist Victor Babes in 1888, and subsequent studies in the USA showed that *Babesia* are transmitted by ticks (Smith and Kilborne, 1893). The discoveries of *T. parva* (Theiler, 1904a) and *T. annulata* (Dschunkowsky and Luhs, 1904) were reported in 1904, and identification of the non-vector-borne apicomplexan parasites, *Toxoplasma* and *Eimeria*, followed several years later (Nicolle and Manceaux, 1909; Splendore, 1909; Fantham, 1910).

T. parva was identified as the causal agent of East Coast fever (ECF) in southern Africa at the beginning of the last century. The discovery of the parasite coincided with a number of major political and cultural upheavals in southern Africa, and the events and people involved had a lasting impact on development of the infrastructure for investigation and control of animal diseases in the region.

This chapter discusses the events leading to discovery of *T. parva*, as well as other related *Theileria* parasites, and presents a brief overview of subsequent advances that were important in our evolving understanding of disease caused by *T. parva*. Most of these topics are covered in greater detail in the chapters that follow.

1.2 Southern Africa at the Beginning of the 20th Century

Towards the end of the 19th century, a devastating pandemic of rinderpest swept through Africa, first appearing in north-eastern Africa in 1889 and reaching the Cape in 1897. In southern Africa, rinderpest is estimated to have resulted in the death of 2.5 million cattle, representing more than 90% of the cattle population (Fig. 1.1; Mack, 1970; Rossiter, 1994). The region had also suffered the ravages of the recent Anglo-Boer war (1899–1902). These events created an acute shortage of cattle in the region, not only for food but also for use as draft animals. Since African horse sickness largely precluded use of horses, haulage of goods throughout the region relied on ox-drawn wagons (Fig. 1.2). To replenish the stock, cattle were imported from a variety of sources, including Argentina, Australia, Britain, the USA and elsewhere in Africa.

The conclusion of the Anglo-Boer war saw the previously Boer-controlled Transvaal and Orange Free State colonies brought together with the Natal and Cape colonies, under British

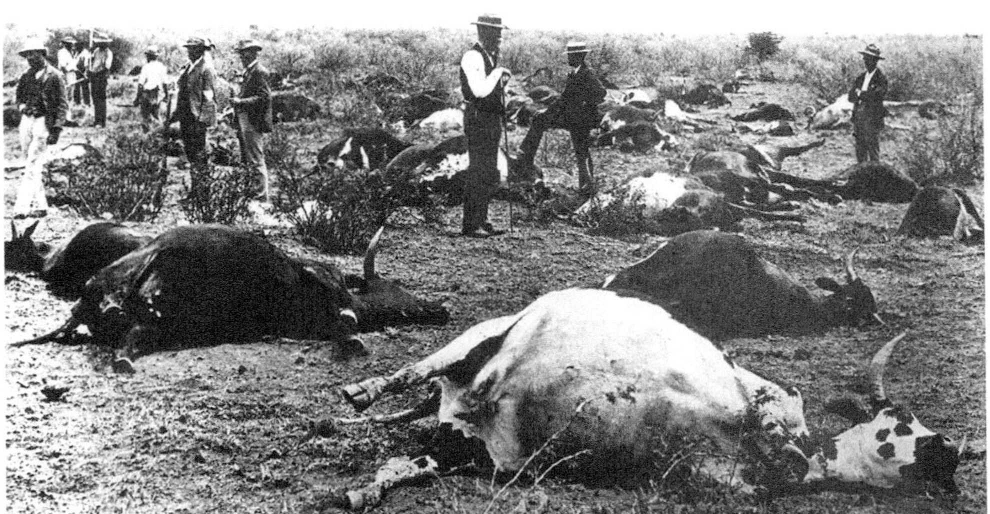

Fig. 1.1. Widespread death of cattle in southern Africa during the rinderpest epidemic. (From National Archives of Zimbabwe.)

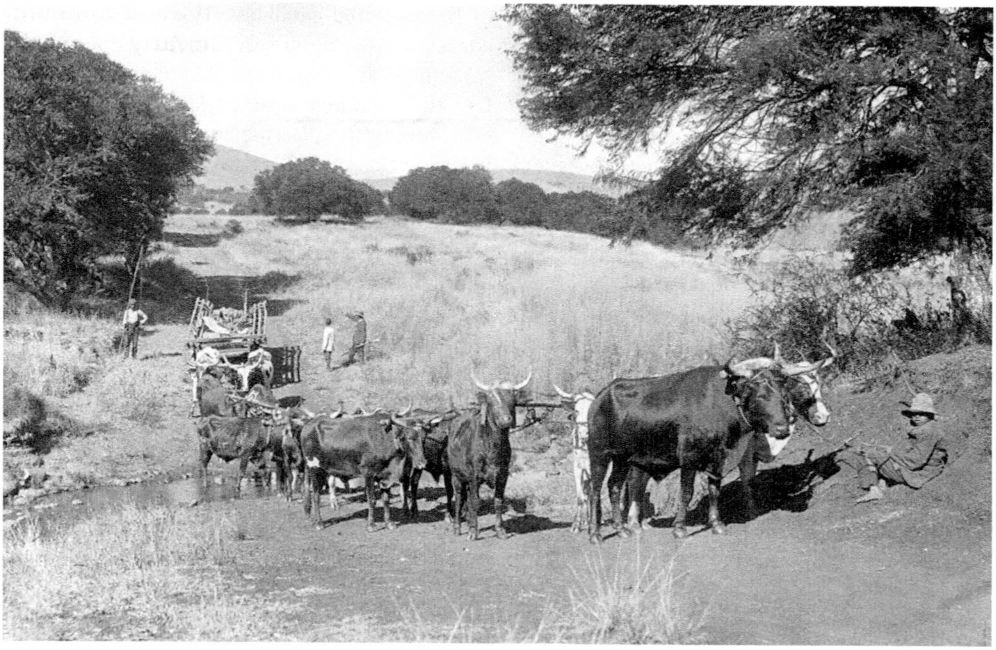

Fig. 1.2. Use of ox-drawn carts to transport goods in southern Africa at the beginning of the 20th century.

rule (subsequently to form the Union of South Africa in 1910). To the north, Rhodesia had been established as a British protectorate in 1889, run by a commercial entity known as the British South African Company (originally headed by Cecil Rhodes), which gradually assumed British colony status over the next decade. Although all under British control at the end of the Anglo-Boer war, these colonies initially retained a degree of independence and had their own administrative organizations.

1.3 Appearance of a New Disease

Towards the end of 1901, an acute disease of cattle (subsequently identified as ECF) was reported in Rhodesia (currently Zimbabwe) and spread rapidly, causing high levels of mortality. Occurring in the wake of the recent devastating impact of rinderpest, the appearance of this disease caused major alarm and led to intensive investigation. Given the limited local infrastructure and rudimentary scientific facilities in southern Africa at that time, it is quite remarkable that the causative organism of the disease and its mode of transmission were identified within the next two years. However, these discoveries were not without controversies and disagreements, which are discussed in detail elsewhere (Cranfield, 1991; Lawrence, 1992) and summarized briefly here.

The new disease was first observed in Rhodesia in December 1901 and in Transvaal about six months later. Its appearance was subsequently attributed to the importation of a shipment of cattle from Tanganyika (now Tanzania). Cattle were offloaded in the port of Beira in Portuguese East Africa (now Mozambique), from where they were moved to Umtali (now Mutare) and then Salisbury (now Harare). The remainder of the shipment was offloaded further south in Laurenco Marques (now Maputo) for transfer to Transvaal. Outbreaks of disease, causing high levels of mortality, occurred following the arrival of these animals. Investigation of affected animals in both Rhodesia and South Africa identified the presence of intra-erythrocytic parasites, similar to but smaller than those of *Babesia*, which had been identified several years earlier (Babes, 1888; Smith and Kilborne, 1893) and was known to be present in the region. A report published jointly by Charles Gray (the Chief Veterinary Officer of Rhodesia) and William Robertson (a bacteriologist in the Cape) in August 1902 provided a detailed description of the disease and proposed that it was an atypical form of babesiosis (Gray and Robertson, 1902). This was despite the absence of haemoglobulinuria (a prominent feature of babesiosis) in most affected animals and detection of other features normally not associated with babesiosis. The conclusions drawn by Gray and Robertson are thought to have been influenced by other recent findings. In December 1901, a shipment of 999 cattle had been imported into Rhodesia from Australia (organized by Cecil Rhodes), and within the first five months all but three of them had died. Many of them showed clinical signs typical of babesiosis, and subsequent enquiries showed that they had been sourced from a *Babesia*-free area in Australia and hence were likely to have been highly susceptible to the disease on their arrival. Nevertheless, suspicions persisted that these animals had been the source of the new disease. Moreover, the association with babesiosis was also linked to a brief report by the eminent bacteriologist Robert Koch of a visit to German East Africa (Tanganyika) in 1897, during which he had observed a disease in cattle similar to the new disease in southern Africa and had suggested that it was an atypical form of babesiosis (Koch, 1898). This conclusion was influenced by findings reported by Smith and Kilborne (1893), who observed small parasites in the erythrocytes of some *Babesia*-infected animals, which they interpreted as immature forms of the *Babesia* parasite.

1.4 Demand for an External Consultant

By April/May 1902, there was growing discontent within the agricultural and mining communities in Rhodesia about the lack of progress in dealing with the disease. Particular pressure came from the mining sector, whose commercial activities had been severely disrupted due to a shortage of draft oxen to provide transport. This led to a request to seek the scientific advice of an external expert and, in view of his previous experience in Tanganyika, Robert Koch was identified as the preferred candidate. However, there was considerable delay in securing his appointment. It required the approval of the Colonial Office in London, but due to strained Anglo-German relations arising from German support of the Boers in the recent Anglo-Boer war, the Colonial Office minister, Joseph Chamberlain, had reservations about appointing a German national. The issue was referred to The Royal Society to identify an alternative, and among those approached were Professor John McFadyean, who at the time was investigating bovine tuberculosis in the UK, and Dr David Bruce, who had recently identified African trypanosomes. However, since these and other suitable British experts were not immediately available, approval to invite Koch was eventually given in October 1902. He did not arrive in Bulawayo until March 1903, having travelled via Tanganyika, where he conducted some further investigations of the disease he had previously observed there. He spent just over a year in Rhodesia, at the end of which he was unable to definitively identify the causal agent. Although he initially considered it to be a variant of the *Babesia* parasite, he eventually accepted that the disease was caused by a novel agent (Koch, 1903), at which point he is likely to have been aware that the parasite had been identified by other workers (discussed below). He also suggested (without any supportive evidence) that the pathogen was probably already present in the coastal regions of Portuguese East Africa (Mozambique) and that the imported Australian cattle had been responsible for the inland spread of the pathogen. Based on this belief, he referred to the disease as African Coast fever. Koch was unable to transmit the disease experimentally using blood from affected animals, although in some recipient animals he observed intra-erythrocyte parasites but no disease, which he interpreted as having induced infection and immunity. However, later studies indicated that these parasites were probably another non-pathogenic species of *Theileria* (*T. mutans* – discussed further below). His unsuccessful attempts to transmit the disease using the blue tick (*Rhipicephalus decoloratus*), the vector of babesiosis, were instigated based on his initial belief that he was dealing with a *Babesia*-like parasite. During the course of his studies, Koch did observe multinucleate bodies within lymphocytes (referred to by others as Koch's blue bodies) (Koch, 1903), which he subsequently described

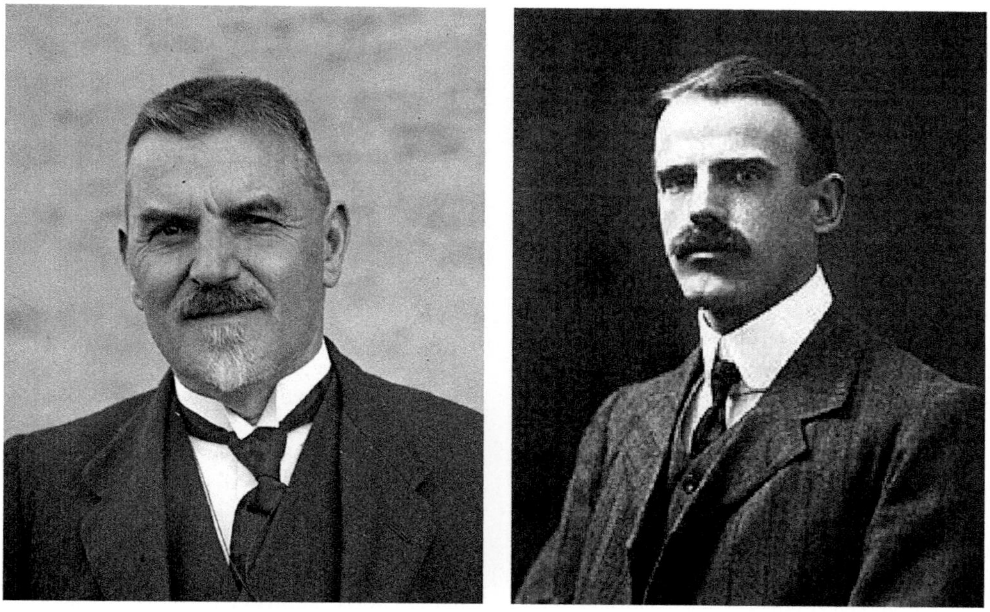

Fig. 1.3. Arnold Theiler (left) and Charles Lounsbury (right).

in greater detail (Koch, 1905, 1906). He suggested correctly that they may represent a site of multiplication of the agent. However, neither Koch nor other early investigators appeared to fully recognize the key role that this stage of the parasite, subsequently called the 'schizont', plays in pathogenesis of the disease.

1.5 Theiler and Lounsbury

In the meantime, during Koch's visit, workers in South Africa had made substantial progress in unravelling the cause of the disease. A number of scientists made important contributions, including Charles Gray and Duncan Hutcheon (the Chief Veterinary Officers in Rhodesia and the Cape Province, respectively), William Robertson, Arnold Theiler and Charles Lounsbury. However, the latter two individuals played a particularly important role in this work (Fig. 1.3).

Arnold Theiler (born 1867) had qualified as a veterinary surgeon in 1889 from the University of Berne in Switzerland and emigrated to Transvaal in 1891. Because of limited opportunities for veterinary employment, he worked for a short period on a large farm. However, having lost his left hand in a farming accident, he decided to set up private veterinary practice in Pretoria but again found little employment. Despite these setbacks, he set about training himself in bacteriology, borrowing money to purchase the necessary equipment. After a brief period of employment to assist in smallpox vaccine production, in 1895 he was appointed as a consultant veterinary surgeon to the Rand Health Board, and shortly thereafter he was sent by the government of Transvaal to Bulawayo to investigate the recently appeared rinderpest epidemic. He clearly made a favourable impression, as on his return the government built and equipped a small laboratory for him near Pretoria. Following the outbreak of the Anglo-Boer war in 1899, he served in the veterinary corps of the Boer army, but by 1901 he had returned to Pretoria and was appointed by the now British authorities as the government's Veterinary Bacteriologist for Transvaal. During this early period in Transvaal, Theiler had studied a number of diseases of cattle and horses (including bovine babesiosis) and, based on studies of biliary cirrhosis in horses, he received a doctorate from the University of Berne in 1901.

Charles Lounsbury (born 1872) had attended the Massachusetts Agricultural College in the USA, as both an undergraduate and a graduate student. While employed as an instructor, he was offered the opportunity in 1895 to take up the position of Government Entomologist in the Department of Agriculture in the Cape Colony, a post created because of the infestation of the Cape vineyards by the arthropod pest *Phylloxera*. His training in the USA had included entomology, and his initial work in the Cape focused on insect pests of plants, but by 1898 he had started to study ticks as vectors of animal diseases. At this time, he was the only qualified entomologist in southern Africa.

Both of these individuals worked in relatively primitive experimental facilities. Construction of a new Department of Agriculture building in Transvaal had just started in 1902, while in the Cape, Lounsbury conducted his initial animal studies in modified builders' sheds. Despite these limitations, they made a number of significant advances. Theiler had observed his first cases of ECF in Transvaal in June 1902 and then visited Rhodesia in October to observe the disease there (Theiler, 1902). In August 1902, he sent a letter and specimens to Laveran, who had reported the first observation of the malaria parasite. Laveran also initially subscribed to the view that the parasites were likely to be forms of *Babesia*. However, contrary to Koch's suggestion, he concluded that the parasites observed in affected animals were distinct from the small parasites observed in some cases of babesiosis by Smith and Kilborne (Laveran, 1903). In the same month, Theiler stated that the disease was not the familiar form of babesiosis and that he was inclined to regard the parasite as a new agent, but in light of Laveran's advice he remained uncommitted. However, following further experiments, Theiler (1903) documented a series of unique characteristics of the parasite and the clinical and pathological features of affected animals, which led him to conclude that the condition was an entirely new disease. He stated that 'knowledge of these facts should surely convince any observer that we have to do with a new disease' (Theiler, 1903, p. 93). The disease had occurred in areas where animals would have been expected to be immune to babesiosis. Experiments initiated by Theiler in October 1902 confirmed that immunity to babesiosis did not protect against the new disease; animals that had recovered naturally from babesiosis or had been immunized by inoculation with *Babesia*-infected blood all succumbed to ECF following field challenge, whereas an animal that had recovered from the new disease survived.

Meanwhile, in the Cape, Lounsbury had carried out a series of experiments with batches of ticks sent to him by Charles Gray in Rhodesia. Consistent with Koch's findings, repeated attempts to transmit the disease with the blue tick were unsuccessful. However, in October 1902 successful transmission was eventually achieved with a batch that contained brown ticks. These brown ticks were identified as *Rhipicephalus appendiculatus*, which had been designated as a new species by L.G. Neumann the previous year, based on examination of ticks sent to him by Lounsbury (Neumann, 1901). *R. appendiculatus* is a three-host tick, meaning that the larva, nymph and adult stages feed on separate hosts. Lounsbury observed that one batch of ticks he received to test transmission of the disease included a few *R. appendiculatus* nymphs, which he allowed to moult, and when the resulting adults were fed on a susceptible animal (only three ticks successfully attached) it developed ECF. Lounsbury went on to confirm these findings over the next few months and also showed that (unlike babesiosis) infection could not be transmitted by ticks that hatched from eggs of infected adult ticks. Lounsbury's initial studies appear to have been conducted largely independently of Theiler, but in March/April 1903 he visited Transvaal and spent four weeks working with Theiler. Although Lounsbury was unable to achieve transmission with nymphal ticks fed as larvae on infected animals, in later experiments Theiler succeeded in transmitting infection with nymphs. Neither Theiler nor Lounsbury were able to transmit infection with ticks that had fed on ECF-recovered animals, leading them to conclude that the parasite does not persist beyond the acute phase of infection, although much later studies in East Africa demonstrated that this was not the case (see below).

Hence, by late 1903 (i.e. before Koch's departure from Rhodesia) Theiler and Lounsbury had identified the agent and the tick vector and demonstrated that it was transmitted trans-stadially (i.e. by nymphs infected as larvae and adults infected as nymphs) by *R. appendiculatus* ticks (Lounsbury, 1904, 1906;

Theiler, 1904a, b, 1905). A formal account of the recognition of the parasite, entitled 'The *Piroplasma bigeminum* of the immune ox' was presented in the 1905 *Report of the Transvaal Department of Agriculture* (Theiler, 1905). The pathogen was later renamed *Theileria parva* in 1907 (Bettencourt *et al.*, 1907). Much later studies showed that *Rhipicephalus zambeziensis*, another tick species found in southern Africa, also acts as an efficient vector of *T. parva* under experimental conditions (Lawrence *et al.*, 1983).

The achievements of Theiler and Lounsbury, identifying the causal agent of ECF and its mode of transmission, laid the groundwork that would allow the formulation of subsequent strategies to control the disease. By implementing a sustained programme involving regular dipping of cattle with acaricides to prevent tick infestation, intensive disease surveillance, slaughter of infected animals following an outbreak and quarantine of affected farms, eradication of ECF was eventually achieved in South Africa in the mid-1950s (reviewed by Lawrence, 1992 and discussed in Chapter 6 of this volume).

1.6 The Impact of Arnold Theiler on Tropical Veterinary Medicine

Theiler's influence in South Africa and his impact on tropical veterinary medicine extended well beyond his work on *T. parva* (reviewed in du Toit and Jackson, 1936; and by his daughter Gertrude Theiler, 1971). He made many important contributions to understanding the aetiology and pathogenesis of a variety of other pathogens of livestock, including two intra-erythrocytic agents encountered during investigations of ECF. In 1906, he identified *Theileria mutans* (Theiler, 1906), a usually non-pathogenic species that is distributed widely in *T. parva*-endemic areas. This parasite could be transmitted experimentally with blood and is believed to have confounded some of Koch's studies on transmission of *T. parva*. A few years later, Theiler identified the aetiological agent of another important disease of cattle, *Anaplasma marginale*, a rickettsial pathogen that infects erythrocytes and causes severe haemolytic anaemia (Theiler, 1910). The small intra-erythrocytic organisms observed by Smith and Kilborne in some of their *Babesia*-infected animals are believed to have been *A. marginale* (rather than immature forms of *Babesia* as suggested by the authors). Aware of previous difficulties in identifying such agents, Theiler organized shipment of cattle from England for his studies of *A. marginale*, to ensure that his investigations were not confounded by the presence of other African pathogens.

In addition to his studies of disease, Theiler was instrumental in setting up the Onderstepoort Research Institute in Pretoria, established in 1908, which he served as Director until 1918. The Institute became an internationally leading centre for research on diseases of African livestock over the following decades. He also played an important role in promoting the need for veterinary education in South Africa, leading to the establishment of a veterinary school, which was initially based in the Onderstepoort Institute before being incorporated into the University of Pretoria in 1920. Theiler was appointed as the first Dean of the Faculty, in which position he continued until his retirement in 1927.

In recognition of his achievements, Arnold Theiler was awarded a knighthood by King George V in 1914. Interestingly, Theiler's son, Max Theiler, became a scientist and emigrated to USA, where he studied Yellow Fever and was awarded the Nobel prize for his work on developing a vaccine for the virus.

1.7 The Pathological Basis of the Disease

Both Gray and Robertson (1902) and Koch (1903) observed enlarged and sometimes haemorrhagic lymph nodes in cases of ECF. Koch also noted the presence of abundant parasites including 'peculiar forms' (Koch's blue bodies) in lymphoid tissues and suggested that the parasite multiplied within these organs. Meyer, who had successfully transmitted infection with *T. parva* by transplanting portions of spleen from infected cattle (Meyer, 1909), presented clear evidence that Koch's blue bodies, now known as 'schizonts', represent a developmental stage of the parasite in lymphocytes (Meyer, 1911). He also established the

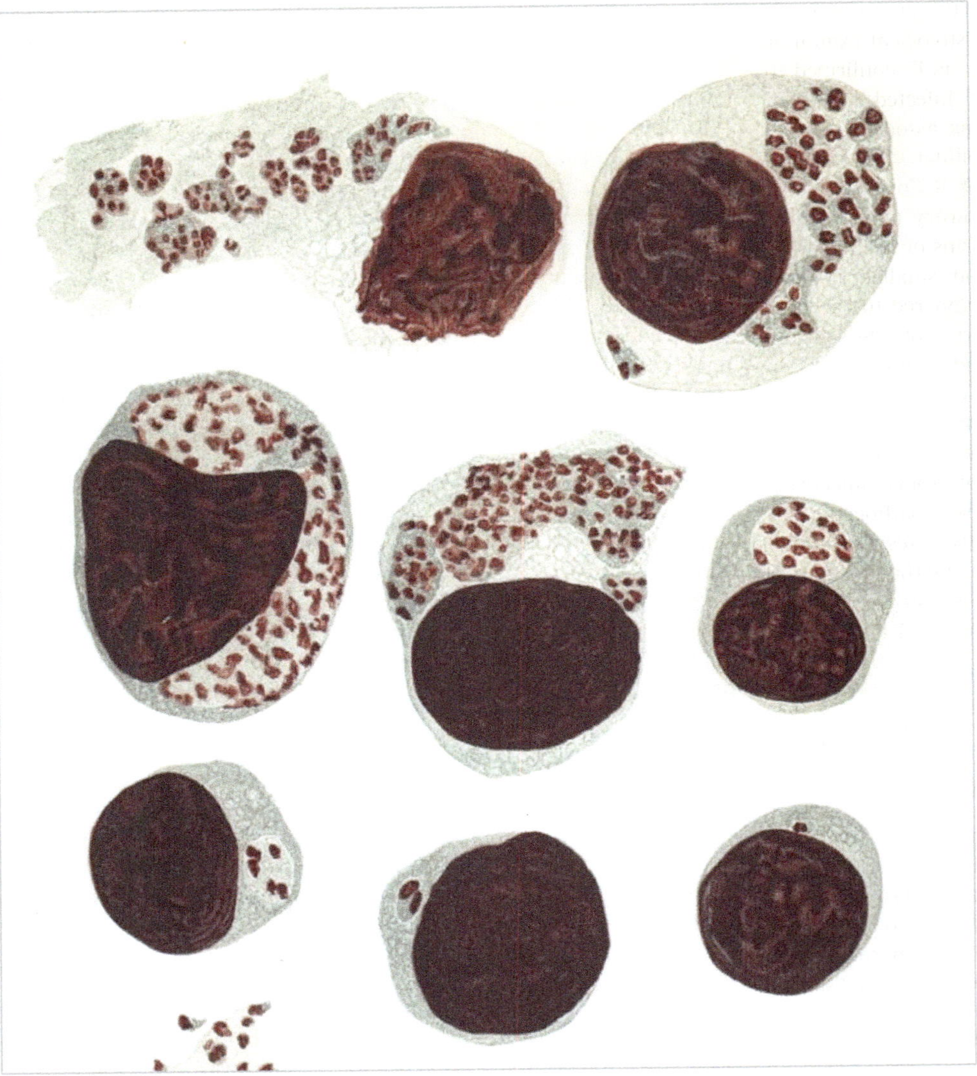

Fig. 1.4. Painting of microscopic images of *T. parva* schizonts in cell aspirates from lymph nodes of an infected animal. (Reproduced from Gonder, 1910.)

method for detecting multinucleate schizonts by examination of needle aspirates from superficial lymph nodes of affected animals, which became an established method for confirming diagnosis of the disease and for monitoring the course of infection in experimental studies. Further studies by Gonder (1910, 1911a), in which he examined the kinetics of development of schizonts in lymphoid tissues, described a progressive increase in schizonts during infection (Fig. 1.4) and proposed correctly that parasite multiplication occurs predominantly in lymphoid cells rather than in erythrocytes, although his theories on how the parasite multiplies subsequently proved incorrect (discussed later). Gonder also suggested that 'the parasite appears only in blood corpuscles (erythrocytes) in order to get into the second host (the tick) where it undergoes sexual development' (Gonder, 1911b, p. 80).

Following these studies, the importance of replication of the parasite in lymphoid tissues in the pathogenesis of ECF gained acceptance. Histological examination of tissues from cases of ECF confirmed that rapid multiplication of infected lymphocytes in lymphoid tissues was associated with extensive cell death and cellular depletion of lymphoid tissues (Steck, 1928; Cowdry and Danks, 1933). The studies by Cowdry and Danks (1933) distinguished later forms of the intra-lymphocytic parasite, which had smaller, more intensely staining nuclei compared to early forms. These early and late forms of the schizont, referred to by Cowdry and Danks as 'agamonts' and 'gamonts', respectively, are now known as 'macroschizonts' and 'microschizonts'. The microschizonts (gamonts) were correctly proposed as the source of the erythrocyte-infective stages. By contrast to the severe pathogenic consequences of infection of leukocytes, these and subsequent studies have shown that infection of erythrocytes by the piroplasm stage of the parasite has relatively minor pathological effects.

1.8 *T. parva* in the African Buffalo (*Syncerus caffer*)

An acute disease in cattle caused by a parasite morphologically similar to *T. parva*, but exhibiting epidemiological differences from ECF, was observed in Rhodesia (Zimbabwe) in 1934 (Lawrence, 1935, 1936). Although the disease showed some features in common with ECF, including acute onset, enlarged lymph nodes and a high level of mortality, affected animals had lower levels of schizont-infected leukocytes in lymphoid tissues and no, or very few, detectable piroplasms in erythrocytes. The disease appeared to be associated with contact of cattle with buffalo. It was noted that when groups of cattle containing animals that had recovered from the disease were removed from buffalo contact to tick-infested pasture, no further cases of the disease occurred, implying that the animals did not represent a source of infection for transmission by ticks. The same disease was reported in South Africa in the 1950s (Neitz *et al.*, 1955) and shown to be transmitted to cattle by *R. appendiculatus* ticks that had fed on buffalo (Neitz, 1955; Neitz *et al.*, 1955). The parasite was named *Theileria lawrencei* and the disease was termed 'Corridor disease', referring to the strip of land between the Hluhluwe and Umfolozi Game Reserves in South Africa where it was initially recognized. Earlier observations suggesting lack of transmission from infected cattle were confirmed by experiments showing that ticks fed on recovered cattle did not transmit the infection (Neitz, 1955). Corridor disease continued to occur in South Africa after the eradication of ECF in the 1950s. Following recognition of the disease, measures to prevent contact between buffalo and cattle were introduced in South Africa and the disease was made notifiable, resulting in quarantine of farms with cases of the disease and slaughter of affected animals, measures that continue to the present day. The role of buffalo as a source of infection for cattle is discussed further in Chapter 5 of this volume, and the eradication of ECF from South Africa is presented in detail in Chapter 6.

1.9 Theileriosis in Eastern and Central Africa

Prior to its appearance in southern Africa, ECF had not been formally identified in eastern and central Africa, although (as noted above) Koch had observed a similar disease in Tanganyika in 1897. The disease was first recorded in Tanganyika and Kenya in 1904 and 1906, respectively, in British East Africa Annual Reports (cited by Norval *et al.*, 1992). However, the first description of the disease was provided by David Bruce in 1910 during his studies of trypanosomiasis in Uganda. He described a disease of indigenous cattle, known locally as 'Amakebe', which was recognized throughout the country and was considered to be the most important disease of cattle in Uganda (Bruce *et al.*, 1910). However, the disease predominantly affected young calves and resulted in lower levels of mortality than ECF as described in southern Africa. Additional reports of the disease in Northern Rhodesia (now Zambia) and Nyasaland (now Malawi) appeared in the following years (Stannus, 1910; Garden, 1912; Turnbull, 1926), although some of these authors expressed uncertainty about the diagnosis of ECF because of the lower levels of mortality and involvement of mainly young calves. Before 1885, settlement of eastern Africa by Europeans was largely confined to the coastal areas, and the cattle in inland areas were mainly indigenous zebu (predominantly *Bos indicus*) or sanga (indigenous breeds containing variable proportions of *Bos taurus* and *Bos indicus*) breeds. Subsequent studies would confirm that the less virulent manifestations of the disease observed in these early studies reflected a degree of genetic resistance of the indigenous cattle residing in tick-infested areas and that the endemic nature of infection with *T. parva* in these cattle resulted in most primary infections occurring in young calves (discussed in Chapter 7 of this volume).

Investigations in Kenya of a disease believed to be ECF were conducted by Montgomery in 1912 (Anon, 1912), who confirmed the identity of the causal agent with *T. parva* studied in South Africa. Cattle that had recovered from the disease in Kenya were found to be immune to challenge with ticks infected with the South African parasite (provided by Arnold Theiler), whereas naïve animals were fully susceptible. Moreover, around the same time, Theiler successfully transmitted ECF with *R. appendiculatus* ticks sent to him from Uganda. By this time, it became apparent that the parasite was present throughout a large part of eastern and central Africa.

In the early part of the 20th century, increased settlement of inland areas was associated with importation of increasing numbers of European cattle. In Kenya and Uganda, this was facilitated by the construction of a railway from Mombasa to Uganda, which commenced in 1896 and reached Lake Victoria in 1901 (described in Miller, 1973). Following these developments, frequent reports appeared of disease typical of ECF, showing high levels of mortality in introduced cattle, which severely constrained development of beef and dairy enterprises in tick-infested areas (discussed in Norval *et al.*, 1992). An early example is cited in the biography of Lord Delamere (Huxley, 1935), who settled in the rift valley of Kenya in 1903, where he intended to establish a dairy enterprise. However, most of the animals he imported died of what was later recognized as ECF, forcing Delamere to move his dairy operation to a region where there was little tick challenge. In a description of ECF in Uganda in 1936, Mettam and Carmichael provided an account of the disease in indigenous cattle and in imported ('grade') cattle. They reported that the disease in indigenous cattle varied in clinical severity and usually resulted in mortality rates of 10–25%, although sometimes higher levels occurred in animals kept in harsh climatic conditions. While this represented a severe disease burden on the indigenous cattle population, the very high levels of mortality caused by the disease in imported cattle completely prohibited their use in many areas. As stated by Mettam and Carmichael, 'repeated attempts to keep pure-bred cattle in 'Amakebe' areas (i.e. ECF-endemic areas) have proved disastrous on every occasion' (Mettam and Carmichael, 1936, p. 279).

Unlike the situation in South Africa, there was no likelihood of ever being able to eradicate ECF, even from localized regions of eastern Africa. Eventually, control programmes involving regular dipping or spraying of cattle with acaricides to prevent tick infestation were developed and became the main means of protecting susceptible cattle against ECF. However, acaricides often needed to be applied up to twice weekly and required considerable infrastructure and organization to be effective. Strict acaricide application also resulted in animals remaining susceptible to ECF, and any interruption in supply of the acaricides risked outbreaks of the disease. Consequently, ECF continued to be seen as one of the most important diseases constraining cattle production.

1.10 Increased Research Activity in Eastern Africa

From the 1960s onwards, the perceived need for more sustainable methods to control the disease led to increased investment in research. Research projects based in East Africa were funded by a number of organizations. Of particular significance was the establishment in 1967 of a large research project on tick-borne diseases funded by the United Nations Development Programme (UNDP) and administered by the Food and Agricultural Organization of the United Nations (FAO), in cooperation with the governments of Kenya, Uganda and Tanzania, which continued until 1976. The project was led by Dr Matt

Cunningham and was based in the East African Veterinary Research Organization's laboratories at Muguga, just outside Nairobi. Although the project had a broad remit, including both laboratory-based and field studies, the ultimate aim was to assess the feasibility of a practical field vaccine for East Coast fever. In addition to its direct activities, this project acted as a focal point for collaboration with many research projects funded by other international organizations, and at the end of the UNDP project some of the investigators obtained further support from other sources to continue working on different aspects of ECF. The principal success of the UNDP project was the development of a method for immunizing cattle against ECF using an 'infection and treatment' protocol (discussed in Chapter 12 of this volume).

The UNDP project and other projects working on *T. parva* in East Africa around this time made a number of other significant observations on the biology of the parasite, which were important in further understanding the epidemiology of ECF and efforts to develop control measures. These observations are discussed further below.

1.10.1 Involvement of the African Buffalo in eastern Africa

The occurrence of disease in cattle caused by *T. lawrencei*, similar to that recognized earlier in southern Africa and arising from transmission by ticks from buffalo, was first reported in eastern Africa by Brocklesby and Barnett (1966), working in Kenya. A subsequent survey of buffalo in different locations in eastern Africa demonstrated that most buffalo residing in *R. appendiculatus*-infested areas are infected with *T. lawrencei* (Young *et al.*, 1978a). As observed in southern Africa, infected cattle displayed lower levels of schizont-infected leukocytes compared to classical ECF and few piroplasms in erythrocytes. Experimental transmission of the parasite by ticks from infected buffalo to naïve buffalo or cattle in Kenya was demonstrated consistently (Young *et al.*, 1973, 1977b), and repeated transmission from the same animals over time confirmed that buffalo remain long-term carriers of the parasite. In one study using a single experimentally infected buffalo held in tick-free accommodation, tick transmission was detected up to 880 days after infection (Grootenhuis *et al.*, 1987).

Despite the observed differences between *T. parva* and *T. lawrencei*, subsequent findings revealed antigenic similarities based on cross-reactivity of antibodies in the serum of recovered animals. Furthermore, experiments involving immunization and challenge of cattle demonstrated cross-protection between some combinations of *T. parva* and *T. lawrencei* isolates (e.g. Radley *et al.*, 1979). Similar to observations in southern Africa, most attempts to transmit infection with ticks fed on cattle infected with buffalo-derived parasites were unsuccessful (e.g. Schreuder *et al.*, 1977). However, in a few instances, transmission was achieved experimentally using large numbers of ticks fed on cattle infected with certain eastern African *T. lawrencei* isolates. Moreover, further tick passage of these isolates through cattle was reported to result in a gradual change in the behaviour of the parasite to eventually resemble *T. parva* (Barnett and Brocklesby, 1966a; Young and Purnell, 1973; Maritim *et al.*, 1992) (discussed further in Chapter 5 of this volume). Consequently, *T. lawrencei* was reclassified as *T. parva*, but the cattle and buffalo parasites were still referred to as *T. parva parva* and *T. parva lawrencei*, respectively (Uilenberg, 1976). *T. parva* parasites in Zimbabwe that caused a less virulent form of disease (Lawrence *et al.*, 1994) were termed *T. parva bovis*. It was pointed out that this trinomial nomenclature did not indicate the existence of subspecies, but merely provided a convenient way of describing different behavioural forms of the same parasite (Uilenberg, 1981; Young, 1981). With further accumulating evidence of antigenic and molecular similarities, support for this subtype nomenclature waned, and more recently the parasites have merely been referred to as *T. parva* of cattle or buffalo origin. It is of interest that Cowdry and Danks (1933), during their discussion of the severe pathology of ECF in cattle, stated that, given the relatively recent introduction of cattle into Africa, 'It is logical to assume the pre-existence of the parasite in some mammal in which it produces few if any symptoms' (Cowdry and Danks, 1933, p. 48). They suggested further investigation of this in wild animal species.

1.10.2 Infection with *T. parva* results in a carrier state

In cattle that have recovered from ECF, parasites are usually not detected microscopically in leukocytes or erythrocytes. Moreover, as discussed above, Theiler and Lounsbury were unable to transmit infection with ticks fed on ECF-recovered animals, and for several decades, cattle that recovered from ECF were considered to have developed a 'sterile immunity' (Neitz, 1957; Barnett, 1968). However, further studies eventually demonstrated that recovered animals develop a persistent infection, referred to as a carrier state, which facilitates transmission by ticks. The first evidence of a carrier state was obtained by Barnett and Brocklesby (1966b), who used *R. appendiculatus* ticks to transmit infection from animals that had been infected experimentally with a field isolate of *T. parva*. However, this parasite appeared to have moderate virulence and it had been isolated from a region apparently grazed only by wildlife, leaving uncertainty about its precise identity. Nevertheless, later studies clearly demonstrated tick transmission of *T. parva* by feeding ticks on cattle that had recovered from natural infection (Young *et al.*, 1986) and also on cattle that had recovered from experimental infection following treatment with the recently developed theilericidal compound parvaquone (Dolan, 1986). The former study demonstrated transmission of infection up to 13 months after the cattle had been removed from field challenge, clearly demonstrating that infection with *T. parva* persists well beyond the acute phase of infection. The failure of early studies to demonstrate persistent infection in recovered animals may have been due to feeding relatively small numbers of ticks, as ticks fed on carrier animals generally have low infection rates. This carrier state is now readily detected using DNA prepared from blood in a polymerase chain reaction (PCR) assay (Skilton *et al.*, 2002). Mathematical modelling of transmission dynamics has indicated that the carrier phase of infection (compared to the acute phase) accounts for a large proportion of the parasite infections in field tick populations in ECF-endemic areas (Medley *et al.*, 1993). Hence, this property is a key parameter in understanding the epidemiology of the disease.

1.10.3 Susceptibility of calves to *T. parva*

As discussed above, early studies of indigenous cattle residing in tick-infested areas demonstrated that calves succumb to disease caused by *T. parva*. This was confirmed in a number of detailed field studies of zebu cattle maintained in endemic areas in the absence of any disease control measures (Barnett, 1957; Moll *et al.*, 1986; Thumbi *et al.*, 2013). In a series of experiments involving challenge of calves and adult animals with different numbers of ticks experimentally infected with *T. parva*, Barnett (1957) showed that a single infected tick was sufficient to produce lethal disease in 100% of adult animals of fully susceptible breeds but lower levels of mortality in indigenous zebu animals. Moreover, 1-month-old calves from indigenous zebu (reared free of tick challenge) suffered lower levels of mortality than older animals (Barnett, 1957). These experiments confirmed a degree of genetic resistance in these zebu animals and suggested that calves were somewhat more resistant compared to adults (although age-related resistance is yet to be confirmed; see Chapter 7 of this volume). However, this difference clearly does not completely prevent losses of calves due to ECF under field challenge. In this regard, *T. parva* differs significantly from the other important tick-borne diseases babesiosis and anaplasmosis, both of which show markedly increased resistance in calves under 6 months of age. This allows animals to acquire immunity as calves, thus creating a situation of endemic stability in endemically infected areas. These issues are discussed more fully in Chapter 7 of this volume.

Maternal antibodies also do not appear to confer significant protection against *T. parva*.

Cunningham *et al.* (1989) showed that calves fed colostral antibody from cows experimentally immunized and repeatedly challenged with *T. parva* remained fully susceptible to parasite challenge. More recently, a survey of levels of maternal antibody to *T. parva* in indigenous zebu calves exposed to field challenge found no correlation of antibody levels with mortality in calves due to *T. parva* (Toye *et al.*, 2013).

1.10.4 Synchronous division of the parasite and host leukocytes

Although the rapid multiplication of infected leukocytes in the lymphoid organs of infected cattle was recognized as a key feature of ECF in early studies, the mechanism of parasite multiplication was not understood. For a long time, it was accepted that this occurred by repeated parasite release and reinvasion of fresh host leukocytes (i.e. similar to what occurs with other apicomplexan parasites). However, in cytological studies conducted by Reichenow (1940), he observed infected cells undergoing mitosis, during which the parasite also appeared to be dividing, suggesting that this may be the mechanism by which at least some parasites multiply.

The development of methods for culturing infected cells *in vitro* in the 1960s and 1970s allowed the mechanism of parasite multiplication to be examined in detail. In the mid-1960s, workers in Israel had developed a system for culturing cells infected with *Theileria annulata in vitro* from tissues of infected cattle (Tsur and Adler, 1962). Initially, such cultures could only be maintained for a few weeks and required the presence of a feeder layer (baby hamster kidney cells were used initially). This system was then used in Kenya to culture *T. parva*-infected cells (Hulliger, 1965).

The use of these cultures to study parasite multiplication confirmed that during mitosis of host leukocytes, the schizont undergoes division at the same time as the host cell, thus remaining within the cell during successive cell divisions (Hulliger *et al.*, 1964; Hulliger, 1965). Thus, multiplication of the parasitized cells occurs by clonal expansion of the cells initially infected by parasites released by the tick, resulting in the parasite being shielded from serum antibodies during this stage of development. Further refinement of culture methods enabled the *T. parva*-infected cells to be cultured in the absence of feeder cells and maintained as continuously growing cell lines (Malmquist *et al.*, 1970). This property of the parasite, to drive proliferation of the host cell while retaining infection in progeny cells, was referred to as transformation, drawing parallels with the behaviour of cancer cells. Studies of *T. annulata* had shown that infected cell lines could be used to immunize cattle against the parasite following passage of the lines *in vitro* to ensure attenuation (Tsur and Pipano, 1966). This method of immunization was deployed successfully in Israel to vaccinate cattle against *T. annulata* (Pipano, 1989). However, a similar approach using cultured *T. parva*-infected cells proved impractical because of the large numbers of cells that were required to induce immunity (Brown, 1981; see Chapter 11 of this volume).

1.10.5 Preservation of parasite isolates *in vitro*

Since *T. parva*-infected lymphocytes do not reproducibly establish infection when administered to cattle, the use of infected ticks was required in early experimental studies of infection in cattle. The production of infected ticks was a costly and time-consuming procedure, and the level of infection varied between different batches of ticks, resulting in difficulties in establishing reproducibility between experiments. Development of methods to cryopreserve the parasite by the UNDP project represented an important technical advance in addressing this problem and helped to underpin the project's research on vaccine development. A protocol for cryopreserving the infectious tick stage of the parasite using homogenized infected ticks was established (Cunningham *et al.*, 1973), which facilitated production of frozen parasite stocks of defined infectivity and virulence (Cunningham *et al.*, 1974). This allowed standardization of parasite challenge in experimental studies and, eventually, production of parasite stocks for the live vaccine. Methods for cryopreserving cell lines of *T. parva*-infected leukocytes were also established. Moreover, it became possible to establish such cell lines by infecting blood leukocytes from naïve animals with parasites harvested from infected ticks (Brown *et al.*, 1973).

This would eventually prove to be invaluable for immunological studies by allowing analyses of cellular immune responses of infected or immunized animals against their own *T. parva*-infected cells *in vitro*.

1.10.6 Vaccination using live parasites reveals antigenic heterogeneity

Studies conducted in South Africa in the 1950s had shown that prophylactic daily treatment of cattle with tetracyclines immediately following parasite challenge prevented development of the disease, although treatment of animals once disease had developed was ineffective (Neitz, 1953). The UNDP group demonstrated that infection of animals with standardized doses of tick-derived sporozoites from cryopreserved stocks and simultaneous treatment with a long-acting formulation of oxytetracycline resulted in a mild transient infection and immunity to subsequent parasite challenge (Radley *et al.*, 1975a).

However, during the course of these studies, although animals subjected to infection and treatment using a single isolate of *T. parva* developed immunity to challenge with the same isolate, some of the animals remained susceptible to experimental challenge with other isolates (Radley *et al.*, 1975b). Further studies revealed that use of a cocktail of three different parasite isolates for immunization provided protection against experimental challenge with several different parasite isolates (Radley *et al.*, 1975c) and against field challenge (Uilenberg *et al.*, 1976). Detailed descriptions of the development and commercialization of this vaccine are provided in Chapters 12 and 13 of this volume.

The findings from these studies highlighted the critical importance of antigenic heterogeneity in *T. parva* with respect to vaccine development and focused attention of subsequent research on the need to understand the antigenic specificity of protective immune responses.

1.11 A New Research Institute to Study Animal Diseases in Africa

By the early 1970s, rapid advances in scientific knowledge, including the recent elucidation of the genetic code and establishment of the basic concepts of humoral and cellular immunity, had created great optimism concerning the potential of research to yield novel methods for the control of infectious diseases. In the field of parasitology, this coincided with an influx of basic immunologists and biochemists, attracted by the challenges of unravelling the intricacies of host–parasite relationships and host immune responses. Growing knowledge of the immune system created confidence that an understanding of protective immune responses could lead to the development of new approaches to vaccination.

In 1970, the Rockefeller Foundation in the USA proposed the establishment of a worldwide network of research institutes aimed at improving food production in developing countries, and, with further support from the World Bank, FAO and UNDP, this led to the establishment of the Consultative Group for International Agricultural Research (CGIAR) in 1971. The CGIAR secured financial support from various national foreign aid programmes, and in 1973 the decision was made to establish a new institute to address important infectious diseases of livestock in Africa. Agreement was reached with the government of Kenya to host the International Laboratory for Research on Animal Diseases (ILRAD) in Nairobi. The remit of ILRAD was to investigate development of improved methods to control important infectious disease, with efforts initially focused on two diseases, ECF and trypanosomiasis, which were considered to be the most important diseases constraining livestock production in sub-Saharan Africa. A major focus of the ECF programme was to gain a better understanding of the immune processes mediating the naturally acquired immunity present in recovered animals, with a view to developing an alternative vaccine. Recruitment of staff to the new institute started in 1975, with an initial cohort of scientists (from eight different countries, including Kenya and Uganda) joining the institute over the next 12 months. Research was conducted in temporary facilities, before moving into purpose-built laboratories in 1978. The institute's activities also included a training programme, which made an important contribution to development of the next generation of African scientists in animal health. As with the earlier UNDP project, ILRAD provided a focal point for collaboration with other research projects, involving countries both within and outside Africa.

In 1994, ILRAD was amalgamated with another CGIAR institute (the International Livestock Centre for Africa – ILCA) to create a new institute, the International Livestock Research Institute (ILRI), which had a wider remit encompassing both animal production and disease and continuing work on ECF. Although ILRAD and ILRI have not succeeded in developing an alternative vaccine for *T. parva*, their work, along with that of others, has extended our knowledge of the biology and immunology of *T. parva* and has laid the groundwork for ongoing research to investigate vaccine development against the parasite. In particular, studies of the immunology of the disease unravelled the immune responses involved in development of natural immunity and identified antigens recognized by these responses, which are the focus of current studies of vaccine development (reviewed in Morrison *et al.*, 2015; Nene and Morrison, 2016). Technical advances in immunology and molecular biology also provided tools to investigate genetic and antigenic diversity in *T. parva* (Conrad *et al.*, 1987; Bishop *et al.*, 2009). Analyses of field populations of the parasite indicated that it frequently undergoes sexual recombination (Oura *et al.*, 2005) and this was subsequently confirmed experimentally (Henson *et al.*, 2012; Katzer *et al.*, 2012). These technologies have been extended by others to provide precise methods for identification of other *Theileria* species and to allow analyses of their host species specificity and genetic diversity (Allsopp *et al.*, 1993; Mans *et al.*, 2015). The advent of genome sequencing also enabled generation of the whole genome sequence of *T. parva* (Gardner *et al.*, 2005), providing a valuable resource for research on the immunobiology of the parasite and a platform for understanding genetic diversity at the level of the whole genome.

Meanwhile, the establishment of robust culture systems coupled with development of molecular technologies enabled a number of laboratories in Europe to initiate studies of the cell biology of *Theileria*-infected leukocytes (Chaussepied and Langsley, 1996; Dobbelaere and Heussler, 1999; Shiels, 1999; Huessler *et al.*, 2006; Shiels *et al.*, 2006; Tajeri *et al.*, 2021). This work, which included studies of both *T. parva* and *T. annulata*, provided the first insight into how the parasite, by driving host cell activation and inhibiting apoptosis, manipulates the behaviour of the infected cell and coordinates parasite and host cell division.

These aspects of the parasite will be discussed in greater detail in subsequent chapters of this volume.

1.12 The Lack of a Laboratory Animal Model

Research on other apicomplexan parasites has made extensive use of laboratory animal models to complement studies of the pathogens in their natural hosts. However, this has not been possible for *T. parva*. Most species of *Theileria* are found in ungulates, and attempts to establish infections in laboratory animals have consistently proved unsuccessful. Moreover, in the case of *T. parva*, the difficulty in establishing infection in the natural host by mechanical transfer of the parasite has necessitated access to tick colonies to generate the infective stages for experimental studies. These features account for the fact that much of the work discussed in this chapter (at least until the most recent advances) was conducted in Africa. The lack of laboratory animal models has constrained studies of some aspects of the immunobiology of the parasites and undoubtedly has limited the extent to which scientists have engaged in studying *T. parva*. The intriguing capacity of the parasite to cause transformation of host leukocytes would undoubtedly have attracted much greater research interest had there been a laboratory animal model. On the other hand, this helped to focus the attention of research on the disease in the natural host, and also resulted in wider benefits. Studies of immunity to *T. parva* required substantial investment of effort to develop reagents and methodologies to study the bovine immune system in order to facilitate identification of protective immune responses and the parasite antigens that they recognize. During the 1970s and 1980s, many of the advances in bovine immunology arose from studies of immunity to *T. parva*. Hence, in addition to contributing to understanding immunity to the parasite, this research has had a wider beneficial impact on the research community studying diseases of cattle.

1.13 Other *Theileria* Species in African Cattle

The *Theileria* genus in now known to include a large number of species that predominantly infect wild and domestic ruminants in tropical and subtropical regions of the world (Uilenberg, 1981; Morrison, 2015). Many of the species found in Africa do not cause disease, or do so infrequently, but detection of their presence is of relevance for differential diagnostic purposes. Unlike *T. parva*, many species multiply predominantly during the intra-erythrocyte stage of development. Since the piroplasm stages of most species are difficult to distinguish morphologically, initial assignment to species frequently relied on the host and/or tick species in which they were detected. Different species names were sometimes used for the same parasites, and some parasites were initially assigned to the incorrect species. Some of the current species assignments may eventually be shown to contain more than one species. A more detailed discussion of definition of the species and the methods used for their detection is provided in Chapter 8 of this volume. The history of discovery of these parasites is summarized here.

1.13.1 *T. annulata*

The other major pathogenic species of *Theileria* in cattle, *T. annulata*, which causes a disease similar to ECF, was first identified in eastern Europe by Dschunkowsky and Luhs in 1904. It is transmitted by different tick vectors than *T. parva* (namely several species of *Hyalomma*) and has a very different geographical distribution. *T. annulata* is present in a broad subtropical zone extending from southern Europe and North Africa through the Middle East into Asia. In Africa, its distribution extends southwards to Sudan (El Hussein *et al.*, 2012) and into South Sudan, where the distribution of *T. parva* and *T. annulata* overlap (Salih *et al.*, 2007). Recently, a report has appeared of the detection of *T. annulata* in *Hyalomma* ticks present in North-east Nigeria (Mamman *et al.*, 2021). However, the findings were based on results of screening by PCR with primers believed to be specific for *T. annulata*, and to date there has been no confirmation by direct detection of the parasite.

1.13.2 *T. mutans* and *T. velifera*

As already discussed, *T. mutans* was first identified by Theiler (1906) who showed that (unlike *T. parva*) infection was transmissible experimentally with blood from infected animals and resulted in mild anaemia. Natural infection usually does not cause overt clinical disease, although occasional instances of clinical disease characterized by anaemia have been reported (Irvin *et al.*, 1972). *T. velifera* was identified as a distinct species in the 1960s, based on the morphology of the piroplasm stage, which includes a veil-like structure (Uilenberg, 1964). It is non-pathogenic in cattle. *T. mutans* and *T. velifera* are both found in African buffalo and are restricted to sub-Saharan Africa, where they are prevalent throughout the regions where *T. parva* is present. They are transmitted by *Amblyoma* sp. ticks (Uilenberg *et al.*, 1974; Young *et al.*, 1978b). Both parasites multiply predominantly during the intra-erythrocytic stage, consistent with their experimental transmissibility with infected blood.

1.13.3 *T. orientalis*

T. orientalis also multiplies predominantly during the intra-erythrocytic stage, but has a much wider global distribution. The nomenclature of this parasite has a complicated history (Uilenberg, 1981; Sugimoto and Fugisaka, 2002). Parasites described as *T. buffeli* were first reported in the Asian buffalo (*Bubalis bubalis*) in South-east Asia (Neveu-Lemaire, 1912), while parasites referred to as *T. sergenti* and *T. orientalis* were reported in the Soviet Union in the 1930s (Yakimov and Dekhterev, 1930; Yakimov and Sudaschenkov, 1931). Parasites under these species names were found to have a widespread global distribution including Africa, where they were found in African buffalo and cattle. These parasites were all shown to be transmitted by *Haemophysalis* sp. ticks. Based on similarities in their morphology, serological reactivities and tick vectors, Uilenberg *et al.* (1985) suggested that they belong to the same species and proposed use of *T. orientalis* as the species name. Some parasites that had been erroneously reported as *T. mutans*, both within and outside Africa, have subsequently been recognized as *T. orientalis*. More recently, molecular studies identified different genotypes of *T. orientalis* (Kawazu *et al.*, 1992; Gubbels *et al.*, 2000), many of which differ in their geographical distribution. Some genotypes found in Asia, Australia and New Zealand produce clinical disease in cattle, manifesting as anaemia and in some cases mortality (Aparna *et al.*, 2011; Islam *et al.*, 2011). Clinical disease has also been reported in Asian buffalo (Vinodkumar *et al.*, 2016). However, the genotypes of *T. orientalis* present in Africa are considered non-pathogenic, and *T. buffeli* is frequently used by some workers in Africa for these parasites (Mans *et al.*, 2015).

1.13.4 *T. taurotragi* and *T.* sp. (buffalo)

These two parasites are more closely related to *T. parva* than those discussed above and therefore pose particular problems for differential diagnosis. Both cause 'transformation' of infected leukocytes enabling infected cells to be cultivated *in vitro* as continuously growing cell lines (Stagg *et al.*, 1976; Zwegarth *et al.*, 2009). *T. taurotragi* was first identified in an eland in 1960 (Martin and Brocklesby, 1960) and was subsequently found to infect cattle (Young *et al.*, 1977a; Grootenhuis *et al.*, 1979). *Rhipicephalus appendiculatus* and several other *Rhipicephalus* tick species act as vectors, and transmission of infection to cattle has been demonstrated both with ticks fed on infected eland and with ticks fed on infected cattle (Young *et al.*, 1977a). A recent study in South Africa detected *T. taurotragi* in cattle, eland, kudu and nyala but not in buffalo, and attempts to transmit the parasite to buffalo were unsuccessful (Pienaar *et al.*, 2018). Clinical disease and mortality due to *T. taurotragi* have been reported in a domesticated herd of eland in Kenya (Grootenhuis *et al.*, 1980) and in mountain bongo that had been bred in the USA and reintroduced to Africa (Bishop *et al.*, 2019), but acute infection of cattle with *T. taurotragi* is generally considered to be non-pathogenic, and there is no evidence of establishment of a carrier state in cattle.

Cerebral theileriosis, often referred to as 'turning sickness', is a sporadic lethal condition in cattle characterized by intravascular accumulation of *Theileria*-infected leukocytes in the brain and meninges of affected animals. Originally described by Mettam and Carmichael (1936) in Uganda, it has been recorded in ECF-endemic areas in both eastern Africa and southern Africa (Flanagan and Le Roux, 1957; Giles *et al.*, 1978; De Vos *et al.*, 1981). Affected animals often have evidence of previous infection with *T. parva*, which led to the belief that the disease occurs either due to reinfection or due to persistence of *T. parva*-infected cells following an earlier acute infection. However, a study in which a series of cases of turning sickness in Tanzania were investigated using *Theileria*-species-specific PCR assays (Catalano *et al.*, 2015), failed to detect *T. parva* in any of the cases but detected *T. taurotragi* in some of them. Hence, *T. taurotragi* is now considered as the likely causal agent of turning sickness.

The first indication of the existence of another parasite closely related to *T. parva* in buffalo came from studies of cloned *Theileria*-infected cell lines isolated from buffalo in East Africa, which revealed some cell lines that showed a distinct pattern of reactivity with *T. parva*-specific monoclonal antibodies and weak hybridization with *T. parva* DNA probes (Conrad *et al.*, 1989). Subsequent studies in South Africa confirmed the presence of parasites in buffalo with a distinct mitochondrial 18S rRNA gene sequence (Allsopp *et al.*, 1993). The parasite was provisionally designated *T.* sp. (buffalo) and was found to have a widespread distribution in buffalo. Evidence of infection in cattle was obtained only recently by examining *Theileria*-infected cell lines isolated from cattle that developed disease following introduction into an area grazed by buffalo; many of the clones derived from these cell lines were found to contain *T.* sp. (buffalo) (Bishop *et al.*, 2015). Since there are no records of infection of cattle with *T.* sp. (buffalo) on its own, the pathogenicity of the parasite for cattle is not known, nor is it known whether it is capable of establishing persistent infection in cattle. The tick vector of *T.* sp. (buffalo) also has not been identified.

1.14 Concluding Remarks

Awareness of the devastating impact of ECF on cattle production was first recognized in southern Africa in the early years of the 20th century, following the introduction of the disease with cattle imported from Tanzania. Importation of cattle had been prompted by acute shortages caused by the recent Anglo-Boer war, coupled with the spread of the pan-African rinderpest epidemic to the Cape. Intensive efforts to investigate the disease led to the identification of the causal agent and its tick vector within a remarkably short period of time, due in large part to contributions by two local scientists, Arnold Theiler and Charles Lounsbury. Although disease (subsequently shown to be caused by *T. parva*) had previously been recognized in indigenous cattle in eastern Africa, it was associated with much lower levels of mortality due to a degree of genetic resistance in the indigenous animals. Subsequent research identified the African buffalo as an important wildlife reservoir of the parasite, but this species does not suffer clinical disease despite being fully susceptible to infection. Sustained application of rigorous control measures in South Africa and Zimbabwe over a 50-year period resulted in clearance of ECF from these countries. However, the disease remained as one of the most important constraints to cattle production throughout a large part of eastern Africa, leading to an increased emphasis of research on the disease in this region. Studies conducted during the latter half of the last century filled in many of the gaps in our knowledge of the epidemiology and pathogenesis of ECF and advanced our understanding of the host–parasite relationship, providing a sound basis for subsequent efforts to develop more effective methods to control the disease.

References

Allsopp, B.A., Baylis, H.A., Allsopp, M.T.E.P., Cavalier-Smith, T., Bishop, R.P. *et al.* (1993) Discrimination between six species of *Theileria* using oligonucleotide probes which detect small subunit ribosomal RNA sequences. *Parasitology* 107(2), 157–165. DOI: 10.1017/s0031182000067263.

Anon (1912) *Annual Report of Department of Agriculture and Veterinary Services, British East Africa*. Government Printers, Nairobi.

Aparna, M., Ravindran, R., Vimalkumar, M.B., Lakshmanan, B., Rameshkumar, P. *et al.* (2011) Molecular characterization of *Theileria orientalis* causing fatal infection in crossbred adult bovines of South India. *Parasitology International* 60(4), 524–529. DOI: 10.1016/j.parint.2011.08.002.

Babes, V. (1888) Sur l'hemoglobinure bactienne des boeuf. *Comptes Rondus Des Seances de l'Acadamie Des Sciences (Paris)* 107, 693–694.

Barnett, S.F. (1957) Theileriasis control. *Bulletin of Epizootic Diseases in Africa* 5, 343–357.

Barnett, S.F. and Brocklesby, D.W. (1966a) The passage of *Theileria lawrencei* (Kenya) through cattle. *British Veterinary Journal* 122, 396–409. DOI: 10.1016/S0007-1935(17)40406-4.

Barnett, S.F. and Brocklesby, D.W. (1966b) Recent investigations into *Theileridae* of cattle and buffalo in Africa. A mild form of East Coast fever (*Theileria parva*) with persistence of infection. *British Veterinary Journal* 122, 361–370.

Barnett, S.F. (1968) Theileriosis. In: Weinman, D. and Ristic, M. (eds) *Infectious Blood Diseases of Man and Animals*, Vol. II. Academic Press, New York, pp. 269–328.

Bettencourt, A., Franca, C. and Borges, I. (1907) Addendum a nota sombre piroplasmose do gamo. *Revista de Medicina Veterinaria Lisbon* 6, 37–40.

Bishop, R.P., Odongo, D.O., Mann, D.J., Pearson, T.W., Sugimoto, C. *et al.* (2009) Theileria. In: Nene, V. and Cole, C. (eds) *Genome Mapping and Genomics in Animal-Associated Microbes*. Springer-Verlag, Berlin, pp. 191–231.

Bishop, R.P., Hemmink, J.D., Morrison, W.I., Weir, W., Toye, P.G. *et al.* (2015) The African buffalo parasite *Theileria* sp. (buffalo) can infect and immortalize cattle leukocytes and encodes divergent orthologues of *Theileria parva* antigen genes. *International Journal for Parasitology: Parasites and Wildlife* 4(3), 333–342. DOI: 10.1016/j.ijppaw.2015.08.006.

Bishop, R.P., Odongo, D.O., Dolan, T.T., Dolan, R.B., Skilton, R.A. *et al*. (2019) Theileriosis in Mountain Bongo repatriated to Kenya: A clinical and molecular investigation. *Journal of Zoo and Wildlife Medicine* 50(2), 342–349. DOI: 10.1638/2018-0110.

Brocklesby, D.W. and Barnett, S.F. (1966) The isolation of *Theileria lawrencei* (Kenya) from a wild buffalo (*Syncerus caffer*) and its serial passage through captive buffalo. *British Veterinary Journal* 122, 387–395. DOI: 10.1016/S0007-1935(17)40405-2.

Brown, C.G.D., Stagg, D.A., Purnell, R.E., Kanhai, G.K. and Payne, R.C. (1973) Infection and transformation of bovine lymphoid cells *in vitro* by infective particles of *Theileria parva*. *Nature* 245(5420), 101–103. DOI: 10.1038/245101a0.

Brown, C.G.D. (1981) Application of *in vitro* techniques to vaccination against theileriosis. In: Irvin, A.D., Cunningham, M.P. and Young, A.S. (eds) *Advances in the Control of Theileriosis. Current Topics in Veterinary Medicine and Animal Science*, Vol. 14. Martinus Nijhoff, The Hague, pp. 104–119.

Bruce, D., Hamerton, A.E., Bateman, H.R. and Mackie, F.P. (1910) Amakebe: A disease of calves in Uganda. *Proceedings of the Royal Society B* 14(5), 467–486.

Catalano, D., Biasibetti, E., Lynen, G., Di Giulio, G. and De Meneghi, D. (2015) "Ormilo disease" a disorder of zebu cattle in Tanzania: Bovine cerebral theileriosis or new protozoan disease? *Tropical Animal Health and Production* 47(5), 895–901. DOI: 10.1007/s11250-015-0805-8.

Chaussepied, M. and Langsley, G. (1996) *Theileria* transformation of bovine leukocytes: A parasite model for the study of lymphoproliferation. *Research in Immunology* 147(3), 127–138. DOI: 10.1016/0923-2494(96)83165-8.

Conrad, P.A., Iams, K., Brown, W.C., Sohanpal, B. and ole-MoiYoi, O.K. (1987) DNA probes detect genomic diversity in *Theileria parva* stocks. *Molecular and Biochemical Parasitology* 25(3), 213–226. DOI: 10.1016/0166-6851(87)90085-5.

Conrad, P.A., ole-MoiYoi, O.K., Baldwin, C.L., Dolan, T.T., O'Callaghan, C.J. *et al*. (1989) Characterization of buffalo-derived *Theilerial* parasites with monoclonal antibodies and DNA probes. *Parasitology* 98(2), 179–188. DOI: 10.1017/S0031182000062089.

Cowdry, E.V. and Danks, W.B.C. (1933) Studies on East Coast Fever. II. Behaviour of the parasite and the development of distinctive lesions in susceptible animals. *Parasitology* 25(1), 1–63. DOI: 10.1017/S003118200001920X.

Cox, F.E.G. (2002) History of human parasitology. *Clinical Microbiology Reviews* 15(4), 595–612. DOI: 10.1128/CMR.15.4.595-612.2002.

Cranfield, P.F. (1991) *Science and Empire: East Coast fever in Rhodesia and Transvaal*. Cambridge University Press, Cambridge, UK, pp. 1–257.

Cunha, C.B. and Cunha, B.A. (2008) Brief history of the clinical diagnosis of malaria: From Hippocrates to Osler. *Journal of Vector Borne Diseases* 45(3), 194–199.

Cunningham, M.P., Brown, C.G.D., Burridge, M.J. and Purnell, R.E. (1973) Cryopreservation of infective particles of *Theileria parva*. *International Journal for Parasitology* 3(5), 583–587. DOI: 10.1016/0020-7519(73)90082-9.

Cunningham, M.P., Brown, C.G.D., Burridge, M.J., Musoke, A.J., Purnell, R.E. *et al*. (1974) East Coast fever: Titration in cattle of suspensions of *Theileria parva* derived from ticks. *British Veterinary Journal* 130(4), 336–345. DOI: 10.1016/S0007-1935(17)35836-0.

Cunningham, M.P., Brown, C.G.D., Burridge, M.J., Morzaria, S.P. and Urquhart, G.M. (1989) *Theileria parva*: The immune status of calves born of dams immunised against East Coast fever. *Research in Veterinary Science* 46(1), 90–94.

De Vos, A.J., Bessenger, R. and Banting, L.F. (1981) *Theileria taurotragi*: A probable agent of bovine cerebral theileriosis. *The Onderstepoort Journal of Veterinary Research* 48(3), 177–178.

Dobbelaere, D. and Heussler, V. (1999) Transformation of leukocytes by *Theileria parva* and *T. annulata*. *Annual Reviews in Microbiology* 53, 1–42. DOI: 10.1146/annurev.micro.53.1.1.

Dolan, T.T. (1986) Chemotherapy of East Coast fever: The long term weight changes, carrier state and disease manifestations of parvaquone treated cattle. *Journal of Comparative Pathology* 96(2), 137–146. DOI: 10.1016/0021-9975(86)90004-6.

Dschunkowsky, E. and Luhs, J. (1904) Die pirplasmen der rinder. *Centralblatt fur Bacteriologie, Parasitenkunde and Infektionskrankheiten* 35, 486–492.

du Toit, P.J. and Jackson, C. (1936) The life and work of Sir Arnold Theiler. *Journal of the South African Veterinary Association* 7, 135–186.

El Hussein, A.M., Hassan, S.M. and Salih, D.A. (2012) Current situation of tropical theileriosis in the Sudan. *Parasitology Research* 111(2), 503–508. DOI: 10.1007/s00436-012-2951-5.

Fantham, H.B. (1910) The morphology and life-history of *Eimeria* (*coccidium*) avium: A sporozoön causing a fatal disease among young grouse. *Proceedings of the Zoological Society of London* 3, 672–691. DOI: 10.1111/j.1096-3642.1910.tb01910.x.

Flanagan, H.O. and Le Roux, J.M.W. (1957) Bovine cerebral theileriosis – a report on two cases occurring in the Union. *Onderstepoort Journal of Veterinary Research* 27, 453–461.

Garden, G. (1912) East coast fever in Nyasaland. *Report of the Department of Agriculture Nyasaland* 29–37.

Gardner, M.J., Bishop, R., Shah, T., de Villiers, E.P., Carlton, J.M. *et al.* (2005) Genome sequence of *Theileria parva*, a bovine pathogen that transforms lymphocytes. *Science* 309(5731), 134–137. DOI: 10.1126/science.1110439.

Giles, N., Davies, F.G., Duffus, W.P.H. and Heinonen, R. (1978) Bovine cerebral theileriosis. *The Veterinary Record* 102(14), 313. DOI: 10.1136/vr.102.14.313.

Gonder, R. (1910) The life cycle of *Theileria parva*: The cause of East Coast fever in cattle in South Africa. *Journal of Comparative Pathology and Therapeutics* 23, 328–335. DOI: 10.1016/S0368-1742(10)80060-8.

Gonder, R. (1911a) Die entwicklung von *Theileria parva* dem erreger des kustenfiebers der rinder in Africa. *Archiv für Protistenkunde* 21, 328–335.

Gonder, R. (1911b) *The Development of Theileria parva, the cause of East Coast Fever in South Africa. First Report of the Director of Veterinary Services, Part II*. Government Printer and Stationery Office, Pretoria, pp. 69–83.

Gray, C.E. and Robertson, W. (1902) Redwater in Rhodesia. *Natal Agricultural Journal* 5, 237–248.

Grootenhuis, J.G., Young, A.S., Dolan, T.T. and Stagg, D.A. (1979) Characteristics of *Theileria* species (eland) infections in eland and cattle. *Research in Veterinary Science* 27(1), 59–68.

Grootenhuis, J.G., Morrison, W.I., Karstad, L., Sayer, P.D., Young, A.S. *et al.* (1980) Fatal theileriosis in Eland (*Taurotragus oryx*): Pathology of natural and experimental cases. *Research in Veterinary Science* 29(2), 219–229.

Grootenhuis, J.G., Leitch, B.L., Stagg, D.A., Dolan, T.T. and Young, A.S. (1987) Experimental induction of *Theileria parva lawrencei* carrier state in an African buffalo (*Syncerus caffer*). *Parasitology* 9(3), 425–431. DOI: 10.1017/s0031182000055773.

Gubbels, M.J., Hong, Y., van der Weide, M., Qi, B., Nijman, I.J. *et al.* (2000) Molecular characterisation of the *Theileria buffeli/orientalis* group. *International Journal for Parasitology* 30(8), 943–952. DOI: 10.1016/s0020-7519(00)00074-6.

Henson, S., Bishop, R.P., Morzaria, S., Spooner, P.R., Pelle, R. *et al.* (2012) High-resolution genotyping and mapping of recombination and gene conversion in the protozoan *Theileria parva* using whole genome sequencing. *BMC Genomics* 13, 503. DOI: 10.1186/1471-2164-13-503.

Huessler, V., Sturm, A. and Langsley, G. (2006) Regulation of host cell survival by intracellular *Plasmodium* and *Theileria parasites*. *Parasitology* 132(S1), 49–60. DOI: 10.1017/S0031182006000850.

Hulliger, L. (1965) Cultivation of three species of *Theileria* in lymphoid cells *in vitro*. *The Journal of Protozoology* 12(4), 649–655. DOI: 10.1111/j.1550-7408.1965.tb03267.x.

Hulliger, L., Wilde, K.H., Brown, C.G. and Turner, L. (1964) Mode of multiplication of *Theileria* in cultures of bovine lymphocytic cells. *Nature* 203, 728–730. DOI: 10.1038/203728a0.

Huxley, E. (1935) *White Man's Country: Lord Delamere and the Making of Kenya*. Chato and Windus, London, pp. 1870–1914.

Irvin, A.D., Brown, C.G., Burridge, M.J., Cunningham, M.P., Musoke, A.J. *et al.* (1972) A pathogenic Theilerial syndrome of cattle in the Narok District of Kenya. I. Transmission studies. *Tropical Animal Health and Production* 4(4), 220–229. DOI: 10.1007/BF02360114.

Islam, M.K., Jabbar, A., Campbell, B.E., Cantacessi, C. and Gasser, R.B. (2011) Bovine theileriosis – an emerging problem in South-Eastern Australia? *Infection, Genetics and Evolution* 11(8), 2095–2097. DOI: 10.1016/j.meegid.2011.08.012.

Katzer, F., Ngugi, D., Oura, C., Bishop, R.P., Taracha, E.L.N. *et al.* (2012) Extensive genotypic diversity in a recombining population of the apicomplexan parasite *Theileria parva*. *Infection and Immunity* 74(10), 5456–5464. DOI: 10.1128/IAI.00472-06.

Kawazu, S., Sugimoto, C., Kamio, T. and Fujisaki, K. (1992) Antigenic differences between Japanese *Theileria sergenti* and other benign *Theileria* species of cattle from Australia (*T. buffalo*) and Britain (*T. orientalis*). *Parasitology Research* 78(2), 130–135. DOI: 10.1007/BF00931654.

Koch, R. (1898) *Reiseberichte uber rinderpest, bubonenpest in Indie und Afrika, tsetse oder surrankrankeit, texasfieber, tropische malaria, Scharzwasserfieber*. Springer, Berlin. DOI: 10.1007/978-3-662-39506-6.

Koch, R. (1903) *Interim Report on Rhodesian Redwater or "African Coast Fever."* Argus Printing and Publishing Co. Ltd, Salisbury, p. 8. *Journal of Comparative Pathology and Therapeutics* 16, 273.

Koch, R. (1905) Vorläufige Mitteilungen über die Ergebnisse einer Forschungsreise nach Ostafriga. *DMW - Deutsche Medizinische Wochenschrift* 31(47), 1865–1869. DOI: 10.1055/s-0029-1188454.

Koch, R. (1906) Beiträge zur Entwicklungsgeschichte der Piroplasmen. *Zeitschrift Für Hygiene Und Infektionskrankheiten* 54(1), 1–9. DOI: 10.1007/BF02141824.

Laveran, A. (1880) Note sur le nouveau parasite trouve dans le sang de plusieurs maladies attients fievre pallustre. *Bulletin de l'Acadamie Nationale de Medicine* 9, 1235–1236.

Laveran, A. (1903) Sur la piroplasme bovine bacilliform. *Comptes Rendus Academie des Sciences* 136, 648–653.

Lawrence, D.A. (1935) *Report of the Director of Veterinary Research, Southern Rhodesia, for the Year 1934*. Rhodesia Printing and Publishing Co. Ltd, Salisbury.

Lawrence, D.A. (1936) *Report of the Director of Veterinary Research, Southern Rhodesia, for the Year 1935*. Rhodesia Printing and Publishing Co. Ltd, Salisbury.

Lawrence, J.A., Norval, R.A. and Uilenberg, G. (1983) *Rhipicephalus zambeziensis* as a vector of theileriidae. *Tropical Animal Health and Production* 15(1), 39–42. DOI: 10.1007/BF02250760.

Lawrence, J.A. (1992) The history of bovine theileriosis in Southern Africa. In: Norval, R.A., Perry, B.D. and Young, A.S. (eds) *The Epidemiology of Theileriosis in Africa*. Academic Press, London, pp. 2–41.

Lawrence, J.A., de Vos, A.J. and Irvin, A.D. (1994) Zimbabwe theileriosis. In: Coetzer, J.A.W., Thomson, G.R. and Tustin, R.C. (eds) *Infectious Diseases of Livestock with Special Reference to Southern Africa*. Oxford University Press, Oxford, UK, pp. 329–330.

Lounsbury, C.P. (1904) Transmission of African Coast fever. *Journal of the Cape of Good Hope* 24, 428–432.

Lounsbury, C.P. (1906) Ticks and African Coast fever. *Agricultural Journal of the Cape of Good Hope* 28, 634–654.

Mack, R. (1970) The great African cattle plague epidemic of the 1890s. *Tropical Animal Health and Production* 2, 210–219. DOI: 10.1007/BF02356441.

Magner, L.N. (2009) *A History of Infectious Diseases and the Microbial World*. Praeger, Connecticut, pp. 19–48. DOI: 10.5040/9798400664915.

Malmquist, W.A., Nyindo, M.B.A. and Brown, C.G.D. (1970) East Coast fever: Cultivation *in vitro* of bovine spleen cell lines infected and transformed by *Theileria parva*. *Tropical Animal Health and Production* 2(3), 139–145. DOI: 10.1007/BF02359680.

Mamman, A.H., Lorusso, V., Adam, B.M., Dogo, G.A., Bown, K.J. *et al.* (2021) First report of *Theileria annulata* in Nigeria: Findings from cattle ticks in Zamfara and Sokoto states. *Parasites & Vectors* 14(1), 242. DOI: 10.1186/s13071-021-04731-4.

Mans, B.J., Pienaar, R. and Latif, A.A. (2015) A review of *Theileria* diagnostics and epidemiology. *International Journal for Parasitology: Parasites and Wildlife* 4(1), 104–118. DOI: 10.1016/j.ijppaw.2014.12.006.

Maritim, A.C., Young, A.S., Lesan, A.C., Ndungu, S.G., Stagg, D.A. *et al.* (1992) Transformation of *Theileria parva* derived from African buffalo (*Syncerus caffer*) by tick passage in cattle and its use in infection and treatment immunization. *Veterinary Parasitology* 43(1–2), 1–14. DOI: 10.1016/0304-4017(92)90043-9.

Martin, H. and Brocklesby, D.W. (1960) A new parasite of eland. *Veterinary Record* 72, 331–332.

Medley, G.F., Perry, B.D. and Young, A.S. (1993) Preliminary analysis of the transmission dynamics of *Theileria parva*. *Parasitology* 106, 251–262. DOI: 10.1017/S0031182000075077.

Mettam, R.W.M. and Carmichael, J. (1936) Turning sickness, a protozoan encephalitis of cattle in Uganda. Its relationship with East Coast fever. *Parasitology* 28(2), 254–283. DOI: 10.1017/S0031182000022447.

Meyer, K.F. (1909) Preliminary note on the transmission of East Coast fever to cattle by intra-peritoneal inoculation of the spleen or portions of the spleen of a sick animal. *Journal of Comparative Pathology and Therapeutics* 22, 213–217. DOI: 10.1016/S0368-1742(09)80048-9.

Meyer, K.F. (1911) Notes on the nature of Koch's granules and their role in the pathogenesis of East Coast fever. In: *Union of South Africa Department of Agriculture. Report of the Government Veterinary Bacteriologist for the Year 1909-1910*. Government Printing and Stationery Office, Pretoria, pp. 56–68.

Miller, C. (1973) *The Lunatic Express*. Ballantine Books, New York.

Moll, G., Lohding, A., Young, A.S. and Leitch, B.L. (1986) Epidemiology of theileriosis in calves in an endemic area of Kenya. *Veterinary Parasitology* 19(3–4), 255–273. DOI: 10.1016/0304-4017(86)90073-7.

Morrison, W.I. (2015) The aetiology, pathogenesis and control of theileriosis in domestic animals. *Revue scientifique et technique (International Office of Epizootics)* 34(2), 599–611. DOI: 10.20506/rst.34.2.2383.

Morrison, W.I., Connelley, T., Hemmink, J.D. and MacHugh, N.D. (2015) Understanding the basis of parasite strain-restricted immunity to *Theileria parva*. *Annual Review of Animal Biosciences* 3(1), 397–418. DOI: 10.1146/annurev-animal-022513-114152.

Neitz, W.O. (1953) Aureomycin in *Theileria parva* infection. *Nature* 171(4340), 34–35. DOI: 10.1038/171034a0.

Neitz, W.O. (1955) Corridor disease: A fatal form of bovine theileriosis encountered in Zululand. *Bulletin of Epizootic Diseases in Africa* 3, 121–123.

Neitz, W.O. (1957) Theileriosis, gonderiosis and cytauxzoonoses: A review. *Onderstepoort Journal of Veterinary Research* 27, 275–430.

Neitz, W.O., Canham, A.S. and Kluge, E.B. (1955) Corridor disease: A fatal form of theileriosis encountered in Zululand. *Journal of South African Veterinary Medical Association* 26, 79–87.

Nene, V. and Morrison, W.I. (2016) Approaches to vaccination against *Theileria parva* and *Theileria annulata*. *Parasite Immunology* 38(12), 724–734. DOI: 10.1111/pim.12388.

Neumann, G. (1901) Revision de la famille des Ixodes (4e mémoire, 1). *Memoires de La Societe Zoologique de France* 14, 249–372.

Neveu-Lemaire, M. (1912) Congrès *Theileria* ou piroplasmes bacilliformes. In: *Parasitologie des animaux domestiques*. J. Lamarre et Cie, Paris, pp. 286–289.

Nicolle, C. and Manceaux, L. (1909) Sur un protozoare nouveau du gondi. *Archive Institut Pasteur* 2, 97–103.

Norval, R.A., Perry, B.D. and Young, A.S. (1992) *The Epidemiology of Theileriosis in Africa*. Academic Press, London.

Oura, C.A.L., Asiimwe, B.B., Weir, W., Lubega, G.W. and Tait, A. (2005) Population genetic analysis and sub-structuring of *Theileria parva* in Uganda. *Molecular and Biochemical Parasitology* 140(2), 229–239. DOI: 10.1016/j.molbiopara.2004.12.015.

Pienaar, R., Latif, A.A. and Mans, B.J. (2018) Investigations into the host specificity of *Theileria taurotragi*. *Veterinary Parasitology* 254, 30–35. DOI: 10.1016/j.vetpar.2018.03.003.

Pipano, E. (1989) Vaccination against *Theileria annulata* theileriosis. In: Wright, I.G. (ed.) *Veterinary Protozoan and Hemoparasite Vaccines*. CRC Press, Boca Raton, Florida, pp. 203–234.

Radley, D.E., Brown, C.G.D., Burridge, M.J., Cunningham, M.P., Kirimi, I.M. *et al.* (1975a) East Coast fever: 1. Chemoprophylactic immunization of cattle against *Theileria parva* (Muguga) and five *Theilerial* strains. *Veterinary Parasitology* 1(1), 35–41. DOI: 10.1016/0304-4017(75)90005-9.

Radley, D.E., Young, A.S., Brown, C.G.D., Burridge, M.J., Cunningham, M.P. *et al.* (1975b) East Coast fever: 2. Cross-immunity trials with a Kenya strain of *Theileria lawrencei*. *Veterinary Parasitology* 1(1), 43–50. DOI: 10.1016/0304-4017(75)90006-0.

Radley, D.E., Brown, C.G.D., Cunningham, M.P., Kimber, C.D., Musisi, F.L. *et al.* (1975c) East Coast fever: 3. Chemoprophylactic immunization of cattle using oxytetracycline and a combination of Theilerial strains. *Veterinary Parasitology* 1(1), 51–60. DOI: 10.1016/0304-4017(75)90007-2.

Radley, D.E., Young, A.S., Grootenhuis, J.G., Cunningham, M.P., Dolan, T.T. *et al.* (1979) Further studies on the immunization of cattle against *Theileria lawrencei* by infection and chemoprophylaxis. *Veterinary Parasitology* 5(2–3), 117–128. DOI: 10.1016/0304-4017(79)90003-7.

Reichenow, E. (1940) Die entwicklungsgang des kunstenfriebererregers im rinde und in der ubertragende zecke. *Archiv für Protistenkunde* 94, 1–56.

Ross, R. (1898) The rôle of the mosquito in the evolution of the malarial parasite. *The Lancet* 152(3912), 488–490. DOI: 10.1016/S0140-6736(01)81400-8.

Ross, R. (1923) *Memoirs with a Full Account of the Great Malaria Problem and its Solution*. John Murray, London, United Kingdom. (Also reprinted as *The Great Malaria Problem and its Solution*. Keynes Press, London, United Kingdom).

Rossiter, P.B. (1994) Rinderpest. In: Coetzer, J.A.W., Thomson, G.R. and Tistin, R.C. (eds) *Infectious Diseases of Livestock with Special Reference to South Africa*. Oxford University Press, Oxford, UK, pp. 735–757.

Salih, D.A., El Hussein, A.M., Seitzer, U. and Ahmed, J.S. (2007) Epidemiological studies on tick-borne diseases of cattle in Central Equatorial State, Southern Sudan. *Parasitology Research* 101(4), 1035–1044. DOI: 10.1007/s00436-007-0583-y.

Schreuder, B.E., Uilenberg, G. and Tondeur, W. (1977) Studies on *Theileriidae* (Sporozoa) in Tanzania. VIII. Experiments with African buffalo (*Syncerus caffer*). *Tropenmedizin Parasitologie* 28, 367–371.

Skilton, R.A., Bishop, R.P., Katende, J.M., Mwaura, S. and Morzaria, S.P. (2002) The persistence of *Theileria parva* infection in cattle immunized using two stocks which differ in their ability to induce a carrier state: Analysis using a novel blood spot PCR assay. *Parasitology* 124(Pt 3), 265–276. DOI: 10.1017/s0031182001001196.

Shiels, B.R. (1999) Should I stay or should I go now? A stochastic model of stage differentiation in *Theileria annulata*. *Parasitology Today* 15(6), 241–245. DOI: 10.1016/S0169-4758(99)01451-9.

Shiels, B., Langsley, G., Weir, W., Pain, A., McKellar, S. *et al.* (2006) Alteration of host cell phenotype by *Theileria annulata* and *Theileria parva*: Mining for manipulators in the parasite genomes. *International Journal for Parasitology* 36(1), 9–21. DOI: 10.1016/j.ijpara.2005.09.002.

Smith, T. and Kilborne, F.L. (1893) Investigations into the nature, causation and prevention of southern cattle fever. In: *US Department of Agriculture, Bureau of Animal Husbandry, Bulletin No. 1*. Government Printing Office, Washington, DC, pp. 177–304.

Splendore, A. (1909) Sur un nouveau protozoaire parasite du lapin, deuxieme note préliminaire. *Bulletin de La Societe de Pathologie Exotique* 2, 462–465.

Stagg, D.A., Kanhai, G.K., Young, A.S. and Brown, C.G.D. (1976) The establishment of *Theileria*-infected cell lines from an eland (*Taurotragus oryx*). *Research in Veterinary Science* 20(2), 122–126.

Stannus, H.S. (1910) Piroplasmosis among cattle in the Mombera District, Nyasaland, 1909. *Parasitology* 3(3), 307–311. DOI: 10.1017/S0031182000002122.

Steck, W. (1928) Histological studies on East Coast fever. *13th and 14th Reports, Union of South Africa Department of Agriculture* Part I, 243–280.

Sugimoto, C. and Fujisaki, K. (2002) Non-transforming *Theileria* parasites of ruminants. In: Dobbelaere, D. and McKeever, D. (eds) *Theileria, World Class Parasites*. Kluwer Academic, Boston, Massachusetts, pp. 93–106.

Tajeri, S., Haidar, M., Sakura, T. and Langsley, G. (2021) Interaction between transforming *Theileria* parasites and their host bovine leukocytes. *Molecular Microbiology* 115(5), 860–869. DOI: 10.1111/mmi.14642.

Theiler, A. (1902) Rhodesian cattle disease and rabies. *Transvaal Agricultural Journal* 1, 37–41.

Theiler, A. (1903) Rhodesian tick fever. *Transvaal Agricultural Journal* 1, 93–110.

Theiler, A. (1904a) East Coast fever. *Journal of the Royal Army Medical Corps* 3(6), 599–620.

Theiler, A. (1904b) Transmission of East Coast fever by ticks. *Journal of Royal Army Medical Corps* 3, 71–86.

Theiler, A. (1905) Report of the veterinary bacteriologist. In: *Report of the Transvaal Department of Agriculture*. 1st July 1903 to 30th June 1904. Pretoria Government Printing and Stationary Office.

Theiler, A. (1906) *Piroplasma mutans* (N. spec.) of South African cattle. *Journal of Comparative Pathology and Therapeutics* 19, 292–300. DOI: 10.1016/S0368-1742(06)80073-1.

Theiler, A. (1910) Gall-sickness in South Africa (Anaplasmosis of cattle). *Journal of Comparative Pathology and Therapeutics* 23, 98–115. DOI: 10.1016/S0368-1742(10)80028-1.

Theiler, G. (1971) Arnold Theiler (1867-1936). His life and times. In: *Commemoration of the Golden Jubilee of the Faculty of Veterinary Science, University of Pretoria*. The University of Pretoria, pp. 1–185.

Thumbi, S.M., Bronsvoort, M.B.M., Kiara, H., Toye, P.G., Poole, J. *et al.* (2013) Mortality in East African shorthorn zebu cattle under one year: Predictors of infectious-disease mortality. *BMC Veterinary Research* 9, 175. DOI: 10.1186/1746-6148-9-175.

Toye, P., Handel, I., Gray, J., Kiara, H., Thumbi, S. *et al.* (2013) Maternal antibody uptake, duration and influence on survival and growth rate in a cohort of indigenous calves in a smallholder farming system in western Kenya. *Veterinary Immunology and Immunopathology* 155(1–2), 129–134. DOI: 10.1016/j.vetimm.2013.06.003.

Tsur, I. and Adler, S. (1962) Cultivation of *Theileria annulata* schizonts in monolayer tissue cultures. *Refuah Veterinarith* 19, 224–225.

Tsur, I. and Pipano, E. (1966) Attenuation of virulence of strains of *Theileria annulata* by growth and passage through tissue culture. *Journal of Protozoology* 13, 33–38.

Turnbull, D.O. (1926) Tropical piroplasmosis in the Fort Jameson District of North-Eastern Rhodesia. *Journal of Comparative Pathology and Therapeutics* 39, 307–311. DOI: 10.1016/S0368-1742(26)80032-3.

Uilenberg, G. (1964) *Haematoxenus velifera*, n.g. n.sp., parasite *incertae cedus* du sang de bovins à Madagascar. *Revue d'Elevage et de Medecin Veterinaire des Pays Tropicaux* 17(4), 655. DOI: 10.19182/remvt.7306.

Uilenberg, G. (1976) Tick-borne disease and their vectors. 2. Epidemiology of tick-borne diseases. *World Animal Review* 17, 8–15.

Uilenberg, G., Robson, J. and Pedersen, V. (1974) Some experiments on the transmission of *Theileria mutans* (Theiler 1906) and *Theileria parva* (Theiler 1904) by the ticks *Amblyoma variegatum* (Fabricius 1794) and *Rhipicephalus appendiculatus* (Neumann 1901) in Uganda. *Zeitschift fur Tropenmedizin und Parasitologie* 25, 207–216.

Uilenberg, G., Schreuder, B.E., Silayo, R.S. and Mpangala, C. (1976) Studies on *Theileriidae* (Sporozoa) in Tanzania. IV. A field trial on immunization against East Coast fever (*Theileria parva* infection of cattle). *Tropenmedizin Parasitologie* 27, 329–336.

Uilenberg, G. (1981) Theilerial species of domestic livestock. In: Irvin, A.D., Cunningham, M.P. and Young, A.S. (eds) *Advances in the Control of Theileriosis. Current Topics in Veterinary Medicine and Animal Science*, Vol. 14. Martinus Nijhoff, The Hague, pp. 3–37.

Uilenberg, G., Perié, N.M., Spanjer, A.A. and Franssen, F.F. (1985) *Theileria orientalis*, a cosmopolitan blood parasite of cattle: Demonstration of the schizont stage. *Research in Veterinary Science* 38(3), 352–360.

Vinodkumar, K., Shyma, V., Justin, D.K., Ashok, S., Anu, J.P. *et al*. (2016) Fatal *Theileria orientalis* N2 genotype infection among asian water buffaloes (*Bubalus bubalis*) in a commercial dairy farm in Kerala, India. *Parasitology* 143(1), 69–74. DOI: 10.1017/S0031182015001468.

Yakimov, W.L. and Dekhterev, N.A. (1930) Zur frage uber die Theileriose in Ost-Sibirien. *Archiv für Protistenkunde* 72, 176–189.

Yakimov, W.L. and Sudaschenkov, W.W. (1931) Zur frage der piroplasmiden der rinder in ost-siberian. *Archiv Für Protistenkuunde* 75, 179–190.

Young, A.S. and Purnell, R.E. (1973) Transmission of *Theileria lawrencei* (Serengeti) by the ixodid tick, *Rhipicephalus appendiculatus*. *Tropical Animal Health and Production* 5(3), 146–152. DOI: 10.1007/BF02251383.

Young, A.S., Brown, C.G.D., Burridge, M.J., Cunningham, M.P., Kirimi, I.M. *et al*. (1973) Observations on the cross-immunity between *Theileria lawrencei* (Serengeti) and *Theileria parva* (Muguga) in cattle. *International Journal for Parasitology* 3(6), 723–728. DOI: 10.1016/0020-7519(73)90063-5.

Young, A.S., Grootenhuis, J.G., Kimber, C.D., Kanhai, G.K. and Stagg, D.A. (1977a) Isolation of a *Theileria species* from eland (*Taurotragus oryx*) infective for cattle. *Tropenmedizin Parasitologie* 27, 185–194.

Young, A.S., Radley, D.E., Cunningham, M.P., Musisi, F.L., Payne, R.C. *et al*. (1977b) Exposure of immunized cattle to prolonged natural challenge of *Theileria lawrencei* derived from African buffalo (*Syncerus caffer*). *Veterinary Parasitology* 3(4), 283–290. DOI: 10.1016/0304-4017(77)90015-2.

Young, A.S., Brown, C.G.D., Burridge, M.J., Grootenhuis, G.K., Kanhau, G.K. *et al*. (1978a) The incidence of *Theilerial parasites* in East African buffalo (*Syncerus caffer*). *Tropenmedizin Parasitologie* 29, 281–288.

Young, A.S., Purnell, R.E., Payne, R.C., Brown, C.G.D. and Kanhai, G.K. (1978b) Studies on the transmission and course of infection of a Kenyan strain of *Theileria mutans*. *Parasitology* 76(1), 99–115. DOI: 10.1017/S0031182000047430.

Young, A.S. (1981) The epidemiology of theileriosis in East Africa. In: Irvin, A.D., Cunningham, M.P. and Young, A.S. (eds) *Advances in the Control of Theileriosis. Current Topics in Veterinary Medicine and Animal Science*, Vol. 14. Martinus Nijhoff, The Hague, pp. 37–55.

Young, A.S., Leitch, B.L., Newson, R.M. and Cunningham, M.P. (1986) Maintenance of *Theileria parva* infection in an endemic area of Kenya. *Parasitology* 93(Pt 1), 9–16. DOI: 10.1017/s0031182000049787.

Zweygarth, E., Koekemoer, O., Josemans, A.I., Rambritch, N., Pienaar, R. *et al*. (2009) *Theileria*-infected cell line from an African buffalo (*Syncerus caffer*). *Parasitology Research* 105(2), 579–581. DOI: 10.1007/s00436-009-1467-0.

2 The Economic and Social Impact of Disease Caused by *Theileria parva*

Gemma Chaters[1]*, Ashley Flynn Railey[2] and Jonathan Rushton[3]
[1]*Lancaster Medical School, University of Lancaster, Lancaster, UK;*
[2]*Oklahoma State University, Oklahoma, USA;* [3]*Roslin Institute, University of Edinburgh, Edinburgh, UK*

2.1 Introduction

The recent description by Hennessy and Marsh (2021) of the economics of animal health as *important*, *broad* and *distinctive* accurately reflects the complex and evolving state of the literature. It is *important* because livestock provide a vital source of protein in the global human diet, because livestock and livestock products are deeply embedded in many cultures and hold tangible and intangible benefits across society, because the livestock industry accounts for a large fraction of global land use and because diseases can cross species barriers. It is *broad* because each disease has its own distinguishing features, in its biology and in the nature of economic damage it inflicts, the availability of mitigation measures and the background investments in education and research. It is *distinctive* because, unlike human health, where the emphasis is on longevity and quality of life (Viscusi and Aldy, 2003; Murray and Lopez, 2013), livestock health is part of the economy. Accordingly, economic analyses of animal health must consider the efficiency with which livestock convert input resources into value-added outputs (Hennessy and Marsh, 2021), and the negative aspects of livestock production, such as greenhouse gas emissions.

Historically, animal health economics has quantified the impact of separate diseases by measuring the monetary value of livestock and their products against losses due to ill health plus the monetary expenditure on preventing or controlling disease. There has also been a tendency to consider the impact of single pathogens or diseases based on data that reflect exposure to an organism with assumptions of impact, rather than carrying out true measurement and attribution of the losses incurred (Thomas *et al.*, 2022). The use of such data as a proxy for losses caused by disease and the reliance on results of studies that have focused on singular pathogens for economic analysis has historically led to inflated estimates of the impact of single pathogens (Rushton, 2017).

To address these issues, studies of the economics of animal health are now moving to include considerations that have traditionally been at the forefront in human health economics. These new metrics will incorporate the impacts of multiple diseases and the impacts beyond direct herd-level production losses and expenditures (e.g. the wider societal impacts of poor animal health, such as food availability and price, and changes to household income, population size and structure and the environmental consequences of this). This is leading to the use

*Corresponding author: g.chaters@lancaster.ac.uk

 East Coast Fever: The Disease, its Impact and Control (eds W.I. Morrison and P. Toye)
DOI: 10.1079/9781800626324.0002

of burden estimations for animal health, which incorporate the farm-level burden (production losses, expenditure on disease abatement measures and gross margins) as well as the societal burden of animal disease (consumer prices and externalities of livestock production, such as greenhouse gas emissions and public health impacts) (Hennessy and Marsh, 2021; Rushton *et al.*, 2021). A further advance is the use of measures that can be applied across populations (e.g. using US$ lost per kilogram of biomass) for comparison between species or geographies. Economic analysis that incorporates the broad and distinct aspects of animal health is a foundation stone in confronting inadequate human, animal and environmental health.

Many of the world's marginalized populations depend on livestock for their livelihoods and social and nutritional security. In the face of a growing human population, poverty indicators continue to increase among livestock-dependent pastoralists (500 million) and smallholders (0.75–1 billion) across sub-Saharan Africa. Improvements to animal health can provide a route out of poverty (Upton, 2004; Otte *et al.*, 2012). Despite the heavy reliance on livestock for livelihoods, investment in livestock health and health services is often minimal, especially across low- and middle-income countries. Within these geographies and production systems, livestock diseases, along with climate shocks and political instability, perpetuate the poverty trap (Blench, 2001; Perry and Grace, 2009; Rich and Perry, 2011; United Nations, 2015; Surve *et al.*, 2023). Through improved understanding of animal health economics and the full impacts of livestock diseases, livestock sectors can generate evidence to guide policy decisions and to advocate for greater investment in animal health and animal health services as both a public and environmental good.

This chapter is concerned with the economic and social impact of the parasitic pathogen *Theileria parva* and the main disease it causes in cattle, East Coast fever (ECF). This disease is of substantial importance as most people in the countries where the parasite is found depend heavily on livestock for their livelihoods and societal well-being (Staal *et al.*, 2009; Thumbi *et al.*, 2015).

2.2 The Burden of *Theileria parva*

T. parva is present in 12 countries that have climatic conditions favouring both large cattle populations and survival of the tick host *Rhipicephalus appendiculatus*. These countries are Burundi, Democratic Republic of the Congo (DRC) (predominantly in the east of the country), Kenya, Malawi, Mozambique, Rwanda, South Africa, South Sudan, Tanzania, Uganda, Zambia and Zimbabwe. In ten of these countries, the pathogen causes the acute and often fatal ECF. As discussed in Chapter 5 of this volume, ECF was eradicated from South Africa and Zimbabwe in the 1950s by government-imposed quarantine and slaughter measures (Thompson *et al.*, 2008; Mbizeni *et al.*, 2013). However, *T. parva* still circulates in buffalo (*Syncerus caffer*) in both countries and occasionally spills over into cattle, causing sporadic outbreaks of a disease known as Corridor disease in areas where cattle graze close to buffalo. Corridor disease also occurs in other countries where buffalo are present. In Zimbabwe, a less virulent form of *T. parva* also remained in cattle after elimination of ECF, causing a disease known as January disease, which results in much lower levels of mortality than ECF.

In this section, we synthesize the extant literature on estimates of the economic cost of *T. parva* infection. We provide a summary of the current economic picture and a conservative estimate for the current burden of ECF. We highlight the similarities and differences of the impact of *T. parva* between cattle of different breeds across agro-ecological areas and different production systems.

2.2.1 Previous estimates of the burden imposed by *T. parva*

The literature on the impact of *T. parva* spans five decades and is largely based on small epidemiological studies focused on subsets of populations, in single countries, and price data are rarely captured. There are methodological problems with using such data and ensuring that estimations of *T. parva* burden include all types of economic loss and expenditure.

Little work has been carried out to establish the economic impact of *T. parva* in the affected region since Mukhebi *et al.* (1992) estimated that disease caused by the parasite costs $168 million annually. The authors acknowledged at the time that there was a need for better data to improve the accuracy of their estimate. The most recent and frequently cited estimate of the economic impact of ECF is $300 million per annum (McLeod and Kristjanson, 1999). However, the data used to generate this estimate are now 25 years old and the study only accounted for the impact of the disease on meat and milk losses in four of the 12 affected countries (Tanzania, Kenya, Zimbabwe and South Africa). More recently, Kivaria (2006), using data from 2000, estimated that ECF was costing around $250 million per year in Tanzania alone. de la Fuente *et al.* (2019) estimated that in 2017 all tick-borne diseases in Uganda, of which *T. parva* is the major contributor, were costing in the region of $700 million per year. These more recent estimates from Tanzania and Uganda suggest that the widely cited $300 million is a significant underestimate of the true burden of ECF. These estimates also do not consider the wider societal impacts of the disease, such as the impact of livestock losses on local food security (higher food prices and less stable supply) and household income and expenditure.

Despite the paucity of evidence on the impacts of ECF, it is still considered one of the leading causes of loss in cattle and cattle products across eastern, central and southern Africa, and contributes to perpetuating the poverty trap (Perry *et al.*, 2002; Carter and Barrett, 2006; Perry and Grace, 2009; Rushton *et al.*, 2017).

2.2.2 Livestock and human population dynamics in the *T. parva*-affected region

The total cattle population in the 12 countries where *T. parva* is present is estimated to be 114 million (FAOSTAT, 2021a), which represents an increase of 90% in the 20 years to 2020 (Table 2.1). Cattle density across continental Africa (Gilbert *et al.*, 2022) is shown in Fig. 2.1, with the *T. parva*-affected countries outlined, excluding South Africa. Outside large commercial beef and dairying operations, cattle are predominantly kept in pastoral, agro-pastoral or smallholder production systems. In essence, pastoral livestock are extensively grazed with herders moving to find pasture and water, often covering great distances. In agro-pastoral systems, there may be some crop production with livestock grazed on land after cropping, as well as moved to access pasture and water. In smallholder settings, livestock can be tethered, often in more densely populated areas, and often brought water or grass/crops (Gachohi *et al.*, 2012; de Glanville *et al.*, 2020).

The estimated increase in the total human population in these countries from 2000 to 2020 is 60%, which is less than the estimated increase of 90% in the cattle population. Consequently, the number of cattle per head of population has increased in all but four countries (DRC, South Africa, Zambia and Zimbabwe), with the figure in Tanzania not having changed. For the seven countries where figures are available, substantial proportions of the human populations are undernourished. The percentage of people considered to be experiencing moderate to severe food insecurity is over 55% in all countries except South Africa (18–20%), with no data available for Burundi and Rwanda (Table 2.1).

With a high reliance on livestock for socio-economic and food security, livestock keepers in the *T. parva*-affected regions face several challenges, most of which are not unique to these regions but are common across sub-Saharan Africa (Countryman *et al.*, 2024). Poor market access and infrastructure contribute to low return to the producer, with livestock often sold first in informal markets and then moved along price gradients towards consumption centres by traders, resulting in poor financial security for livestock keepers (Motta *et al.*, 2017; Chaters *et al.*, 2019; Lysholm *et al.*, 2022). Reduced animal productivity translates into negative consequences for the health and well-being of all persons in the dependent household, particularly women and children, who suffer disproportionately from livestock losses (Haseeb *et al.*, 2019; FAOSTAT, 2021b; Teufel *et al.*, 2021). Improvements in livestock health and production in low-resource systems, however, can improve girls' access to education (Marsh *et al.*, 2016) and lower market prices for livestock-derived products, providing a wider societal benefit (Countryman *et al.*, 2024). Finally, across

Table 2.1. Cattle and human population size in 2000 and 2020, population growth 2000–2020, cattle per capita, nutrition associated poverty indicators, *T. parva* seroprevalence in countries where *T. parva* is present. From FAOSTAT, 2021a, b, c; World Bank, 2021.

Country	Human population (World Bank)			Cattle population (FAOSTAT)			Cattle per capita			Poverty indicators		*Theileria parva* sero-prevalence (%)
	2000	2020	Change 2000–2020 (%)	2000	2020	Change 2000–2020 (%)	2000	2020	Change 2000–2020 (%)	No. of people under-nourished (million) (% population)	Number of people moderately–severely food insecure (million) (% population)	
Burundi	6,307,659	12,220,227	94	358,492	755,145	111	0.057	0.062	9	–	–	67–90[a]
DRC	48,616,317	92,853,164	91	822,355	1,343,889	63	0.017	0.014	–14	35.6 (40%)	63–67M (70–75%)	82–99[b]
Kenya	30,851,606	51,985,780	69	11,444,800	26,765,935	134	0.371	0.515	39	14.4 (27%)	37–38M (68–71%)	22–85[c]
Malawi	11,229,387	19,377,061	73	763,724	1,946,033	155	0.068	0.100	48	3.4 (18%)	15–16M (80–83%)	33–54*[d]
Mozambique	17,768,505	31,178,239	75	780,000	2,183,857	180	0.044	0.070	60	–	22–24M (70–77%)	
Rwanda	8,109,989	13,146,362	62	732,123	1,608,499	120	0.090	0.122	36	4.6 (36%)	–	25–28[e]
South Africa	46,813,266	58,801,927	26	13,600,000	12,297,621	–10	0.263	0.209	–20	4.1 (7%)	11–12M (18–20%)	sporadic[f]
South Sudan	6,114,440	10,606,227	73	11,823,700 (2015)	13,784,065	17	–	1.300	–	–	9–10M (85–88%)	22–77[g]
Tanzania	34,463,704	61,704,518	79	16,713,000	29,971,623	79	0.485	0.486	0	13.5 (23%)	33–36M (55–60%)	5–98.4[h]
Uganda	24,020,697	44,404,611	85	5,965,500	14,515,333	143	0.248	0.327	32	–	32–34M (70–75%)	3–55[i]
Zambia	9,891,136	18,927,715	91	2,620,987	3,814,438	46	0.265	0.202	–24	5.7 (31%)	12–13M (67–72%)	2–40[j]
Zimbabwe	11,834,676	15,669,666	32	6,186,000	5,195,154	–16	0.523	0.332	–37	–	10–12M (69–77%)	12–98[k]
TOTAL	256,021,382	430,875,497	68	59,986,981	114,181,592	90	0.234	0.265	13	–	–	–

*Detection of pathogen by PCR, not seroprevalence (exposure).
[a]Nyabongo *et al.*, 2021
[b]Kalume *et al.*, 2012, Eastern DRC study
[c]Rubaire-Akiiki *et al.*, 2006
[d]Chatanga *et al.*, 2020, 2022
[e]Bazarusanga *et al.*, 2007
[f]Mbizeni *et al.*, 2013
[g]Marcellino *et al.*, 2017; Mohammed *et al.*, 2019
[h]Allan *et al.*, 2021
[i]Kabi *et al.*, 2014; Muhanguzi *et al.*, 2014
[j]Fandamu *et al.*, 2005; Simuunza *et al.*, 2011
[k]Latif *et al.*, 2001

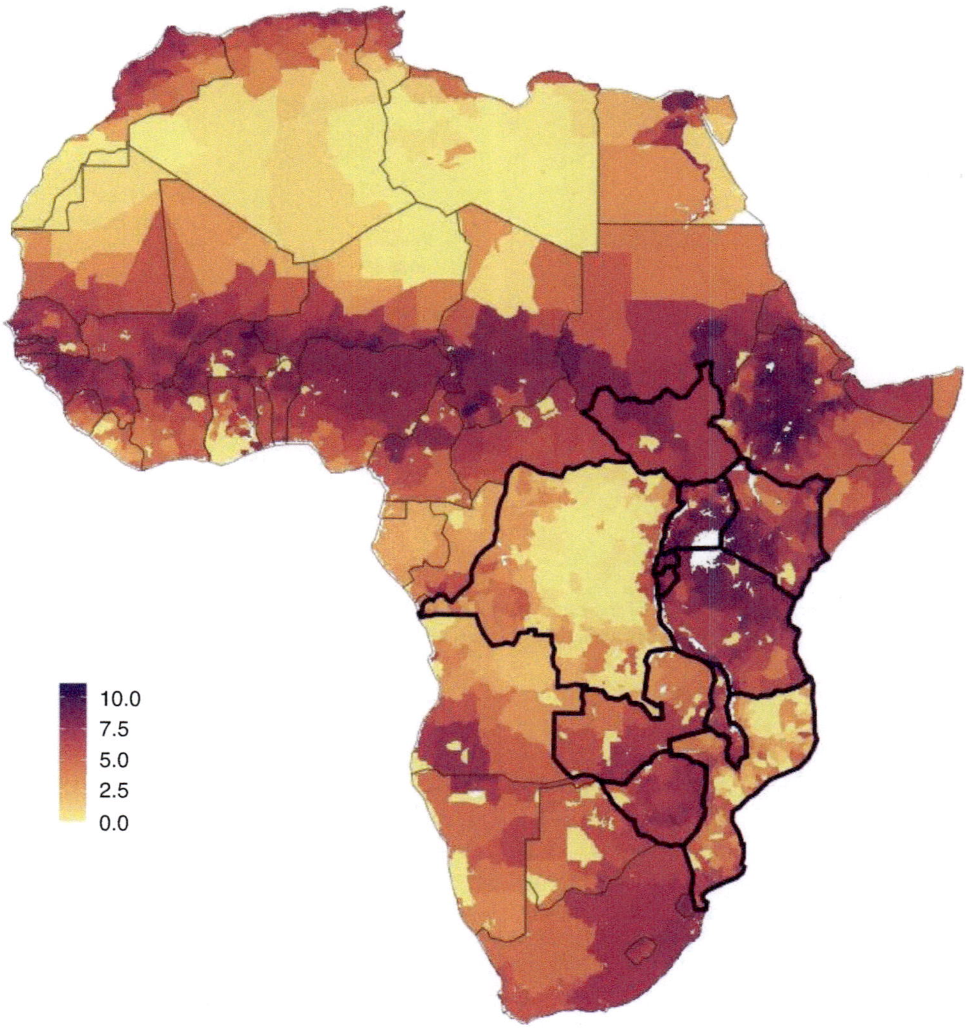

Fig. 2.1. Continental Africa cattle density (log_{10} cattle head per 5 km square) at 5 km square resolution using Gilbert *et al*. (2022). All countries where *T. parva* is found are outlined, except South Africa.

much of the *T. parva*-affected region, livestock hold a value beyond their monetary worth for consumption, in the form of insurance, savings, bride price, draught power and socio-cultural status values (Stroebel *et al.*, 2011; Cullis, 2021; Mwila *et al.*, 2022; Surve *et al.*, 2023). The socio-economic importance of livestock across the *T. parva*-affected region means that estimations of disease burdens based on market prices alone will underestimate the true burden of disease, and this must be considered when interpreting local estimates (Ng'ang'a *et al.*, 2018).

2.2.3 A qualitative analysis of the losses due to *T. parva*

The impacts of livestock disease, in their most basic form, can be split into *direct* and *indirect* losses. *Direct* losses can then be separated into visible losses, such as mortality, and invisible losses, such as lost meat, milk, dung and draught power, which are inherently more difficult to measure. *Indirect* losses can be split into additional costs, including treatments, control of tick infestation, vaccination and healthcare

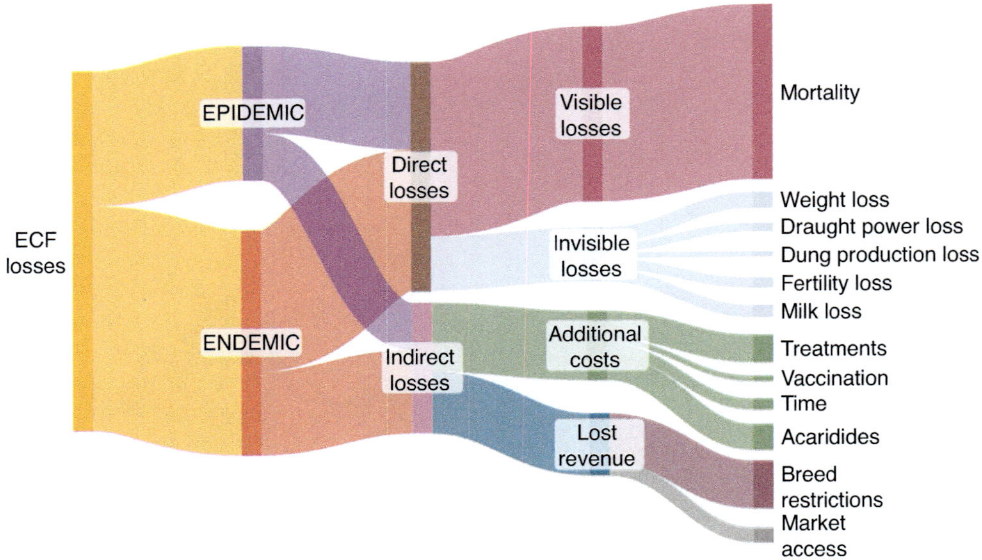

Fig. 2.2. Schematic representation of the direct and indirect losses incurred due to *T. parva* in the endemically stable and epidemic scenarios. Size of flow reflects relative importance of impact but is not proportional.

time, and foregone revenue, such as lack of market access and the inability to use improved breeds due to the frequently fatal nature of ECF in non-indigenous breeds (Rushton *et al.*, 1999; Rushton, 2009). Fig. 2.2 provides a schematic diagram illustrating the direct and indirect losses incurred due to ECF. These are described in more detail in Sections 2.2.3.1 and 2.2.3.2.

The economic impact of *T. parva* also varies between agro-ecological production systems, both within and between countries (Deem *et al.*, 1993; Rubaire-Akiiki *et al.*, 2006; Gachohi *et al.*, 2012). This is due to the multiple differences between production systems, which impact pathogen exposure risk, disease pathology, access to preventive measures and treatment, and local market prices. Different production systems tend to have preferences for different cattle breeds, which vary in their susceptibility to ECF. Taurine cattle of recent European origin are far more susceptible to disease than are indicine cattle, with differences also evident within the latter population (see Chapter 7 of this volume). Husbandry and feeding practices also vary between production systems (zero-grazed, tethered, pastoral), which affects tick challenge and risk of pathogen exposure. Access to markets, effective livestock healthcare advice, preventative medicines such as vaccines (limited), acaricides (often multi-purpose against ticks and biting flies) and effective treatments also varies by geographic location, which is related to the dominant local livestock production system. The economic impact of *T. parva* will also vary between seasons and years as rainfall frequency and duration affects tick activity and thus parasite challenge (Chepkwony *et al.*, 2020). These factors should all be considered when interpreting the estimates of the cost of ECF that are provided later in this chapter for each country and the region (Section 2.2.4).

2.2.3.1 Direct losses

Production losses directly attributable to the presence of a disease in the population are generally classed as mortality and morbidity losses. The estimates of direct losses due to *T. parva* cited in this section are overwhelmingly derived from small research studies in specific cattle subpopulations.

2.2.3.1.1 MORTALITY (VISIBLE LOSSES). Death is a significant outcome with *T. parva* infections and is a major part of the ECF burden. It is the most likely outcome of this disease to be reported and varies drastically by cattle breed, age, production system, geography and history of animals' previous exposure. The case fatality rate due to ECF falls into two distinct categories: endemic and epidemic.

In endemic scenarios, indigenous breeds of cattle show a degree of resistance to *T. parva* and record relatively lower fatality rates compared to non-indigenous breeds (discussed in Chapter 7 of this volume). The mortality rate in calves of indigenous cattle breeds is conservatively estimated to be around 6–8% (Ocaido *et al.*, 2009) but can be as high as 40–60% (Homewood *et al.*, 2006), depending on the breed of cattle and level of challenge (Gitau *et al.*, 1994; Di Giulio *et al.*, 2009). A recent study of 548 indigenous cattle in western Kenya, in which no animal health interventions were allowed, reported an ECF mortality rate of 6% (Bronsvoort *et al.*, 2013; Thumbi *et al.*, 2013).

Non-indigenous cattle not previously exposed to *T. parva* can have epidemic outbreaks of the disease and have recorded fatality rates of up to 100%. The implementation of ECF preventative measures, most notably acaricide treatment, has also reduced recorded mortality rates.

2.2.3.1.2 MORBIDITY (INVISIBLE LOSSES). *T. parva* infection causes weight loss and reduces fertility, milk yield, draught power and dung production in affected animals, all of which contribute to lost household income from cattle across the *T. parva*-affected region. However, evidence of the extent of these losses is not readily available due to the difficulty in recording these losses and directly attributing them to ECF rather than to concurrent infections or environmental stressors. The following text provides a summary of some historical estimates of production loss due to *T. parva* infection. It should be emphasized that these estimates are taken from small-scale studies and are up to three decades old.

The study published by Mukhebi *et al.* in 1992 reported that experts estimated production losses attributable to *T. parva* could include a 25% reduction in milk yield, a 3% reduction in draught power and a 12.5% reduction in manure production per year for affected cattle. It was also estimated that lost draught power would contribute around 13% of the total economic loss due to ECF and weight loss would contribute around 7.5% of the total economic loss (Mukhebi *et al.*, 1992; Rashid *et al.*, 2019).

As indicated above by the figures from Mukhebi *et al.*, milk loss is a major contributor to the overall economic loss due to ECF. A trial of the use of preventative measures in smallholder cattle in Zambia found an increase in milk yield of 0.23l per day (per lactation) in animals that were prevented from getting ECF in comparison to the control group (Minjauw *et al.*, 1997). Minjauw and McLeod (2003) showed losses were highest per head in the smallholder dairy sector ($21.80 per affected animal) compared to the pastoral sector ($8.00 per affected animal). It should be noted that decreased availability of milk is of human health and social significance due to the role increased milk consumption can play in improving child nutrition and development, especially given the level of malnourishment in children across much of the affected region (Table 2.1).

A study by Minjauw and McLeod (2003) compared the *T. parva*-associated losses in the smallholder and pastoralist systems in Tanzania, Kenya and Malawi (Table 2.2). The highest overall losses were estimated to be in the Tanzanian traditional (pastoral) sector, largely driven by the fact that this is the largest sector in the region. In contrast, most losses in Kenya were observed in the smallholder dairy sector.

In summary, it is clear that without extended, longitudinal studies that measure productivity and incidence of infection, it is impossible to provide accurate estimates of the

Table 2.2. Estimates of production loss due to *T. parva* infection in three eastern African countries. Data from 1999 to 2003; extracted from Minjauw and McLeod, 2003.

Country	Smallholder dairy (US$ million)	Traditional (US$ million)
Tanzania	4.41	129.5
Kenya	54.5	34.41
Malawi	0.1	2.5

morbidity-associated losses that are directly attributable to *T. parva* infection.

2.2.3.2 *Indirect losses*

2.2.3.2.1 CONTROL COSTS. *T. parva* infection has traditionally been controlled by frequent application of acaricides to prevent infestation by the tick vector (employing dipping, spraying or pour-ons), chemotherapy to treat clinical cases and, more recently, vaccination using the Infection and Treatment method (ITM). The detailed histories of the development and use of these interventions are presented in more detail elsewhere in this volume (Chapters 15, 14 and 13, respectively). Additional management measures have also been employed that are not based on the use of commercial products. Cattle can be restricted from grazing in heavily tick-infested areas, but this has limited application as areas most suitable for cattle grazing are also often suitable tick habitats. As mentioned above, a further measure is the use of ECF-resistant indigenous cattle, but these tend to be substantially less productive. ECF is thus a major limiting factor in the ability of livestock owners to use more productive breeds of cattle across a large part of eastern and southern Africa, limiting cattle production potential across the region (Murray *et al.*, 1984; Kivaria *et al.*, 2004; Gachohi *et al.*, 2012; Orenge *et al.*, 2012).

2.2.3.2.2 PREVENTATIVE INTERVENTIONS. The two major intervention options to prevent ECF are regular acaricide use to prevent infestation by the tick vector (*R. appendiculatus*) and vaccination against the pathogen (*T. parva*). The most cost-efficient intervention to control the spread and reduce the impact of *T. parva* infection will vary according to access to, and price of, mitigation measures, as well as the type of tick habitat, grazing practices and value of livestock products (Mumba *et al.*, 2017; Rich and Niemi, 2017; de Glanville *et al.*, 2020). Policies that support implementation of interventions must consider the agro-ecological and socio-economic context in which the livestock are kept, as well as the disease epidemiology (Gitau *et al.*, 1999).

2.2.3.2.3 ACARICIDE USE. The frequency of acaricide application to control ECF ranges from weekly to twice weekly during rainy seasons and in areas of high risk (Githaka *et al.*, 2022), and applications occur over the productive life of the animal. The documented costs of applying acaricides in eastern Africa range between \$2.1 and \$36 per adult animal per year (Minjauw and McLeod, 2003; Mugisha *et al.*, 2005; Kivaria, 2006; Lynen *et al.*, 2012; Kwankanaba Bantuzeko *et al.*, 2022). The cost of acaricide application in cattle cannot be wholly attributed to the prevention of ECF, as acaricides are also used to prevent other tick- and tsetse-borne diseases and direct skin damage by ticks. Prevention of these other conditions, however, requires less frequent application. Additionally, although frequent acaricide application can prevent severe ECF disease, it also creates a high-risk environment for selecting acaricide-resistant ticks.

2.2.3.2.4 VACCINATION. Immunization of cattle by ITM offers an effective alternative for *T. parva* control. The most commonly used vaccine stabilate utilizes a trivalent formulation containing three strains of *T. parva* and is known as the Muguga cocktail (MC). It is administered to animals as a single inoculation along with a dose of long-acting oxytetracycline (see Chapters 12 and 13 of this volume). Vaccination results in mild or no clinical signs and induces a broad and long-lasting immunity. Its use leads to substantial cost savings due to the reduction in the frequency of acaricide use (Kivaria, 2006; Kivaria *et al.*, 2007; Lynen *et al.*, 2012).

The first commercial-scale batches of the vaccine were made in 1996, and several batches have been made subsequently. Uptake of the vaccine has, however, been below expectations and is currently averaging 138,000 doses per year. The reasons for this are discussed in depth in Chapter 13 of this volume.

2.2.3.2.5 THERAPEUTIC INTERVENTIONS. The treatment of choice for cases of ECF is buparvaquone, which has superseded the related naphthoquinone parvaquone (see Chapter 14 of this volume for a detailed account of these compounds). Though very effective if administered before clinical signs reach the advanced stage, buparvaquone is expensive (ranging from \$9 to \$27 per dose, depending on body weight) and not always available. Cure rates with buparvaquone and parvaquone of over 80% have been shown in trial conditions (D'Haese *et al.*, 1999; Al-Hosary *et al.*, 2010) and its efficacy has been confirmed in various field trials (see Chapter 14 of this volume). Oxytetracycline is a more widely obtainable and cheaper drug but is ineffective once clinical signs of disease become evident and therefore its use as a treatment for ECF is often a waste of resources. In some areas, traditional plant-based medicines, which are cheaper and more accessible, are also purchased to treat clinical disease (Ezeanya-Esiobu *et al.*, 2021), but evidence on their efficacy is lacking. Animals that have been successfully treated for ECF still lose body condition, drop milk yield and, if pregnant, have a higher risk of abortion (Sitawa *et al.*, 2016). Inadequate access to veterinary services and therapeutic agents across much of the ECF region often leads to delayed treatment, reducing the chance of treatment success and exacerbating the burden of the disease.

2.2.4 A revised assessment of the costs of losses due to *T. parva*

In this section we provide a transparent estimate of the current cost of ECF, using the structure of the schematic diagram in Fig. 2.3. The analysis is in two parts: the economic loss due to mortality from ECF and the costs of disease control. An estimate of the value of production losses is not included in the calculations due to lack of reliable data.

2.2.4.1 Estimated losses due to mortality

To calculate mortality losses, we apply figures of 5 and 10% mortality to the calf population at risk of *T. parva* infection in each country (the *at-risk* population). Because most ECF mortalities occur in the first year of life, the total calf population size is estimated as country cattle population size N^{pop} (FAOSTAT, 2021a) multiplied by 1/life expectancy $\left(\frac{1}{LExp}\right)$ (assumed to be an average of five years for the study population). The lower and upper number of *at-risk* calves is calculated by applying the lower and upper bounds of country-specific seroprevalence values to the total calf population (Table 2.3). In this scenario, we assume that seroprevalence equates to the national cattle populations' risk of pathogen exposure in a year. We accept that this is not a precise measure of disease incidence each year, but it is the closest estimate available. We stress to the reader that these estimates could both over- or underestimate the true incidence and exposure levels and must be interpreted with caution, but can be updated and improved when better estimates of the number of *at-risk* cattle in each country are produced. For Mozambique, there were no seroprevalence data available, so the mean seroprevalence from its neighbouring countries (South Africa, Zimbabwe, Zambia, Malawi, Tanzania) was used to estimate the size of its *at-risk* population. As vaccinated cattle are assumed to be protected from ECF, the number of such cattle was subtracted from the *at-risk* calf population. This assumes that all vaccine doses delivered to each country were used and were administered to calves in high-disease-risk areas of the country. Finally, the lower and upper bounds of the mortality losses were calculated by applying a 5% mortality rate to the lower estimate of the *at-risk* calf population (Eqn 2.1) and a 10% mortality rate to the upper estimate of the *at-risk* calf population (Eqn 2.2), respectively.

$$M^{lower} = \left(\left(N^{pop} \times \left(\frac{1}{LExp}\right) \times SeroPrev^{lower}\right) - N^{vac}\right) \times 0.05 \quad (2.1)$$

$$M^{upper} = \left(\left(N^{pop} \times \left(\frac{1}{LExp}\right) \times SeroPrev^{upper}\right) - N^{vac}\right) \times 0.10 \quad (2.2)$$

We next estimated the monetary cost of the mortality losses (*MV*) using liveweight price data (minimum and maximum values available) from 2024 (FAOSTAT, 2021d) and assumed an average live weight of 250 kg to account for the market value of a growing calf. The lower bound of the price per kilogram ($\$kg^{lower}$) was applied to the minimum expected mortality loss (M^{lower}), and the upper bound of the price per kilogram ($\$kg^{upper}$) was applied to the maximum expected mortality loss (M^{upper}), to generate a range of potential losses incurred due to ECF mortality per country (Eqns 2.3 and 2.4, respectively).

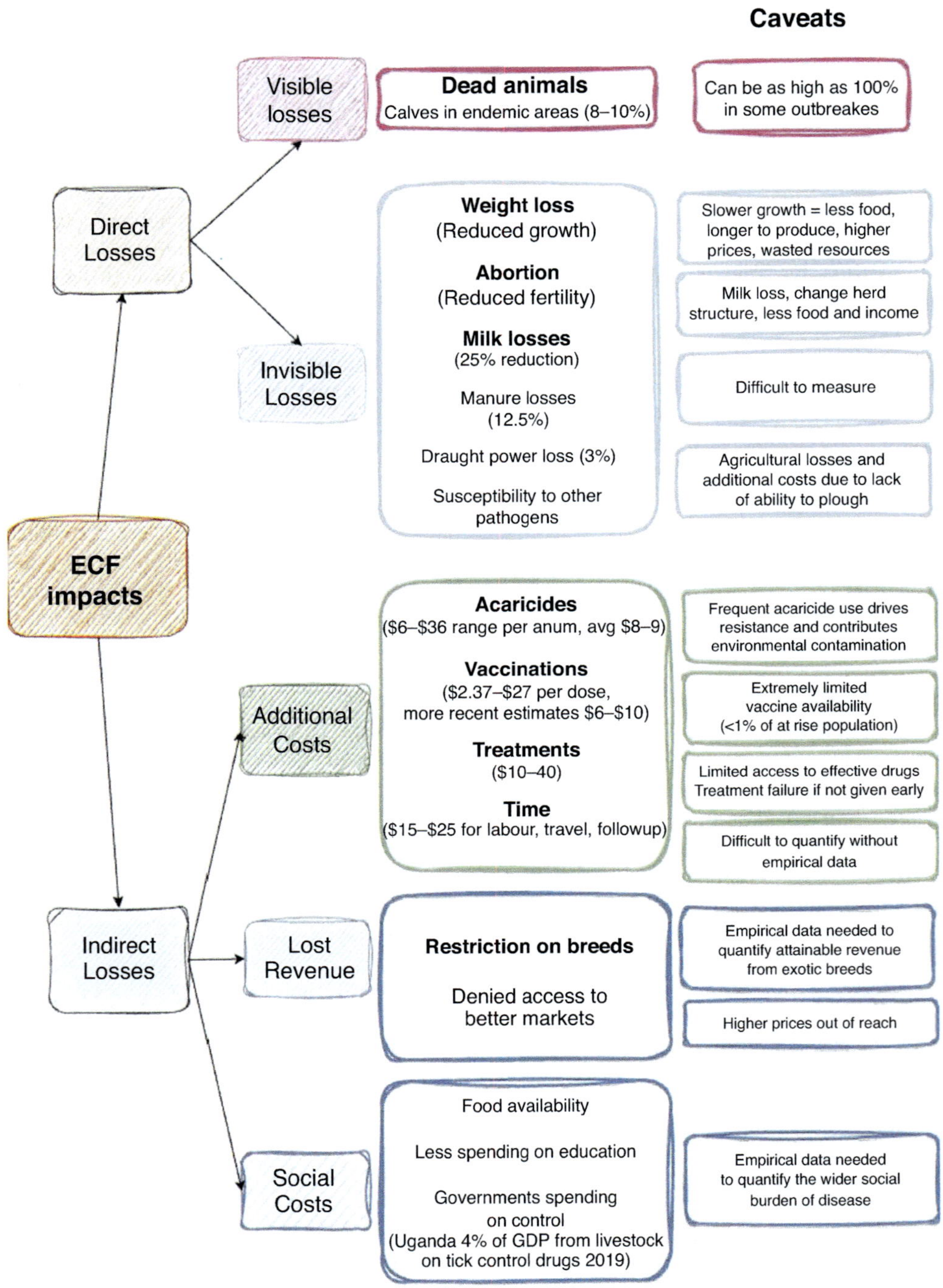

Fig. 2.3. Schematic representation of the costs incurred due to *T. parva*, with values associated with losses and caveats to consider when using these data. (Modified framework from Rushton *et al.*, 1999.)

Table 2.3. Estimated visible losses and control costs for ECF across 12 affected countries in 2020.

Country	Calf population assuming average life expectancy is 5 years (20% of 2020 FAOSTAT cattle population)	*T. parva* Sero-prevalence (range from literature)	Estimated minimum number of calf deaths (5% mortality in minimum at risk calf pop – N vaccinated (M^{lower})	Estimated maximum number of calf deaths (10% mortality in maximum at risk calf pop – N vaccinated (M^{upper})	Price per kg range (US$) (2024 price data)[l]	Mortality loss value (min. $/kg * 250kg * M^{lower}) (US$ million)	Mortality loss value (max $/kg * 250kg * M^{upper}) (US$ million)	Expenditure on vaccine (vaccine doses distributed in 2020 at $8 per dose) (US$ million)	*AcaricideV$* Acaricide expenditure (50% of at-risk cattle treated for US$ 8.5/year/head and 50% of this cost is attributed to ECF prevention (US$ million)	Treatment expenditure assuming 20% of at-risk cattle treated/year with: 10% buparvaquone (US$ 15/dose) 10% oxytetracycline (US$ 5.5/dose) (US$ million)	Total (US$ million)
Burundi	151,029	0.67–0.90[a]	4659	9515	2.0–5.0	2.33	15.99	0.064	1.25	1.21	4.9–19
DRC	268,778	0.82–0.99[b]	11020	18626	1.3–3.4	3.58	22.62	0	2.57	2.48	8.6–28
Kenya	5,353,187	0.22–0.85[c]	58635	318515	2.0–2.50	29.32	284.08	0.040	30.15	29.08	89–343
Malawi	389,207	0.33–0.54[d*]	6396	14712	0.96–1.0	1.54	5.19	0.004	1.78	1.72	5.0–8.7
Mozambique	436,771	0.35**	7643	10701	3.96	7.57	15.13	0	1.86	1.79	11–19
Rwanda	321,700	0.25–0.28[e]	3727	6305	2.9–4.0	2.68	8.48	0.047	0.91	0.87	4.5–10
South Africa	2,459,524	0.05[f]***	6149	8608	2.0–3.0	3.07	9.22	0	1.31	1.26	5.6–12
South Sudan	2,756,813	0.22–0.77[g]	30325	148592	4.4–5.8	33.36	307.80	0	13.03	12.57	59–333
Tanzania	5,994,325	0.05–0.98[h]	11686	411211	2.8–4.1	8.18	595.36	0.528	32.48	31.34	73–660
Uganda	2,903,067	0.03–0.55[i]	1355	111768	2.0–5.0	0.68	192.09	0.480	8.95	8.63	19–210
Zambia	762,888	0.02–0.40[j]	763	21361	0.6–1.0	0.11	7.63	0	1.70	1.64	3.5–11
Zimbabwe	1,039,031	0.12–0.98[k]	6234	71278	4.2–5.8	6.55	147.65	0	6.07	5.86	18–160
Total			148,592	1,630,019		98.6–1,611.2		1.163	102.05	98.45	300–1812

Continued

Table 2.3. Continued

*Detection of pathogen by PCR, not seroprevalence (exposure).
**Mean seroprevalence from neighbouring countries.
***Assumption 5% of population are at risk based on sporadic outbreaks from buffalo migration. At risk cattle = midpoint of seroprevalence × total cattle pop. (FAOSTAT, 2021a). Lower bound of at-risk calves = lower bound of seroprevalence × (0.2 × total cattle pop.) (FAOSTAT, 2020). Upper bound of at-risk calves = upper bound of seroprevalence × (0.15 × total cattle pop.) (FAOSTAT, 2021a)
[a](Nyabongo *et al.*, 2021; FAOSTAT, 2021a)
[b](Kalume *et al.*, 2012) Eastern DRC study
[c](Rubaire-Akiiki *et al.*, 2006)
[d](Chatanga *et al.*, 2020, 2022)
[e](Bazarusanga *et al.*, 2007)
[f](Mbizeni *et al.*, 2013)
[g](Marcellino *et al.*, 2017; Mohammed *et al.*, 2019)
[h](Allan *et al.*, 2021)
[i](Kabi *et al.*, 2014; Muhanguzi *et al.*, 2014)
[j](Fandamu *et al.*, 2005; Simuunza *et al.*, 2011)
[k](Latif *et al.*, 2001)
[l](FAOSTAT, 2021d)

$$MV^{lower} = M^{lower} \times 250 \times \$kg^{lower} \quad (2.3)$$

$$MV^{upper} = M^{upper} \times 250 \times \$kg^{upper} \quad (2.4)$$

Using these data and assumptions, we calculated that the direct loss due to ECF-related mortality each year ranges from $98 million to $1611 million (Table 2.3). These estimates of mortality loss have a wide range and can only be improved by using more accurate data on numbers of livestock and mortality rates for the production systems within each country.

2.2.4.2 *Estimated expenditure on disease control interventions*

2.2.4.2.1 ACARICIDES. The cost of acaricide use was calculated by estimating that 50% of the *at-risk* cattle population ($0.5 \times N^{pop} \times SeroPrev^{mean}$) have regular acaricide application costing $8.5/year (taken from a summary of the literature described above) multiplied by 0.5 on the conservative assumption that half the cost of acaricide use should be attributed to ECF prevention and half to other tick- and tsetse-borne diseases (Eqn 2.5).

$$AcaricideV = \left(0.5 \times N^{pop} \times SeroPrev^{mean} \times 8.5\right) \times 0.5 \quad (2.5)$$

Applied across all countries and based on the cattle population size in 2020, this equation estimates that around $102 million are spent each year in the region on acaricide use to prevent ECF.

An alternative estimate can be calculated based on the purchase of acaricides by the Ugandan government ($81 million – which was equal to 4% of Uganda's livestock-derived GDP in 2020). Extrapolation of these figures across all countries in the region comes to $1194 million, and attributing half to the control of ECF means that governments could be spending in the region of $0.6 billion each year on acaricide acquisition to prevent ECF losses.

2.2.4.2.2 VACCINATION. Cattle require one dose of the MC vaccine for lifelong protection from ECF. Broadly, the ECF literature assumes the cost of ITM vaccine to be between $6 and $10 per dose (Lynen *et al.*, 2012; Perry, 2016), with larger animals requiring a higher dose of the oxytetracycline antibiotic. In Tanzania in 2010, farmers paid approximately $7 for the ITM vaccine, an anthelmintic and an ear tag (J. Rushton, UK, 2025, personal communication). Household survey data from Tanzania in 2019 shows the household cost per calf dose was $4–4.5, regardless of the numbers of calves treated (Auty, 2023, personal communication). The costs appear low in relation to the value of individual animals in the region and the potential scale of loss due to ECF disease.

Expenditure on vaccination was calculated using the number of vaccine doses (N^{doses}) (total = 145,400) data from 2020 (see Chapter 13 of this volume, Tables 13.7 and 13.8) and $8 per dose (taken from a summary of the literature described above) and was estimated to be $1.163 million per year (Eqn 2.6).

$$VaccinationV = N^{doses} \times \$8 \quad (2.6)$$

This value is similar to that presented in Chapter 13 of this volume, as the current (2025) sales of the MC vaccine are slightly lower, with a mean value of 138,000 doses per year and using the same conservative vaccination cost of $8 per animal.

2.2.4.2.3 TREATMENT. Longitudinal data from Tanzania covering 2019/20 shows the cost of a single dose of buparvaquone ranged from $12 to $20, depending on body weight (Auty, 2023, personal communication), and in Zambia in 1997 a buparvaquone dose ranged from $9 to $27, including delivery costs. The cost of a dose of oxytetracycline used to treat ECF ranged from $4.5 to $6.5 per dose in Tanzania in 2019/20 (Auty, 2023, personal communication). The cost of treatments was estimated by assuming 10% of the *at-risk* cattle population are treated for ECF disease symptoms each year with buparvaquone at $15 per dose and 10% are treated with oxytetracycline at $5.5 per dose (Eqns 2.7–2.9).

$$TreatmentV^{bup} = N^{pop} \times SeroPrev^{mean} \times \times 0.1 \times \$15 \quad (2.7)$$

$$TreatmentV^{oxy} = N^{pop} \times SeroPrev^{mean} \times \times 0.1 \times \$5.5 \quad (2.8)$$

$$TreatmentV = TreatmentV^{bup} + TreatmentV^{oxy} \quad (2.9)$$

Applying Eqns 2.7–2.9 to the 2020 regional cattle population, using mean seroprevalence to estimate the *at-risk* population for each country, the total cost of treatment was estimated to be \$98.45 million. This could be considered an overestimate due to the limited availability of buparvaquone in the region but could also be an underestimate as we use the mean seroprevalence to estimate the *at-risk* cattle, and the number actually affected and identified as needing treatment could be much higher than the mean seroprevalence each year.

2.2.4.2.4 TOTAL. In summary, the total estimated range of the cost of ECF for each country in the region is the sum of the lower/upper bound of the mortality cost, the acaricide cost, the vaccination cost and the treatment costs (Eqns 2.10 and 2.11) (Table 2.3).

$$ECFV^{lower} = MV^{lower} + AcaricideV + TreatmentV + VaccinationV \quad (2.10)$$

$$ECFV^{upper} = MV^{upper} + AcaricideV + TreatmentV + VaccinationV \quad (2.11)$$

These calculations produce an estimated range of the annual ECF cost across the region of \$0.3–1.8 billion for 2020. The calculations do not include the invisible losses (milk, meat, dung and draught power losses), which are significant due to the levels of food and social insecurity across the region, and the other societal costs of disease. The estimate also does not include the foregone revenue for cattle keepers across the region due to limitations in the breeds of cattle that can be kept and areas available for grazing.

It could be argued that the width of the estimated range of the cost of ECF is suboptimal. As stated before, this can only be rectified by the acquisition of more precise and representative data. Nevertheless, the available estimates provide considerable confidence that ECF remains a predominant cause of economic loss in the livestock sectors of the countries where *T. parva* is present.

2.2.5 Country-specific analyses

T. parva is widely recognized as the disease of greatest significance to livestock keepers across eastern and southern Africa. However, the impact of the disease varies between the affected countries, due to the size of the cattle populations, the breeds of cattle and types of cattle production systems, the availability of disease control measures and other socio-economic factors. A summary of current knowledge of these features in the individual countries and estimates of the overall economic burden of disease caused by *T. parva* in each country is provided in Appendix 2.1. Table 2.4 and Figs 2.4 and 2.5 present an overview of factors relevant to ECF in individual countries.

2.3 Costs and Benefits of Theileriosis Control Options

2.3.1 Elimination

As described in detail in Chapter 6 of this volume, ECF was first recognized in South Africa in 1902 and was eliminated by 1955 through sustained application of strict control of cattle movement, surveillance and slaughter of infected cattle. It is estimated that 5.5 million cattle were lost during the elimination campaign.

Attempted elimination of the disease in the rest of Africa is very unlikely to be successful for a variety of reasons. Firstly, the diagnosis and necessary slaughter of large numbers of infected cattle is unacceptable for financial, implementation and social reasons. Secondly, restrictions on cattle movement and interaction with buffalo will be challenging to establish and maintain. Thirdly, the lack of seasonal tick activity in areas close to the equator may make eradication more difficult than experienced in southern Africa. Thus, repeating the success of South Africa in eliminating ECF is not a feasible control option.

Table 2.4. Country-specific social and economic factors associated with the livestock sector and *T. parva* control.

Country	GDP US$ billion 2020	% Population in rural areas	% GDP from livestock	Livestock derived GDP (US$ billion)	Calf population size (20% of 2020 cattle pop. FAOSTAT)	Vaccine available 2020	Proportion of *at risk** calves vaccinated (2020)	Mean loss** per *at-risk* calf ($/calf)
Burundi	3.62	86	4.60[a]	0.17	151,029	8000	0.068	99
DRC	45.3	54	10[b]	4.53	268,778	0	0	75
Kenya	101	72	> 13[c]	13.13	5,353,187	5000	0.002	76
Malawi	11.8	83	6.60[d]	0.78	389,207	520	0.003	41
Mozambique	14.2	63	1.65[e]	0.23	436,771	0	0	86
Rwanda	10.2	83	3[f]	0.31	321,700	5880	0.069	87
South Africa	338	33	1[g]	3.38	2,459,524	0	0	71
South Sudan	4.22	80	23[h]	0.97	2,756,813	0	0	160
Tanzania	38.1	75	7[i]	2.67	5,994,325	66000	0.022	120
Uganda	67.7	65	3[j]	2.03	2,903,067	60000	0.071	136
Zambia	18.1	55	1.70[k]	0.31	762,888	0	0	45
Zimbabwe	21.7	68	6–6.5[l]	1.36	1,039,031	0	0	156
Total				29.86				

*At risk calves estimated using mid-point seroprevalence from literature (Table 2.3).
**Loss estimated in Table 2.3 based on mortalities, vaccination, treatment and acaricide application costs only.
[a](Hatungumukama *et al.*, 2007)
[b](Cox, 2012)
[c](Behnke and Muthami, 2011; Lengesse, 2014)
[d](Matchaya *et al.*, 2012; National Statistical Office (NSO), 2020)
[e](Trading Economics, 2022)
[f](Makoni *et al.*, 2014; Claire *et al.*, 2017)
[g](MacroTrends, 2022)
[h](IGAD Center for Pastoral Areas & Livestock Development (ICPALD), 2016)
[i](Ministry of Livestock and Fisheries, 2022)
[j](Ministry of Agriculture, Animal Industry and Fisheries (MAAIF), 2020)
[k](Dutilly *et al.*, 2020)
[l](FAO, 2022)

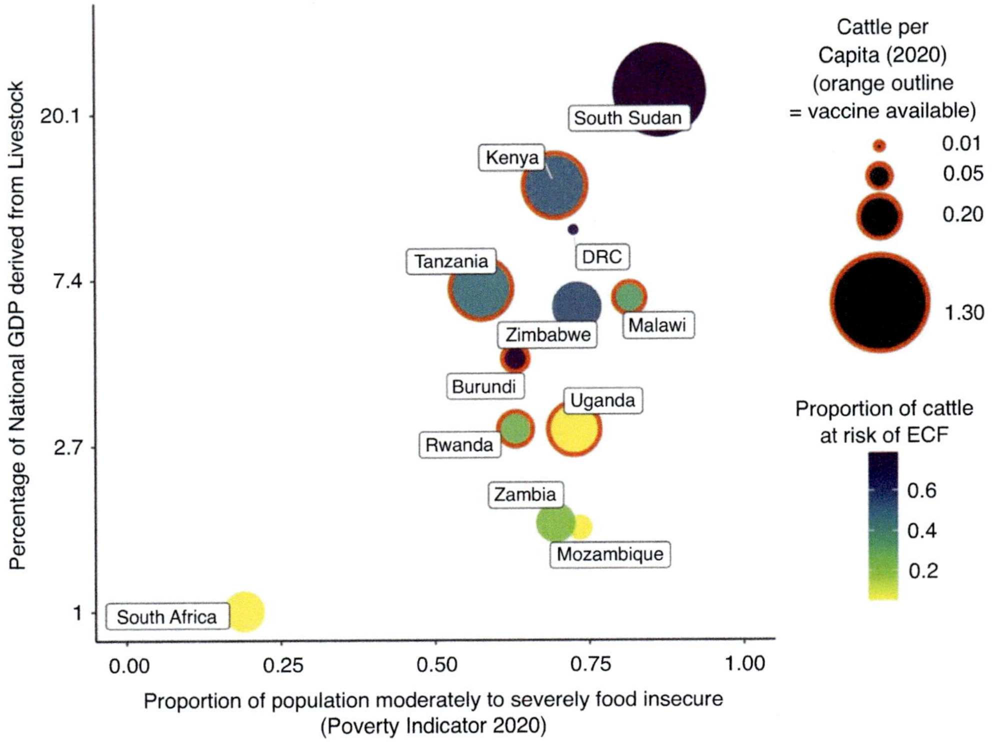

Fig. 2.4. Poverty indicator (FAOSTAT, 2021c) and % of national GDP from livestock (FAOSTAT, 2021b). The size of the circle reflects the number of cattle per capita (2020). The colour of the circle indicates the number of cattle at risk based on ECF seroprevalence, and the orange border reflects vaccine availability in 2020.

2.3.2 Acaricide use versus vaccination with ITM

Most economic analyses of *T. parva* control strategies are derived from farm budget data and the studies tend to focus on the relative benefits of adopting ITM compared to acaricide use. Not surprisingly, the study results vary by location, cattle breed and production system. Nevertheless, there have been several studies comparing the economic benefits of acaricide use and vaccination. In both Kenya and Zambia, use of the ITM vaccine in traditionally managed cattle was found to be more profitable when compared to regular acaricide treatment and allowing natural infection and immunity to develop (Minjauw *et al.*, 1999; Sitawa *et al.*, 2016). An analysis from Uganda comparing a range of scenarios in which ITM vaccination, acaricide application or a combination of both were adopted found that ITM in non-indigenous cattle was always most profitable, but in indigenous cattle ITM was only profitable if applied along with a reduction in acaricide use of at least 50% (Laker, 1993). ITM use in Kenya was associated with reduction in acaricide use and contributed a net benefit of $6.5 per head (Marsh *et al.*, 2016). A simulation model study in Kenya also showed that the use of ITM would be profitable irrespective of the herd size (Nyangito *et al.*, 1995). In Tanzania, the profit gain for immunized pastoral calves was estimated to be up to $5.6 per calf (Babo Martins *et al.*, 2010). This profit came from increased sale of calves, increased value of immunized calves in the market and higher milk production.

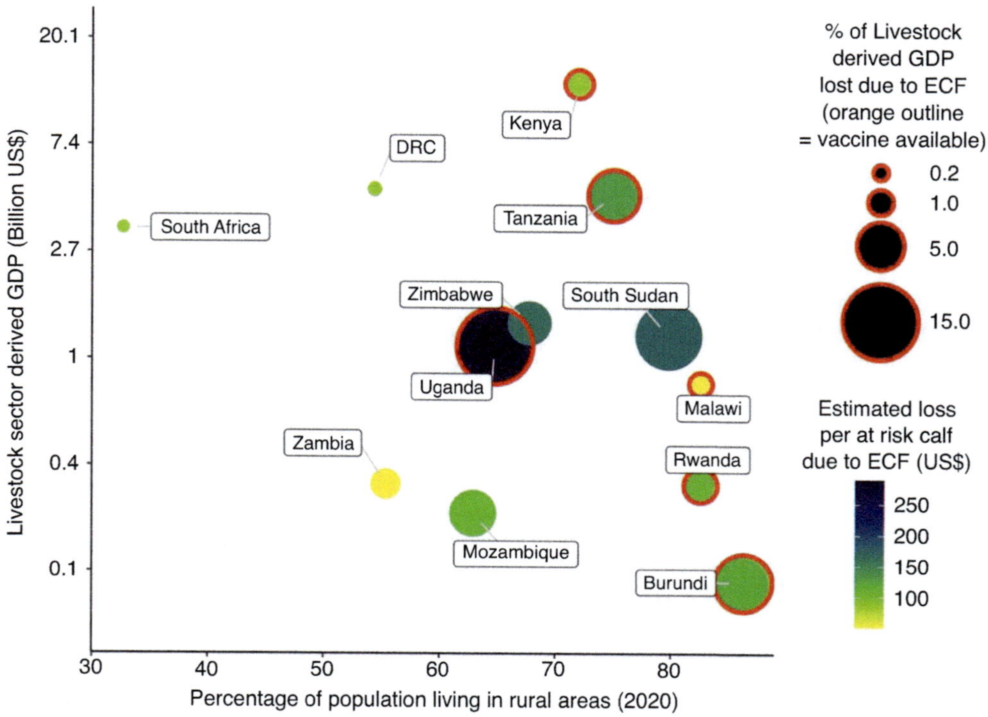

Fig. 2.5. Country-specific livestock sector relative importance and ECF burden; proportion of people living in rural areas and livestock sector-derived GDP ($ billion) (FAOSTAT, 2021b, c). The X axis shows the percentage of the country's population that lives in rural areas, the Y axis shows the absolute value of GDP that is derived from the livestock sector, the size of the circle represents the estimated proportion of livestock-derived GDP that is lost due to ECF, the orange border reflects vaccine availability in country and the colour of the circle represents the estimated ECF losses per *at-risk* calf due to ECF.

Few studies have evaluated the national impacts of ECF control. An analysis of the livestock sector in Kenya, which included crop production and livestock-derived products (e.g. feed, draught power, manure) found that using the ITM vaccine allowed a reduction of acaricide use by 75% and had a benefit–cost ratio of 5.2 (for every $1 spent $5.2 were gained) (Nyangito *et al.*, 1995). Extending this analysis across livestock systems, Toye *et al.* (2020) found the use of ITM increased the value of the agricultural sector by around 12% compared to no-vaccination scenarios. The difference was attributed to increases in revenue through expanded livestock production and lower food expenditures. These results align with farm-level analyses (Marsh *et al.*, 2016).

In summary, these studies reveal that, compared to use of acaricides alone, adopting ITM provides benefits, by improving both livestock productivity and profitability. Additional benefits, not captured in many of these studies, come from reduced use of acaricides when using the ITM vaccine. In addition to financial savings, this reduces the local selection pressure for acaricide-resistance in the tick population and decreases the negative environmental impacts of acaricides, thus prolonging their lifespan (De Meneghi *et al.*, 2016).

Local variation in tick density and parasite challenge, as well as the breed of cattle, affect the magnitude of the benefits from ITM. The variation in values from the cost–benefit analysis from different countries, years and using different input and output values highlights the need for applying a standardized approach to data collection and analysis across the at-risk population (Gilbert *et al.*, 2024).

2.4 Public–Private Considerations of Control

Deciding on the control option with the highest net benefits should be accompanied by considerations for the likelihood of private adoption, potential for (efficient) distribution, technical feasibility, and local motives and demand for control measures. Producer disease priorities, access to financial resources (particularly for women and low-income diversity groups) and trust in, or access to, external animal health services all affect uptake of control measures (Homewood *et al.*, 2006). For example, poor marketing and information dissemination about the vaccine has resulted in a lack of knowledge on its effects (Jumba *et al.*, 2020), as highlighted in Chapter 13 of this volume. In the past 15 years of commercial availability of the ITM, pastoralist systems have disproportionately adopted the vaccine compared to smallholder dairy and agro-pastoral systems (Toye *et al.*, 2020). To ensure adequate and equitable control of ECF, targeted and locally relevant information dissemination and knowledge exchange on the protective properties of the vaccines and the impacts of other available control measures is needed.

2.5 Alternative Approaches to Assess the Economic Impact of *T. parva*

As illustrated above, it is difficult to obtain an accurate estimate of the burden of *T. parva*. This problem stems from the lack of production, attribution and expenditure data from across the affected region, a problem shared with most of the world's livestock production sectors (Rushton *et al.*, 2018).

The key information that is required to improve the estimate of losses due to ECF includes the effect on production due to mortality and morbidity and the household expenditures on ECF prevention and control. However, it is recognized that robust empirical data will not be available from across the region in the near future, due to inadequately funded animal health services, poor market infrastructure and climatic and political barriers in the *T. parva*-affected region.

Where empirical data are not available, a 'hierarchies of evidence' approach can be used to parameterize models (Burns *et al.*, 2011; Clough *et al.*, 2025), and data from, potentially multiple, locally relevant sources can be synthesized through structured meta-analysis. Where all formal data are lacking, approaches such as formal expert elicitation can be used to fill data gaps (Colson and Cooke, 2018; Larkins *et al.*, 2023). When synthesizing data from multiple secondary sources to parameterize economic models, estimates of uncertainty around point values are essential when communicating any results (Oberkampf *et al.*, 2004).

As reliable production system data become available, a framework for determining the Global Burden of Animal Diseases (GBAD), presented in Box 2.1, can be used to estimate country- and production-system losses attributable to *T. parva*.

2.6 Conclusion

Estimates of the burden of infectious diseases of livestock are needed to aid with farm and political decision making and advocacy for investments in livestock health to reduce the burden of disease across society (Pradère, 2014; Rushton *et al.*, 2018). This chapter presents a transparent process that has estimated the annual loss due to *T. parva* to be between $300 million and $1.8 billion for 2020. This does not include lost production of meat, milk, dung and draught power, or the forgone revenue due to the disease-induced breed restrictions.

Despite the paucity of precise up-to-date data with which to estimate the losses caused by the disease, the conservative estimates presented herein, coupled with the clearly visible social impact of the disease, indicate that *T. parva* continues to be one of the most important constraints to cattle production in Africa and that the allocation of additional resources devoted to enhancing the control of this disease is fully justified.

Box 2.1. The Global Burden of Animal Diseases programme

Aligning with the logic of the burden approach to measuring animal health loss, we describe a framework from the Global Burden of Animal Diseases programme used to consider the burden of animal disease. The framework measures the burden of loss in a livestock herd, population or sector and relates it to its specific causes. Importantly, the framework sets a ceiling, or envelope, which allows multiple pathogens or diseases to have multiple effects on production without double-counting. This allows specific diseases or causes of loss to be measured in relative terms and in the context of other locally relevant causes of loss (such as feed shortage or predation as well as more commonly described infectious disease causes) to allow the wider social and economic impacts of diseases to be quantified. The framework is based on the basic model for production animals in Hennessy and Marsh (2021) and adapted for the Global Burden of Animal Diseases programme (Gilbert *et al*., 2024). Here we reproduce the model equation and discuss considering *T. parva*:

$$Y = F(z, \theta)\, x\, [1 - L(b_0 * (1 - C(x, \theta))]$$

where Y is the total output from the production livestock system and F(z,θ) captures the production function during normal production with regular inputs z and exogenous parameters θ. The exogenous parameters facilitate the application of the model to distinct regulations, social norms or environmental changes that occur outside of the farm production system. The regular inputs are those applied in the absence of disease and include the measures that producers regularly employ with their animals, such as selecting on genetics, shelter and feed. Including these here introduces a potential production baseline level that is comparable to the 'perfect' health considerations in human disease and comes from the crop-loss literature (Lichtenberg and Zilberman, 1986; Marsh *et al*., 2000).

The loss function $L(0 \leq L \leq 1)$ describes the disease damage *b_0* on the total production *Y* and the control approaches, which are measured through the control function $C(x,\theta)(0 \leq C \leq 1)$ and increase with control inputs x (vaccines, acaricides, treatments) to reduce the effects of *b_0*. When *b_0* = 0, there is no loss of output, and 'ideal' production exists, which is defined by regular inputs and the absence of disease. The burden of disease is then retrieved by comparing to this 'ideal' case through the combined value of lost output when *Y* is less than *F(z,θ)*, added any expenditure on control where x > 0. Through this basic model, disease loss can be seen as it relates to the severity of morbidity outcomes as a continuous measure and the occurrence of mortality as binary. As production occurs over time, outputs from animal production are adjusted to reflect disease-specific management changes (such as through culling rates and declining physical conditions). For *T. parva*, mortality rates account for a significant portion of the direct losses and morbidity is characterized by reduced physical condition, milk yield, dung production and draught power. Additional specifications are provided in Hennessy and Marsh (2021) and considerations in Gilbert *et al*. (2024). This approach can be applied to estimate the burden of ECF in affected countries and production systems if data to parameterize the model equation can be generated. It has been demonstrated in Senegal for the impact of Peste des petits ruminants in small ruminants (Meyer *et al*., 2025).

References

Al-Hosary, A., Abdel-Redy, A., Ahmed, L.S. and Mohamed, A. (2010) Comparison between using of Bupaquone® and other compounds in treatment of bovine theileriosis. *International Journal for Agro-Veterinary and Medical Sciences* 4, 3–7.

Allan, F.K., Sindoya, E., Adam, K.E., Byamungu, M., Lea, R.S. *et al*. (2021) A cross-sectional survey to establish *Theileria parva* prevalence and vector control at the wildlife-livestock interface, Northern Tanzania. *Preventive Veterinary Medicine* 196(98 Pt 2), 105491. DOI: 10.1016/j.prevetmed.2021.105491.

Anon (2013) National Dairy Strategy. Republic of Rwanda, Ministry of Agriculture and Animal Resources (MINAGRI). FAO. Available at: https://faolex.fao.org/docs/pdf/rwa149681.pdf (accessed 3 December 2025).

Anon (2015) Second National Development Plan (NDP II): Strengthening Uganda's Competitiveness for Sustainable Wealth Creation, Employment and Inclusive Growth. Republic of Uganda. FAO. Available at: https://faolex.fao.org/docs/pdf/uga151369.pdf (accessed 3 December 2025).

Anon (2020) *Fifth Integrated Household Survey 2019–2020*. National Statistical Office and World Bank Development Data Group, Malawi. DOI: 10.48529/yqn3-zv74.

Babo Martins, S., Di Giulio, G., Lynen, G., Peters, A. and Rushton, J. (2010) Assessing the impact of East Coast Fever immunisation by the infection and treatment method in Tanzanian pastoralist systems. *Preventive Veterinary Medicine* 97(3–4), 175–182. DOI: 10.1016/j.prevetmed.2010.09.018.

Bazarusanga, T., Vercruysse, J., Marcotty, T. and Geysen, D. (2007) Epidemiological studies on *Theileriosis* and the dynamics of *Theileria parva* infections in Rwanda. *Veterinary Parasitology* 143(3–4), 214–221. DOI: 10.1016/j.vetpar.2006.09.009.

Bazarusanga, T., Vercruysse, J. and Geysen, D. (2008) Epidemiological studies on East Coast Fever in Rwanda. *Afrika Focus* 21(2), 107–109. DOI: 10.1163/2031356X-02102008.

Behnke, R. and Muthami, D. (2011) The contribution of livestock to the Kenyan economy. IGAD Livestock Policy Initiative. Available at: https://cgspace.cgiar.org/server/api/core/bitstreams/ae8118f4-cb42-4240-954f-27653e83f4a4/content (accessed 2 December 2025).

Benson, T. and Mugarura, S. (2013) Livestock development planning in Uganda: Identification of areas of opportunity and challenge. *Land Use Policy* 35, 131–139. DOI: 10.1016/j.landusepol.2013.05.013.

Blench, R. (2001) 'You can't go home again'. Pastoralism in the new millennium. Overseas Development Institute, London. Available at: https://media.odi.org/documents/6329.pdf (accessed 3 December 2025).

Bronsvoort, B.M. de C., Thumbi, S.M., Poole, E.J., Kiara, H., Auguet, O.T. *et al.* (2013) Design and descriptive epidemiology of the Infectious Diseases of East African Livestock (IDEAL) project, a longitudinal calf cohort study in western Kenya. *BMC Veterinary Research* 9(1), 171. DOI: 10.1186/1746-6148-9-171.

Bundervoet, T. (2006) Livestock, activity choices and conflict: Evidence from Burundi. *Households in Conflict Network Working Paper* no.24. Available at: https://hicn.org/wp-content/uploads/2012/06/wp24.pdf (accessed 3 December 2025).

Burns, P.B., Rohrich, R.J. and Chung, K.C. (2011) The levels of evidence and their role in evidence-based medicine. *Plastic and Reconstructive Surgery* 128(1), 305–310. DOI: 10.1097/PRS.0b013e318219c171.

Carter, M.R. and Barrett, C.B. (2006) The economics of poverty traps and persistent poverty: An asset-based approach. *Journal of Development Studies* 42(2), 178–199. DOI: 10.1080/00220380500405261.

Catley, A. (2018) *Livestock and Livelihoods in South Sudan, K4D Helpdesk Report*. Institute of Development Studies, Brighton, UK. Available at: https://assets.publishing.service.gov.uk/media/5c6ebda7ed915d4a33065327/Livestock.pdf (accessed 3 December 2025).

Chatanga, E., Hayashida, K., Muleya, W., Kusakisako, K., Moustafa, M.A.M. *et al.* (2020) Genetic diversity and sequence polymorphism of two genes encoding *Theileria parva* antigens recognized by $CD8^+$ T cells among vaccinated and unvaccinated cattle in Malawi. *Pathogens* 9(5), 334. DOI: 10.3390/pathogens9050334.

Chatanga, E., Maganga, E., Mohamed, W.M.A., Ogata, S., Pandey, G.S. *et al.* (2022) High infection rate of tick-borne protozoan and rickettsial pathogens of cattle in Malawi and the development of a multiplex PCR for *Babesia* and *Theileria* species identification. *Acta Tropica* 231, 106413. DOI: 10.1016/j.actatropica.2022.106413.

Chaters, G.L., Johnson, P.C.D., Cleaveland, S., Crispell, J., de Glanville, W.A. *et al.* (2019) Analysing livestock network data for infectious disease control: An argument for routine data collection in emerging economies. *Philosophical Transactions of the Royal Society B* 374(1776), 20180264. DOI: 10.1098/rstb.2018.0264.

Chepkwony, R., Castagna, C., Heitkönig, I., van Bommel, S. and van Langevelde, F. (2020) Associations between monthly rainfall and mortality in cattle due to East Coast fever, anaplasmosis and babesiosis. *Parasitology* 147(14), 1743–1751. DOI: 10.1017/S0031182020001638.

Claire, D.H., Donald, R.K., Tiba, M., Jean, D.R., Aline, K. *et al.* (2017) Management and phenotypic features of indigenous cattle in Rwanda. *International Journal of Livestock Production* 8(7), 95–112. DOI: 10.5897/IJLP2017.0362.

Clough, H.E., Chaters, G.L., Havelaar, A.H., McIntyre, K.M., Marsh, T.L. *et al.* (2025) A framework for handling uncertainty in a large-scale programme estimating the global burden of animal diseases. *Frontiers in Veterinary Science* 12, 1459209. DOI: 10.3389/fvets.2025.1459209.

Colson, A.R. and Cooke, R.M. (2018) Expert elicitation: Using the classical model to validate experts' judgments. *Review of Environmental Economics and Policy* 12(1), 113–132. DOI: 10.1093/reep/rex022.

Countryman, A.M., de Menezes, T.C., Pendell, D.L., Rushton, J. and Marsh, T.L. (2024) Economic effects of livestock disease burden in Ethiopia: A computable general equilibrium analysis. *PLoS ONE* 19(12), e0310268. DOI: 10.1371/journal.pone.0310268.

Cox, T.P. (2012) Farming the battlefield: The meanings of war, cattle and soil in South Kivu, Democratic Republic of the Congo. *Disasters* 36(2), 233–248. DOI: 10.1111/j.1467-7717.2011.01257.x.

Cullis, A. (2021) Understanding the livestock economy in South Sudan: Field study findings. Tana Copenhagen ApS. Available at: https://tanacopenhagen.com/wp-content/uploads/2021/04/Field-Report.pdf (accessed 3 December 2025).

de Glanville, W.A., Davis, A., Allan, K.J., Buza, J., Claxton, J.R. *et al.* (2020) Classification and characterisation of livestock production systems in Northern Tanzania. *PloS ONE* 15(12), e0229478. DOI: 10.1371/journal.pone.0229478.

de la Fuente, J., Contreras, M., Kasaija, P., Gortazar, C., Ruiz-Fons, J. *et al.* (2019) Towards a multidisciplinary approach to improve cattle health and production in Uganda. *Vaccines* 7(4), 165. DOI: 10.3390/vaccines7040165.

De Meneghi, D., Stachurski, F. and Adakal, H. (2016) Experiences in tick control by acaricide in the traditional cattle sector in Zambia and Burkina Faso: Possible environmental and public health implications. *Frontiers in Public Health* 4, 239. DOI: 10.3389/fpubh.2016.00239.

Deem, S.L., Perry, B.D., Katende, J.M., McDermott, J.J., Mahan, S.M. *et al.* (1993) Variations in prevalence rates of tick-borne diseases in Zebu cattle by agroecological zone: Implications for East Coast Fever immunization. *Preventive Veterinary Medicine* 16(3), 171–187. DOI: 10.1016/0167-5877(93)90064-Z.

D'Haese, L., Penne, K. and Elyn, R. (1999) Economics of *Theileriosis* control in Zambia. *Tropical Medicine & International Health* 4(9), A49–A57. DOI: 10.1046/j.1365-3156.1999.00451.x.

Di Giulio, G., Lynen, G., Morzaria, S., Oura, C. and Bishop, R. (2009) Live immunization against East Coast fever – Current status. *Trends in Parasitology* 25(2), 85–92. DOI: 10.1016/j.pt.2008.11.007.

Direito, B. (2021) Livestock and veterinary health in Southern Mozambique in the beginning of the twentieth century: The case of the fight against East Coast fever. *Historia, Ciencias, Saude – Manguinhos* 28(4), 939–959. DOI: 10.1590/S0104-59702021000400003.

Dube, T., Homann-Kee Tui, S., Rooyen, A. and Rodriguez, D. (2014) Baseline and situation analysis report: Integrating crop and livestock production for improved food security and livelihoods in rural Zimbabwe. *International Crops Research Institute for the Semi-Arid Tropics Socioeconomics Discussion Paper Series 29*. Hyderabad, India. Available at: https://hdl.handle.net/10568/56935 (accessed 3 December 2025).

Dutilly, C., Alary, V., Bonnet, P., Lesnoff, M., Fandamu, P. *et al.* (2020) Multi-scale assessment of the livestock sector for policy design in Zambia. *Journal of Policy Modeling* 42(2), 401–418. DOI: 10.1016/j.jpolmod.2019.07.004.

Ermyas, S. (2023) Conservation Agriculture Techniques Are Improving Agricultural Productivity in Zimbabwe's Drylands. *ILRI News*. Available at: https://www.ilri.org/news/conservation-agriculture-techniques-are-improving-agricultural-productivity-zimbabwes-drylands (accessed 3 December 2025).

Ezeanya-Esiobu, C., Oguamanam, C. and Ndungutse, V. (2021) Marginalisation of Indigenous knowledge in African education: The case of Rwandan traditional medicinal treatments for livestock. *Open African Innovation Research Working Paper 24*. Available at: https://openair.africa/wp-content/uploads/2021/02/WP-24-Marginalisation-of-Indigenous-Knowledge-in-African-Education.pdf (accessed 3 December 2025).

Fandamu, P., Duchateau, L., Speybroeck, N., Marcotty, T., Mbao, V. *et al.* (2005) *Theileria parva* seroprevalence in traditionally kept cattle in southern Zambia and El Niño. *International Journal for Parasitology* 35(4), 391–396. DOI: 10.1016/j.ijpara.2004.12.011.

FAO (2022) Zimbabwe at a Glance. Available at: https://www.fao.org/zimbabwe/fao-in-zimbabwe/zimbabwe-at-a-glance/es/ (accessed 1 December 2025).

FAOSTAT (2020) FAOSTAT database. Available at: https://www.fao.org/faostat/en/#data/QCL (accessed 1 December 2025).

FAOSTAT (2021a) FAOSTAT Crops and Livestock Products. Available at: https://www.fao.org/faostat/en/#data/QCL (accessed 2 December 2025).

FAOSTAT (2021b) FAOSTAT Macro Indicators. Available at: https://www.fao.org/faostat/en/#data/MK (accessed 2 December 2025).

FAOSTAT (2021c) FAOSTAT Suite of Food Security Indicators. Available at: https://www.fao.org/faostat/en/#data/FS (accessed 2 December 2025).

FAOSTAT (2021d) FAOSTAT Value of Agricultural Production. Available at: https://www.fao.org/faostat/en/#data/QV (accessed 2 December 2025).

Fransen, S., Ruiz, I. and Vargas-Silva, C. (2017) Return migration and economic outcomes in the conflict context. *World Development* 95, 196–210. DOI: 10.1016/j.worlddev.2017.02.015.

Gachohi, J., Skilton, R., Hansen, F., Ngumi, P. and Kitala, P. (2012) Epidemiology of East Coast fever (*Theileria parva* infection) in Kenya: Past, present and the future. *Parasites & Vectors* 5(1), 194. DOI: 10.1186/1756-3305-5-194.

Gilbert, M., Cinardi, G., Da Re, D., Wint, W.G.R., Wisser, D. *et al.* (2022) Global cattle distribution in 2015 (5 minutes of arc). Harvard Dataverse. DOI: 10.7910/DVN/LHBICE.

Gilbert, W., Marsh, T.L., Chaters, G., Jemberu, W.T., Bruce, M. *et al.* (2024) Quantifying cost of disease in livestock: A new metric for the global burden of animal diseases. *The Lancet Planetary Health* 8(5), e309–e317. DOI: 10.1016/S2542-5196(24)00047-0.

Gitau, G.K., O'Callaghan, C.J., McDermott, J.J., Omore, A.O., Odima, P.A. *et al.* (1994) Description of smallholder dairy farms in Kiambu district, Kenya. *Preventive Veterinary Medicine* 21(2), 155–166. DOI: 10.1016/0167-5877(94)90004-3.

Gitau, G.K., Perry, B.D. and McDermott, J.J. (1999) The incidence, calf morbidity and mortality due to *Theileria parva* infections in smallholder dairy farms in Murang'a district, Kenya. *Preventive Veterinary Medicine* 39(1), 65–79. DOI: 10.1016/s0167-5877(98)00137-8.

Githaka, N.W., Kanduma, E.G., Wieland, B., Darghouth, M.A. and Bishop, R.P. (2022) Acaricide resistance in livestock ticks infesting cattle in Africa: Current status and potential mitigation strategies. *Current Research in Parasitology & Vector-Borne Diseases* 2, 100090. DOI: 10.1016/j.crpvbd.2022.100090.

Haseeb, A., Jonathan, Y., William, A. de G., Alicia, D., Tito, J.K. *et al.* (2019) Economic burden of livestock disease and drought in Northern Tanzania. *Journal of Development and Agricultural Economics* 11(6), 140–151. DOI: 10.5897/JDAE2018.1028.

Hatungumukama, G., Hornick, J.-L. and Detilleux, J. (2007) Zootechnical aspects of bovine breeding in Burundi: Present and future. *Annales de Médecine Vétérinaire* 151, 150–165.

Hennessy, D.A. and Marsh, T.L. (2021) Economics of animal health and livestock disease. *Handbook of Agricultural Economics* 5, 4233–4330. DOI: 10.1016/bs.hesagr.2021.10.005.

Homewood, K., Trench, P., Randall, S., Lynen, G. and Bishop, B. (2006) Livestock health and socio-economic impacts of a veterinary intervention in Maasailand: Infection-and-treatment vaccine against East Coast fever. *Agricultural Systems* 89(2–3), 248–271. DOI: 10.1016/j.agsy.2005.09.004.

Idris, I. (2018) Livestock and Conflict in South Sudan. *K4D Helpdesk Report 484*. Institute of Development Studies, Brighton, UK. Available at: https://hdl.handle.net/20.500.12413/14316 (accessed 1 December 2025).

IGAD Center for Pastoral Areas & Livestock Development (ICPALD) (2016) The Contribution of Livestock to the South Sudan Economy. Available at: https://icpald.org/wp-content/uploads/2019/08/Policy-Brief-on-the-Contribution-of-Livestock-to-South-Sudan-National-GDP-Jan-2016.pdf (accessed 3 December 2025).

Johnson, N., Njuki, J., Waithanji, E., Nhambeto, M., Rogers, M. *et al.* (2015) The gendered impacts of agricultural asset transfer projects: Lessons from the Manica smallholder dairy development program. *Gender, Technology and Development* 19(2), 145–180. DOI: 10.1177/0971852415578041.

Jumba, H., Kiara, H., Owuor, G. and Teufel, N. (2020) Are there gender differences in access to and demand for East Coast fever vaccine? Empirical evidence from rural smallholder dairy farmers in Kenya. *Journal of Agriculture and Rural Development in the Tropics and Subtropics* 121, 219–231. DOI: 10.17170/KOBRA-202010191970.

Juvenal, N. and Edward, M. (2010) Seasonal dynamics and distribution of ticks in Rwanda: Implications for tick control strategy in Rwanda. *International Journal of Animal and Veterinary Advances* 2, 21–25.

Kabi, F., Masembe, C., Muwanika, V., Kirunda, H. and Negrini, R. (2014) Geographic distribution of non-clinical *Theileria parva* infection among indigenous cattle populations in contrasting agro-ecological zones of Uganda: Implications for control strategies. *Parasites & Vectors* 7(1), 414. DOI: 10.1186/1756-3305-7-414.

Kalume, M.K., Saegerman, C., Marcotty, T., Duchatel, J.-P. and Losson, B. (2012) Statut épidémiologique de l'East Coast fever dans deux troupeaux de bovins issus de systèmes d'élevage distincts au nord-Kivu, République Démocratique du Congo. *Annales de Médecine Vétérinaire* 156, 99–108.

Kaumbata, W., Nakimbugwe, H., Nandolo, W., Banda, L.J., Mészáros, G. *et al*. (2021) Experiences from the implementation of community-based goat breeding programs in Malawi and Uganda: A potential approach for conservation and improvement of indigenous small ruminants in smallholder farms. *Sustainability* 13(3), 1494. DOI: 10.3390/su13031494.

Kivaria, F.M. (2006) Estimated direct economic costs associated with tick-borne diseases on cattle in Tanzania. *Tropical Animal Health and Production* 38(4), 291–299. DOI: 10.1007/s11250-006-4181-2.

Kivaria, F.M., Heuer, C., Jongejan, F., Okello-Onen, J., Rutagwenda, T. *et al*. (2004) Endemic stability for *Theileria parva* infections in Ankole calves of the Ankole ranching scheme, Uganda. *Onderstepoort Journal of Veterinary Research* 71(3), 189–195. DOI: 10.4102/ojvr.v71i3.259.

Kivaria, F.M., Ruheta, M.R., Mkonyi, P.A. and Malamsha, P.C. (2007) Epidemiological aspects and economic impact of bovine theileriosis (East Coast fever) and its control: A preliminary assessment with special reference to Kibaha district, Tanzania. *The Veterinary Journal* 173(2), 384–390. DOI: 10.1016/j.tvjl.2005.08.013.

Kwankanaba Bantuzeko, F., Ciza Mushagalusa, A., Barume, C.A., Mugumaarhahama, Y. and Sefu, A.G. (2022) Farmers' perceptions on technical controls and risk factors of East Coast Fever caused by *Theileria parva* in mountainous Kivu, Democratic Republic of Congo. *Journal of Animal and Plant Sciences* 51, 9213–9226.

Laker, C.D. (1993) The economics of East Coast Fever immunization in Uganda. MSc thesis, University of Nairobi. Available at: https://hdl.handle.net/10568/79645 (accessed 1 December 2025).

Larkins, A., Temesgen, W., Chaters, G., Di Bari, C., Kwok, S. *et al*. (2023) Attributing Ethiopian animal health losses to high-level causes using expert elicitation. *Preventive Veterinary Medicine* 221, 106077. DOI: 10.1016/j.prevetmed.2023.106077.

Latif, A.A., Hove, T., Kanhai, G.K. and Masaka, S. (2001) Laboratory and field investigations into the *Theileria parva* carrier-state in cattle in Zimbabwe. *Onderstepoort Journal of Veterinary Research* 68(3), 203–208.

Lichtenberg, E. and Zilberman, D. (1986) The econometrics of damage control: Why specification matters. *American Journal of Agricultural Economics* 68(2), 261–273. DOI: 10.2307/1241427.

Lynen, G., Yrjö-Koskinen, A.E., Bakuname, C., Di Giulio, G., Mlinga, N. *et al*. (2012) East Coast fever immunisation field trial in crossbred dairy cattle in Hanang and Handeni districts in Northern Tanzania. *Tropical Animal Health and Production* 44(3), 567–572. DOI: 10.1007/s11250-011-9936-8.

Lysholm, S., Lindahl, J.F., Munyeme, M., Misinzo, G., Mathew, C. *et al*. (2022) Crossing the line: Seroprevalence and risk factors for transboundary animal diseases along the Tanzania–Zambia border. *Frontiers in Veterinary Science* 9, 809128. DOI: 10.3389/fvets.2022.809128.

MacroTrends (2022) South Africa GDP Per Capita. Available at: https://www.macrotrends.net/global-metrics/countries/zaf/south-africa/gdp-per-capita (accessed 3 December 2025).

Makoni, N., Mwai, R., Redda, T., Zijpp, A. van der and Lee, J. van der (2014) White gold: Opportunities for dairy sector development collaboration in East Africa. *CDI report CDI-14-006*. Centre for Development Innovation, Wageningen UR (University & Research Centre), Wageningen, The Netherlands. Available at: https://edepot.wur.nl/307878

Marcellino, W.L., Salih, D.A., Njahira, M.N., Ndiwa, N., Araba, A. *et al*. (2017) The emergence of *Theileria parva* in Jonglei state, South Sudan: Confirmation using molecular and serological diagnostic tools. *Transboundary and Emerging Diseases* 64(4), 1229–1235. DOI: 10.1111/tbed.12495.

Marsh, T.L., Huffaker, R.G. and Long, G.E. (2000) Optimal control of vector-virus-plant interactions: The case of potato leafroll virus net necrosis. *American Journal of Agricultural Economics* 82(3), 556–569. DOI: 10.1111/0002-9092.00046.

Marsh, T.L., Yoder, J., Deboch, T., McElwain, T.F. and Palmer, G.H. (2016) Livestock vaccinations translate into increased human capital and school attendance by girls. *Science Advances* 2(12), e1601410. DOI: 10.1126/sciadv.1601410.

Matchaya, G., Phiri, A., Chilonda, P. and Musaba, E. (2012) *Agricultural Growth Trends and Outlook Report: Trends in Agricultural Sector Performance, Growth and Poverty in Malawi*. ReSAKSS–SA Annual Trends and Outlook Report 2012. International Food Policy Research Institute (IFPRI) and the International Water Management Institute (IWMI). Available at: https://www.resakss.org/sites/default/files/pdfs/resakss_malawi_ator.pdf (accessed 1 December 2025).

Mazibe, M. and Lopes Pereirat, C. (1988) Theileriosis in Mozambique. In: Dolan, T.T. (ed.) *Theileriosis in Eastern, Central and Southern Africa: Proceedings of a Workshop on East Coast Fever Immunization, Held in Lilongwe, Malawi*, ILRAD, Nairobi, Kenya, pp. 17–19.

Mazimpaka, E., Mbuza, F., Michael, T., Gatari, E.N., Bukenya, E.M. *et al.* (2017) Current status of cattle production system in Nyagatare district, Rwanda. *Tropical Animal Health and Production* 49(8), 1645–1656. DOI: 10.1007/s11250-017-1372-y.

Mbizeni, S., Potgieter, F.T., Troskie, C., Mans, B.J., Penzhorn, B.L. *et al.* (2013) Field and laboratory studies on Corridor disease (*Theileria parva* infection) in cattle population at the livestock/game interface of Uphongolo-Mkuze area, South Africa. *Ticks and Tick-Borne Diseases* 4(3), 227–234. DOI: 10.1016/j.ttbdis.2012.11.005.

McLeod, R. and Kristjanson, P. (1999) Economic Impact of Ticks and Tick-Borne Diseases on Livestock in Africa, Asia and Australia. *Report to the International Livestock Research Institute*, Nairobi, Kenya.

Melesse, M.B., Tirra, A.N., Homann-Kee Tui, S., Van Rooyen, A.F. and Hauser, M. (2023) Production decisions and food security outcomes of smallholders' livestock market participation: Empirical evidence from Zimbabwe. *Frontiers in Sustainable Food Systems* 7, 1222509. DOI: 10.3389/fsufs.2023.1222509.

Meyer, A., Ndiaye, B., Larkins, A., Chaters, G., Gilbert, W. *et al.* (2025) Economic assessment of animal disease burden in Senegalese small ruminants. *Preventive Veterinary Medicine* 234, 106382. DOI: 10.1016/j.prevetmed.2024.106382.

Michael, S., Mbwambo, N., Mruttu, H., Dotto, M.M., Ndomba, C. *et al.* (2018) *Tanzania Livestock Master Plan*. ILRI, Nairobi, Kenya. Available at: https://hdl.handle.net/10568/92405 (accessed 1 December 2025).

Ministry of Agriculture, Animal Industry and Fisheries (MAAIF) (2020) Roll Out of National Traceability System Under Way. Available at: https://www.agriculture.go.ug/2020/01/13/roll-out-of-national-traceability-system-under-way/ (accessed 3 December 2025).

Ministry of Livestock and Fisheries (2022) *The United Republic of Tanzania Ministry of Livestock and Fisheries, Livestock Sector Transformation Plan (LSTP) 2022/23 – 2026/27*. Available at: https://faolex.fao.org/docs/pdf/tan223748.pdf (accessed 2 December 2025).

Minjauw, B. and McLeod, A. (2003) *Tick-Borne Diseases and Poverty. The Impact of Ticks and Tick-Borne Diseases on the Livelihood of Small-Scale and Marginal Livestock Owners in India and Eastern and Southern Africa*. Research report. DFID Animal Health Programme, Centre for Tropical Veterinary Medicine, University of Edinburgh. UK, pp. 59–60.

Minjauw, B., Otte, J., James, A.D., de Castro, J.J. and Sinyangwe, P. (1997) Effect of different East Coast Fever control strategies on fertility, milk production and weight gain of Sanga cattle in the Central province of Zambia. *Experimental & Applied Acarology* 21(12), 715–730. DOI: 10.1023/A:1018417004323.

Minjauw, B., Rushton, J., James, A.D. and Upton, M. (1999) Financial analysis of East Coast Fever control strategies in traditionally managed Sanga cattle in Central province of Zambia. *Preventive Veterinary Medicine* 38(1), 35–45. DOI: 10.1016/s0167-5877(98)00128-7.

Mohammed, A.A., Al Shaekh, A.I., Saaid, A.A. and Salih, D.A. (2019) The spreading of East Coast Fever into Greater Bahr-el-Ghazal region, north-west of South Sudan. *Tanzanian Veterinary Journal* 34, 1–8.

Mosites, E.M., Rabinowitz, P.M., Thumbi, S.M., Montgomery, J.M., Palmer, G.H. *et al.* (2015) The relationship between livestock ownership and child stunting in three countries in Eastern Africa using national survey data. *PLoS ONE* 10(9), e0136686. DOI: 10.1371/journal.pone.0136686.

Motta, P., Porphyre, T., Handel, I., Hamman, S.M., Ngu Ngwa, V. *et al.* (2017) Implications of the cattle trade network in Cameroon for regional disease prevention and control. *Scientific Reports* 7, 43932. DOI: 10.1038/srep43932.

Mugisha, A., McLeod, A., Percy, R. and Kyewalabye, E. (2005) Strategies, effectiveness and rationale of vector-borne disease control in the pastoralist system of south-western uganda. *Tropical Animal Health and Production* 37(6), 479–489. DOI: 10.1007/s11250-005-2174-1.

Mugumaarhahama, Y., Ayagirwe, R.B.B., Mutwedu, V.B., Cirezi, N.C., Wasso, D.S. *et al.* (2021) Characterization of smallholder cattle production systems in South-Kivu province, Eastern Democratic Republic of Congo. *Pastoralism* 11(1), 1–15. DOI: 10.1186/s13570-020-00187-w.

Muhanguzi, D., Picozzi, K., Hatendorf, J., Thrusfield, M., Welburn, S. *et al.* (2014) Prevalence and spatial distribution of *Theileria parva* in cattle under crop-livestock farming systems in Tororo district, Eastern Uganda. *Parasites & Vectors* 7(1), 91. DOI: 10.1186/1756-3305-7-91.

Mukhebi, A.W., Wathanga, J., Perry, B.D., Irvin, A.D. and Morzaria, S.P. (1989) Financial analysis of East Coast fever control strategies on beef production under farm conditions. *Veterinary Record* 125(18), 456–459. DOI: 10.1136/vr.125.18.456.

Mukhebi, A.W., Perry, B.D. and Kruska, R. (1992) Estimated economics of theileriosis control in Africa. *Preventive Veterinary Medicine* 12(1–2), 73–85. DOI: 10.1016/0167-5877(92)90070-V.

Mumba, C., Skjerve, E., Rich, M. and Rich, K.M. (2017) Application of system dynamics and participatory spatial group model building in animal health: A case study of East Coast Fever interventions in Lundazi and Monze districts of Zambia. *PloS ONE* 12(12), e0189878. DOI: 10.1371/journal.pone.0189878.

Murray, C.J.L. and Lopez, A.D. (2013) Measuring the global burden of disease. *New England Journal of Medicine* 369(5), 448–457. DOI: 10.1056/NEJMra1201534.

Murray, M., Trail, J.C.M., Davis, C.E. and Black, S.J. (1984) Genetic resistance to African trypanosomiasis. *The Journal of Infectious Diseases* 149(3), 311–319. DOI: 10.1093/infdis/149.3.311.

Mutwedu, V.B., Buuma, B.K., Mushagalusa, A.C., Bisimwa, N.P., Cirezi, N.C. *et al.* (2019) Prevalence and economic losses of calf fetal wastage in ELAKAT public slaughterhouse of Bukavu, democratic republic of Congo. *Veterinary World* 12(10), 1644–1649. DOI: 10.14202/vetworld.2019.1644-1649.

Mwila, N., Mumba, C., Salih, O., Sichibalo, K., Simulundu, E.S. *et al.* (2022) Modeling the non-monetary societal burden of tick-borne diseases for cattle: A case study of East Coast fever in the traditional cattle-keeping households of Namwala district of Zambia. *University of Zambia Journal of Agricultural and Biomedical Sciences* 6(2), 60–78. DOI: 10.53974/unza.jabs.6.2.877.

Nambota, A., Samui, K., Sugimoto, C., Kakuta, T. and Onuma, M. (1994) Theileriosis in Zambia: Etiology, epidemiology and control measures. *The Japanese Journal of Veterinary Research* 42(1), 1–18.

National Statistical Office (NSO) (2020) *Fifth integrated household survey 2019-2020* [data set]. World Bank, Development Data Group. DOI: 10.48529/MPYK-DS48.

Ng'ang'a, S.K., Ritho, C., Herrero, M. and Fraval, S. (2018) Household-oriented benefits largely outweigh commercial benefits derived from cattle in Mabalane district, Mozambique. *The Rangeland Journal* 40(6), 565–576. DOI: 10.1071/RJ17115.

Nkonki-Mandleni, B., Ogunkoya, F. and Omotayo, A.O. (2018) Socioeconomic factors influencing livestock production among smallholder farmers in the free state province of South Africa. *International Journal of Entrepreneurship* 22, 1939–4675.

Nwafor, C.U., Ogundeji, A.A. and van der Westhuizen, C. (2020) Adoption of ICT-based information sources and market participation among smallholder livestock farmers in South Africa. *Agriculture* 10(2), 44. DOI: 10.3390/agriculture10020044.

Nyabongo, L., Odongo, D.O., Milton, G., Machuka, E., Vudriko, P. *et al.* (2021) Molecular survey of cattle ticks in Burundi: First report on the presence of the invasive *Rhipicephalus microplus* tick. *PLoS One* 16(12), e0261218. DOI: 10.1371/journal.pone.0261218.

Nyangito, H.O., Richardson, J.W., Mukhebi, A.W., Mundy, D.S., Zimmel, P. *et al.* (1995) Whole farm economic evaluation of East Coast fever immunization strategies on farms in the Uasin Gishu district of Kenya. *Computers and Electronics in Agriculture* 12(1), 19–33. DOI: 10.1016/0168-1699(94)00035-O.

Oberkampf, W.L., Helton, J.C., Joslyn, C.A., Wojtkiewicz, S.F. and Ferson, S. (2004) Challenge problems: Uncertainty in system response given uncertain parameters. *Reliability Engineering & System Safety* 85(1–3), 11–19. DOI: 10.1016/j.ress.2004.03.002.

Ocaido, M., Muwazi, R.T. and Opuda, J.A. (2009) Disease incidence in ranch and pastoral livestock herds around lake Mburo National Park, in South Western Uganda. *Tropical Animal Health and Production* 41, 1299–1308. DOI: 10.1007/S11250-009-9315-X/TABLES/9.

Ombeni, J.B., Babe, T., Munyuli, T.M., Kashosi, T.M. and Mwangi, T.B. (2018) Hygienic quality assessment of fresh beef meat in Bukavu urban slaughter houses, South Kivu province of the long sale chain; potential health risks for consumers eastern DR Congo. *Bacterial Empire* 1(1), 1. DOI: 10.36547/be.2018.1.1.1-9.

Orenge, C.O., Munga, L., Kimwele, C.N., Kemp, S., Korol, A. *et al.* (2012) Trypanotolerance in n'Dama x Boran crosses under natural trypanosome challenge: Effect of test-year environment, gender, and breed composition. *BMC Genetics* 13, 1–15. DOI: 10.1186/1471-2156-13-87/FIGURES/2.

Otte, J., Costales, A., Dijkman, J., Pica-Ciamarra, U., Robinson, T. *et al.* (2012) *Livestock Sector Development for Poverty Reduction: An Economic and Policy Perspective – Livestock's Many Virtues*. FAO/Cambridge University Press, Cambridge, UK. Available at: http://www.fao.org/docrep/015/i2744e/i2744e00.pdf (accessed 1 December 2025).

Paling, R.W., Mpangala, C., Luttikhuizen, B. and Sibomana, G. (1991) Exposure of Ankole and crossbred cattle to theileriosis in Rwanda. *Tropical Animal Health and Production* 23(4), 203–214. DOI: 10.1007/BF02357101.

Perry, B.D. (2016) The control of East Coast fever of cattle by live parasite vaccination: A science-to-impact narrative. *One Health* 2, 103–114. DOI: 10.1016/j.onehlt.2016.07.002.

Perry, B. and Grace, D. (2009) The impacts of livestock diseases and their control on growth and development processes that are pro-poor. *Philosophical Transactions of the Royal Society B* 364(1530), 2643–2655. DOI: 10.1098/rstb.2009.0097.

Perry, B.D., Randolph, T.F., McDermott, J.J., Sones, K.R. and Thornton, P.K. (2002) *Investing in Animal Health Research to Alleviate Poverty*. ILRI (International Livestock Research Institute), Nairobi, Kenya.

Pradère, J.-P. (2014) Improving animal health and livestock productivity to reduce poverty. *Revue Scientifique et Technique (International Office of Epizootics)* 33, 735–744.

Rashid, M., Rashid, M.I., Akbar, H., Ahmad, L., Hassan, M.A. *et al.* (2019) A systematic review on modelling approaches for economic losses studies caused by parasites and their associated diseases in cattle. *Parasitology* 146(2), 129–141. DOI: 10.1017/S0031182018001282.

Rawlins, R., Pimkina, S., Barrett, C.B., Pedersen, S. and Wydick, B. (2014) Got milk? The impact of Heifer International's livestock donation programs in Rwanda on nutritional outcomes. *Food Policy* 44, 202–213. DOI: 10.1016/j.foodpol.2013.12.003.

Rich, K.M. and Perry, B.D. (2011) The economic and poverty impacts of animal diseases in developing countries: New roles, new demands for economics and epidemiology. *Preventive Veterinary Medicine* 101(3–4), 133–147. DOI: 10.1016/j.prevetmed.2010.08.002.

Rich, K.M. and Niemi, J.K. (2017) The economic impact of a new animal disease: Same effects in developed and developing countries? *Revue Scientifique et Technique de l'OIE* 36(1), 115–124. DOI: 10.20506/rst.36.1.2615.

Rossi, L., Hoerz, T., Thouvenot, V., Pastore, G. and Michael, M. (2006) Evaluation of health, nutrition and food security programmes in a complex emergency: The case of Congo as an example of a chronic post-conflict situation. *Public Health Nutrition* 9(5), 551–556. DOI: 10.1079/phn2005928.

Rubaire-Akiiki, C.M., Okello-Onen, J., Musunga, D., Kabagambe, E.K., Vaarst, M. *et al.* (2006) Effect of agro-ecological zone and grazing system on incidence of East Coast Fever in calves in Mbale and Sironko districts of Eastern Uganda. *Preventive Veterinary Medicine* 75(3–4), 251–266. DOI: 10.1016/j.prevetmed.2006.04.015.

Rushton, J. (2009) *The Economics of Animal Health and Production*. CAB International, Wallingford, UK.

Rushton, J. (2017) Improving the use of economics in animal health – Challenges in research, policy and education. *Preventive Veterinary Medicine* 137(Pt B), 130–139. DOI: 10.1016/j.prevetmed.2016.11.020.

Rushton, J., Thornton, P.K. and Otte, M.J. (1999) Methods of economic impact assessment. *Revue Scientifique et Technique de l'OIE* 18(2), 315–342. DOI: 10.20506/rst.18.2.1172.

Rushton, J., Uggla, A. and Magnusson, U. (2017) Animal health in development – Its role for poverty reduction and human welfare. *EBA – Rapporter* 2017:3. Expertgruppen for Bistandsanalys. Available at: https://eba.se/app/uploads/2017/03/2017-03_Djurh%C3%A4lsa_webb_Tillganp.pdf (accessed 1 December 2025).

Rushton, J., Bruce, M., Bellet, C., Torgerson, P., Shaw, A. *et al.* (2018) Initiation of global burden of animal diseases programme. *Lancet* 392(10147), 538–540. DOI: 10.1016/S0140-6736(18)31472-7.

Rushton, J., Huntington, B., Gilbert, W., Herrero, M., Torgerson, P.R. *et al.* (2021) Roll-out of the global burden of animal diseases programme. *Lancet* 397(10279), 1045–1046. DOI: 10.1016/S0140-6736(21)00189-6.

Simuunza, M., Weir, W., Courcier, E., Tait, A. and Shiels, B. (2011) Epidemiological analysis of tick-borne diseases in Zambia. *Veterinary Parasitology* 175(3–4), 331–342. DOI: 10.1016/j.vetpar.2010.09.027.

Sitawa, R., Mbogoh, S.G., Gathuma, J.M. and Kairu, S. (2016) An evaluation of economic returns from East Coast Fever control through infection and treatment method at household level in Nandi and Uasin-Gishu counties of Kenya. *International Journal of Agricultural Policy and Research* 4(8), 149–156. DOI: 10.15739/IJAPR.16.019.

Staal, S.J., Poole, E.J., Baltenweck, I., Mwacharo, J.M., Notenbaert, A.M.O. *et al.* (2009) Targeting strategic investment in livestock development as a vehicle for rural livelihoods. Bill and Melinda Gates Foundation – ILRI Knowledge Generation Project Report. ILRI, Nairobi, Kenya. Available at: https://hdl.handle.net/10568/35206 (accessed 3 December 2025).

Stroebel, A., Swanepoel, F.J.C. and Pell, A.N. (2011) Sustainable smallholder livestock systems: A case study of Limpopo province, South Africa. *Livestock Science* 139(1–2), 186–190. DOI: 10.1016/j.livsci.2011.03.004.

Surve, A.A., Hwang, J.Y., Manian, S., Onono, J.O. and Yoder, J. (2023) Economics of East Coast fever: A literature review. *Frontiers in Veterinary Science* 10, 1239110. DOI: 10.3389/FVETS.2023.1239110/BIBTEX.

Taruvinga, A., Kambanje, A., Mushunje, A. and Mukarumbwa, P. (2022) Determinants of livestock species ownership at household level: Evidence from rural OR Tambo District Municipality, South Africa. *Pastoralism* 12(1), 1–11. DOI: 10.1186/s13570-021-00220-6.

Teufel, N., Korir, L., Hammond, J., van Wijk, M. and Kiara, H. (2021) Farm and livelihood characteristics after ITM vaccination against East Coast fever in Tanzania. *Frontiers in Veterinary Science* 8, 889. DOI: 10.3389/FVETS.2021.639762/BIBTEX.

Thomas, K.M., Kibona, T., Claxton, J.R., de Glanville, W.A., Lankester, F. *et al.* (2022) Prospective cohort study reveals unexpected aetiologies of livestock abortion in northern Tanzania. *Scientific Reports* 12(1), 11669. DOI: 10.1038/s41598-022-15517-8.

Thompson, B.E., Latif, A.A., Oosthuizen, M.C., Troskie, M. and Penzhorn, B.L. (2008) Occurrence of *Theileria parva* infection in cattle on a farm in the Ladysmith district, KwaZulu-Natal, South Africa. *Journal of the South African Veterinary Association* 79(1), 31–35. DOI: 10.4102/jsava.v79i1.237.

Thumbi, S.M., Bronsvoort, M., Kiara, H., Toye, P.G., Poole, J. *et al.* (2013) Mortality in East African shorthorn zebu cattle under one year: Predictors of infectious-disease mortality. *BMC Veterinary Research* 9(1), 175. DOI: 10.1186/1746-6148-9-175.

Thumbi, S.M., Njenga, M.K., Marsh, T.L., Noh, S., Otiang, E. *et al.* (2015) Linking human health and livestock health: A "One-Health" platform for integrated analysis of human health, livestock health, and economic welfare in livestock dependent communities. *PloS ONE* 10(3), e0120761. DOI: 10.1371/journal.pone.0120761.

Toye, P., Kiara, H., ole-MoiYoi, O., Enahoro, D. and Rich, K.M. (2020) The management and economics of East Coast fever. In: McIntire, J. and Grace, D. (eds) *The Impact of the International Livestock Research Institute. ILRI, Nairobi, Kenya*. CAB International, Wallingford, UK, pp. 239–273.

Trading Economics (2022) Mozambique GDP From Agriculture. Available at: https://tradingeconomics.com/mozambique/gdp-from-agriculture (accessed 3 December 2025).

Tschirley, D.L. and Weber, M.T. (1994) Food security strategies under extremely adverse conditions: The determinants of household income and consumption in rural Mozambique. *World Development* 22(2), 159–173. DOI: 10.1016/0305-750X(94)90067-1.

United Nations (2015) Sustainable Development Goals. Department of Economic and Social Affairs. Available at: https://sdgs.un.org/goals/goal2 (accessed 3 December 2025).

Upton, M. (2004) The role of livestock in economic development and poverty reduction. *Prio-Poor Livestock Policy Initiative Working Paper 23783*. DOI: 10.22004/AG.ECON.23783.

USAID, A. (2016) *Feed the Future Innovation Lab for Livestock Systems Rwanda: Animal Source Foods Production and Marketing Brief*. Available at: https://livestocklab.ifas.ufl.edu/media/livestocklabifasufledu/pdf-/pdfs-by-country-pre2019/Rwanda_Brief_ASFProdMkt_final.pdf (accessed 3 December 2025).

Vernooji, A., dos Anjos, M. and van Mierlo, J. (2016) *Livestock Development in the Zambezi Valley, Mozambique: Poultry, Dairy and Beef Production: Description of the current situation and emerging opportunities*. Wageningen UR (University and Research) Centre for Development Innovation, Report CDI-16-027. Wageningen. Available at: https://edepot.wur.nl/406337 (accessed 2 December 2025).

Viscusi, W.K. and Aldy, J.E. (2003) The value of a statistical life: A critical review of market estimates throughout the world. *Journal of Risk and Uncertainty* 27(1), 5–76. DOI: 10.1023/A:1025598106257.

Wild, H., Jok, J.M. and Patel, R. (2018) The militarization of cattle raiding in South Sudan: How a traditional practice became a tool for political violence. *Journal of International Humanitarian Action* 3(1), 2. DOI: 10.1186/s41018-018-0030-y.

World Bank (2021) Population Estimates and Projections. Available at: https://databank.worldbank.org/source/population-estimates-and-projections (accessed 3 December 2025).

Wurzinger, M., Ndumu, D., Baumung, R., Drucker, A., Okeyo, A.M. *et al.* (2006) Comparison of production systems and selection criteria of Ankole cattle by breeders in Burundi, Rwanda, Tanzania and Uganda. *Tropical Animal Health and Production* 38, 571–581. DOI: 10.1007/S11250-006-4426-0/METRICS.

Appendix 2.1. Country-Specific Assessments

Burundi

The majority of the population in Burundi live rurally, with 14% of households owning some cattle and 90% of the population dependent on livestock and agriculture for income. Prolonged civil war has left livestock keepers in Burundi poorer and less secure than in other parts of the region (Bundervoet, 2006; Fransen *et al.*, 2017).

Democratic Republic of Congo (DRC)

The livestock sector in DRC is unstable (Cox, 2012); veterinary services are insufficient (Ombeni *et al.*, 2018; Mutwedu *et al.*, 2019), perpetuating low levels of food production and poverty (Rossi *et al.*, 2006; Mugumaarhahama *et al.*, 2021). Pastoralism is the predominant means of keeping cattle in DRC, with the majority (70%) of cattle kept in small herds (< 9), often co-grazed with small ruminants along roadsides and on communal lands. Large herds are grazed on paddocks at higher altitude.

Kenya

In Kenya, the majority (75%) of livestock are kept in the pastoral sector, which supplies 20% of the milk and 28% of the meat consumed in the country. ITM immunized subgroups of cattle have long since been recognized as more profitable through increased milk yields and reduced mortality in Kenya (Mukhebi *et al.*, 1989).

Malawi

Malawi has some of the most extreme poverty globally. The majority of households rely on income from livestock, but the agriculture sector receives < 0.8% of annual government funding. Livestock are used to buffer external shocks, and poorer households generate less income from livestock because they have less produce to sell (Matchaya *et al.*, 2012; Anon, 2020). There is significant scope to improve livestock health and productivity in Malawi, especially through use of the ITM vaccine, to increase social and nutritional security (Anon, 2020; Kaumbata *et al.*, 2021; Chatanga *et al.*, 2022).

Mozambique

Around 95% of food consumed in Mozambique comes from small-scale producers, and people predominantly rely on their own farm-based production, but food insecurity remains rife (Tschirley and Weber, 1994). Improved veterinary services and investment in extension services are identified as key areas needed to improve livestock production in Mozambique; multiple projects have been initiated to try to increase production across the country (primary focus on meat and dairy) (Johnson *et al.*, 2015; Vernooji *et al.*, 2016). There is a paucity of data in the literature on the impact of ECF on cattle production in Mozambique, but it has been circulating endemically since the early 1900s and remains a primary constraint on livestock production (Mazibe and Lopes Pereirat, 1988; Direito, 2021).

Rwanda

The national herd in Rwanda consists predominantly of indigenous breeds (67%), with 28% cross-bred and 5% exotic. The government encourages cross-breeding of less ECF-susceptible cattle for meat and milk production (Paling *et al.*, 1991). The government of Rwanda recognizes the importance of production from the livestock sector to improve child nutrition, so they have initiated national action plans to improve milk availability in schools (Girinka is a government programme which has provided over 400,000 dairy animals to poor households) (Anon, 2013; Rawlins *et al.*, 2014; USAID, 2016). The majority of cattle (60%) are kept in small sedentary herds, fenced or tethered due to land restrictions, for subsistence production, and the remaining cattle graze openly (Wurzinger *et al.*, 2006; Mazimpaka *et al.*, 2017). The intensity of *T. parva* challenge in Rwanda is highly correlated with management practices, agro-ecological conditions and breed, so targeted control and treatment options are needed (Bazarusanga *et al.*, 2008; Juvenal and Edward, 2010).

South Africa

In South Africa, rural households, the poorest households and women-headed households predominantly rely on livestock for income and intangible social benefits (loans, insurance, social capital). Cattle productivity in the country is reportedly declining, with poor access to markets and veterinary services (Stroebel *et al.*, 2011; Nkonki-Mandleni *et al.*, 2018; Nwafor *et al.*, 2020; Taruvinga *et al.*, 2022).

Since ECF has been eliminated from South Africa, costs of disease relate to losses due to occasional outbreaks of Corridor disease and government measures to prevent its spread and to maintain ECF-free status. Chemotherapy and vaccination against *T. parva* are prohibited. In 1999, infections with *T. parva* were estimated to be costing $50 million in South Africa ($4 per head of cattle) (McLeod and Kristjanson, 1999).

South Sudan

Cattle supply around 65% of meat eaten in South Sudan. Due to continual political unrest, cattle are targets for violent rustling attacks, with larger herds more susceptible and cattle raiding events negatively impacting cattle production and survivability. There is also limited access to treatment from veterinary services in South Sudan (Cullis, 2021). War and ongoing conflict have been responsible for the collapse of livestock markets and infrastructure, which will take considerable time to rebuild (Idris, 2018). Stability of the livestock sector and reliance on livestock as a route out of poverty seem like a distant vision in South Sudan (Idris, 2018; Wild *et al.*, 2018). Better market integration and rebuilding of market access, infrastructure and improved livestock health services are desperately needed (Catley, 2018; Cullis, 2021).

T. parva is circulating at relatively high levels in South Sudan (28–77%), with the pathogen moving north over recent years (Marcellino *et al.*, 2017; Mohammed *et al.*, 2019).

Tanzania

Tanzania has the second largest cattle population in Africa, with 35% of the 4.6 million livestock-dependent households keeping cattle. The Tanzanian government has made investment plans to improve livestock health and productivity. This was largely driven by the political will to increase livestock's contribution to GDP (7% in 2020) through improved productivity, but also because livestock hold intangible worth, beyond their monetary value, across many societies in Tanzania (Michael *et al.*, 2018). Cattle are predominantly kept in low-input pastoral (herded free grazing) or agro-pastoral (some grazing over finished crop areas) production systems, with a small percentage kept in smallholder (tethering) and peri-urban dairy production systems (de Glanville *et al.*, 2020).

In 1999, McLeod estimated that ECF was costing around $50 million ($4 per head) a year in Tanzania (McLeod and Kristjanson, 1999), but in 2006 (using data from 2000), Kivaria estimated the national annual losses due to ECF were more likely five times greater than this ($250 million, or $205 per head). This latter estimate was presented in six component parts: mortality 49% ($121 million), chemotherapy 21% ($52 million), acaricide use 14% ($35 million), weight loss 9% ($22.5 million), milk loss 6% ($15 million) and ITM vaccination 1% ($2.5 million) (Kivaria, 2006).

Uganda

Increased productivity from the livestock sector in Uganda is a priority for development and strengthening the economy (Anon, 2015). There is a mix of farming types, from extensive pastoralists to intensive dairy, with smallholder production supporting most livelihoods (Benson and Mugarura, 2013) and keeping improved dairy breeds, associated with improved child nutrition (Mosites *et al.*, 2015).

T. parva is endemic in Uganda. Seroprevalence varies across agro-ecological zones, with a *T. parva* seroprevalence 95% confidence interval of 3–55% (Kabi *et al.*, 2014). The disease is often controlled by restricting calf grazing access and using tick control in draught animals (Muhanguzi *et al.*, 2014). A national report from 2017 estimated the losses due to tick-borne diseases, of which *T. parva* is a major contributor, to be in the region of $700 million ($187 million for lost milk, $472 million for lost meat production and $26 million for lost blood (nutritional product consumed from cattle)) (de la Fuente *et al.*, 2019).

Zambia

In Zambia, cattle-keeping households derive 60–90% of their income from livestock and are separated into three categories: grassland (23%), mixed (72%) and commercial (5%). The smaller mixed and grassland herd households have a high incidence of poverty (73%) and represent some of the country's poorest households (Dutilly *et al.*, 2020). National policies to support the development of sustainable, stable cattle markets have been suggested in the country to support smallholder and mixed farm enterprises and increase economic growth (Mumba *et al.*, 2017)

Seroprevalence for *T. parva* infection varies between seasons and provinces in Zambia and is as low as 14% in the dry season and up to 40% in the wet season (Simuunza *et al.*, 2011). In 1994, Zambia had 3 million cattle, with an estimated 1.4 million at risk of infection with *T. parva* and annual mortality attributed to *T. parva* estimated at 10,000 cattle (Nambota *et al.*, 1994). Use of models to test the cost–benefit of different *T. parva* control options in Zambia in 1999 indicated that immunization of cattle against *T. parva* could cost up to $26 per animal before profitability was affected (Minjauw *et al.*, 1999). If the disease epidemiology and other control options remain similar, then this figure was likely higher 20 years later, showing the high value of, and benefits to be gained from, vaccination.

Zimbabwe

In Zimbabwe, 60% of rural households own some livestock, mainly smallholders keeping small numbers of cattle (average herd size 4–7, varies between districts) (Dube *et al.*, 2014). Livestock provide social security, but survival and production is threatened by drought, soil infertility and lack of infrastructure as well as disease (Ermyas, 2023). Most livestock keepers in Zimbabwe, and indeed most across the *T. parva*-affected region, are needs driven – this means that non-price factors such as a *need* to buy household goods or pay school fees or medical bills drives most livestock sales (92%) (Melesse *et al.*, 2023). This demonstrates that other household and family needs overshadow purely economic reasons for livestock keeping and sales. Farmers who engage in market activities have improved income and nutritional security, but poorer smallholders are prevented from engaging in market-orientated production due to lack of market access, information and capital for investment in the additional inputs required (Melesse *et al.*, 2023).

Infection with the form of *T. parva* that causes January disease is widespread in Zimbabwe (7/10 provinces, seroprevalence 12–98%) and the impact on production varies by farm location, province and production system (communal grazing associated with higher seroprevalence) (Latif *et al.*, 2001).

3 Development of *Theileria parva* in the Tick and Mammalian Hosts

W. Ivan Morrison*
Roslin Institute, University of Edinburgh, Edinburgh, UK

3.1 Introduction

Understanding the epidemiology of *T. parva* and the pathogenesis of the diseases it produces depends on knowledge of the processes involved in development and replication of the parasite in its mammalian and arthropod hosts. Although many aspects of the development of *T. parva* are shared with other apicomplexan parasites, the parasite displays a number of unique features in its mammalian hosts, which fundamentally influence how it is able to cause disease and how it interacts with the host's immune system. This brief chapter presents a summary of current knowledge of the development of *T. parva* in its tick and mammalian hosts, in order to provide a context for discussions in subsequent chapters.

3.2 Development of *T. parva* in the Tick Vector

The tick vectors of *T. parva* are discussed in Chapter 15 of this volume. The principal vector, *Rhipicephalus appendiculatus*, is a three-host tick, such that the larval, nymphal and adult stages feed on separate hosts. Transmission of *T. parva* occurs trans-stadially, i.e. infections acquired by feeding larvae and nymphs are transmitted to new hosts, following moulting of the ticks, by the nymph and adult stages, respectively. Unlike *Babesia* species, there is no transmission from the adult stage to eggs in female ticks. Early morphological studies of development of *T. parva* in *R. appendiculatus* ticks, employing light microscopy, provided a remarkably accurate general picture of the developmental stages of the parasites in the tick (Cowdry and Ham, 1932). In the 1970s and 1980s, application of electron microscopy yielded more detailed information on the processes involved in differentiation of the parasite in the tick (Mehlhorn *et al.*, 1978; Fawcett *et al.*, 1982; Mehlhorn and Schein, 1984).

3.2.1 Life cycle stages in the tick

Parasites ingested by ticks feeding on a *T. parva*-infected animal undergo a series of developmental stages following detachment of the tick from the host, which are illustrated in Fig. 3.1.

All stages of the parasite in the mammalian host are haploid, but development in the tick vector includes a sexual stage during which recombination between genotypically different parasite strains can occur (Katzer *et al.*, 2011; Henson *et al.*, 2012). Piroplasms ingested by feeding ticks are released following lysis of infected erythrocytes in the tick gut and differentiate within a few days to form

*Corresponding author: Ivan.Morrison@ed.ac.uk

 East Coast Fever: The Disease, its Impact and Control (eds W.I. Morrison and P. Toye)
DOI: 10.1079/9781800626324.0003

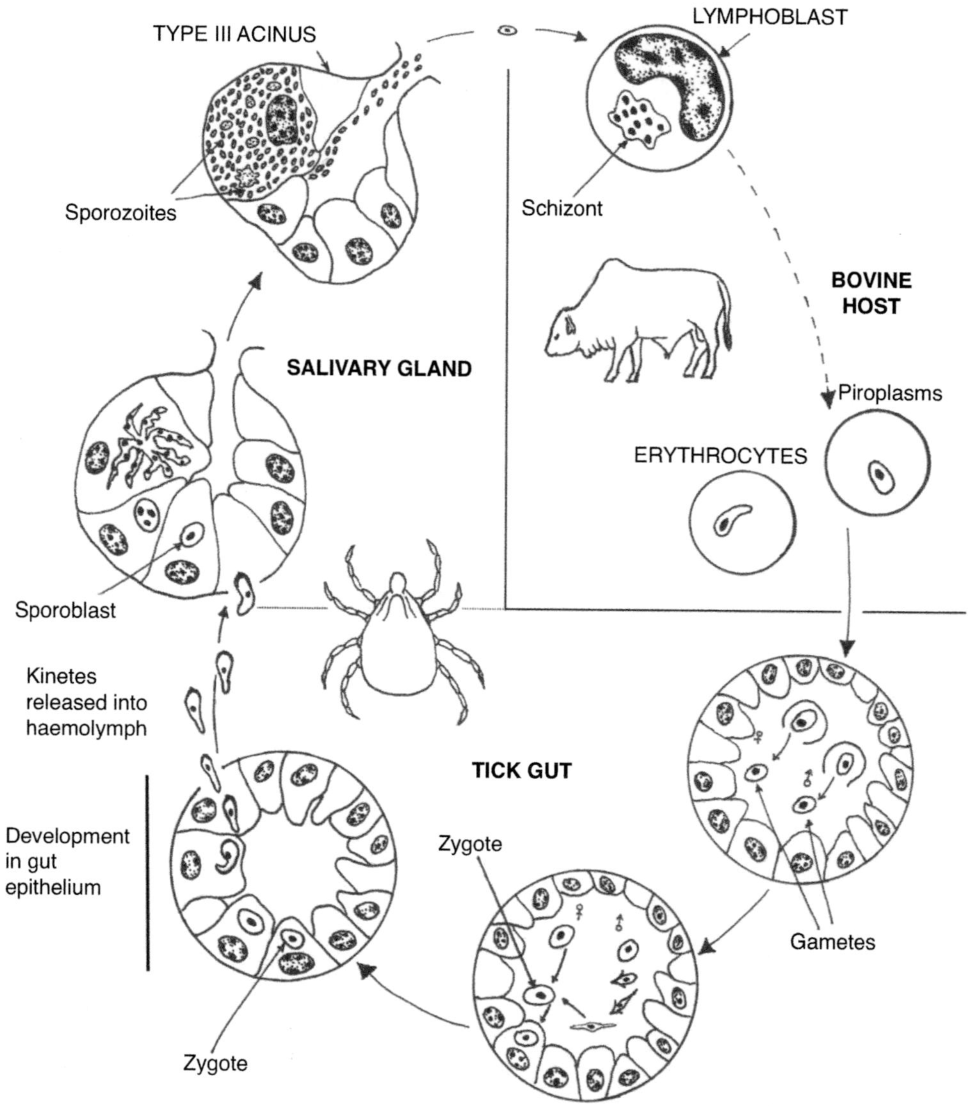

Fig. 3.1. Schematic representation of the stages of development of *T. parva* in the tick and mammalian hosts. (Figure prepared by Karen Cryer.)

distinct morphological forms considered to be either micro- or macro-gametes (Mehlhorn and Schein, 1984). Fusion of pairs of gametes results in formation of zygotes, which invade gut epithelial cells and differentiate into kinetes. Measurement of DNA content of these stages to determine their ploidy (Gauer *et al.*, 1995) confirmed that the early zygotes are diploid, but with further development they become tetraploid. The demonstration that the progeny kinetes are haploid led the authors to propose that they are generated by two meiotic divisions of the mature zygotes. Unlike most other developmental forms of *T. parva*, kinetes are motile and, following their release from the gut epithelium into the haemolymph, they migrate to the salivary glands (Mehlhorn *et al.*, 1978). The motility of kinetes is consistent with the presence of cytoplasmic organelles referred to as micronemes, which are associated with motility in other apicomplexan parasites (Tomley and Soldati, 2001). In ticks infected as nymphs, kinete production occurs just after the ticks moult to the adult stage, about 3 weeks after detachment under laboratory conditions.

Kinetes enter the salivary glands, which have become metabolically inactive and greatly reduced in size following cessation of tick feeding on the mammalian host. The kinetes invade epithelial cells of type III acini, usually one kinete per acinar cell. These acini contain three cell types (d, e and f), of which only the d and e cells can be invaded by *T. parva* kinetes and support their development. As with other developmental stages of *T. parva*, the parasite is found free within the cytoplasm of the tick cells. Kinetes appear to undergo a few nuclear divisions shortly after invasion of the salivary gland cells, but further development is delayed until the tick commences feeding on a new host (Mehlhorn and Schein, 1984). Feeding stimulates metabolic activity and enlargement of the salivary glands and provokes rapid differentiation of the internalized kinetes to eventually generate sporozoites, in a process known as sporogony (Fawcett *et al.*, 1982). Initially, there is rapid division of the parasite nuclei, and the body of the parasite forms a complex labyrinthine syncytium leading to swelling of the infected cells, which can be observed by light microscopy in stained histological sections of salivary glands (Fig. 3.2).

After 3–5 days, this multinucleate structure undergoes fission to generate the uninucleate sporozoites that are released into the saliva. Prior to and following fission, electron-dense bodies appear in the parasite cytoplasm and take on the typical shape of rhoptries (discussed further for sporozoites in Section 3.3.2). A second organelle, the dense body erroneously referred to by Fawcett *et al.* as the microneme, is found in very small numbers in fully formed sporozoites within the salivary glands, and subsequently increases in number with further maturation of the sporozoites (Fawcett *et al.*, 1982).

The level of infection in ticks, measured by examining dissected salivary glands, varies between individual ticks fed on the same animal (Purnell *et al.*, 1974; Büscher and Otim, 1986; Büscher and Tangus, 1986). In batches of ticks fed on cattle experimentally infected with *T. parva*, some ticks may contain over 100 infected salivary gland acini, whereas others remain

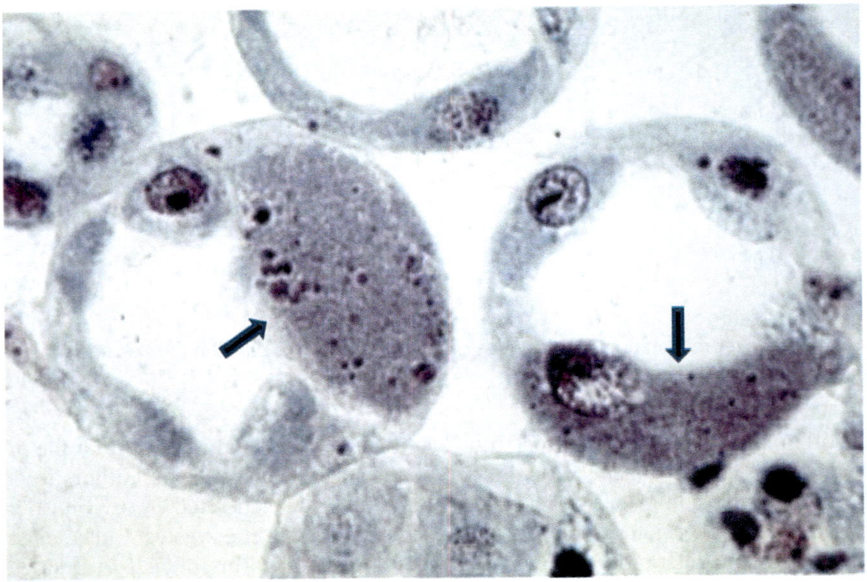

Fig. 3.2. Histological section of a salivary gland from a *T. parva*-infected *R. appendiculatus* tick stained with methylgreen pyronin, showing two infected salivary gland cells (arrows). (Photomicrograph provided by Dr Gottfried Buscher.).

uninfected. Experimental studies to examine the heritability of susceptibility of ticks to infection have indicated that at least some of this variation has a genetic basis (Young *et al.*, 1995). The level of infection is somewhat lower in male ticks compared to females, which Büscher and Otim (1986) reported was largely due to fewer ticks with large numbers of infected acini rather than a lower percentage of infected ticks. The level of infection in nymphal ticks fed as larvae is approximately one third of that in adults (Purnell *et al.*, 1971).

Based on ultrastructural observations, a single infected tick epithelial cell has been estimated to contain up to 4.8×10^4 sporozoites (Jarrett *et al.*, 1969). The rate at which sporozoites develop in different acinar cells in an infected tick varies, so that sporozoites are released into the saliva gradually over several days (Shaw and Young, 1995), with maximal numbers usually released 4–5 days after commencement of tick feeding (Purnell, 1977).

Although sporogony usually commences only when infected ticks begin feeding, initiation of sporogony has been reported in some infected ticks incubated *in vitro* at 28°C or 37°C; small numbers of sporozoites were produced, which were infective for cattle (Young *et al.*, 1984). Sporozoite development could only be heat-induced in young ticks, up to 41 days after completion of feeding. Similar findings have also been obtained with infected ticks placed on pasture where maximal monthly temperatures were 27–32°C (Young *et al.*, 1987).

Climatic conditions influence the duration of the life cycle in the tick. Studies of infected ticks in an experimental paddock in Kenya showed that the minimum time required for transmission of infection acquired by nymphal ticks was 30 days during the warm season but 62 days during the cold season, where the mean temperature differed by 4°C (Young *et al.*, 1981). In southern Africa, adult *R. appendiculatus* ticks have a seasonal diapausing behaviour, i.e. ticks overwinter in a low metabolic state of suspended development, during which adult ticks delay host-seeking and feeding (Randolph, 1997; see Chapter 6 of this volume). Eastern African *R. appendiculatus* ticks do not exhibit diapause when exposed to a South African environment (Madder *et al.*, 2002). Diapause is regulated primarily by changes in photoperiod (i.e. daily length of daylight), with humidity and ambient temperature also playing a role.

3.2.2 Sexual recombination

The occurrence of recombination in *T. parva* during development in the tick has been confirmed experimentally by genotyping of parasites produced in ticks fed on calves co-infected with two genotypically distinct cloned *T. parva* populations (Katzer *et al.*, 2011; Henson *et al.*, 2012). Using a series of 79 genetic markers to analyse 35 cloned progeny, Katzer *et al.* (2011) detected frequent cross-over events and estimated a rate of recombination for each meiotic generation of 0.22 centimorgans per 10 kb, a rate that is similar to that reported for other *Apicomplexa*. Results of studies involving genotyping of field populations of *T. parva* in endemically infected cattle in Uganda and Kenya, using a panel of satellite DNA markers, indicated that the parasite populations were panmictic (i.e. characterized by random mating within the populations), which is consistent with the occurrence of frequent sexual recombination (Oura *et al.*, 2005; Odongo *et al.*, 2006). The results of these studies also revealed that most infected cattle harbour parasites of several genotypes, most likely originating from multiple infection events. This epidemiological state is highly favourable for ingestion of mixed parasite genotypes by feeding ticks and hence provides ample opportunity for sexual recombination during transmission.

3.3 Infection of Bovine Cells

Early studies by Cowdry and Danks (1933) employing light microscopy provided an accurate general account of the developmental stages of *T. parva* in the bovine host. The application of electron microscopy in a series of later studies yielded a much more detailed picture of the events involved in invasion of and development within bovine cells (Fawcett *et al.*, 1984; Webster *et al.*, 1985; Shaw, 1997, 2003). These studies were greatly aided by development of culture systems to infect bovine leukocytes with *T. parva* sporozoites and propagate them *in vitro* (Brown *et al.*, 1973), allowing the development of the parasite in bovine cells to be

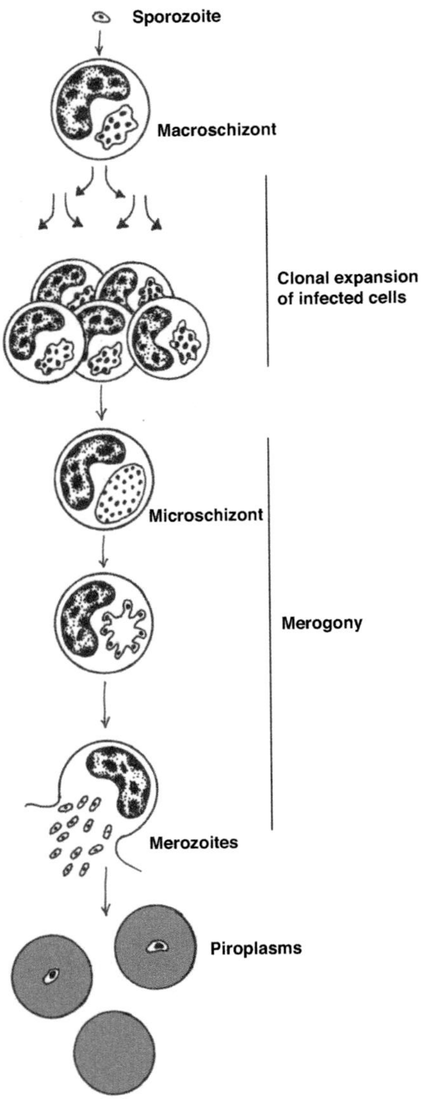

Fig. 3.3. Schematic representation of the stages of development of *T. parva* in the bovine host. (Figure prepared by Karen Cryer.)

examined in greater detail than had been possible in the tick vector. The main steps in development are illustrated in Fig. 3.3.

3.3.1 Cell types infected by the parasite

By incubation of sporozoites with purified populations of different cell types *in vitro*, it has been possible to show that both B and T lymphocytes are susceptible to infection by *T. parva* (Baldwin *et al.*, 1988). Ultrastructural studies have shown that monocytes and dendritic cells can also bind and internalize sporozoites in a similar manner to lymphocytes, but the parasites fail to develop beyond this early intracytoplasmic stage (Shaw *et al.*, 1993). Sporozoites are unable to bind to other cell types such as neutrophils and fibroblasts. The influence of the phenotype of cells infected with *T. parva* on their ability to cause disease in cattle is discussed further in Chapter 4 of this volume.

3.3.2 Morphological features of host cell invasion

Apicomplexan parasites are so named because the infective stages contain a set of cytoplasmic structures and organelles known as the apical complex. In the sporozoites of most apicomplexan parasites, the apical complex includes a structure known as a 'conoid' associated with cytoplasmic organelles. The conoid is positioned at the apical end of the parasite, and in most *Apicomplexa* the apical complex is polarized towards the site of attachment to and entry into host cells during cell invasion. However, *T. parva* sporozoites have a less structured apical complex and lack a conoid or equivalent structure. They contain two types of apical organelles, namely pear-shaped structures known as 'rhoptries' and smaller, spherical, dense granules (Shaw *et al.*, 1991; Shaw, 1996). *Theileria* sporozoites are oval in shape and much smaller than those of many other apicomplexan parasites – approximately 1 micron in diameter compared to, for example, the highly motile, crescent-shaped *Plasmodium* sporozoites, which are 8–14 microns in length (Frischknecht and Matuschewski, 2017). Cell entry by *T. parva* sporozoites differs in several respects from that of most other apicomplexan parasites: they can enter host cells in any orientation, there is no obvious release of the contents of rhoptries and dense granules during the entry process and they do not possess a subpellicular complex of microtubules and are non-motile (Shaw, 1996, 1997). Lack of sporozoite motility is consistent with the absence of a third type of organelle, micronemes, which are associated

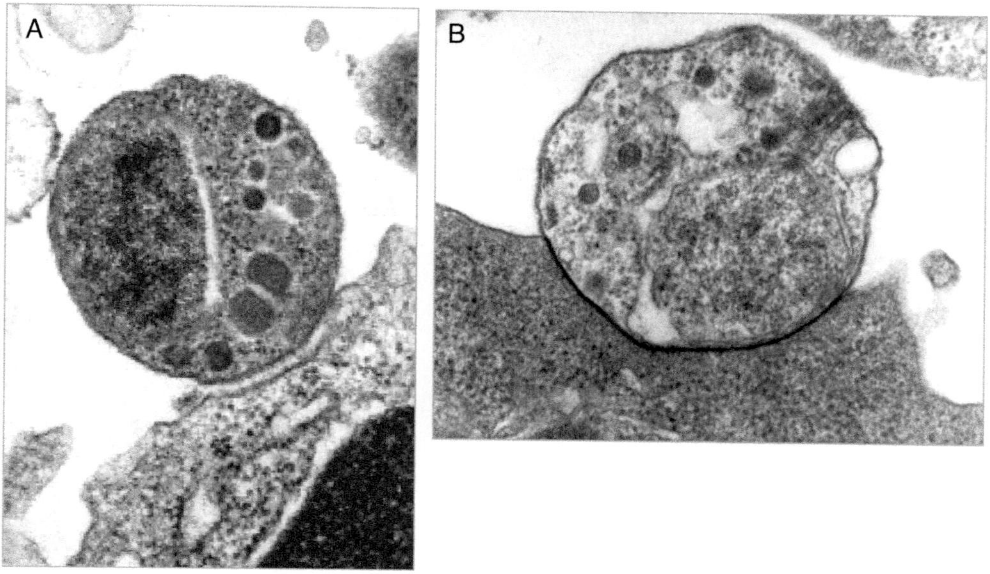

Fig. 3.4. Attachment of *T. parva* sporozoites to bovine lymphocytes: (A) Initial loose attachment, followed by (B) an intimate attachment of the parasite and host cell membranes. (Figure reproduced by permission of Rockefeller University Press from Shaw *et al.*, 1991).

with motility in other *Apicomplexa* (Mehlhorn *et al.*, 1978; Tomley and Soldati, 2001). These features suggest that the apicomplexan organelles do not play a significant role in cell entry by *T. parva*, as they do in other *Apicomplexa*.

T. parva sporozoites are covered by a 20–25 nm-thick surface coat, which upon initial contact with bovine target cells binds to the host cell membrane (Fig. 3.4A). This is followed by establishment of a more intimate association of the sporozoite and lymphocyte cell membranes (Fig. 3.4B), during which all or most of the sporozoite surface coat is cleaved and shed (Webster *et al.*, 1985). Rapid circumferential zippering of the parasite and host cell membranes results in internalization of the parasite into the host cell. Binding and internalization of the sporozoite occurs within 2–3 min of initial contact. Following internalization, dissolution of the surrounding host cell membrane occurs, so that within 15 min the parasite lies free within the cytosol. This process is initiated by focal separation of the parasite and host membranes and discharge of the contents of rhoptries and dense granules into the inter-membrane spaces (Fig. 3.5A,B), suggesting their involvement in dissolution of the host membrane. The role of these organelles appears to have evolved differently from that of other apicomplexan parasites, which discharge the contents of their apical complex organelles during cell entry. *T. parva* sporozoites that remain within the endocytic vacuole beyond 15–30 min die. Following escape into the host cell cytosol, arrays of host cell microtubules assemble close to the parasite surface (Fig. 3.5C), and their presence remains a consistent feature throughout the macroschizont stage of development.

3.3.3 Mechanisms involved in cell invasion

Although initial cell binding of sporozoites to bovine lymphocytes can occur at 4°C, internalization is temperature-dependent and requires both intact viable sporozoites and viable host cells (Shaw, 1996, 1999). Sporozoite binding depends on the integrity of the host actin cytoskeleton, presumably to facilitate cross-linking of host receptor proteins. However, entry of sporozoites into the host cell is independent of the host cytoskeleton (Shaw, 2003), as

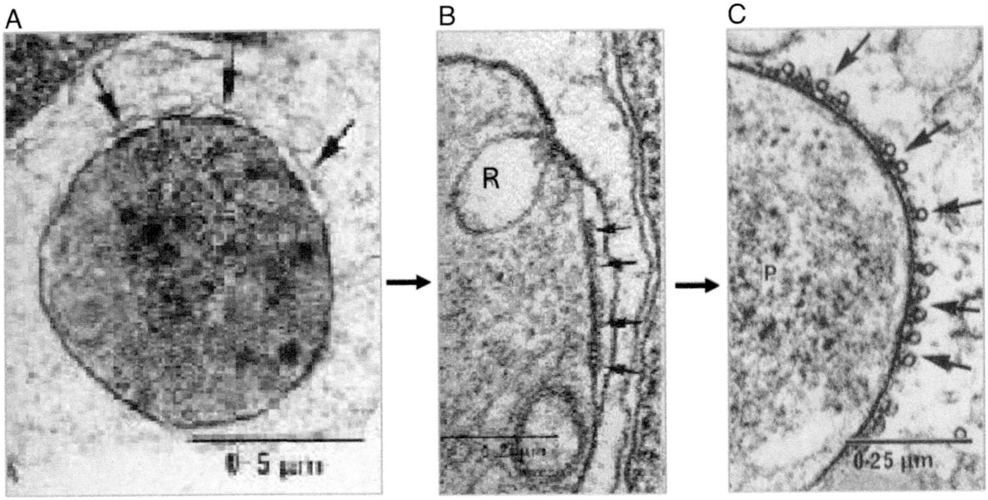

Fig. 3.5. Internalization of *T. parva* sporozoites into the lymphocyte cytoplasm: (A) Initial separation of the sporozoite and surrounding host cell membrane (arrows). (B) The presence of electron-dense material in the inter-membrane space (arrows), in close proximity to an empty parasite rhoptry. (C) Formation of host microtubules around the sporozoite membrane. R = rhoptry; P = parasite. (Figure reproduced by permission of Rockefeller University Press from Shaw *et al*., 1993).

indicated by the absence of accumulation of microfilaments beneath the cell membrane and no obvious remodelling of the host cell surface and formation of pseudopodia, as occur during phagocytosis. These observations, coupled with the lack of motility of *T. parva* sporozoites, indicated that internalization of the sporozoite is essentially a passive process on the part of the parasite, and, given the small size of the sporozoite, both Fawcett *et al.* (1984) and Shaw (2003) have suggested that the observed circumferential zippering process is the main driving force in drawing the sporozoite into the host cell. Additional studies with pharmacological inhibitors have shown that pre-treatment of sporozoites or host cells with certain protease inhibitors blocked cell entry, implying that the process may involve both parasite and host cell surface enzymatic activities (Shaw, 1997). Pre-treatment of sporozoites with agents that inhibit ATP synthesis or mitochondrial activity was found to inhibit cell invasion, whereas pre-treatment of the host cells with these agents had little or no effect on invasion. Inhibitors of cell signalling pathways in either the sporozoite or the host cell also inhibit cell invasion by sporozoites (Shaw, 1996).

While these findings have provided a detailed picture of the morphology of host cell invasion by *T. parva* sporozoites and an indication of the cellular activities involved, the precise nature of the sequential steps in cell invasion and the identity of the parasite and lymphocyte proteins involved remain incompletely understood (see further detailed discussion by Shaw, 1997). It seems likely that initial host cell binding by sporozoites and/or cleavage of the sporozoite surface coat triggers signalling events that lead to a sequence of processes culminating in delivery of the sporozoite into the host cell cytoplasm, as well as priming the cell to undergo transformation by the parasite.

3.3.4 Proteins involved in invasion by sporozoites

Although the molecular interactions that mediate host cell invasion by sporozoites are poorly defined, some of the proteins involved have been identified. Their identification has come mainly from studies aimed at investigating the use of parasite antigens for vaccination, which are discussed in further detail in Chapter 11 of this volume. A 67 kDa protein (p67), identified using monoclonal antibodies raised against sporozoites, was shown to be a component of the sporozoite surface coat (Dobbelaere *et al.*, 1984, 1985; Musoke *et al.*, 1984). Some of the p67-specific monoclonal antibodies inhibit host cell binding and infectivity of sporozoites *in vitro*, and immuno-electron microscopy has demonstrated that the surface coat shed during cell invasion contains p67 (Webster *et al.*, 1985). Incubation of cells with recombinant p67 protein also competitively inhibits cell surface binding of sporozoites and cell invasion, provided it remains present in the culture medium (Shaw, 1997). However, pre-exposure of lymphocytes to recombinant p67 and its subsequent omission from the culture medium fails to neutralize infectivity, indicating that the affinity of monomeric p67 for its ligand is weak. The multimeric ligand binding of intact sporozoites resulting from the high density of p67 on the sporozoite surface is likely to allow binding of much higher avidity to lymphocytes.

Mouse monoclonal antibodies specific for a second parasite protein, the polymorphic immunodominant molecule (PIM), have also been shown to reduce the ability of sporozoites to infect bovine lymphocytes *in vitro* (Toye *et al.*, 1995). Similar inhibition was also observed with rat antisera raised against recombinant PIM. The mouse antibodies reduce the numbers of sporozoites that bind to host cells but do not affect the internalization of the sporozoites that attach (Toye *et al.*, 2014). It was also observed that pre-incubation of lymphocytes with recombinant PIM reduced both the binding and internalization of sporozoites. The PIM protein is found in the dense granule organelles of sporozoites (Toye *et al.*, 2014), but it is not readily detectable on the surface of free sporozoites, although one monoclonal antibody detected PIM on about 10% of sporozoites. However, expression of PIM on the sporozoite surface is detected during host cell invasion by the parasite, although it remains unclear why some PIM-specific antibodies are able to neutralize infectivity. It may reflect low-level expression of the protein on the surface of sporozoites, not detectable by the methods used to examine expression.

It might be argued that the inhibition reported above is due not to specific disruption of p67 or PIM with their respective ligands, but to steric interference affecting nearby molecules that are the true ligands. However, the ability of recombinant versions of both molecules to reduce infection and the observation that some monoclonal antibodies specific for p67 (Nene *et al.*, 1999) and PIM (Toye *et al.*, 2014) do not affect sporozoite entry undermine this argument.

A more recent study, which investigated recombinant fragments of a number of other *T. parva* proteins expressed by sporozoites and predicted to have a GPI (glycosyl-phosphatidyl-inositol) membrane anchor, demonstrated that antisera raised against two of the proteins (encoded by genes 01g00876 and 01g00939) neutralized the infectivity of sporozoites *in vitro* to a level similar to that obtained with p67-specific antibodies (Nyagwange *et al.*, 2018), supporting the view that cell invasion involves multiple parasite proteins.

On the host side, monoclonal antibodies specific for a variety of leukocyte surface proteins have been tested for their ability to inhibit sporozoite binding to target cells and/or sporozoite infectivity. Somewhat surprisingly, a number of antibodies specific for major histocompatibility complex (MHC) class I proteins were found to inhibit host cell binding and infectivity of sporozoites (Shaw *et al.*, 1991, 1995). MHC-deficient *T. parva*-infected cells, which had been generated by mutagenesis and subsequent selection of cells lacking expression of MHC class I proteins, showed substantial reduction in their ability to bind sporozoites (Shaw *et al.*, 1995). Previous studies had shown that sporozoites could invade and infect previously infected cells (Stagg *et al.*, 1984). These findings indicate that the neutralizing activity of class I-specific antibodies is not merely due to indirect effects on the cell surface. However, the inability of sporozoites to bind to and infect cell types such as neutrophils and fibroblasts that express class I MHC clearly indicates that these molecules do not on their own act as receptors for the parasite. Rather, the findings suggest that binding and entry of sporozoites into bovine cells involve a complex of host and parasite proteins.

3.3.5 Development of the schizont stage

Following invasion of host cells, the sporozoites increase in size over the first 2–3 days, with

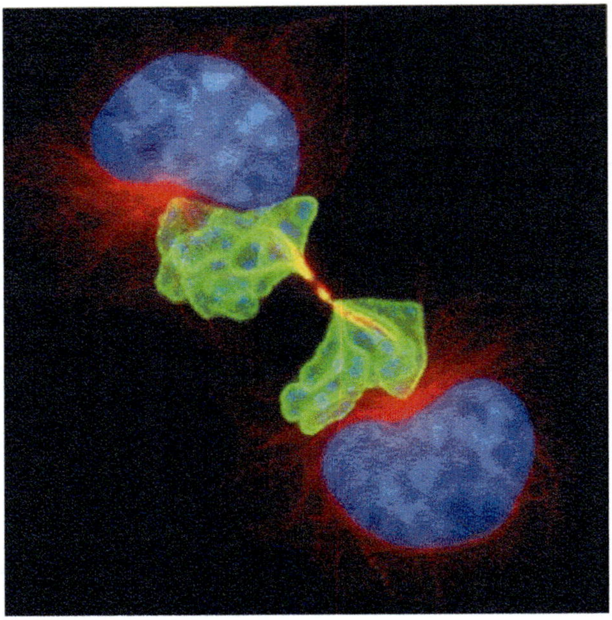

Fig. 3.6. Dividing *T. annulata*-infected cell stained by immunofluorescence, showing synchronous division of the parasite and host cell. Host cell nucleus shown in blue; macroschizont shown in green. (From Molloy, 2010. Micrograph provided by Conrad von Schubert, with permission of *Nature Reviews Microbiology*.).

expansion of their cytoplasm, and nuclear division commences. By the third day, typical multinuclear macroschizonts are detected (Stagg *et al.*, 1981), with most host cells containing schizonts with 3–7 nuclei (Jarrett *et al.*, 1969). During this time the host cell becomes activated and starts to divide. The close relationship with host microtubules enables the parasite to associate with the mitotic apparatus of the cell, resulting in simultaneous division of the schizont and the host cell, with schizont nuclei randomly distributed to both daughter cells (Hulliger *et al.*, 1964). This is illustrated in Fig. 3.6 for *Theileria annulata*, which employs the same mechanism to synchronize division with that of the host cells.

The intimate relationship of the parasite with the host cell enables rapid proliferation of the parasitized cells and ensures that the parasite is not exposed to the extracellular environment during this stage of development. Macroschizont-infected cells can be established as continuously growing cell lines *in vitro*, which can be maintained indefinitely without addition of growth factors or feeder cells (Brown *et al.*, 1973). Such cells are referred to as 'transformed', because of the similarity of their behaviour to that of cancer cells. However, the transformed state is reversible, as shown by return of the cells to a non-transformed state following treatment of the cultures with a theilericidal drug (Dobbelaere *et al.*, 1988). The macroschizont-infected cells in *in vitro* cultures have a population doubling time of 18–24 h. This is similar to the estimated growth rate of infected cells *in vivo* reported by Jarrett *et al.* (1969), who observed an exponential expansion of infected cells resulting in a tenfold increase every 3 days. A subsequent study (Morrison *et al.*, 1981) confirmed a period of exponential growth once infection reached 1% in lymphoid tissues but observed a more rapid growth rate prior to this and a reduced growth rate in the late stages of infection (discussed further in Chapter 4 of this volume).

The molecular basis of host cell transformation and the synchronous division of the parasite and host cell are discussed in further detail in Chapter 10 of this volume.

3.4 Development of the Erythrocyte-Infective Stages

3.4.1 Merogony within infected lymphocytes

Production of the erythrocyte-infective stages of *T. parva* occurs by a process of merogony involving differentiation of the schizonts within infected leukocytes. From about 10–11 days after infection, the schizonts in some of the infected cells show an increase in the number of nuclei, with many containing 15–30 nuclei (Jarrett *et al.*, 1969), which are reduced in size and show condensation in their chromatin. This stage of the parasite, referred to as the 'microschizont', is where merogony occurs and is associated with cessation of proliferation of the host cell. Low levels of merogony occur within the first 6 weeks after establishment of *in vitro* cultures of macroschizont-infected cells (Madder *et al.*, 2003), but there is no reliable experimental system for infecting erythrocytes *in vitro* with merozoites. Detailed ultrastructural studies of these developmental stages have, therefore, relied largely on multiple observations on samples of tissues collected from infected cattle, in which parasites can be present in >30% of lymphocytes and up to 70% of erythrocytes. The early events in merogony involve a series of structural changes within the schizont, including the development of a prominent endoplasmic reticulum (which is not discernible in the macroschizont), the appearance of rhoptries in the cytoplasm and the formation of an obvious coat on the outer surface of the schizont (Shaw and Tilney, 1992). These changes are also associated with disappearance of the host microtubules previously associated with the surface of the schizont. A few microspheres appear in the cytoplasm later during development. Each schizont nucleus becomes interconnected with a complement of cytoplasmic organelles and relocates to contact the periphery of the schizont. A process of budding of each of the parasite nuclei and associated organelles from the surface of the schizonts occurs, leading to release of free uninucleate merozoites within the cytoplasm of the host cell (Fig. 3.7A, B). The mature merozoites are liberated by the breakdown of the cell membrane.

Jarrett *et al.* (1969) observed that the onset of merogony, as indicated by detection of microschizonts and initial detection of infected erythrocytes in infected cattle, appeared to be time-dependent rather than dependent on the infective dose of parasites. The authors proposed that this may reflect occurrence of merogony after a fixed number of divisions of the infected cells, although there has been no further evidence to support this suggestion.

A B

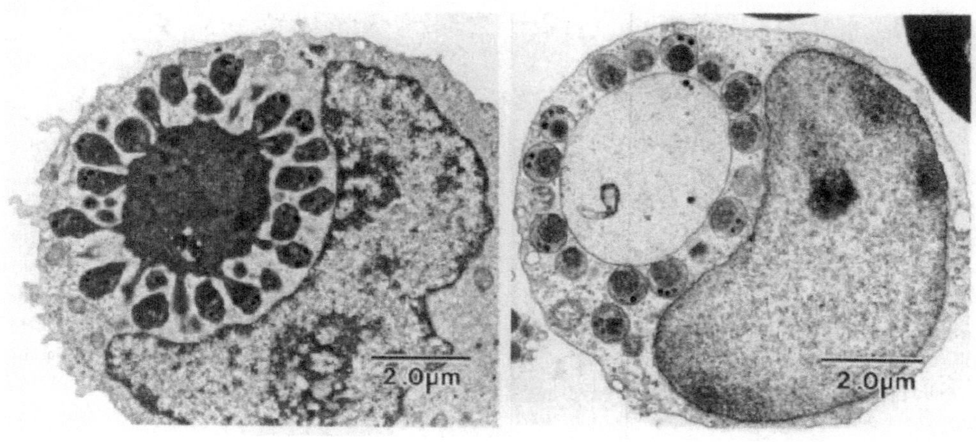

Fig. 3.7. Merogony in *T. parva*-infected bovine lymphocytes: (A) Budding of merozoites from the body of the parasite schizont. (B) Free merozoites released into the cytoplasm of the infected cell. (Figure reproduced from Shaw and Tilney, 1992. Used with permission.)

3.4.2 Infection of erythrocytes

The free merozoites measure approximately 1 μm in diameter and are covered by a distinct 20–25 nm surface coat. Similar to sporozoites, they do not have a clearly defined apical complex and can invade erythrocytes in any orientation. Each merozoite contains a set of 3–6 rhoptries and a small number of structures similar to the dense granules found in sporozoites. Morphologically, the events involved in merozoite invasion of erythrocytes are almost identical to the process of sporozoite invasion of lymphocytes (Shaw and Tilney, 1995). Following erythrocyte binding by the merozoite surface coat, internalization is achieved by a zippering process between the parasite and erythrocyte membranes, and dissolution of the surrounding erythrocyte membrane results in the parasite, now referred to as a 'piroplasm', lying free within the erythrocyte. The piroplasm stage of *T. parva* undergoes little if any multiplication, consistent with long-standing evidence that infection cannot readily be established by adoptive transfer of blood from infected animals (Theiler, 1903, 1911). Therefore, infection of erythrocytes is entirely dependent on generation of merozoites. There is no evidence of extensive parasite-mediated lysis of erythrocytes, and hence anaemia is not a prominent clinical sign in disease caused by *T. parva*, unlike other haemoparasites. Piroplasms are presumably removed along with the normal removal of erythrocytes, although little is known of the effect of the piroplasm on the lifespan of the erythrocyte.

3.4.3 Obstacles to completing the life cycle *in vitro*

As indicated above, merogony in *in vitro* cultures of *T. parva*-infected cells is only detected transiently in early cultures (Madder *et al.*, 2003). However, studies of both *T. parva* and *T. annulata* have shown that incubation of established cultures of macroschizont-infected cells at elevated temperatures (41–42°C) results in differentiation to microschizonts in a proportion of the cells (Hulliger *et al.*, 1966; Glascodine *et al.*, 1990). Merozoites were also found in the *T. annulata* cultures. These conditions mimicked the high body temperatures produced by infections with the parasites *in vivo*. Danskin and Wilde (1976), working with *T. parva*-infected cultures, also found that incubation of the cells in 20% foetal bovine serum plus 10% bovine lymph resulted in differentiation to microschizonts and production of merozoites; small numbers of piroplasms developed in erythrocytes added to these cultures. However, since *T. parva* piroplasms undergo little if any proliferation, there is little prospect of cultivating this stage of the parasite *in vitro*. Moreover, although there has been some progress in feeding *R. appendiculatus* ticks *in vitro* on artificial membranes (Waladde *et al.*, 1995; Musyoki *et al.*, 2004; Vimonish *et al.*, 2021; Asri *et al.*, 2023), there is as yet no robust *in vitro* system that would facilitate transfer of infections into the tick vector.

3.5 Persistence of Infection

T. parva can persist in the mammalian host well beyond the acute phase of the infection and the resolution of clinical signs. This persistent infection is referred to as the carrier state. Although the parasite is usually undetectable microscopically, infection can be transmitted by feeding ticks (Young *et al.*, 1986). Persistence of infected lymphocytes is required to generate merozoites for infection of erythrocytes. The tissue sites where the infected cells persist and how they avoid elimination by host immune responses are not understood. The significance of the carrier state with respect to the epidemiology of the parasite is discussed in further detail elsewhere in this book.

3.6 Concluding Remarks

A particularly distinctive feature of the life cycle of *T. parva* that distinguishes it from most other apicomplexan parasites is that all of the intracellular stages in both the mammalian and arthropod hosts lie free within the cytoplasm of the host cells. Thus, there is no requirement for the processes employed by other apicomplexan parasites, such as *Plasmodium* and *Toxoplasma* species, to create a modified endocytic vacuole in which the parasites reside. There is also no obvious mechanism by which the *Theileria* parasites can express parasite proteins on the surface of host lymphocytes or erythrocytes, apart from parasite peptides associated with the MHC molecules on the surface of infected lymphocytes. The unique capacity of *T. parva* to activate and transform the infected lymphocyte and to synchronize its division with that of the host cell facilitates rapid multiplication of the macroschizont stage of the parasite while remaining in an intracellular location. These properties of *T. parva* have important implications for how the parasite can cause disease and the nature of the immune responses it induces, which will be discussed in further detail in Chapters 4 and 11 of this volume. Several important questions regarding the process by which the parasite invades host lymphocytes and the parasite proteins involved remain unresolved. For example, despite the discoveries over 30 years ago that the p67 sporozoite antigen and host class I MHC proteins are involved in entry of the parasite into host cells, there have been no concerted efforts to identify the ligands of these proteins. It will have become apparent to the reader of this chapter that almost all of the studies on aspects of the development of the parasite in host and tick tissues were published before the mid-1990s. Much of this research was conducted by scientists at the International Laboratory for Research on Animal Diseases (ILRAD) in Nairobi, which unfortunately was discontinued following ILRAD's incorporation into the International Livestock Research Institute (ILRI).

Acknowledgements

I wish to pay tribute to the late Dr Michael Shaw and his colleagues Professors Lewis Tilney and Don Fawcett, whose excellent work provided a large part of the information presented in this chapter.

References

Asri, B., Tahir, D., Evans, A., Meyer, L.N., Rhalem, A. *et al.* (2023) Assessment of an *in vitro* tick feeding system for the successful feeding of adult *Rhipicephalus appendiculatus* ticks. *Parasitologia* 3(2), 101–108. DOI: 10.3390/parasitologia3020012.

Baldwin, C.L., Black, S.J., Brown, W.C., Conrad, P.A., Goddeeris, B.M. *et al.* (1988) Bovine T cells, B cells, and null cells are transformed by the protozoan parasite *Theileria parva*. *Infection and Immunity* 56(2), 462–467. DOI: 10.1128/iai.56.2.462-467.1988.

Brown, C.G., Stagg, D.A., Purnell, R.E., Kanhai, G.K. and Payne, R.C. (1973) Infection and transformation of bovine lymphoid cells *in vitro* by infective particles of *Theileria parva*. *Letter. Nature* 245(5420), 101–103. DOI: 10.1038/245101a0.

Büscher, G. and Otim, B. (1986) Quantitative studies on *Theileria parva* in the salivary glands of *Rhipicephalus appendiculatus* adults: Quantitation and prediction of infection. *International Journal for Parasitology* 16(1), 93–100. DOI: 10.1016/0020-7519(86)90071-8.

Büscher, G. and Tangus, J. (1986) Quantitative studies on *Theileria parva* in the salivary glands of *Rhipicephalus appendiculatus* adults: Search for conditions for high infections. *International Journal for Parasitology* 16(2), 121–129. DOI: 10.1016/0020-7519(86)90097-4.

Cowdry, E.V. and Ham, A.W. (1932) Studies on East Coast fever. I. The life cycle of the parasite in ticks. *Parasitology* 24(1), 1–49. DOI: 10.1017/S0031182000020394.

Cowdry, E.V. and Danks, W.B.C. (1933) Studies on East Coast fever. II. Behaviour of the parasite and the development of distinctive lesions in susceptible animals. *Parasitology* 25(1), 1–63. DOI: 10.1017/S003118200001920X.

Danskin, D. and Wilde, J.K.H. (1976) Stimulation *in vitro* of bovine host cycle of *Theileria parva*. *Nature* 261(5558), 311–312. DOI: 10.1038/261311a0.

Dobbelaere, D.A., Spooner, P.R., Barry, W.C. and Irvin, A.D. (1984) Monoclonal antibody neutralizes the sporozoite stage of different *Theileria parva* stocks. *Parasite Immunology* 6, 361–370. DOI: 10.1111/j.1365-3024.1984.tb00808.x.

Dobbelaere, D.A.E., Webster, P., Leitch, B.L., Voigt, W.P. and Irvin, A.D. (1985) *Theileria parva*: Expression of a sporozoite surface coat antigen. *Experimental Parasitology* 60(1), 90–100. DOI: 10.1016/S0014-4894(85)80026-6.

Dobbelaere, D.A.E., Coquerelle, T.M., Roditi, I.J., Eichhorn, M. and Williams, R.O. (1988) *Theileria parva* infection induces autocrine growth of bovine lymphocytes. *Proceedings of the National Academy of Sciences* 85(13), 4730–4734. DOI: 10.1073/pnas.85.13.4730.

Fawcett, D., Musoke, A. and Voigt, W. (1984) Interaction of sporozoites of *Theileria parva* with bovine lymphocytes *in vitro*. I. Early events after invasion. *Tissue and Cell* 16(6), 873–884. DOI: 10.1016/0040-8166(84)90068-5.

Fawcett, D.W., Büscher, G. and Doxsey, S. (1982) Salivary gland of the tick vector of East Coast fever. III. The ultrastructure of sporogony in *Theileria parva*. *Tissue and Cell* 14(1), 183–206. DOI: 10.1016/0040-8166(82)90017-9.

Frischknecht, F. and Matuschewski, K. (2017) Plasmodium sporozoite biology. *Cold Spring Harbor Perspectives in Medicine* 7(5), a025478. DOI: 10.1101/cshperspect.a025478.

Gauer, M., Mackenstedt, U., Mehlhorn, H., Schein, E., Zapf, F. *et al.* (1995) DNA measurements and ploidy determination of developmental stages in the life cycles of *Theileria annulata* and *T. parva*. *Parasitology Research* 81(7), 565–574. DOI: 10.1007/BF00932023.

Glascodine, J., Tetley, L., Tait, A., Brown, D. and Shiels, B. (1990) Developmental expression of a *Theileria annulata* merozoite surface antigen. *Molecular and Biochemical Parasitology* 40(1), 105–112. DOI: 10.1016/0166-6851(90)90084-y.

Henson, S., Bishop, R.P., Morzaria, S., Spooner, P.R., Pelle, R. *et al.* (2012) High-resolution genotyping and mapping of recombination and gene conversion in the protozoan *Theileria parva* using whole genome sequencing. *BMC Genomics* 13(1), 503. DOI: 10.1186/1471-2164-13-503.

Hulliger, L., Wilde, K.H., Brown, C.G. and Turner, L. (1964) Mode of multiplication of *Theileria* in cultures of bovine lymphocytic cells. *Nature* 203, 728–730. DOI: 10.1038/203728a0.

Hulliger, L., Brown, C.G.D. and Wilde, J.K.H. (1966) Transition of developmental stages of *Theileria parva in vitro* at high temperature. *Nature* 211(5046), 328–329. DOI: 10.1038/211328a0.

Jarrett, W.F.H., Crighton, G.W. and Pirie, H.M. (1969) *Theileria parva*: Kinetics of replication. *Experimental Parasitology* 24(1), 9–25. DOI: 10.1016/0014-4894(69)90215-X.

Katzer, F., Lizundia, R., Ngugi, D., Blake, D. and McKeever, D. (2011) Construction of a genetic map for *Theileria parva*: Identification of hotspots of recombination. *International Journal for Parasitology* 41(6), 669–675. DOI: 10.1016/j.ijpara.2011.01.001.

Madder, M., Speybroeck, N., Brandt, J., Tirry, L., Hodek, I. *et al.* (2002) Geographic variation in diapause response of adult *Rhipicephalus appendiculatus* ticks. *Experimental & Applied Acarology* 27(3), 209–221. DOI: 10.1023/A:1021694207456.

Madder, M., Speybroeck, N., Berkvens, D., Baudoux, V., Marcotty, T. *et al.* (2003) Merogony in *in vitro* cultures of *Theileria parva*. *Veterinary Parasitology* 114(3), 195–203. DOI: 10.1016/s0304-4017(03)00142-0.

Mehlhorn, H. and Schein, E. (1984) The piroplasms: Life cycle and sexual stages. *Advances in Parasitology* 23, 37–103. DOI: 10.1016/s0065-308x(08)60285-7.

Mehlhorn, H., Schein, E. and Warnecke, M. (1978) Electron microscopic studies on the development of kinetes of *Theileria parva* (Theiler 1904) in the gut of the vector ticks *Rhipicephalus appendiculatus*. *Revue Scientifique et Technique, Office International Des Epizooties* 34, 599–611.

Molloy, S. (2010) Theileria survival and the spindle. *Nature Reviews Microbiology* 8(11), 757–757. DOI: 10.1038/nrmicro2468.

Morrison, W.I., Buscher, G., Murray, M., Emery, D.L., Masake, R.A. *et al.* (1981) *Theileria parva*: Kinetics of infection in the lymphoid system of cattle. *Experimental Parasitology* 52(2), 248–260. DOI: 10.1016/0014-4894(81)90080-1.

Musoke, A.J., Nantulya, V.M., Rurangirwa, F.R. and Buscher, G. (1984) Evidence for a common protective antigenic determinant on sporozoites of several *Theileria parva* strains. *Immunology* 52(2), 231–238.

Musyoki, J.M., Osir, E.O., Kiara, H.K. and Kokwaro, E.D. (2004) Comparative studies on the infectivity of *Theileria parva* in ticks fed *in vitro* and those fed on cattle. *Experimental and Applied Acarology* 32(1–2), 51–67. DOI: 10.1023/B:APPA.0000018159.47700.e4.

Nene, V., Gobright, E., Bishop, R., Morzaria, S. and Musoke, A. (1999) Linear peptide specificity of bovine antibody responses to p67 of *Theileria parva* and sequence diversity of sporozoite-neutralizing epitopes: Implications for a vaccine. *Infection and Immunity* 67(3), 1261–1266. DOI: 10.1128/IAI.67.3.1261-1266.1999.

Nyagwange, J., Nene, V., Mwalimu, S., Henson, S., Steinaa, L. *et al.* (2018) Antibodies to *in silico* selected GPI-anchored *Theileria parva* proteins neutralise sporozoite infection *in vitro*. *Veterinary Immunology and Immunopathology* 199, 8–14. DOI: 10.1016/j.vetimm.2018.03.004.

Odongo, D.O., Oura, C.A.L., Spooner, P.R., Kiara, H., Mburu, D. *et al.* (2006) Linkage disequilibrium between alleles at highly polymorphic mini- and micro-satellite loci of *Theileria parva* isolated from cattle in three regions of Kenya. *International Journal for Parasitology* 36(8), 937–946. DOI: 10.1016/j.ijpara.2006.01.008.

Oura, C.A.L., Asiimwe, B.B., Weir, W., Lubega, G.W. and Tait, A. (2005) Population genetic analysis and sub-structuring of *Theileria parva* in Uganda. *Molecular and Biochemical Parasitology* 140(2), 229–239. DOI: 10.1016/j.molbiopara.2004.12.015.

Purnell, R.E. (1977) East Coast fever: Some recent research in East Africa. *Advances in Parasitology* 15, 83–132. DOI: 10.1016/s0065-308x(08)60527-8.

Purnell, R.E., Boarer, C.D. and Pierce, M.A. (1971) *Theileria parva*: Comparative infection rates of adult and nymphal *Rhipicephalus appendiculatus*. *Parasitology* 62(2), 349–353. DOI: 10.1017/s0031182000071584.

Purnell, R.E., Ledger, M.A., Omwoyo, P.L., Payne, R.C. and Peirce, M.A. (1974) *Theileria parva*: Variation in the infection rate of the vector tick *Rhipicephalus appendiculatus*. *International Journal for Parasitology* 4(5), 513–517. DOI: 10.1016/0020-7519(74)90069-1.

Randolph, S.E. (1997) Abiotic and biotic determinants of the seasonal dynamics of the tick *Rhipicephalus appendiculatus* in South Africa. *Medical and Veterinary Entomology* 11(1), 25–37. DOI: 10.1111/j.1365-2915.1997.tb00286.x.

Shaw, M.K. (1996) *Theileria parva* sporozoite entry into bovine lymphocytes involves both parasite and host cell signal transduction processes. *Experimental Parasitology* 84(3), 344–354. DOI: 10.1006/expr.1996.0123.

Shaw, M.K. (1997) The same but different: The biology of *Theileria* sporozoite entry into bovine cells. *International Journal for Parasitology* 27(5), 457–474. DOI: 10.1016/s0020-7519(97)00015-5.

Shaw, M.K. (1999) *Theileria parva*: Sporozoite entry into bovine lymphocytes is not dependent on the parasite cytoskeleton. *Experimental Parasitology* 92(1), 24–31. DOI: 10.1006/expr.1998.4393.

Shaw, M.K. (2003) Cell invasion by *Theileria* sporozoites. *Trends in Parasitology* 19(1), 2–6. DOI: 10.1016/s1471-4922(02)00015-6.

Shaw, M.K. and Tilney, L.G. (1992) How individual cells develop from a syncytium: Merogony in *Theileria parva (Apicomplexa)*. *Journal of Cell Science* 101(Pt 1), 109–123. DOI: 10.1242/jcs.101.1.109.

Shaw, M.K. and Tilney, L.G. (1995) The entry of *Theileria parva* merozoites into bovine erythrocytes occurs by a process similar to sporozoite invasion of lymphocytes. *Parasitology* 111(Pt 4), 455–461. DOI: 10.1017/s0031182000065951.

Shaw, M.K. and Young, A.S. (1995) Differential development and emission of *Theileria parva* sporozoites from the salivary gland of *Rhipicephalus appendiculatus*. *Parasitology* 111(Pt 2), 153–160. DOI: 10.1017/s0031182000064891.

Shaw, M.K., Tilney, L.G. and Musoke, A.J. (1991) The entry of *Theileria parva* sporozoites into bovine lymphocytes: Evidence for MHC class I involvement. *The Journal of Cell Biology* 113(1), 87–101. DOI: 10.1083/jcb.113.1.87.

Shaw, M.K., Tilney, L.G. and McKeever, D.J. (1993) Tick salivary gland extract and interleukin-2 stimulation enhance susceptibility of lymphocytes to infection by *Theileria parva* sporozoites. *Infection and Immunity* 61(4), 1486–1495. DOI: 10.1128/iai.61.4.1486-1495.1993.

Shaw, M.K., Tilney, L.G., Musoke, A.J. and Teale, A.J. (1995) MHC class I molecules are an essential cell surface component involved in *Theileria parva* sporozoite binding to bovine lymphocytes. *Journal of Cell Science* 108(Pt 4), 1587–1596. DOI: 10.1242/jcs.108.4.1587.

Stagg, D.A., Dolan, T.T., Leitch, B.L. and Young, A.S. (1981) The initial stages of infection of cattle cells with *Theileria parva* sporozoites *in vitro*. *Parasitology* 83(Pt 1), 191–197. DOI: 10.1017/s0031182000050150.

Stagg, D.A., Fawcett, D.W., Young, A.S. and Leitch, B.L. (1984) Superinfection of established *Theileria*-infected bovid cell lines with *Theileria parva* sporozoites. *Annals of Tropical Medicine and Parasitology* 78(3), 335–337. DOI: 10.1080/00034983.1984.11811827.

Theiler, A. (1903) The Rhodesian tick fever. *Transvaal Agricultural Journal* 1, 93–110.

Theiler, A. (1911) *The artificial transmission of East Coast fever*. Report of the Government Veterinary Bacteriologist. Pretoria: Government Printer and Stationery Office.

Tomley, F.M. and Soldati, D.S. (2001) Mix and match modules: Structure and function of microneme proteins in apicomplexan parasites. *Trends in Parasitology* 17(2), 81–88. DOI: 10.1016/s1471-4922(00)01761-x.

Toye, P., Musoke, A.J. and Naessens, J. (2014) Role of the polymorphic immunodominant molecule in entry of *Theileria parva* sporozoites into bovine lymphocytes. *Infection and Immunity* 82(5), 1786–1792. DOI: 10.1128/IAI.01029-13.

Toye, P.G., Metzelaar, M.J., Wijngaard, P.L., Nene, V., Iams, K. *et al.* (1995) Characterisation of the gene encoding the polymorphic immunodominant molecule, a neutralising antigen of *Theileria parva*. *Journal of Immunology* 155(3), 1370–1381. DOI: 10.4049/jimmunol.155.3.1370.

Vimonish, R., Dinkel, K.D., Fry, L.M., Johnson, W.C., Capelli-Peixoto, J. *et al.* (2021) Isolation of infectious *Theileria parva* sporozoites secreted by infected *Rhipicephalus appendiculatus* ticks into an *in vitro* tick feeding system. *Parasites & Vectors* 14(1), 616. DOI: 10.1186/s13071-021-05120-7.

Waladde, S.M., Young, A.S., Mwaura, S.N., Njihia, G.N. and Mwakima, F.N. (1995) Optimization of the *in vitro* feeding of *Rhipicephalus appendiculatus* nymphae for the transmission of *Theileria parva*. *Parasitology* 111(Pt 4), 463–468. DOI: 10.1017/s0031182000065963.

Webster, P., Dobbelaere, D.A. and Fawcett, D.W. (1985) The entry of sporozoites of *Theileria parva* into bovine lymphocytes *in vitro*: Immunoelectron microscopic observations. *European Journal of Cell Biology* 36(2), 157–162.

Young, A.S., Leitch, B.L. and Newson, R.M. (1981) The occurrence of a *Theileria parva* carrier state in cattle from an East Coast fever endemic area of Kenya. In: Irvin, A.D., Cunningham, M.P. and Young, A.S. (eds) *Advances in the Control of Theileriosis. Current Topics in Veterinary Medicine and Animal Science*. Springer, Dordrecht, The Netherlands, pp. 60–62.

Young, A.S., Leitch, B.L. and Mutugi, J.J. (1984) Some factors controlling the stimulation of sporogony of *Theileria parva* in its tick vector *Rhipicephalus appendiculatus*. *International Journal for Parasitology* 14(1), 97–102. DOI: 10.1016/0020-7519(84)90018-3.

Young, A.S., Leitch, B.L., Newson, R.M. and Cunningham, M.P. (1986) Maintenance of *Theileria parva* infection in an endemic area of Kenya. *Parasitology* 93(Pt 1), 9–16. DOI: 10.1017/s0031182000049787.

Young, A.S., Leitch, B.L., Morzaria, S.P., Irvin, A.D., Omwoyo, P.L. *et al.* (1987) Development and survival of *Theileria parva* parva in *Rhipicephalus appendiculatus* exposed in the Trans-Mara, Kenya. *Parasitology* 94(Pt 3), 433–441. DOI: 10.1017/s0031182000055785.

Young, A.S., Dolan, T.T., Mwakima, F.N., Ochanda, H., Mwaura, S.N. *et al.* (1995) Estimation of heritability of susceptibility to infection with *Theileria parva* in the tick *Rhipicephalus appendiculatus*. *Parasitology* 111(Pt 1), 31–38. DOI: 10.1017/s003118200006457x.

4 The Pathogenesis of East Coast Fever

W. Ivan Morrison* and Jorge Del-Pozo
Roslin Institute, University of Edinburgh, Edinburgh, UK

4.1 Introduction

Theileria parasites are characterized by their ability to undergo sequential development in leukocytes and erythrocytes. The different species of *Theileria* that infect cattle vary markedly in their pathogenicity, resulting in infections that range from being asymptomatic to highly virulent, causing high levels of mortality (Uilenberg, 1981; Morrison, 2015). In Africa, *Theileria parva* is overwhelmingly the most important species in cattle, causing an acute lymphoproliferative disease known as East Coast fever (ECF) that can kill the host within 4 weeks of infection (Irvin and Morrison, 1987). The distribution of the disease follows that of the main tick vector *Rhipicephalus appendiculatus*, which is found throughout a large area of eastern and southern Africa (Norval *et al.*, 1992), where ECF results in severe economic losses. In addition to its direct impact on cattle production, limitations in available methods used to control the disease have imposed constraints on the ability to genetically improve the productivity of cattle in affected areas.

Multiplication of *T. parva* in the mammalian host occurs predominantly during the intra-lymphocytic stage of development. Following invasion of leukocytes by sporozoites deposited in tick saliva, the parasite establishes an intimate intracellular relationship with the host cell involving activation and induction of proliferation, which allows rapid multiplication of the infected cells. This proliferation of infected leukocytes plays a central role in the pathogenesis of the disease. There are a number of early detailed descriptions of the pathology of ECF, which document the pathological effects of the parasite (Steck, 1928; Cowdry and Danks, 1933; De Kock, 1957; Barnett, 1960). These studies correctly highlighted the impact that infection has on lymphoid tissues, although functional interpretation of their findings was hampered by a lack of understanding of the life cycle of lymphocytes and their immunological functions at the time the studies were undertaken. This point was acknowledged in the excellent study by Cowdry and Danks (1933), who stated that: 'Our information is superficial and leaves out of account what is probably the key problem, namely the disturbance of lymphocyte function resulting from the direct action of the parasites' (Cowdry and Danks, 1933, p. 44).

This chapter aims to provide an account of our understanding of the pathogenesis of the disease, taking into consideration current knowledge of the functions of the immune system. Most of the information discussed is derived from experimental studies using the Muguga isolate of *T. parva* and includes not only pathological and clinical findings from animals examined at different stages of the disease but also quantitative data on the kinetics of infection, including information

*Corresponding author: Ivan.Morrison@ed.ac.uk

 East Coast Fever: The Disease, its Impact and Control (eds W.I. Morrison and P. Toye)
DOI: 10.1079/9781800626324.0004

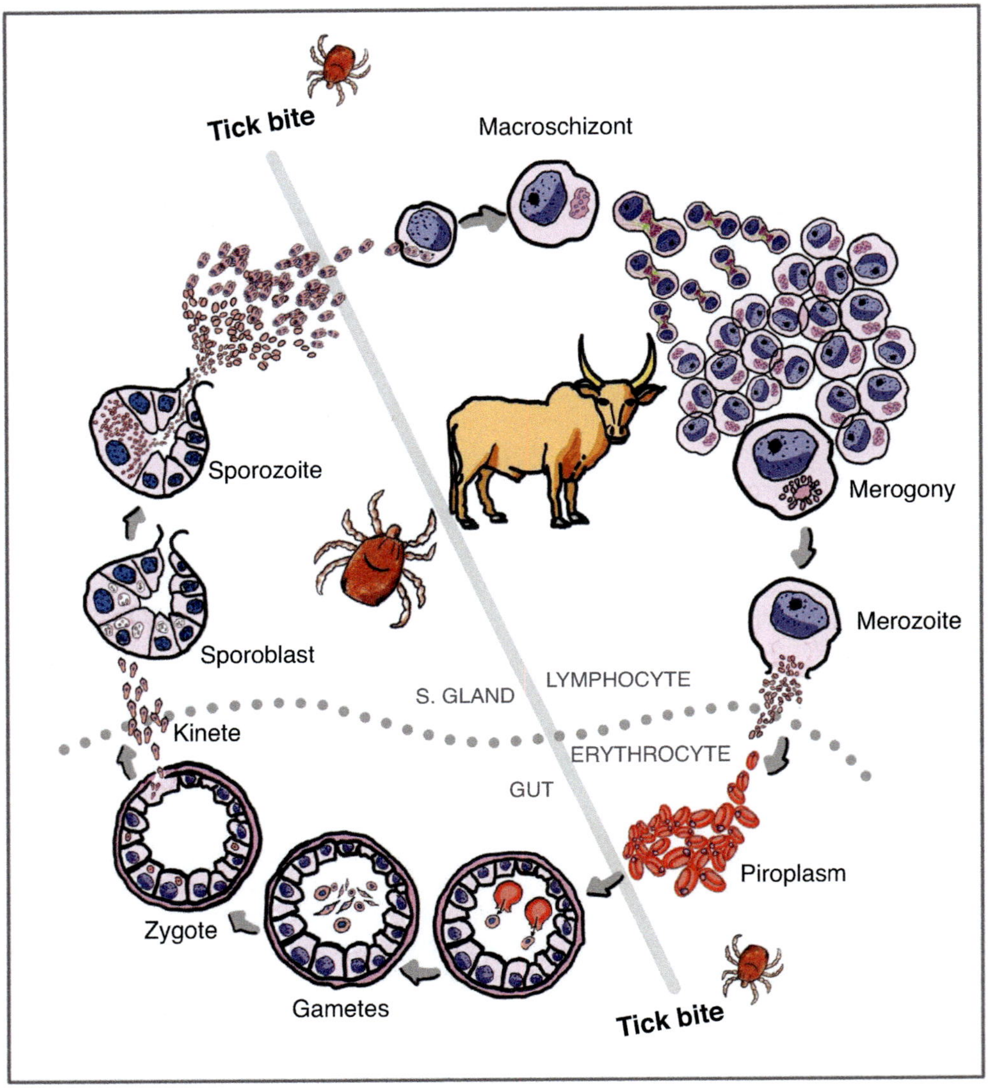

Fig. 4.1. The life cycle of *T. parva*. (Prepared by J. Del Pozo.)

derived from use of lymph duct cannulation procedures.

the key features relevant to the parasite's ability to cause disease in cattle.

4.2 Infection of the Bovine Host by *T. parva*

The developmental stages of *T. parva* in the tick and bovine hosts are discussed in detail in Chapter 3 of this volume and illustrated in Fig. 4.1. Herein, we provide a brief summary of

4.2.1 Development of the parasite in bovine cells

Infection is initiated by sporozoites emitted in the saliva of feeding ticks. Sporozoites invade leukocytes in which they escape from the endocytic vacuole and lie free within the cytoplasm of the infected cell (Fawcett *et al.*, 1984; Shaw, 1997; Shaw, 2003). Within 2–3 days, the parasite develops into a multinucleate stage, the macroschizont, which induces activation of the infected host cells leading to proliferation. By closely associating with the mitotic apparatus of the host cell, the macroschizont divides synchronously with it, resulting in parasite nuclei being distributed to both daughter cells (Hulliger *et al.*, 1964). This relationship facilitates rapid multiplication of the infected cells and ensures that the parasite remains in an intracellular location throughout this stage of development. It also allows parasitized cells to be cultivated *in vitro* as continuously growing cell lines (Brown *et al.*, 1973). This property of *T. parva* is referred to as 'transformation', drawing parallels between the behaviour of the infected cells and that of cancer cells. The mechanisms involved in parasite-induced transformation of the host cells are discussed by Woods *et al.* (2021) and in Chapter 10 of this volume.

In infected animals, some of the macroschizonts undergo merogony during the second week of infection. Initially, they differentiate to microschizonts, which have increased numbers of densely stained nuclei, and merozoites are then generated from the microschizonts by a budding process. Development of merogony is associated with cessation of proliferation of the host cells and eventually results in disruption of the infected cells and release of merozoites (Shaw and Tilney, 1992). Invasion of erythrocytes by merozoites gives rise to the piroplasm stage, which is infective for ticks (Shaw and Tilney, 1995). The piroplasms of *T. parva* undergo little if any proliferation.

4.2.2 Cell lineages infected by the parasite

Although some investigators have suggested that *T. parva* infects monocytes and endothelial cells (e.g. Moulton *et al.*, 1984), most have described infected cells as resembling medium-sized lymphocytes. The generation of monoclonal antibody reagents specific for subsets of bovine leukocytes in the early 1980s enabled studies to determine the cell types infected with *T. parva*. Parasitized cell lines isolated from infected cattle and the majority of those established by infection of peripheral blood mononuclear cells (PBM) *in vitro* were found to be T cells (Morrison *et al.*, 1996). However, experiments in which purified subsets of cells were cultured *in vitro* at limiting dilution with sporozoites demonstrated that infected cell lines could be established from T lymphocytes and B lymphocytes at similar efficiency and that CD4, CD8 and γδ T cell subsets are all susceptible to infection (Baldwin *et al.*, 1988). Around the same time, studies of the other major pathogenic species of *Theileria*, *T. annulata*, using a similar *in vitro* system, showed that this species infects monocytes and B lymphocytes, but not T lymphocytes (Spooner *et al.*, 1989).

A further study, which investigated the phenotype of *T. parva*-infected cells in cultures established by *in vitro* infection of peripheral blood mononuclear cells with sporozoites, revealed that during the first 10 days a large proportion of the infected cells were B cells, but infected T cells gradually dominated the cultures during the subsequent 10 days (Morrison *et al.*, 1996). Since infected T cells and B cells cultured on their own appear to grow at similar rates, this finding indicated that in mixed cell populations, infected T cells have other properties that confer a competitive advantage.

In contrast to results obtained with lymphocytes, infected cell lines could not be established from purified monocytes or neutrophils (Shaw *et al.*, 1993). Ultrastructural studies revealed that sporozoites bind to and invade monocytes and macrophages, some by phagocytosis and others by the receptor-mediated process described for infection of lymphocytes. However, internalized parasites did not undergo further development in these cell types. Binding and receptor-mediated uptake of sporozoites by dendritic cells isolated from afferent lymph was also observed, and in this cell type, early development of the internalized sporozoites occurred but did not progress to nuclear division and establishment of infection (Shaw *et al.*, 1993). These findings demonstrate that susceptibility of host cells to infection with *T. parva* depends not only on the ability to invade target cells but also on other, as yet unidentified, post-invasion interactions that are required for further parasite development.

A more recent study identified a *T. parva* isolate of low virulence (*T. parva* Chitongo) that readily infects and transforms CD8T cells but not CD4 and γδ T cells (Tindih *et al.*, 2012). Sporozoites failed to bind to non-CD8 T cells despite the finding that the major surface coat protein p67, which acts as a ligand for binding to host target cells (Shaw, 1997), is identical in sequence to that of other *T. parva* isolates. The reason for this discrepancy has not been determined, but the finding illustrates the complexity of the surface ligands involved in host cell invasion. The restriction of the target population to CD8 cells essentially reduces the effective dose, which the authors suggested may be responsible for the low pathogenicity of this isolate.

Analyses of the phenotypes of infected cells *in vivo* have revealed that cell types shown to be susceptible to infection *in vitro* differ in their pathogenicity *in vivo*. First, phenotyping of infected cells in cattle undergoing lethal infection showed that the vast majority of infected cells are T cells, including both $CD4^+$ and $CD8^+$ T cells and also cells that co-express CD4 and CD8 (Emery *et al.*, 1988). Secondly, inoculation of cattle with purified autologous T cells or B cells that had been incubated *in vitro* with sporozoites for 48 hour resulted in lethal infections in animals receiving T cells but mild transient infections in those receiving B cells (Morrison *et al.*, 1996). These experiments included one animal that received a tenfold higher number of B cells, which also experienced a mild transient infection. These findings demonstrated that although purified T cells and B cells are infected and transformed by *T. parva* at similar frequency *in vitro*, they differ in their ability to cause disease.

4.3 Cellular Changes in the Tick Bite Site

The responses in the skin of cattle at the site of attachment of *R. appendiculatus* ticks have not been studied in detail. However, available data from one study of *R. appendiculatus* (Walker and Fletcher, 1986) and from studies of related tick species (Tatchell and Moorhouse, 1968; Theis and Budwiser, 1974) have indicated the main changes following tick attachment. The tick becomes anchored into the skin by a layer of cement secreted around the embedded mouthparts, and secretion of saliva stimulates an inflammatory response in the dermis. The tick saliva contains enzymes that prevent coagulation of blood and cause breakdown of collagen in the dermis, creating a more open reticular structure containing serous fluid and inflammatory cells. There is an increase in the permeability of blood and lymph vessels and some damage to the vessels, which after 2–3 days results in leakage of blood into the feeding site. An increase in infiltration of granulocytes and mononuclear cells occurs between 2 and 6 days after attachment (Walker and Fletcher, 1986). Development of sporozoites in *T. parva*-infected ticks does not occur until the ticks commence feeding, so that sporozoites are not released in the saliva until 3–5 days after commencement of feeding (Purnell, 1977). Thus, by the time sporozoites are introduced by feeding ticks, there is a substantial increase in numbers of lymphocytes in the feeding site, potentially favouring establishment of infection. These changes also result in an increase in the flow of afferent lymph and cells from the attachment site into the draining lymph node.

4.4 The Quantum of Infection

For some diseases, the infective dose of the pathogen has a strong influence on the severity of disease. Establishment of methods to cryopreserve *T. parva* sporozoites in the 1970s (Cunningham *et al.*, 1973) enabled studies to explore whether infection of cattle with small doses of parasites could be used to induce mild infections from which animals reproducibly recover and develop immunity. However, experiments involving titration of the infective dose of sporozoite suspensions administered to groups of cattle demonstrated that this was not the case. Thus, for example in the study reported by Cunningham *et al.* (1974), the smallest dose of parasites that reproducibly infected all animals resulted in lethal infection in some animals and mild infection in others. In another study, which reported the numbers of ticks used to prepare a fresh batch of tick homogenate, two out of four animals that received 0.01 ml of the homogenate, equivalent to 0.16 of a tick, developed lethal infections (Radley *et al.*, 1974). These findings indicated that small numbers of parasites are sufficient to produce a lethal infection.

The level of infection with *T. parva* in populations of ticks can be determined by enumeration of cells containing sporoblasts in dissected salivary glands of partially fed ticks (Büscher and Otim, 1986). Only a small proportion of parasites ingested by ticks successfully establish infections in the tick salivary glands. Purnell (1977) has estimated that individual ticks fed on experimentally infected cattle may ingest up to 10^7 *T. parva*-infected erythrocytes; yet some ticks fed on such animals fail to become infected. The level of infection in batches of infected ticks fed on experimentally infected animals varies, usually ranging from 40 to 80% of the ticks being infected, with an average of 10–60 infected salivary gland acini per tick (Purnell *et al.*, 1974). Moreover, the distribution of infection is invariably over-dispersed, that is, only a small number of the ticks have large numbers of infected acini, many contain only one or two and others are uninfected (Büscher and Otim, 1986; Norval *et al.*, 1992). Genetic variability in susceptibility of ticks to infection with *T. parva* has been demonstrated and is believed to contribute to this variation (Young *et al.*, 1995). The infection rate in ticks collected from the field in ECF-endemic areas is usually less than 4%, and again many of the infected ticks contain only one or two sporoblasts (Moll *et al.*, 1986; Gitau *et al.*, 2000). Studies conducted in the 1950s, in which a large number of animals were challenged with single experimentally infected ticks, showed that most susceptible animals developed severe infection with a lethal outcome (Barnett, 1957). Collectively, these data indicate that sporozoites from a single salivary gland cell are sufficient to produce a lethal infection. Although each infected cell has been estimated to accommodate up to 4.8×10^4 sporozoites (Jarrett *et al.*, 1969), the proportion of these sporozoites that are capable of infecting and transforming bovine lymphocytes is not known.

Studies involving inoculation of cattle with autologous cells infected *in vitro* with sporozoites have also provided information on the numbers of infected cells required to produce severe disease (Morrison *et al.*, 1996). Cells isolated from the blood of individual animals were incubated *in vitro* for 48 hour with freshly prepared homogenates of infected tick salivary glands, at which time no infective sporozoites remained in the extracellular medium, and defined numbers of cells were then administered to the autologous animals. Doses ranging from 3×10^4 to 3×10^5 of unfractionated PBM or highly purified CD4 or CD8T cells all resulted in severe infections with high levels of infected cells in the draining and contralateral lymph nodes, persisting to day 16, when the animals were euthanazed. Since separate studies had indicated that infection only establishes in a proportion of the cells in such cultures, these results support the evidence that the number of infective units required to establish a severe infection is within that estimated for a single infected salivary gland cell.

It should be noted that sporozoite suspensions prepared in the form of homogenized partially fed ticks will contain significantly fewer sporozoites per sporoblast than are produced by natural tick feeding. Some of the sporozoites will have been emitted prior to collection of the ticks on day four and other sporozoites will be immature at the time of collection. There will also be some loss of sporozoites during the process used to prepare the sporozoite suspensions, and freezing of sporozoites in cryoprotectant to produce frozen stabilates also results in a more than tenfold reduction in infectivity when they are thawed, compared to the fresh sporozoite suspensions (Wilkie *et al.*, 2002). Irrespective of whether infection is initiated using tick homogenates or by feeding ticks, the number of infective units that successfully establish infected cells *in vivo* is likely to be substantially lower than the number of inoculated sporozoites. Some sporozoites will be taken up by monocytes and dendritic cells, and others may fail to make contact with a susceptible target cell. The observed narrow margin in dosage between production of a lethal infection and failure to establish infection in animals given diluted sporozoite suspensions suggests that indeed only a fraction of the sporozoites successfully establish infection.

4.5 Variation in Virulence of *T. parva* in Cattle?

It should be borne in mind that the majority of detailed experimental studies of the pathogenesis of infection with *T. parva* have been conducted with the Muguga isolate of the parasite. Work with other isolates, such as those used in the studies carried out in the course of development of the Infection and Treatment Method (ITM) of vaccination, indicated that they were similarly virulent. The finding that the majority of susceptible animals introduced into endemically infected areas suffer severe disease also implies that most of the challenge parasites in the field are highly virulent. However, the virulence of different isolates may vary dependent on infective dose. As discussed earlier, *in vivo* titration of the Muguga isolate in cattle showed that this parasite remains highly virulent at low doses (Cunningham *et al.*, 1974). However, other parasite isolates have not been subjected to similar titrations to assess virulence in relation to infectivity and, therefore, it is possible that different parasites show a range of virulence dependent on infective dose. Most laboratory-maintained isolates of *T. parva* have been obtained by tick pick-up from clinical cases of ECF, which would have biased against isolation of low-virulence parasites. There have been occasional reports of isolates of *T. parva* that produce less severe disease (Barnett and Brocklesby, 1966; Tindih *et al.*, 2012). Hence, it remains possible that parasites of low or moderate virulence are present among the highly pathogenic populations found in the field. In this regard, it is of interest that a less severe disease caused by *T. parva*, known as January disease, emerged in Zimbabwe following the eradication of classical ECF from that country. As discussed in Chapter 6 of this volume, the progressive elimination of all animals suffering from severe disease may have allowed selection of this less pathogenic form of the parasite from the starting *T. parva* population. Although clearly less virulent than the parasites causing classical ECF, infection of calves with larger doses of the parasite caused more severe (non-lethal) clinical reactions (Koch *et al.*, 1988). Irvin *et al.* (1989) also reported more severe reactions, resulting in a few mortalities, in calves inoculated with parasites that had undergone one or two additional cattle/tick passages, which they attributed to higher concentrations of sporozoites in these stabilates compared to that of the parent stabilate. They proposed that the observed less severe clinical nature of January disease compared to classical ECF is due to the ability of the causal agent to induce mild clinical reactions over a wider infectious dose range, resulting in most animals in the field receiving a non-lethal dose of the parasite.

4.6 The Kinetics of Infection

The course of infection with *T. parva* in infected cattle can be monitored by detection of infected cells in stained smears prepared with needle aspirates from superficial lymph nodes. Such smears often contain extracellular schizonts released during preparation of the smear. Therefore, a schizont index, defined as the total number of intracellular and extracellular parasites expressed as a percentage of the number of intact leukocytes, is often used as a quantitative measure of parasitosis.

Initial detection of parasitized cells in the lymph node draining the site of infection is influenced by the infective dose of parasites. Parasites have been detected as early as 4 days after infection with large doses of sporozoite suspensions and progressively later with smaller parasite doses. Wilde (1967) presented evidence that infection spreads rapidly from the site of feeding of infected ticks in the skin. He reported that removal of the feeding ticks and amputation of the tick attachment sites on the ear 5 days after the ticks had been applied (i.e. coinciding with maximal release of sporozoites by the ticks) had no significant effect on subsequent development of infection. The detection of infection in the draining lymph node 2–3 days earlier than in other distant lymph nodes is consistent with other evidence that infection is transported from the site of infection to the regional lymph node in afferent lymph. There is also rapid dissemination of infection to other distant lymphoid tissues, as indicated by the finding that surgical removal of the lymph node draining the site of infection as early as 2 days after challenge of cattle with sporozoites had little effect on the subsequent course of infection (Emery, 1981).

The first detailed quantitative analysis of the kinetics of infection was reported by Jarrett *et al.* (1969), based on studies of groups of cattle infected by application of 10, 100 or 1000 experimentally infected ticks. Ticks were fed on the ears of the animals, and the schizont index was monitored in smears prepared daily from a prescapular lymph node. The results provided evidence of exponential growth of the parasite, with similar rates of growth recorded in groups infected with different numbers of ticks. Parasitized cells were estimated to increase approximately tenfold every 3 days, a figure that is consistent with the observed cell doubling time (18–24 hour) of cells in parasitized cell lines *in vitro*. In contrast to the influence of challenge dose on the time to initial detection of macroschizonts, Jarrett *et al.* (1967) observed that the time to initial detection of schizonts undergoing merogony (microschizonts) and to initial detection of piroplasms in erythrocytes was similar in animals receiving different doses of parasites, leading the authors to propose that merogony occurs after a defined number of divisions of infected lymphocytes.

A later study (Radley *et al.*, 1974) of animals infected with different doses of infected tick homogenate gave broadly similar results, although small differences were obtained in the calculated growth rate of parasitized cells in animals receiving different doses of parasites, smaller doses resulting in more rapid multiplication.

The studies reported by Jarrett *et al.* (1969) and Radley *et al.* (1974) relied on measurement of percentages of infected cells and therefore did not take account of changes in total numbers of cells in the lymphoid tissues. Morrison *et al.* (1981) reported the findings from experiments in which total content of cells and parasitized cells were determined for several lymphoid tissues harvested from pairs of animals slaughtered at 2-day intervals after infection with a lethal dose of sporozoites. Two groups of animals were used, Borans (*Bos indicus*) aged 10 months and Holsteins (*B. taurus*) aged 6 months. Data from these studies are summarized in Fig. 4.2.

The findings revealed a dramatic sudden increase in the weight and total cell content of the lymph node (Fig. 4.2A and 4.2B)

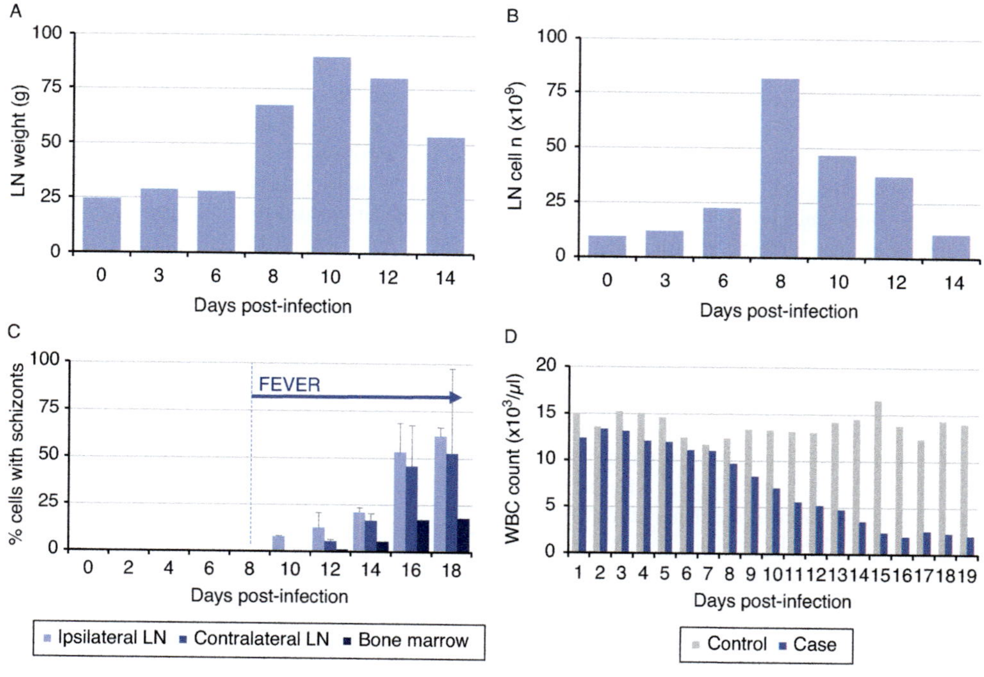

Fig. 4.2. Kinetics of infection in cattle infected with *T. parva*. A and B: Bar charts illustrating the temporal changes in organ weight and cellularity, respectively, of the prefemoral lymph node draining the site of infection. C: Temporal changes in the % of infected cells in the draining and contralateral prescapular lymph nodes, and in the bone marrow. D: Changes in blood leukocyte counts compared to uninfected control animals (*n*=2 per group at all time point; LN = lymph node).

draining the site of infection, coinciding with initial detection of parasites and the onset of fever. Cell numbers increased approximately eightfold in the Friesian animals and fourfold in the Borans, between days 6 and 8 after infection. Similar increases in cellularity, but of lower magnitude, were detected in other lymph nodes coinciding with initial detection of parasites. From day 12 onwards, there was a gradual decrease in cellularity of all lymphoid organs, leading to cellular depletion below normal levels in the later stages of the disease. Similar to results obtained in previous studies (Jarrett *et al.*, 1969; Radley *et al.*, 1974), the numbers of parasitized cells in all lymphoid tissues increased progressively following initial detection of parasites (Fig. 4.2c), and there was a phase of linear exponential growth during a period of about 6 days after the levels of parasitized cells reached 1%. However, a much more rapid increase in parasitized cells during the 2 days following initial detection of parasites was consistently observed in all four lymph nodes examined, indicating a more rapid multiplication of parasitized cells during this early period, equivalent to a doubling time for parasitized cells of <12 hour. There was also a decrease in the rate of parasite multiplication during the later stages of the infection, which is consistent with the occurrence of merogony in some infected cells accompanied by cessation of host cell proliferation. This trend towards a convex growth profile can also be discerned in the data on parasite levels shown by Jarrett *et al.* (1969) and would have compromised attempts by these authors to obtain an accurate estimate of the initial infective dose of parasites based on extrapolation of the parasite growth curves.

In separate experiments employing lymph duct cannulation techniques in animals infected with the same dose of parasites used by Morrison *et al.* (1981), efferent lymph draining from the regional lymph node showed cellular changes similar to those in the parent node (Emery, 1981). There was an abrupt increase in lymph flow and lymphocyte output in efferent lymph, which included numerous infected cells, in the period following initial detection of parasites. Depletion in the cell content of the lymph below resting levels was observed from day 16 onwards, and cannulation of the thoracic duct in infected animals revealed a similar profound progressive depletion of cellular content in the late stages of the infection.

4.7 Histological Changes in the Tissues of Infected Animals

The pathogenesis of ECF is linked fundamentally to the properties of the infected lymphocytes and their impact on the function and structural integrity of the lymphoid and haematopoietic tissues. The following discussion draws largely on findings from histological examination of samples obtained from the study reported by Morrison *et al.* (1981), some of which have been presented by Fry *et al.* (2016).

Immuno-staining of tissues from infected animals for parasites confirms a progressive increase in the numbers of infected cells in lymphoid tissues and in some non-lymphoid tissues, notably the lungs and intestinal mucosa, during the course of infection (Fig. 4.3).

Based on the cellular kinetics discussed above and histological findings, the disease resulting from infection with a lethal dose of *T. parva* can be considered to progress through three phases: 1. A preclinical phase during which parasites are undetectable and infected animals remain clinically normal. 2. A lymphoproliferative phase characterized by the onset of fever and initial detection of parasites followed by their dissemination throughout the lymphoid system. 3. A final phase of disorganization and cellular depletion of lymphoid tissues. As referred to above, the precise timing of these phases depends on the infective dose of parasites. The main histological and clinical findings during these phases of the infection are summarized in Fig. 4.4.

4.7.1 Secondary lymphoid tissues

4.7.1.1 The preclinical period

The difficulty in detecting parasites during the early stages of infection has precluded direct studies of the events occurring between inoculation of sporozoite by the tick and initial detection of macroschizonts. Early development

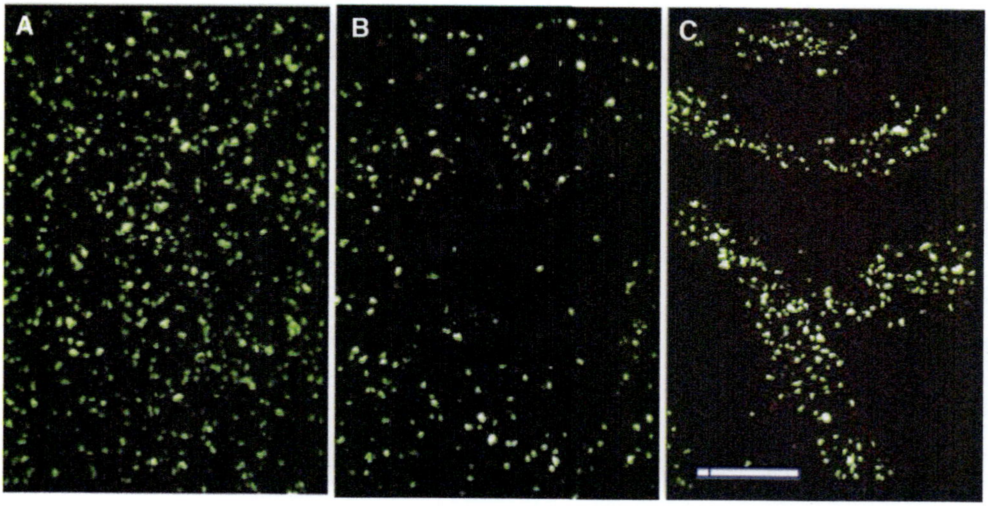

Fig. 4.3. Detection of *T. parva*-infected cells by immunofluorescence in tissue sections of lymph node (A), lung (B) and intestinal lamina propria (C), examined 16 days after infection. Scale bar (A, B and C): 100 μm at × 20.

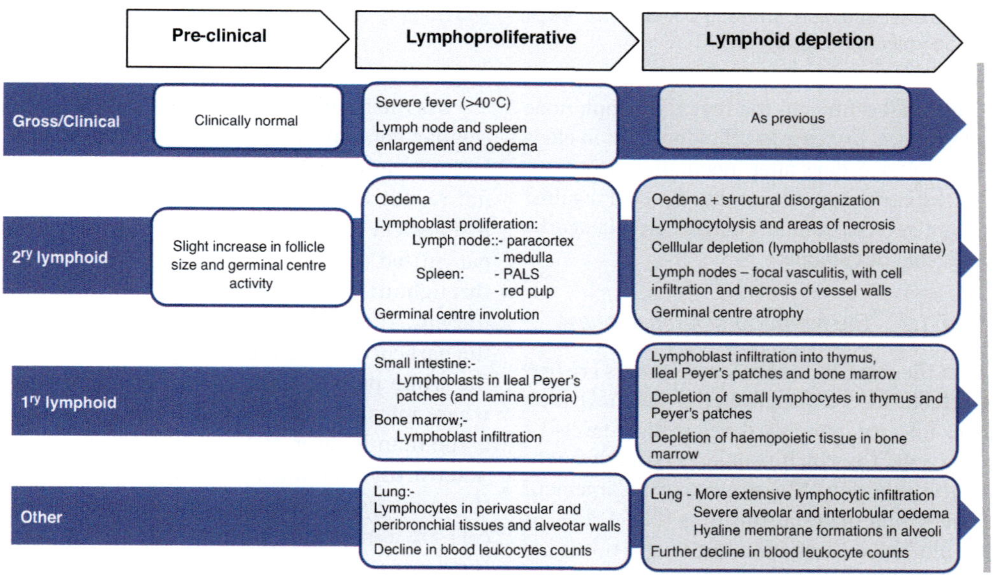

Fig. 4.4. Summary of the development of clinical and pathological changes in cattle during the different stages of infection with *T. parva*. (PALS = periarteriolar lymphocytic sheath.)

of the parasite after host cell invasion has been described in an *in vitro* study involving microscopic examination of lymphocytes over several days following incubation with saturating concentrations of sporozoites (Stagg *et al.*, 1981). During the first 48 h following invasion, sporozoites increased in size, with expansion of their cytoplasm and appearance of binucleate forms on the second day. Typical multinucleate schizonts were then detected on the third day.

In animals infected using tick homogenate, there is a moderate blast response with formation

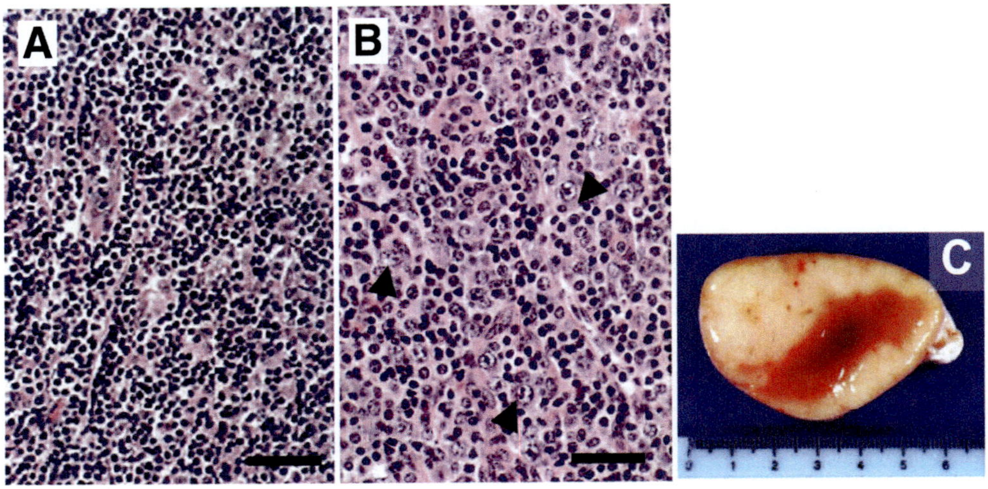

Fig. 4.5. Gross and histological images of lesion development in the lymph nodes after infection with *T. parva*. A: The paracortex of a lymph node from an uninfected animal, which is populated mostly by small lymphocytes. B: The paracortex of an animal at 9 days post-infection with *T. parva,* showing widespread presence of large lymphoblasts (arrowheads). (Haemotoxylin and eosin (H&E) stained section, scale bars: 50 um at × 40.) C: A transverse cut section of a prescapular lymph node examined 10 days after infection, showing oedematous swelling and bulging of cortical regions from the cut surface (ruler unit: 1 cm).

of germinal centres in the regional lymph node and a modest increase in cellular output in efferent lymph 4–5 days after inoculation. However, this response appears to be directed against tick antigens as similar changes are elicited by uninfected tick stabilate.

4.7.1.2 The lymphoproliferative phase

About the same time as macroschizonts are first detectable microscopically in the regional lymph node, infected animals develop high levels of fever (> 40°C), which usually persists throughout the infection. There is rapid enlargement of the lymph nodes at this time (Fig. 4.2A). At post-mortem examination, the lymph nodes are oedematous and the pale cortical areas bulge from cut surfaces of the nodes (Fig. 4.5C). A similar oedematous appearance with prominent white pulp follicles is observed in the spleen. Histologically, the increase in cellularity of the lymph nodes is associated with a progressive increase in the numbers of lymphoblasts, which are found throughout the paracortical areas (Fig. 4.5B, compared to healthy lymph node, Fig. 4.5A) and slightly later in the medullary cords.

As the numbers of blast cells increase, the cellular content of the sinuses increases and includes numerous lymphoblasts. Parasites are not readily detected in conventionally stained histological sections but immuno-labelling of parasitized cells reveals that they are present throughout the lymph nodes and spleen. Initially, they tend to be more numerous in the paracortical areas of the lymph nodes and the white pulp of the spleen. The one region where infected cells are much less numerous is the mantle layer of the B cell follicles. It is noteworthy that during the early stages when the numbers of parasites are low, the infected cells are disseminated individually throughout the tissues, rather than appearing as clusters, indicating that they are motile within the lymphoid organs. Comparison of the histological and immuno-histological findings at each time point indicates that the lymphoblasts detected by conventional histology substantially outnumber the infected cells detected by immunohistology, demonstrating that there is a strong cellular response to the infection (discussed further below). Histological evidence of a proliferative response of uninfected cells was also reported by DeMartini and Moulton (1973). Despite this indication of an immunological response within the lymph nodes, there is little evidence of a germinal centre response in the B cell follicles, which might be expected given the obvious antigenic challenge of the infection. Resting lymph nodes of cattle often contain numerous large active germinal centres, and this is apparent in *T. parva*-infected animals during the preclinical phase of infection. However, following detection of parasites, there is a striking decrease in the size of the B cell follicles, and the germinal centres are smaller and less active.

Similar changes are observed in the spleen, in which there is a progressive increase in the number of lymphoblasts in the periarteriolar lymphocytic sheath compartment of the white pulp, and a decrease in the size of B cell follicles and germinal centres. The numbers of lymphoblasts in the red pulp also progressively increase.

4.7.1.3 Lymphoid disorganization and depletion

Once parasitized cells reach levels of 5–10% in the lymph nodes and spleen (approximately 4–5 days after initial detection of parasites in the regional node), there is a progressive disruption of the normal cellular organization of the tissues. The percentage of parasitized cells continues to increase, reaching levels that may exceed 50%, and lymphoblasts gradually become the predominant cell type in the lymph nodes and spleen. At the same time, there is a gradual decrease in total cellularity of the tissues, eventually leading to severe cellular depletion during the later stages of the infection (Fig. 4.2B). Focal areas of lymphocytolysis are detectable 4–5 days after initial detection of parasites, becoming more extensive later, and in the terminal stages some lymph nodes contain focally extensive areas of oedema and liquefactive necrosis with fibrin deposition, which clearly involves non-parasitized resident cells as well as infected cells (Figs 4.6 and 4.7).

There is infiltration of mononuclear cells into the walls of some blood vessels, which appears to have occurred by invasion from the perivascular spaces. In areas of lymphocytolysis and cellular depletion, intramural infiltration of mononuclear cells in some small-calibre arterioles is accompanied by the presence of eosinophilic material, which stains red with Martius Scarlet Blue (indicating fibrinoid necrosis) (Fig. 4.8). These lesions are likely the result of impaired regional vascular supply causing hypoxia, which may contribute to the areas of fibrinoid necrosis within the lymph nodes.

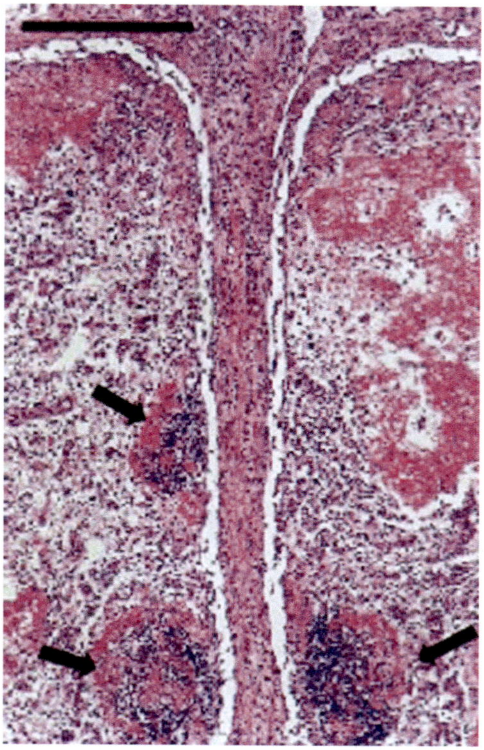

Fig. 4.6. Outer cortex of lymph node examined 17 days after infection with *T. parva*, showing profound cellular depletion and extensive areas of necrosis. Arrows indicate remnants of B cell follicles. Scale bar: 100 μm at × 20.

There is continued involution of the B cell follicles, which in terminal cases are often no longer distinguishable from the surrounding areas. Some lymph nodes at this stage remain structurally intact, but different regions of the node are largely indistinguishable and sparsely

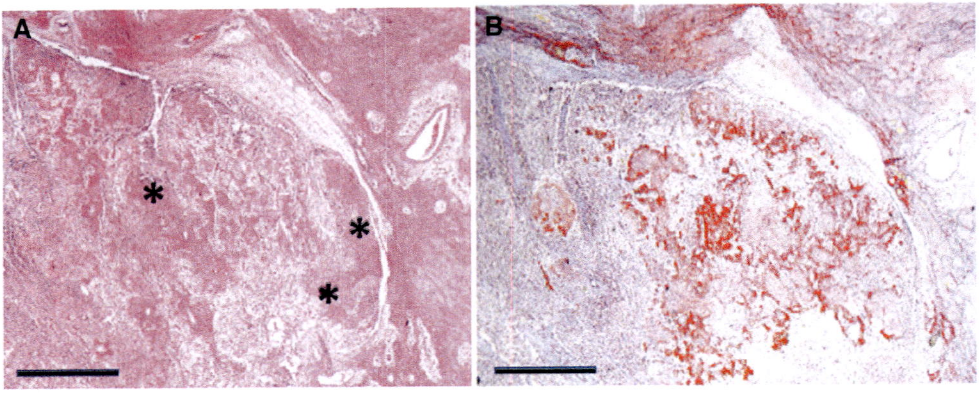

Fig. 4.7. Histological images of the cortex of a lymph node from an animal infected with *T. parva* examined 16 days post-infection. A: Marked cellular depletion and large areas of necrosis (*) in a section stained by H&E. B: A section from the same lymph node, showing intralesional fibrin deposits, stained red with Martius Scarlet Blue stain. Scale bar: 500 µm at × 4.

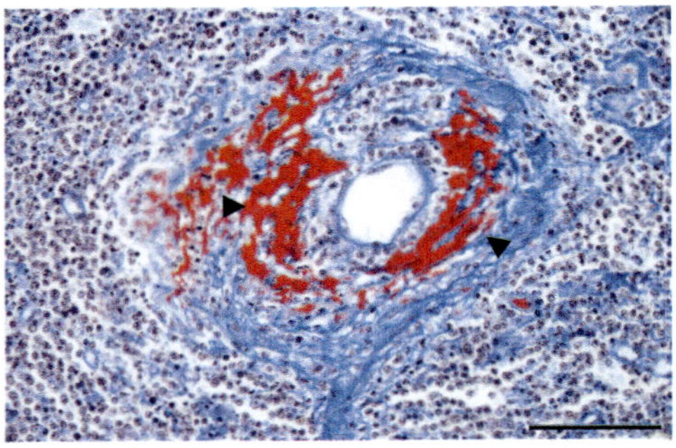

Fig. 4.8. Histological image of a blood vessel in the lymph node cortex of an animal infected with *T. parva* at 19 days post-infection, illustrating extensive cellular infiltration and fibril deposits (arrowheads) in the vessel wall. Martius Scarlet Blue stain, scale bar: 50 µm at × 40.

populated by lymphoblasts interspersed with macrophages throughout the tissue.

4.7.2 Primary lymphoid tissues

Infection with *T. parva* has a profound impact on primary as well as secondary lymphoid tissues. A number of early studies reported a progressive decrease in blood leukocyte counts in infected cattle (Steck, 1928; Wilde, 1967). This finding was confirmed in studies reported by Morrison *et al.* (1981) and Maxie *et al.* (1982), who showed that blood leukocyte counts started to decline just after initial detection of parasites, eventually resulting in levels at least fourfold below normal levels in the terminal stages of the disease (Fig. 4.2D). Leukopaenia involved both mononuclear and granulocytic lineages.

A number of early studies reported changes in bone marrow of infected cattle (Cowdry and Danks, 1933; Barnett, 1957; De Kock, 1957), including the detection of infected lymphocytes. Morrison *et al.* (1981) detected infected cells in bone marrow from day 10 onwards, reaching >10% in the late stages of the disease (Fig. 4.2C), and histological sections from the same animals revealed areas of bone marrow devoid of erythroid and granulocyte precursors and containing predominantly lymphoblast-like cells. Wilde (1966) examined the cytological profiles of bone marrow cells from a series of experimentally infected animals. His findings showed an increase in the percentages of lymphoid cells in the marrow and a relative decrease in more mature granulocytic cells, suggesting arrested maturation of the granulocytic lineage. As reported by Mbassa *et al.* (2006), cell lysis and profound involution of thymic tissue also occur during the patent phases of infection, and in the later stages, the thymus is completely devoid of the small lymphocytes that normally populate the organ (Fig. 4.9).

In ruminants, the ileal Peyer's patch, found in the terminal ileum, is considered to be a

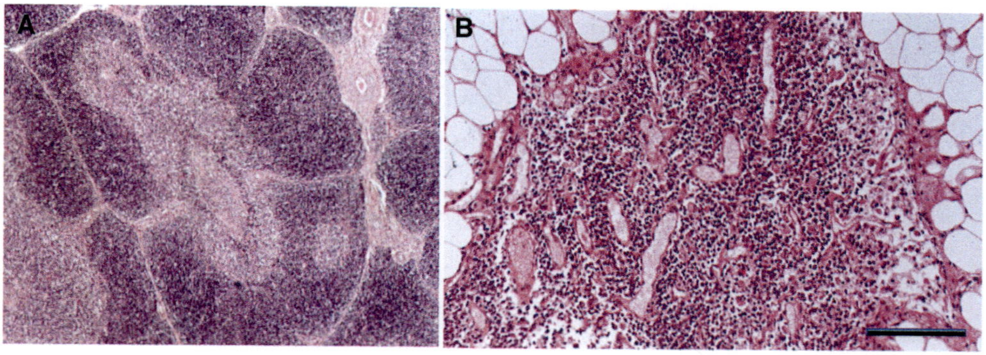

Fig. 4.9. Histological sections of thymus stained by H&E. A: Low magnification image of thymus from a healthy animal, showing large darkly stained cortical areas densely populated by small lymphocytes. B: A thymic lobe examined 18 days post-infection with *T. parva* showing marked cellular depletion and no distinction between cortical and medullary areas. Scale bar: 50 µm at × 20.

primary lymphoid tissue in which diversification of the B cell immunoglobulin repertoire occurs (Reynaud *et al.*, 1991; Yasuda *et al.*, 2006). The Peyer's patch follicles are infiltrated by *T. parva*-infected cells and become progressively disorganized and depleted as the disease progresses. Cell lysis and necrosis of some follicles are also observed.

These changes in primary haemopoietic tissues account for the observed early decline in blood leukocyte counts. Although infected animals show a small decrease in packed red cell volume, anaemia is not a significant clinical feature of the disease. The longer half-life of erythrocytes compared to leukocytes probably accounts for the more limited impact of bone marrow changes on erythrocyte counts.

4.7.3 Non-lymphoid tissues

A key property of normal lymphocytes is their ability to recirculate through lymphoid tissues, enabling them to respond to antigenic challenge, and to migrate as effector cells into peripheral tissues. *T. parva*-infected cells appear to retain these properties, since they rapidly disseminate throughout the lymphoid system and are found in abundance in other tissues through which lymphocytes frequently migrate. Organs of particular significance are the gastrointestinal tract and the lungs, the latter being centrally involved in the pathogenesis of ECF.

There is diffuse infiltration by infected lymphoblasts into the *lamina propria* of the intestines and the Peyer's patches and, in common with other lymphoid tissues, the Peyer's patches undergo severe lymphocyte depletion during the later stages of the disease.

In the lungs, parasitized cells infiltrate alveolar walls and the peribronchiolar and perivascular connective tissue. The numbers of infected cells increase over time, and in the later stages they are also found infiltrating perivascular tissues and interlobular septae. Pulmonary oedema is a prominent feature of the late stages of the disease, with exudation of proteinaceous fluid into the alveolar spaces and the pulmonary interstitium. In the terminal stages, there is often widespread hyaline membrane formation in the alveolar spaces, which, coupled with the intra-alveolar oedema, accounts for the respiratory distress suffered by affected animals (Fig. 4.10).

The course of clinical respiratory symptoms is variable; it may occur acutely within the last 24 h before death of the animal or develop progressively over several days. It is the latter cases that frequently show intra-alveolar hyaline membrane formation, with occasional superimposed multifocal hyperplasia of type II pneumocytes (epithelialization of the alveolar epithelium). Animals that have died from ECF usually present a characteristic picture of copious frothy fluid exuding from the nostrils (Fig. 4.11A). At post-mortem examination, the trachea and bronchi are filled with this frothy fluid and there is massive

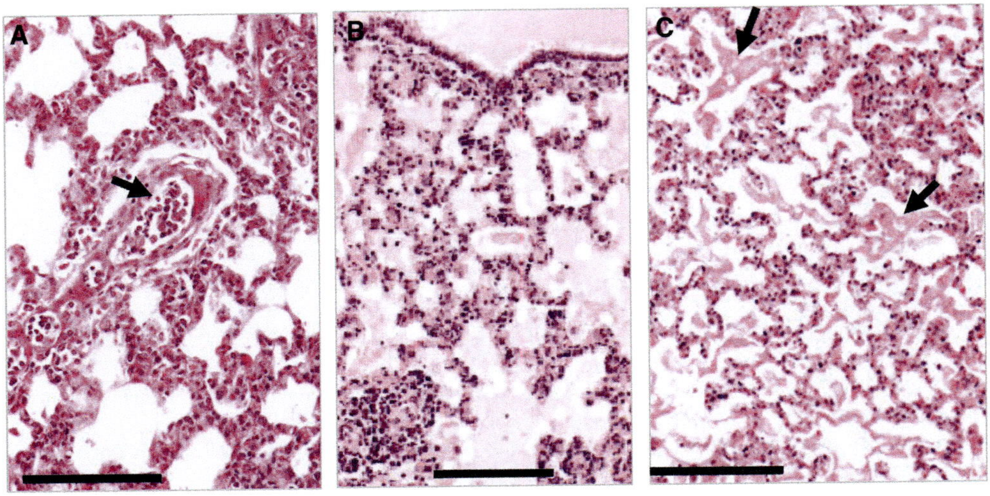

Fig. 4.10. Illustration of the pathological changes in the lungs of animals infected with *T. parva* at 18 days post-infection. A: Thickening of alveolar walls due to infiltration by lymphoblasts and intravascular accumulations of lymphoblasts. B: Extensive (pink) oedema fluid within the lung alveoli. C: Widespread intra-alveolar hyaline membrane formation (arrows). (H&E stain, scale bars: A and B: 50 µm at × 40; C: 100 µm at × 20.)

oedema throughout the lungs, with pronounced separation of the interlobular septae with oedema fluid and copious fluid in the thoracic cavity (Fig. 4.11B and 4.11C).

Lesions have been reported in other tissues, including the kidneys, liver, eyes and skin (Cowdry and Danks, 1933; Uilenberg and Zwart, 1979). However, the degree to which they are involved varies between animals and they do not appear to play a major role in development of the clinical disease. As discussed earlier, parasitized cells tend to follow the migration patterns of normal lymphocytes and therefore the occurrence of lesions in some of these tissues may arise partly from infiltration of infected cells into pre-existing sites of inflammation.

4.8 The Clinical Disease

4.8.1 Clinical features

In susceptible breeds of cattle introduced into ECF-endemic areas in the absence of any preventative measures, the morbidity rate due to ECF may approach 100% and mortality can exceed 90%, although these figures are often lower in areas where parasite challenge is lower. As indicated in the above discussion, the main clinical signs of disease are elevated body temperature and enlargement of lymph nodes, which are apparent as soon as parasites become detectable, followed later by respiratory signs (Irvin and Mwamachi, 1983). In the field, fever and lymph node enlargement may be detectable 12–14 days after exposure to tick challenge and, since *R. appendiculatus* ticks have a predilection to feed on the ears of cattle, lymph node enlargement is usually first apparent in the local draining parotid nodes. Enlargement of other superficial lymph nodes (prescapular and prefemoral) follows a few days later. Fever often exceeds 41°C and is sustained until the terminal stages of the disease. An increase in respiratory rate occurs, usually 5–7 days after fever develops, and thereafter progresses to respiratory distress. Auscultation of the thorax reveals harsh respiratory sounds and evidence of pulmonary oedema. Animals may die after a brief acute respiratory episode or may survive for 2–5 days before succumbing. Terminally, oedema fluid may drip from the nostrils, and animals that have died are often found with frothy oedema fluid exuding from the nostrils.

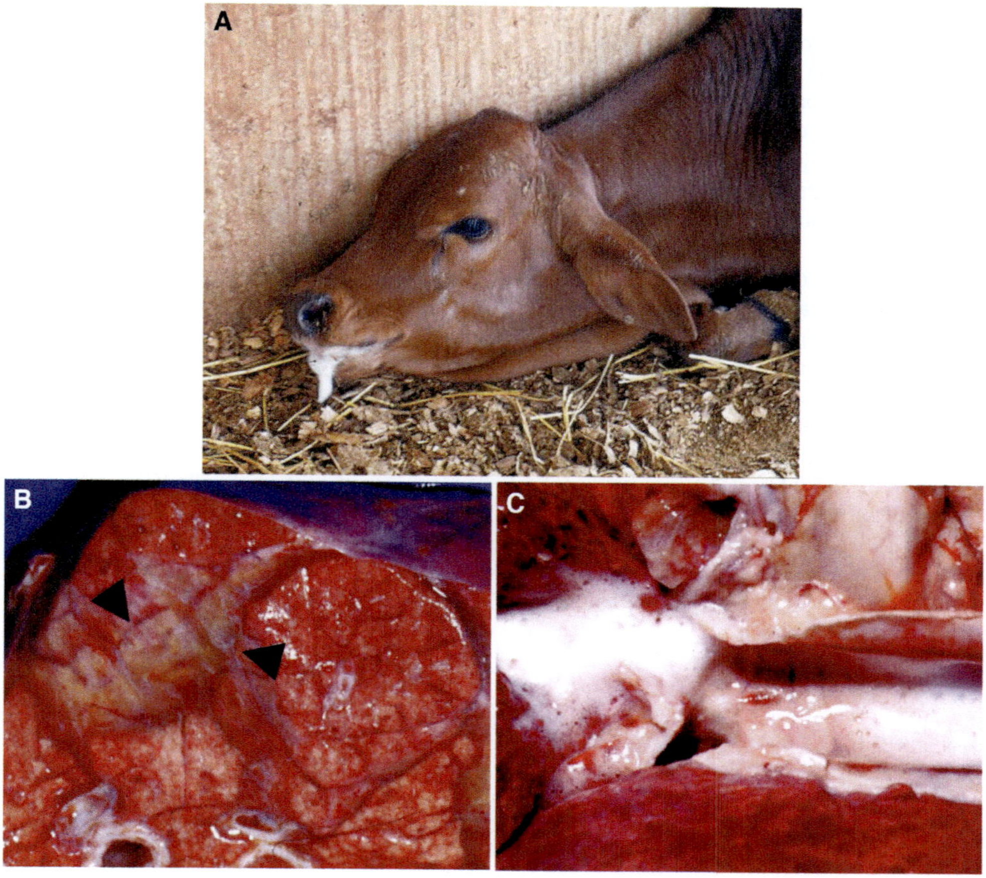

Fig. 4.11. Clinical and gross changes in the respiratory tract of animals in the advanced stages of infection with *T. parva*. A. Frothy fluid exuding from nostrils and mouth of an animal in the terminal stages of the disease. B. Greyish-pink consolidation of the lung tissue, with extensive oedema of the interlobular septae (arrowheads). C. Copious amounts of white, frothy fluid in the airways.

During the febrile phase of the disease, affected animals show a progressive loss of appetite and eventually become dull and listless, accompanied by loss of bodily condition and depressed milk yield in lactating animals. Some animals develop diarrhoea during the later stages of the disease. Examination of blood samples reveals a severe leukopoenia affecting both mononuclear and granulocytic cells.

4.8.2 The cause of death

The cause of death in the majority of cases of ECF is respiratory failure due to pulmonary oedema. However, if infected animals were not to develop respiratory symptoms, they would almost certainly succumb as a result of destruction of their immune system rendering them susceptible to secondary infections. As evidence of loss of immune competence, failure to induce an antibody response to rinderpest vaccination has been observed in animals vaccinated following infection with a lethal dose of *T. parva* (Wagner *et al.*, 1975). Since animals residing in tick-infested areas frequently develop carrier infections with other tick-borne pathogens such as *Babesia* and *Anaplasma*, the immunocompromised state of animals suffering ECF may facilitate recrudescence of these and other infections, complicating the pathology of the disease. In this regard, some accounts of ECF describe jaundice as a symptom of the disease. However, in the authors' experience, using animals screened prior to infection as free from other tick-borne diseases, jaundice has never been observed as a feature of the disease caused by *T. parva* alone.

The immunocompromised state of *T. parva*-infected animals is also an important issue in the application of chemotherapy. The theilericidal compound buparvaquone is the treatment of choice for ECF (Dolan, 1986; Muraguri *et al.*, 1999). Although effective when applied during the early clinical stages of the disease, it is often ineffective in the later stages because of the destructive nature of the disease on the immune system. The authors have observed deaths due to fungal pneumonia and infectious bovine rhinotracheitis in cases of ECF undergoing treatment with buparvaquone.

4.9 The Nature of the Early Cellular Response to Infection

Histological findings have indicated that the early cellular changes in the lymph nodes of infected animals reflect not only rapid expansion of the infected cell population but also a potent blastogenic response by uninfected lymphocytes. However, relatively little research effort has been directed to investigating this aspect of the disease. An analysis of the phenotype of cells aspirated from the regional lymph node of animals infected with *T. parva* has demonstrated that infection induces a strong early T cell response in the regional lymph node coinciding with initial detection of parasites (Houston *et al.*, 2008). By day 9 after infection, when the level of infected cells had reached about 1%, the regional node contained 15–25% lymphoblasts. There was a dramatic increase in the content of CD8$^+$ T cells, which represented 60–70% of the total cells by day 9, resulting in a decrease in the CD4:CD8 T cell ratio. In contrast to the cytotoxic T cell responses detected in lymph node cells from immune cattle undergoing parasite challenge, the lymph node cells from naïve animals did not exhibit any specific cytotoxic activity against autologous *T. parva*-infected cells (Houston *et al.*, 2008). This early cellular response exhibited a number of unusual features. First, the CD8$^+$ population included ~70% of cells that lacked expression of CD2, a phenotype that is uncommon in resting or antigen-specific T cell populations. Purified populations of these cells were unresponsive *in vitro* to stimulation with autologous *T. parva*-infected cells, with or without added cytokines, and also failed to respond to non-specific stimulation with phorbol myristyl acetate (PMA) and ionomycin. By contrast, purified CD2$^+$ CD8$^+$ T cells proliferated in these assays, although the stimulated cells did not display cytotoxic activity against *T. parva*-infected cells (Houston *et al.*, 2008). Thus, a large population of activated CD8$^+$cells in the regional lymph node appear to be anergic (as assessed by *in vitro* stimulation), suggesting that there is dysregulation of the immune response to the parasite. Given that the presence of these responding T cells coincides with a period of rapid multiplication of the infected cells, they clearly lack any effector activity against the parasitized cells.

The same study detected expression of interferon-gamma (IFNγ) and IL-10 by lymph node cells 7–9 days after infection (Houston *et al.*, 2008). The CD2$^-$ CD8$^+$ and CD2$^+$ CD8$^+$ populations both produced IFNγ. Although IFNγ is an important effector against viral infections and some other intracellular parasites (Schofield *et al.*, 1987; Nishiyama *et al.*, 2020), it has no obvious inhibitory effect on the viability or growth of *T. parva* or the infected host cells (DeMartini and Baldwin, 1991), and indeed some parasitized cells themselves produce IFNγ (Ahmed *et al.*, 1993; McKeever *et al.*, 1997). The cellular source of IL-10 detected by Houston *et al.* (2008) was not identified. Despite the presence of large numbers of activated T cells in the lymph node, there was no discernible increase in IL-2 expression above control levels. A similar absence of an IL-2 response in PBM from *T. parva*-infected animals has also been reported (Yamada *et al.*, 2009).

The expression of cytokines by *T. parva*-infected cells in the tissues of infected animals has not been investigated. However, infected cell lines established *in vitro* have been shown to express a number of cytokines. In a study using a panel of 19 *T. parva*-infected cell lines, which included CD4, CD8 and γδ T cells and B cells, McKeever *et al.* (1997) examined transcripts for seven cytokines (IL-1β, IL-2, IL-4, IL-6, IL-10, TNFα and IFNγ). Overall, different cell lines showed variable cytokine expression profiles: IL-1β and IL-4 were not detected in any of the lines, abundant IL-10 transcripts were found in all of the lines and the other cytokines were detected in only some of the lines. There was no obvious correlation of cytokine profiles with the lineage of the infected cells. Studies of soluble mediators that influence the growth of infected cells have shown that addition of recombinant IL-2 enhances the growth of infected cell lines *in vitro* (DeMartini and Baldwin, 1991), particularly when cells are seeded at low cell densities. IL-2 has also been shown to increase the efficiency of infection of PBM with sporozoites *in vitro* (Shaw *et al.*, 1995). Earlier studies had identified IL-2-like activity in supernatants of some infected cell lines and detected expression of the IL-2 receptor on infected cells (Brown and Logan, 1986; Dobbelaere *et al.*, 1988), leading the authors to propose that IL-2 may act in an autocrine manner to potentiate the growth of infected cells. However, although some cell lines express low levels of transcripts for IL-2, production of IL-2 protein has not been confirmed (discussed in Ahmed *et al.*, 1999). Evidence that enhanced proliferation of *T. parva*-infected cells by cytokines can occur via an autocrine loop has been obtained for TNF-β (Guergnon *et al.*, 2003) and GM-CSF (Baumgartner *et al.*, 2000). In both cases, production of the cytokine was confirmed for the cell lines studied, and suppression of expression of the cytokines was shown to result in decreased proliferation of the cells. While these and other cytokines may well act in an autocrine manner to enhance growth of the infected cells *in vivo*, particularly during the early stages of infection, exogenous cytokines generated from the initial T cell response to the parasite are likely to have a greater impact on potentiating the growth of the infected cells, as suggested by the observed phase of very rapid growth of infected cells coinciding with the early vigorous T cell response in the lymph nodes.

More detailed information is required on the role of cytokines in modulating the growth of cells infected with *T. parva*. The most striking finding from the available data is the consistent expression of abundant IL-10 by infected cell lines and by lymph node cells from infected animals. IL-10 is a regulatory cytokine produced in a feedback response to strong IFN-γ and IL-12 responses, which has been shown to suppress Th1 T cell responses (Jankovic *et al.*, 2010), and is therefore likely to have a role in modulating the effector immune response to *T. parva*.

4.10 Mechanisms Involved in Late-Stage Pathology

Given the complexity of the pathological changes during the advanced stages of ECF, it is difficult to draw clear-cut conclusions regarding the underlying mechanisms. There has also been a paucity of research directed to dissecting this stage of the disease process.

4.10.1 Cellular depletion

The profound cellular depletion in lymphoid tissues involves involution of primary haemopoietic tissues as well as destruction of lymphocytes. The early decline of blood leukocytes, coupled with detection of parasitized cells in the bone marrow and evidence of curtailed granulopoiesis, indicates that the presence of infected cells imposes a suppressive effect on haemopoiesis. However, the factors that mediate this effect have not been investigated. While the development of merogony in infected lymphoid cells results in some destruction of cells within the lymphoid tissues, there is clearly also extensive cell death of uninfected lymphocytes. PBM harvested from infected cattle 14–18 days after infection have been shown to display non-specific killer cell (NK-like) cytotoxic activity (Emery *et al.*, 1981), and infected cells have been shown to stimulate activation of NK cells *in vitro* (Longhi, 2009). However, the contribution that these cells make to the cell death observed *in vivo* remains to be determined. As discussed above, there is evidence that a component of the early T cell response to the parasite may be driven into terminal differentiation, which may also contribute to the loss of cells from lymphoid tissues.

4.10.2 Impairment of immune responses

Despite the early potent T cell proliferative response to the infection, there is no evidence of induction of an effective immune response capable of restraining growth of the parasite. Available data also indicate that animals suffering fatal ECF rarely generate antibody responses to the parasite (Shitakha *et al.*, 1983) and also fail to respond to rinderpest vaccination (Wagner *et al.*, 1975). There is clear histological evidence of impairment of B cell function, visible as progressive profound involution of B cell follicles and disappearance of active germinal centres in the lymph nodes and spleen. While the mechanisms underlying these defects remain to be investigated, the production of IL-10 in infected lymph nodes, including expression by the infected cells, is likely to be involved in modulating immune responses. IL-10 can be produced by different cell types, including subsets of macrophages and lymphocytes, and has an important role in regulating pro-inflammatory responses. It is produced in a feedback response to strong Th1-type T cell responses, but, in addition to counteracting potentially damaging inflammatory effects, can suppress T cell responses (Jankovic *et al.*, 2010; Cyktor and Turner, 2011). Strong IL-10 responses are induced by several other intracellular parasites, including *Toxoplasma* and *Leishmania*, and have been implicated in suppression of the specific immune responses and favouring persistence of infection (Suzuki *et al.*, 2000; Nylén and Sacks, 2007). Fry *et al.* (2016) have described numerous CD163$^+$ macrophages in the lungs of cattle in the terminal stages of ECF. The human scavenger receptor, CD163, is expressed at high levels on mature actively phagocytic tissue macrophages found in sites of chronic inflammation and in some tumour tissues (Fabriek *et al.*, 2005). It is one of the markers expressed on the M2 subset of human macrophages, which have been shown to have immunosuppressive activity and have been described in some chronic protozoal infections (Tomioka *et al.*, 2012; Pinto *et al.*, 2019). Interestingly, IL-10 is involved in upregulating expression of CD163 (Buechler *et al.*, 2000).

4.10.3 An inflammatory response

Although there is evidence of a strong inflammatory response leading to extensive vascular permeability and oedema during the later stages of ECF, almost nothing is known about the factors that are responsible. Depressed levels of total complement and C3 have been reported, but no *T. parva*-specific antibody or immune complexes were detected (Shitakha *et al.*, 1983). It is possible that parasite products or the products of dying cells may be responsible for direct stimulation of inflammatory responses. The study by Fry *et al.* (2016) referred to above detected expression of the pro-inflammatory cytokine IL-17 in some of the CD163$^+$ macrophages found in ECF lungs. This cytokine has been detected in the alveolar macrophages of human asthma patients, in which it is implicated as a mediator of the inflammatory response (Song *et al.*, 2008). While these responses may all contribute to the pathology observed in advanced cases of ECF, they may represent the secondary consequences of other earlier events.

4.11 Concluding Remarks

The capacity of *T. parva* to induce transformation of infected cells is an important factor in the ability of the parasite to cause disease, and some early studies suggested that rapid multiplication of parasitized cells simply outpaces the ability to mount an effective immune response. However, it is now clear that host cell transformation on its own is not sufficient to account for pathogenicity of the parasite. Firstly, although *T. parva* efficiently transforms bovine T cells and B cells, infected B cells do not appear to play an important role in the disease, and purified B cells infected *in vitro* with *T. parva* produce a transient self-limiting infection when administered to autologous animals (Morrison *et al.*, 1996). Secondly, *T. parva* readily infects and transforms buffalo cells, but infection is non-pathogenic in that species (Morrison *et al.*, 2020). Baldwin *et al.* (1986) showed that sporozoites bind to similar percentages of bovine and buffalo PBM and, by comparing the level of transformation in cultures of cattle and buffalo cells infected at limiting dilution with cattle-derived or buffalo-derived isolates, showed that although the levels of transformation were significantly higher with parasite isolates of the homologous species origin, the level of transformation of buffalo and cattle cells with their respective parasites was similar. The different disease outcomes in the two host species must therefore be due to differences in the nature of the host responses to the parasite.

Analyses of the cellular changes in the lymph nodes of infected cattle have demonstrated a strong early T cell response, but this response lacks effector function and appears to be highly dysregulated. Dysregulation of the primary immune response to the parasite, by allowing unrestrained growth of parasitized cells, appears to be a key determinant of the pathogenesis of the disease, dictating the subsequent pathological consequences of infection. However, if growth of the parasitized cells is curtailed, as occurs in cattle vaccinated by infection and treatment, recovery from infection occurs and results in development of robust immunity (Radley *et al.*, 1975). Unlike many other intracellular pathogens, which attempt to 'hide' from the immune response within infected cells, *T. parva*-infected cells display strong immunostimulatory properties. Surface expression of class I and class II MHC proteins, as well as co-stimulatory proteins such as CD80 and CD40, are upregulated on *Theileria*-infected cells (DeMartini *et al.*, 1993; Hart *et al.*, 2011), and infected cells have been shown to be efficient antigen-presenting cells *in vitro* (Goddeeris and Morrison, 1988; Hart *et al.*, 2011). They can be used as stimulator cells to recall parasite-specific T cells *in vitro* from the blood of immune cattle, in the absence of added antigen-presenting cells (Taracha *et al.*, 1997). Thus, the parasite is able to dictate the type of immune response it induces and, at least in cattle, is able to dysregulate the immune response.

The properties of *T. parva* that result in modulation of the immune response must have evolved to provide a selective advantage for survival in the parasite. Primary exposure of the natural buffalo host results in a mild transient infection and development of immunity, although a carrier state is established with persistence of low levels of parasites (Grootenhuis *et al.*, 1987). Further challenge of immune animals also results in the challenge parasites establishing infections resulting in carrier infections containing mixed *T. parva* genotypes (Hemmink *et al.*, 2018). Such persistent infections, by allowing frequent tick transmission, are required to ensure maintenance of parasite populations in the field, and they facilitate sexual recombination between genotypically different strains in feeding ticks (Katzer *et al.*, 2011). The immunomodulatory activity of *T. parva* may have co-evolved with the buffalo to subtly modify the immune response in order to delay development of immunity and facilitate establishment of carrier infections. However, since cattle have been introduced relatively recently into Africa (Hanotte *et al.*, 2002), they have not had sufficient time to adapt to co-existing with the parasite and therefore generate an unbalanced and inappropriate immune response to infection.

References

Ahmed, J.S., Wiegers, P., Steuber, S., Schein, E., Williams, R.O. *et al.* (1993) Production of interferon by *Theileria annulata*- and *T. parva*-infected bovine lymphoid cell lines. *Parasitology Research* 79(3), 178–182. DOI: 10.1007/BF00931888.

Ahmed, J.S., Schnittger, L. and Mehlhorn, H. (1999) Review: *Theileria* schizonts induce fundamental alterations in their host cells. *Parasitology Research* 85(7), 527–538. DOI: 10.1007/s004360050592.

Baldwin, C.L., Malu, M.N., Kinuthia, S.W., Conrad, P.A. and Grootenhuis, J.G. (1986) Comparative analysis of infection and transformation of lymphocytes from African buffalo and boran cattle with *Theileria parva subsp. parva* and *T. parva* subsp. lawrencei. *Infection and Immunity* 53(1), 186–191. DOI: 10.1128/iai.53.1.186-191.1986.

Baldwin, C.L., Black, S.J., Brown, W.C., Conrad, P.A., Goddeeris, B.M. *et al.* (1988) Bovine T cells, B cells, and null cells are transformed by the protozoan parasite *Theileria parva*. *Infection and Immunity* 56(2), 462–467. DOI: 10.1128/iai.56.2.462-467.1988.
Barnett, S.F. (1957) Theileriasis control. *Bulletin of Epizootic Diseases in Africa* 5, 343–357.
Barnett, S.F. (1960) Connective tissue reactions in acute fatal East Coast fever (*Theileria parva*) of cattle. *The Journal of Infectious Diseases* 107, 253–282. DOI: 10.1093/infdis/107.3.253.
Barnett, S.F. and Brocklesby, D.W. (1966) Recent investigations into *Theileridae* of cattle and buffalo in Africa: A mild form of East Coast fever (*Theileria parva*) with persistence of infection. *British Veterinary Journal* 122, 361–371. DOI: 10.1016/S0007-1935(17)40402-7.
Baumgartner, M., Chaussepied, M., Moreau, M.-F., Werling, D., Davis, W.C. *et al.* (2000) Constitutive PI3-K activity is essential for proliferation but not survival of *Theileria parva*-transformed B cells. *Cellular Microbiology* 2, 329–339. DOI: 10.1046/j.1462-5822.2000.00062.x.
Brown, W.C. and Logan, K.S. (1986) Bovine t-cell clones infected with *Theileria parva* produce a factor with IL 2-like activity. *Parasite Immunology* 8(2), 189–192. DOI: 10.1111/j.1365-3024.1986.tb00844.x.
Brown, C.G., Stagg, D.A., Purnell, R.E., Kanhai, G.K. and Payne, R.C. (1973) Infection and transformation of bovine lymphoid cells *in vitro* by infective particles of *Theileria parva*. *Letter. Nature* 245(5420), 101–103. DOI: 10.1038/245101a0.
Buechler, C., Ritter, M., Orsó, E., Langmann, T., Klucken, J. *et al.* (2000) Regulation of scavenger receptor CD163 expression in human monocytes and macrophages by pro- and antiinflammatory stimuli. *Journal of Leukocyte Biology* 67(1), 97–103.
Büscher, G. and Otim, B. (1986) Quantitative studies on *Theileria parva* in the salivary glands of *Rhipicephalus appendiculatus* adults: Quantitation and prediction of infection. *International Journal for Parasitology* 16(1), 93–100. DOI: 10.1016/0020-7519(86)90071-8.
Cowdry, E.V. and Danks, W.B.C. (1933) Studies on East Coast fever. II. Behaviour of the parasite and the development of distinctive lesions in susceptible animals. *Parasitology* 25(1), 1–63. DOI: 10.1017/S003118200001920X.
Cunningham, M.P., Brown, C.G., Burridge, M.J. and Purnell, R.E. (1973) Cryopreservation of infective particles of *Theileria parva*. *International Journal for Parasitology* 3(5), 583–587. DOI: 10.1016/0020-7519(73)90082-9.
Cunningham, M.P., Brown, C.G., Burridge, M.J., Musoke, A.J., Purnell, R.E. *et al.* (1974) East coast fever: Titration in cattle of suspensions of *Theileria parva* derived from ticks. *The British Veterinary Journal* 130(4), 336–345. DOI: 10.1016/s0007-1935(17)35836-0.
Cyktor, J.C. and Turner, J. (2011) Interleukin-10 and immunity against prokaryotic and eukaryotic intracellular pathogens. *Infection and Immunity* 79(8), 2964–2973. DOI: 10.1128/IAI.00047-11.
De Kock, G. (1957) Studies on the lesions and pathogenesis of East Coast fever (*Theileria parva* infection) in cattle with special reference to the lymphoid tissue. *Onderstepoort Journal of Veterinary Research* 27, 431–452.
DeMartini, J.C. and Moulton, J.E. (1973) Responses of the bovine lymphatic system to infection by *Theileria parva*. *Journal of Comparative Pathology* 83(3), 299–306. DOI: 10.1016/0021-9975(73)90054-6.
DeMartini, J.C. and Baldwin, C.L. (1991) Effects of gamma interferon, tumor necrosis factor alpha, and interleukin-2 on infection and proliferation of *Theileria parva*-infected bovine lymphoblasts and production of interferon by parasitized cells. *Infection and Immunity* 59(12), 4540–4546. DOI: 10.1128/iai.59.12.4540-4546.1991.
DeMartini, J.C., MacHugh, N.D., Naessens, J. and Teale, A.J. (1993) Differential *in vitro* and *in vivo* expression of MHC class II antigens in bovine lymphocytes infected by *Theileria parva*. *Veterinary Immunology and Immunopathology* 35(3–4), 253–273. DOI: 10.1016/0165-2427(93)90038-6.
Dobbelaere, D.A., Coquerelle, T.M., Roditi, I.J., Eichhorn, M. and Williams, R.O. (1988) *Theileria parva* infection induces autocrine growth of bovine lymphocytes. *Proceedings of the National Academy of Sciences USA* 85(13), 4730–4734. DOI: 10.1073/pnas.85.13.4730.
Dolan, T.T. (1986) Chemotherapy of east coast fever: The long term weight changes, carrier state and disease manifestations of parvaquone treated cattle. *Journal of Comparative Pathology* 96(2), 137–146. DOI: 10.1016/0021-9975(86)90004-6.
Emery, D.L. (1981) Kinetics of infection with *Theileria parva* (East Coast Fever) in the central lymph of cattle. *Veterinary Parasitology* 9(1), 1–16. DOI: 10.1016/0304-4017(81)90002-9.
Emery, D.L., Eugui, E.M., Nelson, R.T. and Tenywa, T. (1981) Cell-mediated immune responses to *Theileria parva* (East Coast Fever) during immunization and lethal infections in cattle. *Immunology* 43(2), 323–336.

Emery, D.L., MacHugh, N.D. and Morrison, W.I. (1988) *Theileria parva* (Muguga) infects bovine T-lymphocytes *in vivo* and induces coexpression of BoT4 and BoT8. *Parasite Immunology* 10(4), 379–391. DOI: 10.1111/j.1365-3024.1988.tb00228.x.

Fabriek, B.O., Dijkstra, C.D. and Berg, T.K. (2005) The macrophage scavenger receptor CD163. *Immunobiology* 210(2–4), 153–160. DOI: 10.1016/j.imbio.2005.05.010.

Fawcett, D., Musoke, A. and Voigt, W. (1984) Interaction of sporozoites of *Theileria parva* with bovine lymphocytes *in vitro*. 1. Early events after invasion. *Tissue and Cell* 16(6), 873–884. DOI: 10.1016/0040-8166(84)90068-5.

Fry, L.M., Schneider, D.A., Frevert, C.W., Nelson, D.D., Morrison, W.I. *et al.* (2016) East Coast fever caused by *Theileria parva* is characterized by macrophage activation associated with vasculitis and respiratory failure. *PLoS ONE* 11(5), e0156004. DOI: 10.1371/journal.pone.0156004.

Gitau, G.K., McDermott, J.J., Katende, J.M., O'Callaghan, C.J., Brown, R.N. *et al.* (2000) Differences in the epidemiology of theileriosis on smallholder dairy farms in contrasting agro-ecological and grazing strata of highland Kenya. *Epidemiology and Infection* 124(2), 325–335. DOI: 10.1017/s0950268800003526.

Goddeeris, B.M. and Morrison, W.I. (1988) Techniques for the generation, cloning, and characterization of bovine cytotoxic T cells specific for the protozoan *Theileria parva*. *Journal of Tissue Culture Methods* 11(2), 101–110. DOI: 10.1007/BF01404140.

Grootenhuis, J.G., Leitch, B.L., Stagg, D.A., Dolan, T.T. and Young, A.S. (1987) Experimental induction of *Theileria parva* lawrencei carrier state in an African buffalo (*Syncerus caffer*). *Parasitology* 94(Pt 3), 425–431. DOI: 10.1017/s0031182000055773.

Guergnon, J., Chaussepied, M., Sopp, P., Lizundia, R., Moreau, M.-F. *et al.* (2003) A tumour necrosis factor alpha autocrine loop contributes to proliferation and nuclear factor-κB activation of *Theileria parva*-transformed B cells. *Cellular Microbiology* 5(10), 709–716. DOI: 10.1046/j.1462-5822.2003.00314.x.

Hanotte, O., Bradley, D.G., Ochieng, J.W., Verjee, Y., Hill, E.W. *et al.* (2002) African pastoralism: Genetic imprints of origins and migrations. *Science* 296(5566), 336–339. DOI: 10.1126/science.1069878.

Hart, J., MacHugh, N.D. and Morrison, W.I. (2011) *Theileria annulata*-transformed cell lines are efficient antigen-presenting cells for *in vitro* analysis of CD8 T cell responses to bovine herpesvirus-1. *Veterinary Research* 42(1), 119–127. DOI: 10.1186/1297-9716-42-119.

Hemmink, J.D., Sitt, T., Pelle, R., de Klerk-Lorist, L.-M., Shiels, B. *et al.* (2018) Ancient diversity and geographical sub-structuring in African buffalo *Theileria parva* populations revealed through metagenetic analysis of antigen-encoding loci. *International Journal for Parasitology* 48(3–4), 287–296. DOI: 10.1016/j.ijpara.2017.10.006.

Houston, E.F., Taracha, E.L., Brackenbury, L., MacHugh, N.D., McKeever, D.J. *et al.* (2008) Infection of cattle with *Theileria parva* induces an early CD8 T cell response lacking appropriate effector function. *International Journal for Parasitology* 38(14), 1693–1704. DOI: 10.1016/j.ijpara.2008.05.014.

Hulliger, L., Wilde, K.H., Brown, C.G. and Turner, L. (1964) Mode of multiplication of *Theileria* in cultures of bovine lymphocytic cells. *Nature* 203, 728–730. DOI: 10.1038/203728a0.

Irvin, A.D. and Mwamachi, D.M. (1983) Clinical and diagnostic features of east coast fever (*Theileria parva*) infection of cattle. *The Veterinary Record* 113(9), 192–198. DOI: 10.1136/vr.113.9.192.

Irvin, A.D. and Morrison, W.I. (1987) Immunopathology, immunology and immunoprophylaxis of *Theileria* infections. In: Soulsby, E.J.L. (ed.) *Immune Responses in Parasitic Infections: Immunology, Immunopathology and Immunoprophylaxis*, Vol. III. Baton Rouge, Florida: Protozoa. CRC Press, pp. 223–274.

Irvin, A.D., Morzaria, S.P., Munatswa, F.C. and Norval, R.A.I. (1989) Immunization of cattle with a *Theileria parva* bovis stock from Zimbabwe protects against challenge with virulent *T. p. parva* and *T. p. lawrencei* stocks from Kenya. *Veterinary Parasitology* 32(4). DOI: 10.1016/0304-4017(89)90037-x.

Jankovic, D., Kugler, D.G. and Sher, A. (2010) IL-10 production by CD4+ effector T cells: A mechanism for self-regulation. *Mucosal Immunology* 3(3), 239–246. DOI: 10.1038/mi.2010.8.

Jarrett, W.F.H., Crighton, G.W. and Pirie, H.M. (1967) Quantitative and ultrastructural studies on the replication of *Theileria parva:* Veterinary medical review. In: Soulsby, E.J.L. (ed.) *The Reaction of the Host to Parasitism: Proceedings of the third International Conference of the World Association for the Advancement of Veterinary Parasitology, Lyons, France, 1967*, pp. 280–287.

Jarrett, W.F.H., Crighton, G.W. and Pirie, H.M. (1969) *Theileria parya*: Kinetics of replication. *Experimental Parasitology* 24(1), 9–25. DOI: 10.1016/0014-4894(69)90215-X.

Katzer, F., Lizundia, R., Ngugi, D., Blake, D. and McKeever, D. (2011) Construction of a genetic map for *Theileria parva*: Identification of hotspots of recombination. *International Journal for Parasitology* 41(6), 669–675. DOI: 10.1016/j.ijpara.2011.01.001.

Koch, H.T., Ocama, J.G.R., Munatswa, F.C., Byrom, B., Norval, R.A.I. *et al.* (1988) Isolation and characterization of bovine *Theileria* parasites in Zimbabwe. *Veterinary Parasitology* 28(1–2), 19–32. DOI: 10.1016/0304-4017(88)90015-5.

Longhi, C.W. (2009) *In vitro* generation and characterization of bovine NKp46+ populations using *Theileria*-infected cell lines. MSc Thesis, University of, Edinburgh, UK.

Maxie, M.G., Dolan, T.T., Jura, W.G.Z., Tabel, H. and Flowers, M.J. (1982) A comparative study of the diseases in cattle caused by *Theileria parva* or *T. lawrencei*: II. Hematology, clinical chemistry, coagulation studies and complement. *Veterinary Parasitology* 10, 1–19. DOI: 10.1016/0304-4017(82)90002-4.

Mbassa, G.K., Kipanyula, M.J., Mellau, L.S.B., Mwamakali, E.D., Bulegeya, F.R. *et al.* (2006) *Theileria parva* infection in calves causes massive lymphocyte death in the thymus, spleen and lymph nodes without initial proliferation. *Veterinary Parasitology* 142(3–4), 260–270. DOI: 10.1016/j.vetpar.2006.07.010.

McKeever, D.J., Nyanjui, J.K. and Ballingall, K.T. (1997) *In vitro* infection with *Theileria parva* is associated with IL10 expression in all bovine lymphocyte lineages. *Parasite Immunology* 19(7), 319–324. DOI: 10.1046/j.1365-3024.1997.d01-214.x.

Moll, G., Lohding, A., Young, A.S. and Leitch, B.L. (1986) Epidemiology of theileriosis in calves in an endemic area of Kenya. *Veterinary Parasitology* 19(3–4), 255–273. DOI: 10.1016/0304-4017(86)90073-7.

Morrison, W.I. (2015) The aetiology, pathogenesis and control of theileriosis in domestic animals. *Revue Scientifique et Technique, Office International Des Epizooties* 34(2), 599–611. DOI: 10.20506/rst.34.2.2383.

Morrison, W.I., Büscher, G., Murray, M., Emery, D.L., Masake, R.A. *et al.* (1981) *Theileria parva*: Kinetics of infection in the lymphoid system of cattle. *Experimental Parasitology* 52(2), 248–260. DOI: 10.1016/0014-4894(81)90080-1.

Morrison, W.I., MacHugh, N.D. and Lalor, P.A. (1996) Pathogenicity of *Theileria parva* is influenced by the host cell type infected by the parasite. *Infection and Immunity* 64(2), 557–562. DOI: 10.1128/iai.64.2.557-562.1996.

Morrison, W.I., Hemmink, J.D. and Toye, P.G. (2020) *Theileria parva*: A parasite of african buffalo, which has adapted to infect and undergo transmission in cattle. *International Journal for Parasitology* 50(5), 403–412. DOI: 10.1016/j.ijpara.2019.12.006.

Moulton, J., Büscher, G., Bovell, D. and Doxsey, S. (1984) Blast transformation of adherent macrophages infected *in vitro* with sporozoites of *Theileria parva*. *American Journal of Veterinary Research* 45(4), 678–684.

Muraguri, G.R., Kiara, H.K. and McHardy, N. (1999) Treatment of East Coast Fever: A comparison of parvaquone and buparvaquone. *Veterinary Parasitology* 87(1), 25–37. DOI: 10.1016/s0304-4017(99)00154-5.

Nishiyama, S., Pradipta, A., Ma, J.S., Sasai, M. and Yamamoto, M. (2020) T cell-derived interferon-γ is required for host defense to *Toxoplasma gondii*. *Parasitology International* 75, 102049. DOI: 10.1016/j.parint.2019.102049.

Norval, R.A., Perry, B.D. and Young, A.S. (1992) *The Epidemiology of Theileriosis in Africa*. London: Academic Press.

Nylén, S. and Sacks, D. (2007) Interleukin-10 and the pathogenesis of human visceral leishmaniasis. *Trends in Immunology* 28(9), 378–384. DOI: 10.1016/j.it.2007.07.004.

Pinto, M.L., Rios, E., Durães, C., Ribeiro, R., Machado, J.C. *et al.* (2019) The two faces of tumor-associated macrophages and their clinical significance in colorectal cancer. *Frontiers in Immunology* 10, 1875. DOI: 10.3389/fimmu.2019.01875.

Purnell, R.E. (1977) East Coast fever: Some recent research in East Africa. *Advances in Parasitology* 15, 83–132. DOI: 10.1016/s0065-308x(08)60527-8.

Purnell, R.E., Ledger, M.A., Omwoyo, P.L., Payne, R.C. and Peirce, M.A. (1974) *Theileria parva*: Variation in the infection rate of the vector tick, *Rhipicephalus appendiculatus*. *International Journal for Parasitology* 4(5), 513–517. DOI: 10.1016/0020-7519(74)90069-1.

Radley, D.E., Brown, C.G.D., Burridge, M.J., Cunningham, M.P., Peirce, M.A. *et al.* (1974) East Coast fever: Quantitative studies of *Theileria parva* in cattle. *Experimental Parasitology* 36(2), 278–287. DOI: 10.1016/0014-4894(74)90067-8.

Radley, D.E., Brown, C.G.D., Burridge, M.J., Cunningham, M.P., Kirimi, I.M. *et al.* (1975) East Coast fever: 1. Chemoprophylactic immunization of cattle against *Theileria parva* (Muguga) and five theilerial strains. *Veterinary Parasitology* 1(1), 35–41. DOI: 10.1016/0304-4017(75)90005-9.

Reynaud, C.-A., Mackay, C.R., Müller, R.G. and Weill, J.-C. (1991) Somatic generation of diversity in a mammalian primary lymphoid organ: The sheep ileal Peyer's patches. *Cell* 64(5), 995–1005. DOI: 10.1016/0092-8674(91)90323-Q.

Schofield, L., Villaquiran, J., Ferreira, A., Schellekens, H., Nussenzweig, R. *et al.* (1987) Gamma interferon, CD8 T cells and antibodies required for immunity to malaria sporozoites. *Nature* 330(6149), 664–666. DOI: 10.1038/330664a0.

Shaw, M.K. (1997) The same but different: The biology of *Theileria sporozoite* entry into bovine cells. *International Journal for Parasitology* 27(5), 457–474. DOI: 10.1016/S0020-7519(97)00015-5.

Shaw, M.K. (2003) Cell invasion by *Theileria* sporozoites. *Trends in Parasitology* 19(1), 2–6. DOI: 10.1016/s1471-4922(02)00015-6.

Shaw, M.K. and Tilney, L.G. (1992) How individual cells develop from a syncytium: Merogony in *Theileria parva* (Apicomplexa). *Journal of Cell Science* 101(Pt 1), 109–123. DOI: 10.1242/jcs.101.1.109.

Shaw, M.K. and Tilney, L.G. (1995) The entry of *Theileria parva* merozoites into bovine erythrocytes occurs by a process similar to sporozoite invasion of lymphocytes. *Parasitology* 111(4), 455–461. DOI: 10.1017/S0031182000065951.

Shaw, M.K., Tilney, L.G. and McKeever, D.J. (1993) Tick salivary gland extract and interleukin-2 stimulation enhance susceptibility of lymphocytes to infection by *Theileria parva* sporozoites. *Infection and Immunity* 61(4), 1486–1495. DOI: 10.1128/iai.61.4.1486-1495.1993.

Shaw, M.K., Tilney, L.G., Musoke, A.J. and Teale, A.J. (1995) MHC class 1 molecules are an essential cell surface component involved in *Theileria parva* sporozoite binding to bovine lymphocytes. *Journal of Cell Science* 108(4), 1587–1596. DOI: 10.1242/jcs.108.4.1587.

Shitakha, V.M., Natulya, V.M., Musoke, A.J., Ramasamy, R. and Büscher, G. (1983) Complement activation and fibrinolysis during infection with *Theileria parva* (East Coast fever) in cattle. *Veterinary Immunology and Immunopathology* 4(3), 361–373. DOI: 10.1016/0165-2427(83)90046-6.

Song, C., Luo, L., Lei, Z., Li, B., Liang, Z. *et al.* (2008) IL-17-producing alveolar macrophages mediate allergic lung inflammation related to asthma. *The Journal of Immunology* 181(9), 6117–6124. DOI: 10.4049/jimmunol.181.9.6117.

Spooner, R.L., Innes, E.A., Glass, E.J. and Brown, C.G. (1989) *Theileria annulata* and *T. parva* infect and transform different bovine mononuclear cells. *Immunology* 66(2), 284–288.

Stagg, D.A., Dolan, T.T., Leitch, B.L. and Young, A.S. (1981) The initial stages of infection of cattle cells with *Theileria parva* sporozoites *in vitro*. *Parasitology* 83(Pt 1), 191–197. DOI: 10.1017/s0031182000050150.

Steck, W. (1928) Histological studies of East Coast fever. *Report of the Director of Veterinary Education and Research, Part I*. Government Printer and Stationery Office, Pretoria, pp. 243–280.

Suzuki, Y., Sher, A., Yap, G., Park, D., Neyer, L.E. *et al.* (2000) IL-10 is required for prevention of necrosis in the small intestine and mortality in both genetically resistant BALB/c and susceptible C57BL/6 mice following peroral infection with *Toxoplasma gondii*. *The Journal of Immunology* 164(10), 5375–5382. DOI: 10.4049/jimmunol.164.10.5375.

Taracha, E.L., Awino, E. and McKeever, D.J. (1997) Distinct CD4+ T cell helper requirements in *Theileria parva*-immune and -naive bovine CTL precursors. *The Journal of Immunology* 159(9), 4539–4545. DOI: 10.4049/jimmunol.159.9.4539.

Tatchell, R.J. and Moorhouse, D.E. (1968) The feeding processes of the cattle tick *Boophilus microplus* (Canestrini). *Parasitology* 58(2), 441–459. DOI: 10.1017/S0031182000069468.

Theis, J.H. and Budwiser, P.D. (1974) *Rhipicephalus sanguineus*: Sequential histopathology at the host-arthropod interface. *Experimental Parasitology* 36(1), 77–105. DOI: 10.1016/0014-4894(74)90115-5.

Tindih, H.S., Geysen, D., Goddeeris, B.M., Awino, E., Dobbelaere, D.A.E. *et al.* (2012) A *Theileria parva* isolate of low virulence infects a subpopulation of lymphocytes. *Infection and Immunity* 80(3), 1267–1273. DOI: 10.1128/IAI.05085-11.

Tomioka, H., Tatano, Y., Maw, W.W., Sano, C., Kanehiro, Y. *et al.* (2012) Characteristics of suppressor macrophages induced by mycobacterial and protozoal infections in relation to alternatively activated macrophages. *Clinical and Developmental Immunology* 635451. DOI: 10.1155/2012/635451.

Uilenberg, G. and Zwart, D. (1979) Skin nodules in East Coast fever. *Research in Veterinary Science* 26(2), 243–245. DOI: 10.1016/S0034-5288(18)32925-4.

Uilenberg, G. (1981) Theilerial species of domestic livestock. In: Irvin, A.D., Cunningham, M.P. and Young, A.S. (eds) *Advances in the Control of Theileriosis. Current Topics in Veterinary Medicine and Animal Science*, Vol. 14. Martinus Nijhoff, The Hague, The Netherlands, pp. 3–37.

Wagner, G.G., Jessett, D.M., Brown, C.G.D. and Radley, D.E. (1975) Diminished antibody response to rinderpest vaccination in cattle undergoing experimental East Coast fever. *Research in Veterinary Science* 19(2), 209–211.

Walker, A.R. and Fletcher, J.D. (1986) Histological study of the attachment sites of adult *Rhipicephalus appendiculatus* on rabbits and cattle. *International Journal for Parasitology* 16(4), 399–413. DOI: 10.1016/0020-7519(86)90121-9.

Wilde, J.K.H. (1966) Changes in bovine bone marrow during the course of East Coast fever. *Research in Veterinary Science* 7(2), 213–226. DOI: 10.1016/S0034-5288(18)34701-5.

Wilde, J.K.H. (1967) East Coast fever. *Advances in Veterinary Sciences* 11, 223–274.

Wilkie, G.M., Kirvar, E. and Brown, C.G.D. (2002) Validation of an *in vitro* method to determine infectivity of cryopreserved sporozoites in stabilates of *Theileria* spp. *Veterinary Parasitology* 104(3), 199–209. DOI: 10.1016/s0304-4017(01)00630-6.

Woods, K., Perry, C., Brühlmann, F. and Olias, P. (2021) *Theileria*'s strategies and effector mechanisms for host cell transformation: From invasion to immortalization. *Frontiers in Cell and Developmental Biology* 9, 662805. DOI: 10.3389/fcell.2021.662805.

Yamada, S., Konnai, S., Imamura, S., Simuunza, M., Chembensofu, M. *et al*. (2009) Quantitative analysis of cytokine mRNA expression and protozoan DNA load in *Theileria parva*-infected cattle. *Journal of Veterinary Medical Science* 71(1), 49–54. DOI: 10.1292/jvms.71.49.

Yasuda, M., Jenne, C.N., Kennedy, L.J. and Reynolds, J.D. (2006) The sheep and cattle Peyer's patch as a site of B cell development. *Veterinary Research* 37(3), 401–415. DOI: 10.1051/vetres:2006008.

Young, A.S., Dolan, T.T., Mwakima, F.N., Ochanda, H., Mwaura, S.N. *et al*. (1995) Estimation of heritability of susceptibility to infection with *Theileria parva* in the tick *Rhipicephalus appendiculatus*. *Parasitology* 111(1), 31–38. DOI: 10.1017/S003118200006457X.

5 *Theileria parva* in the African Buffalo (*Syncerus caffer*)

W. Ivan Morrison[1]*, Liam J. Morrison[1], Olivier Hanotte[2] and Philip Toye[3]
[1]Roslin Institute, University of Edinburgh, Edinburgh, UK; [2]International Livestock Research Institute, Addis Ababa, Ethiopia; [3]International Livestock Research Institute, Nairobi, Kenya

5.1 Introduction

The African buffalo (*Syncerus caffer*) is found only in Africa, where it is the largest bovid species in the African savannah ecosystem. It is now the closest wild bovid relative of domestic cattle (*Bos taurus*) on the African continent, following the extinction of the African auroch (*Bos primigenius mauretanicus*), which may have survived up to around 1000 BC in Egypt (Beierkuhnlein, 2015). The common ancestor of African buffalo and domestic cattle remains disputed, but existed at least several million years ago (Caron *et al.*, 2023; Prins *et al.*, 2023). Unlike the Asian water buffalo (*Bubalus bubalis*), which is extensively used as a domestic animal, the African buffalo has never been domesticated due to its aggressive temperament. It is present throughout a large part of sub-Saharan Africa and can survive and prosper in areas where many of the most important pathogens of cattle are endemic. Its habitat includes areas infested with arthropod vectors, most notably ticks and tsetse flies, the vectors of East Coast fever (ECF) and African trypanosomosis, respectively. The buffalo also acts as a carrier of several serotypes of foot and mouth disease virus. These pathogens establish infections in the buffalo, but in contrast to the often devastating diseases caused in cattle, infections in the buffalo do not appear to cause significant disease.

As discussed elsewhere in this book (see Chapters 1 and 6), *Theileria parva* was first identified in cattle in 1902, but the presence of the parasite in the buffalo was not recognized until much later. An acute disease in cattle caused by *Theileria* parasites transmitted from buffalo was recognized in Zimbabwe in 1934 (Lawrence, 1935) and subsequently reported in South Africa in the 1950s (Neitz, 1955). Although the clinical disease was similar to ECF, including acute onset and a high level of mortality, affected animals had lower levels of schizont-infected leukocytes in lymphoid tissues and no, or very few, detectable piroplasms in erythrocytes. Because of these differences, the parasite was initially named *Theileria lawrencei* and the disease was referred to as Corridor disease (CD), relating to the local region in South Africa where it was initially recognized. A similar disease in cattle caused by *T. lawrencei*, also arising from transmission by ticks from buffalo, was later recognized in East Africa (Brocklesby and Barnett, 1966). Despite the observed differences between *T. parva* and *T. lawrencei*, subsequent findings revealed antigenic similarities, and experiments

*Corresponding author: Ivan.Morrison@ed.ac.uk

 East Coast Fever: The Disease, its Impact and Control (eds W.I. Morrison and P. Toye)
DOI: 10.1079/9781800626324.0005

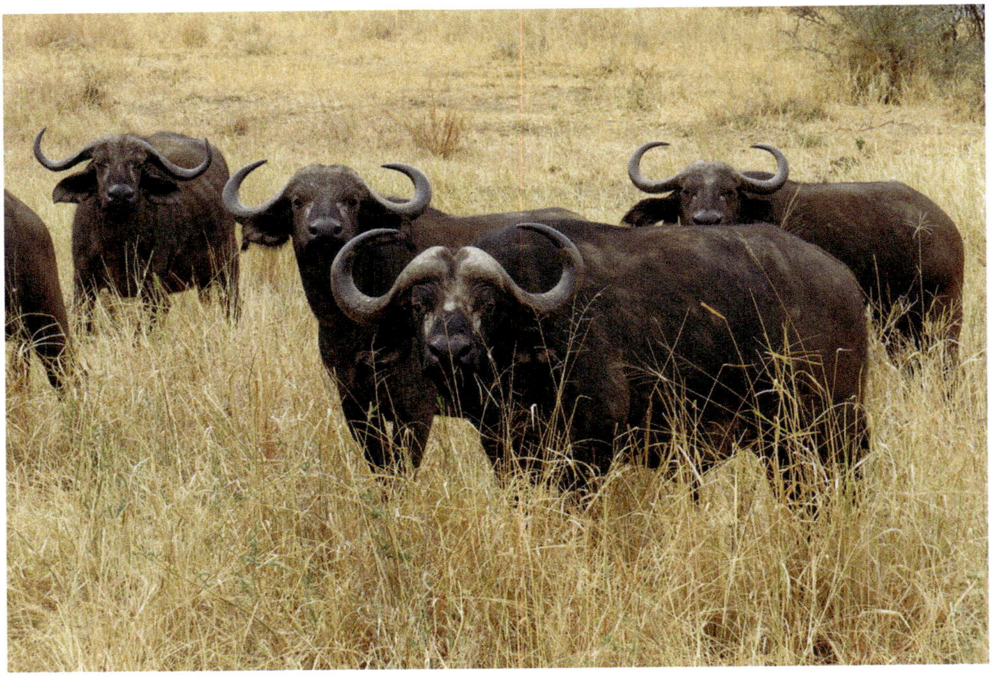

Fig. 5.1. The African buffalo (*Syncerus caffer*). (Photograph provided by Liam Morrison.)

involving immunization and challenge of cattle demonstrated cross-protection between some combinations of *T. parva* and *T. lawrencei* isolates (Young *et al.*, 1973). Therefore, the two parasites were considered to represent the same species and *T. lawrencei* was reclassified as *T. parva*. It is now widely accepted that most buffalo residing in *R. appendiculatus*-infested areas are infected with *T. parva* (Young *et al.*, 1978).

This chapter will briefly review the evolutionary history of buffalo and cattle in Africa and discuss differences in the *T. parva* parasites found in the two species and the nature of the infections they produce in cattle.

5.2 The African Buffalo

The African buffalo (*S. caffer*) is a member of the Bovidae (characterized by one or two pairs of unforked horns), within the subfamily *Bovinae* and tribe *Bovini* (Prins *et al.*, 2023) (Fig. 5.1).

The evolutionary history is complex and not fully understood; African buffalo and Asian water buffalo (*B. bubalis*) last had a common ancestor approximately 8 million years ago, and while there is a reasonable consensus about the ancestry of *B. bubalis*, that of *S. caffer* remains unclear due to a fragmented and incomplete fossil record. While *S. caffer* is the most closely related wild bovid to domestic cattle in Africa, as with *B. bubalis*, it is not possible to produce hybrid offspring between *S. caffer* and cattle (unlike, for example, between cattle and American bison, yak or banteng, where hybrid offspring can be generated).

Historically, the species range has effectively spanned almost all of sub-Saharan Africa, occupying most habitat types, with the exception of semi-desert, desert and high mountain. The present-day distribution is significantly fragmented, with population numbers in many cases being substantially reduced and ranges becoming discontinuous, with some populations isolated, due to human-induced activities and loss of habitat.

S. caffer is currently described (by the International Union for Conservation of Nature) as comprising four subspecies, namely *S. c. caffer* (the East and Southern African savannah

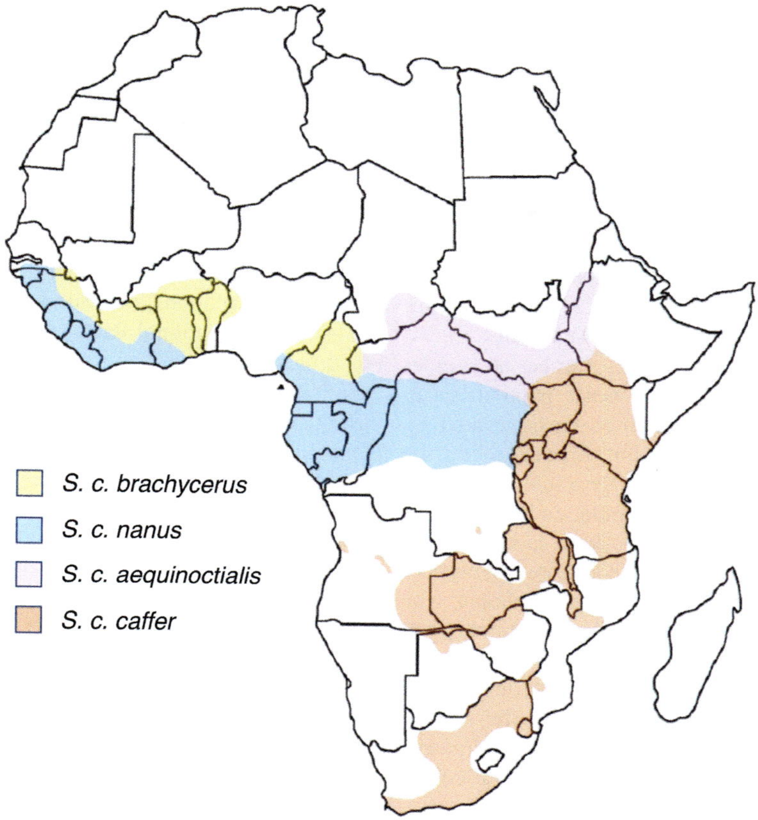

Fig. 5.2. Distribution of different subspecies of *Syncerus caffer* in Africa.

buffalo), *S. c. aequinoctialis* (Central African savannah buffalo), *S. c. brachyceros* (West African savannah buffalo) and *S. c. nanus* (West/Central African forest buffalo). The distribution of these subspecies in Africa is illustrated in Fig. 5.2.

S. c. caffer is by far the most numerous, with an estimated 540,000 individuals across the range, whereas much lower numbers exist for *S. c. aequinoctialis* (34,000) and *S. c. brachyceros* (20,500). The practical difficulty in assessing numbers for *S. c. nanus* means there is no reliable current estimate for this subspecies (Cornelis *et al.*, 2023).

Historically, taxonomic status has been based on morphology, behaviour, habitat and geographical distribution. This is exemplified by the forest buffalo *S. c. nanus* being much smaller, a different colour (rufous as opposed to black) and with horn shape and other features that substantially differ from its savannah buffalo counterparts. Such distinct differences made it reasonable to assume that genetic relatedness would mirror classification based on morphology. However, genetic analyses, using either low-resolution markers (mitochondrial D-loop sequences, microsatellites and mitochondrial genomes) or high-resolution genome-wide approaches (single nucleotide polymorphisms or whole genome sequences), have provided very little support for the four described subspecies (Heller *et al.*, 2012; Smitz *et al.*, 2013, Smitz *et al.*, 2014; de Jager *et al.*, 2021; Michaux *et al.*, 2023; Talenti *et al.*, 2024). Instead, the data suggest that there is a very strong correlation between genetic distance (a measure of the genetic divergence between two populations) and geographic distance – a phenomenon known as 'isolation-by-distance' (see Michaux *et al.*, 2023; Talenti *et al.*, 2024). This indicates that historically buffalo have effectively existed as one continuous meta-population, with the genetic differentiation largely being driven by probability of mating between two individuals reducing with increasing geographic distance. There are some exceptions to this isolation-by-distance effect, and this arises where populations have particularly elevated inbreeding coefficients (indicated by the F statistic or F_{ST}). Perhaps the best characterized of these is the *S. c. caffer* population in Hluhluwe-Umfolozi National Park in South Africa (de Jager *et al.*, 2021; Quinn *et al.*, 2023; Talenti *et al.*, 2024), which is known to derive from a very small number of founder animals. Similarly, *S. c. nanus* populations in Gabon have been shown to have elevated F_{ST} (Michaux *et al.*, 2023), but this may reflect the ease of gene flow in forest ecosystems compared to savannah. Effective population size analyses indicated that for the savannah species (where there was sufficient power in terms of number of samples for such analyses), despite the fragmented nature of extant populations, there is limited evidence for inbreeding depression (i.e. reduced biological fitness that has the potential to result from inbreeding) across the species, with the exception of the Hluhluwe-Umfolozi NP population (Talenti *et al.*, 2024 – as discussed above).

While genetic and genomic data are increasing, further representation is required from populations that are currently not sampled or are under-sampled. This is particularly the case for West African populations, and especially *S. c. nanus*, for which genetic data are only available for a small number of individuals and locations. Improving the resolution of genetic/genomic data will greatly aid the characterization of the continent-wide genetic landscape, and also potentially contribute to informing conservation and management strategies. For example, if there is a desire to maintain genetic integrity (or diversity) of particular populations or subpopulations, genetic information can provide a route to informing translocations, and indeed how any future integration of the large number of buffalo managed in private ownership (an estimated 75,000 animals – located mainly in Southern Africa) with current wild populations should be managed (see e.g. Smitz *et al.*, 2014; Cornelis *et al.*, 2023).

With respect to *T. parva*, the current distribution of *R. appendiculatus* means that it is only *S. c. caffer* populations that act as the primary host reservoir of the parasite (although it probably cannot be formally ruled out that some members of the eastern-most *S. c. aequinoctialis* and *S. c. nanus* populations are exposed/infected). Interestingly, within the range of *S. c. caffer* there are clearly both populations that are endemic and populations that are free from *T. parva* exposure/infection, and indeed within Uganda it has been shown that northern populations (the Murchison Falls and Kidepo Valley National Parks) are not exposed to *R. appendiculatus* (and therefore *T. parva*, as confirmed by polymerase chain reaction (PCR) assay), whereas the southern parks are endemic for both *R. appendiculatus* and *T. parva* (Obara *et al.*, 2020). This scenario, with both *T. parva*-positive and *T. parva*-negative populations in a relatively restricted geographic area, raises the possibility of identifying genetic factors that enable *S. caffer* to tolerate infections that cause significant disease in domestic cattle. However, this relies on sufficient sample numbers in endemic and non-endemic areas. Additionally, when analysing genetic signatures of selection, a caveat is that historical tick/pathogen distribution cannot be inferred based upon current distribution, given that *S. caffer* and *T. parva* have co-evolved for millennia. Nonetheless, as outlined above, genetic and genomic information and resources for *S. caffer* are advancing, with a good quality reference genome having been generated and an increasing number of genomes available (de Jager *et al.*, 2021; Quinn *et al.*, 2023; Talenti *et al.*, 2024), which now should allow us to address the intriguing question of how buffalo tolerate infection with *T. parva*.

5.3 The Introduction of Cattle into Africa

The history of African cattle pastoralism is complex (see for example Hanotte *et al.*, 2002; Gifford-Gonzalez and Hanotte, 2011; Kim *et al.*, 2023). Cattle have been introduced at various times from both of the recognized centres of cattle domestication, in the Near East (humpless taurine *Bos taurus taurus*) and the Indian subcontinent (*B. t. indicus*) (Fig. 5.3; Hanotte *et al.*, 2002). Subsequent interbreeding of the

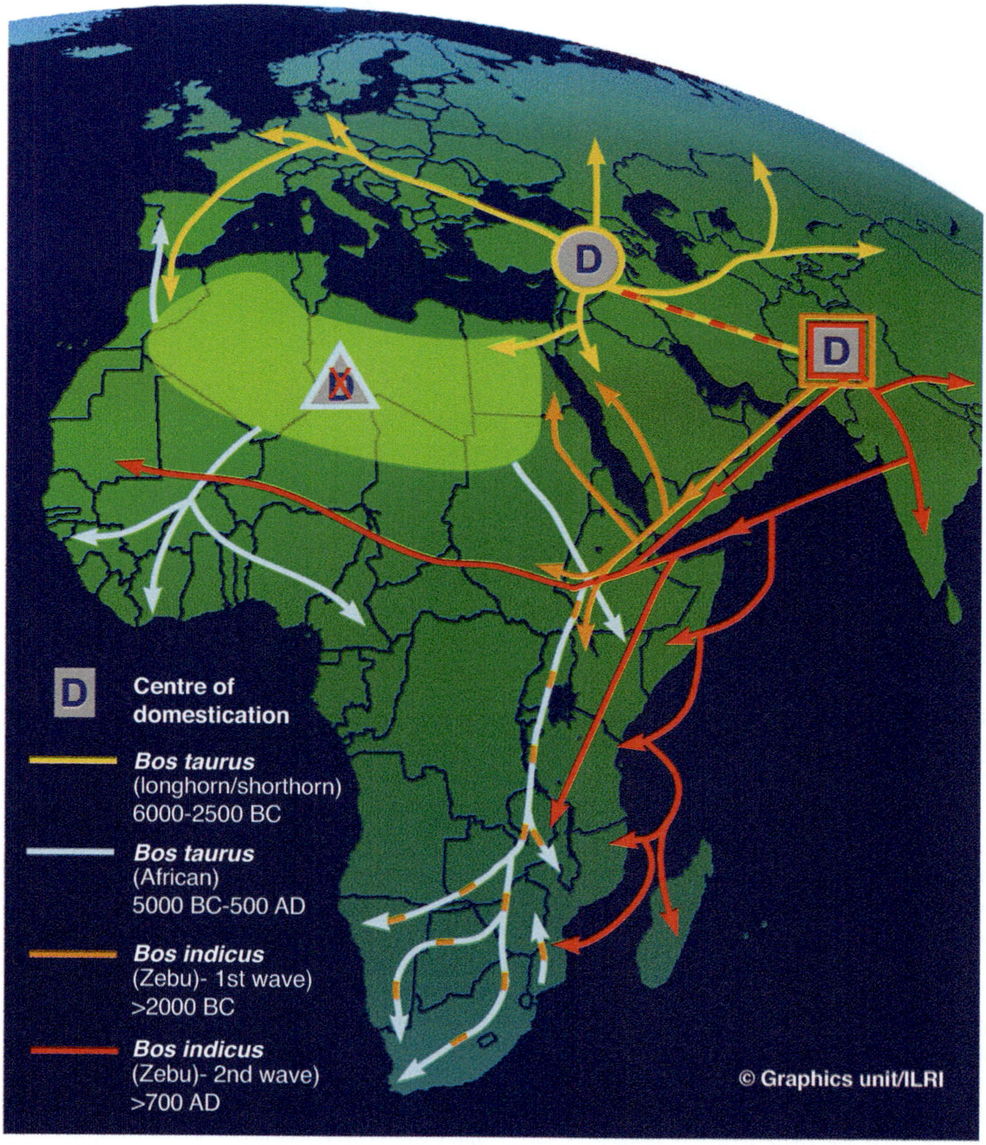
D
D
D
Centre of domestication
Bos taurus
(longhorn/shorthorn)
6000-2500 BC
Bos taurus
(African)
5000 BC-500 AD
Bos indicus
(Zebu)- 1st wave)
>2000 BC
Bos indicus
(Zebu)- 2nd wave)
>700 AD
© Graphics unit/ILRI

Fig. 5.3. Illustration showing the entry and migration of domestic cattle into Africa, with estimated dates, from the centres of domestication in the Near East and the Indian subcontinent. A centre of domestication in North Africa was initially proposed, but recent evidence does not support this. (Illustration prepared by O. Hanotte and D. Elsworth, copyright held by the International Livestock Research Institute, Nairobi, Kenya, and used with permission.)

descendants of these cattle populations has resulted in the many indigenous breeds of cattle now present in Africa.

The first cattle to reach the African continent were *B. t. taurus* that entered Africa about 8000 years ago through what is now known as Egypt and the Sinai. The auroch (*Bos primigenius*), a wild ancestor of modern cattle, was already present in North Africa, but there is no evidence that it was locally domesticated (Pitt *et al.*, 2018). Nevertheless, genome-wide analyses, including of ancient DNA genomes,

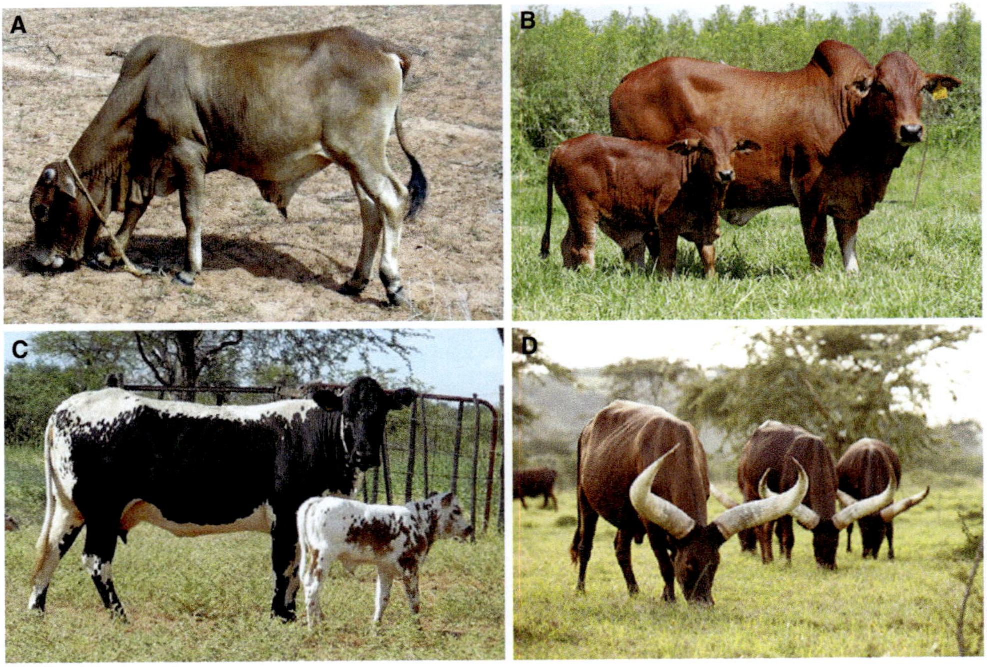

Fig. 5.4. Examples of *Bos indicus* and sanga cattle breeds in Africa. Top row – East African *Bos indicus*: Indigenous East African zebu (A), Boran (B). Bottom row – sanga breeds: South African Nguni (C), Ugandan Ankole (D).

have increasingly revealed introgression of an archaic cattle population and/or African aurochs among the West African taurine domestic cattle (Ginja *et al.*, 2023; Kim *et al.*, 2023).

The humped *B. t. indicus*, also referred to as zebu or indicine cattle, reached the African continent later, with several introductions beginning about 4000 years ago. Although they were likely present initially in low numbers, the onset of Swahili civilization and its maritime trading network favoured their arrival in large numbers about 1400 years ago. Already adapted to a drier environment than taurine animals, they rapidly spread west and south within Africa (Kim *et al.*, 2020). Hybridization with local taurine in the continent's southern region gave rise to today's African sanga cattle.

Today, cattle with different proportions of taurine and indicine genome admixture are found in geographic areas under the challenge of *T. parva* transmission. They are mainly grouped as African zebu (e.g. Kenyan Boran) and African sanga (e.g. Ankole in eastern Africa, Nguni in southern Africa), according to their morphology of a thoracic or cervicothoracic hump, respectively (illustrated in Fig. 5.4). Typically, the proportion of indicine genome is higher in African zebu than in African sanga, and it is higher in the Horn of Africa, the main entry point of Asian indicine cattle on the continent, than in the southern African region (Hanotte *et al.*, 2002).

Taurine mitochondrial DNA haplotypes are found in all African indigenous cattle (taurine, zebu, sanga and their cross-bred offspring; Kwon *et al.*, 2022), indicating that indicine genes have been introduced predominantly by male lines. Apart from the recently introduced taurine cattle of European descent, no humpless cattle are found in eastern, central and southern Africa. The African sanga of eastern and southern Africa are geographically separated.

The detailed history of the eastern and southern African admixed zebu–taurine cattle populations that reside in areas where *T. parva* and its tick vector (*R. appendiculatus*) are found is still fragmentary. While the first cattle in eastern Africa might have been taurine, the successful

Table 5.1. Species of *Theileria* detected by high-throughput sequencing of PCR amplicons of the 18S rRNA gene from blood samples of 14 buffalo. Summary of data reported by Hemmink *et al.* (2018).

Number of buffalo positive for each species					
T. parva	*T. sp.* (buffalo)	*T. velifera*	*T. mutans*	*T. orientalis*	*T. sinensis*
13	14	13	8	2	3

dispersion of cattle in these regions might have been associated with the early arrival of indicine cattle, cross-breeding and human migrations. Taurine–indicine cross-breeding has likely contributed to the rapid adaptation of cattle populations to new environmental challenges (Kim *et al.*, 2020), particularly for infectious diseases. For example, African taurine cattle in western Africa are well known for their trypanotolerance (Hanotte *et al.*, 2003), while eastern African indigenous zebu from endemic regions show a degree of resistance to ECF (see Chapter 7 of this volume).

5.4 *Theileria* Species Found in Buffalo

The vast majority of buffalo residing in areas infested with *R. appendiculatus* are persistently infected with *T. parva*. In addition, most buffalo carry infections with other *Theileria* species that infect cattle. An example of the species detected in 14 buffalo, six from South Africa and eight from Kenya, is shown in Table 5.1. Detection was based on high-throughput sequencing of PCR amplicons of a fragment of the 18S rRNA gene from a blood sample of each animal (Hemmink *et al.*, 2018). *T.* sp. (Buffalo) was detected in all 14 animals, *T. parva* and *T. velifera* in 13 of the animals, *T. mutans* in eight of the animals, and *T. senensis* and *T. orientalis* in three and two of the animals, respectively. These species infect cattle but apart from *T. parva* they do not cause clinical disease in cattle, although their presence is of relevance for differential diagnosis.

5.5 The Disease in Cattle Caused by Buffalo-Derived *T. parva*

The clinical signs presented in ECF and CD are very similar, and the diseases are difficult to distinguish in the field (Neitz, 1955; Irvin and Mwamachi, 1983; Cook *et al.*, 2021). A detailed summary of such signs of CD can be found, for example, in a recently published study of a closely monitored group of 46 *B. indicus* cattle exposed in the field to buffalo-derived parasites (Cook *et al.*, 2021). The mortality rate in this study was 91% (42/46), which is similar to the mortality rate reported by Neitz in 1955. Interestingly, the four animals that survived harboured the C→T single nucleotide polymorphism (three heterozygotes and one homozygote) that is significantly associated with resistance to *T. parva* infection (Wragg *et al.*, 2022; Chapter 7 of this volume).

As noted elsewhere, the major distinguishing feature between ECF and CD is the relatively low parasitosis detected in the latter, in both the schizont and particularly the piroplasm stages. It has also been suggested that CD progresses more rapidly. Cook *et al.* (2021) reported that the mean time from first detection of pyrexia to death was 4.8 days in the 42 *B. indicus* cattle exposed to buffalo-derived parasites in the field. Irvin and Mwamachi (1983) noted that cattle suffering from ECF may die within 'five to six days' of pyrexia, but more commonly the clinical course lasts '10–14 days'. However, in an experimental setting using animals infected with stabilates of *T. parva*, there was no difference in the mean time-to-death of animals challenged with buffalo-derived or cattle-derived parasites (Jura and Losos, 1980). These results reflect the difficulty in comparing the disease in field cases of ECF and CD, as the progression of the disease is dose-dependent and will vary in different epidemiological settings.

Although some reduction in packed red cell volume (PCV) is frequently observed in animals with ECF, anaemia is not a significant clinical feature of the disease. Cook *et al.* (2021) observed a gradual decline in the PCV in all of the animals naturally infected with buffalo-derived parasites over the course of infection, with about half of the animals developing a mild clinical anaemia. Anaemia in haemoparasitic infections is often partially due to destruction of red blood cells during the emergence of the erythrocytic stage of the pathogen. However, there are very few if any piroplasms present during CD. Hence, it is likely that the reduced PCV is a consequence of the effects of parasitized cells on erythropoiesis, as described for ECF (see Chapter 4 of this volume).

There are no detailed accounts of the pathology in cases of CD. However, unpublished histopathological findings in terminal cases of the disease from the study conducted by Cook *et al.* (2021) have indicated that the pulmonary changes are essentially similar to those observed in ECF. The main difference from ECF was much less severe lesions in lymphoid tissues, although the severity varied between animals (E.A.J. Cook, Nairobi, and W.I. Morrison, Edinburgh, 2025, personal communication).

5.6 Tick Transmission of Cattle and Buffalo *T. parva*

5.6.1 Tick transmission of buffalo *T. parva* in cattle

The capacity to undergo tick transmission is a key factor that distinguishes infections in cattle with cattle-maintained and buffalo-derived *T. parva*. Infection with *T. parva* is transmitted trans-stadially, meaning that infections acquired by the larval and nymphal stages of the tick are transmitted to other hosts by the nymph and adult stages, respectively. *T. parva* undergoes a complex life cycle in the tick (Mehlhorn and Schein, 1984), which includes a sexual stage when recombination can occur between different parasite strains (Katzer *et al.*, 2011; further detail in Chapter 3 of this volume).

Infections with *T. parva* in buffalo and infections with cattle-maintained *T. parva* in cattle are both efficiently transmitted by ticks, and both establish a carrier state, enabling transmission to occur from animals harbouring very low levels of parasites. The efficiency of this transmission is particularly apparent in carrier cattle, which usually do not have microscopically detectable parasites in their blood. By contrast to the efficient transmission of parasites from infected buffalo, ticks fed on cattle infected with the same buffalo-derived parasites usually fail to transmit infection (Fig. 5.5; e.g. Schreuder *et al.*, 1977). This is associated with detection of no, or very low levels of, piroplasms in cattle infected with buffalo-derived parasites.

For example, a study conducted by Sitt *et al.* (2015), which involved introduction of naïve and vaccinated calves into an area previously grazed only by buffalo, reported that all animals developed infection with *T. parva* but only two of the 24 animals had detectable piroplasms. It should be noted, however, that these piroplasms could have been from other *Theileria* species, since the piroplasms of most species are morphologically indistinguishable. The parasitological

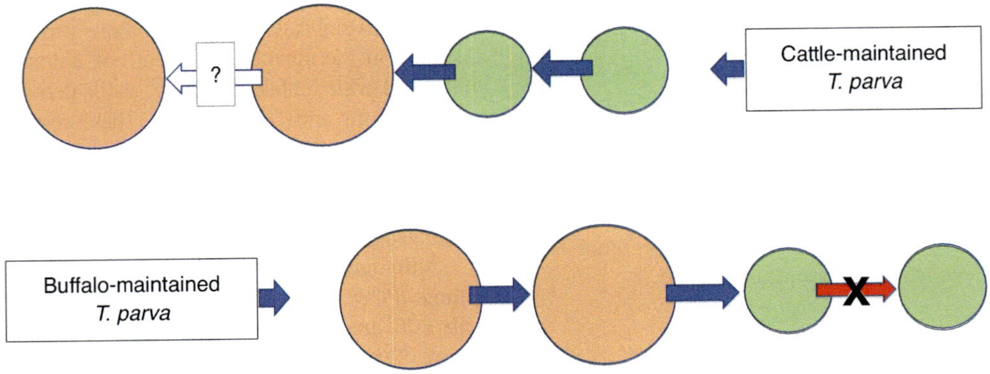

Fig. 5.5. Diagrammatic representation of transmission of cattle- and buffalo-maintained *T. parva* in cattle and buffalo. The orange and green circles represent buffalo and cattle populations, respectively.

findings are consistent with early observations that cattle that had recovered from infections with buffalo parasites failed to transmit infection when moved to fresh tick-infested pasture (Neitz *et al.*, 1955). The lack of transmission by ticks appears to be due to a failure of schizonts in infected lymphocytes to undergo merogony, consistent with the observation that microschizonts (i.e. schizonts undergoing merogony) are rarely detected in lymphoid tissues in cases of CD (Lawrence, 1937; Young *et al.*, 1977b). Hence, there is a failure to generate the erythrocyte-infective stages.

5.6.2 Experimental studies of transmission in buffalo

There are only a few detailed studies of experimental infection of buffalo with cattle-maintained *T. parva* (Lewis, 1943; Barnett and Brocklesby, 1966b) and these yielded variable results. Successful transmission from occasional animals was observed. However, Grootenhuis *et al.* (1987b) reported that attempts to demonstrate a carrier state in buffalo infected with cattle *T. parva* proved unsuccessful. Given the inconsistency of these limited studies and the uncertain infection status of the animals used in some of the experiments, it is difficult to be certain of their conclusions. Hence (as indicated in Fig. 5.5), the transmissibility of cattle *T. parva* to buffalo and their ability to establish persistent infections in buffalo are not clearly defined. Further experimental studies are needed to address these questions.

5.6.3 Transmission barriers in other *Theileria* species

A number of other *Theileria* species are also able to infect non-definitive hosts, but infection is not maintained in these hosts. These include infections of cattle with *T.* sp. (buffalo) and *T. taurotragi*, which are parasites closely related to *T. parva* found in African buffalo and antelopes, respectively, which infect cattle but do not appear to be maintained by tick transmission in cattle. The cattle parasite *T. annulata* has been shown to infect sheep, both naturally and experimentally, but (as with buffalo-derived *T. parva* in cattle) *T. annulata* does not differentiate to the tick-infective piroplasm stage in sheep (Leemans *et al.*, 1999a, Leemans *et al.*, 1999b). In this regard, it has been suggested that the closely related sheep parasite *T. lestoquardi* may have evolved by adaptation of *T. annulata* to sheep. Thus, the ability to undergo differentiation to tick-infective stages appears to be a key parameter in determining the host specificity of *Theileria* parasites.

5.7 Behavioural 'Transformation' of Buffalo *T. parva* in Cattle

While numerous attempts have failed to transmit buffalo-derived parasites from cattle, a few instances of transmission of such parasites have been reported in East Africa, and serial tick transmission was found to result in altered behaviour of the parasites to resemble that of cattle-maintained *T. parva*. This so-called 'transformation' was first reported by Barnett and Brocklesby (1966a), who infested susceptible cattle with ticks that had fed on a *Theileria*-infected buffalo, and then conducted tick passages to further naïve cattle. Although the first and second passages usually did not result in microscopically detectable parasites, transmission was successful in a proportion of the tick feeds. Further tick passages resulted in progressively increasing levels of parasites in both erythrocytes and lymphocytes and severe, fatal disease in some animals, which by the fourth and sixth passages resembled disease produced by cattle-maintained *T. parva*. Unfortunately, methods to cryopreserve the parasites were not available at that time and therefore further studies of this parasite are not possible. In 1973, Young and Purnell also reported successful tick transmission of a buffalo isolate of *T. parva* in cattle and observed progressively increasing levels of piroplasm parasitaemia upon serial tick passage. This cattle-adapted parasite, *T. parva* (Serengeti), was subsequently used as one of the components of a live vaccine against *T. parva* (discussed in Chapter 12 of this volume). A third instance of adaptation of a Kenyan buffalo isolate of *T. parva* to tick transmission between cattle was reported by Maritim *et al.* in 1992. Again, the levels of piroplasm parasitaemia and the efficiency of transmission progressively increased during five tick passages through cattle. Significantly, in this study, examination of the parasites using a panel of monoclonal antibodies demonstrated that they retained a similar antibody profile during passage, including reactivity with an antibody that usually only reacts with buffalo-derived parasites. It is of note that one of the cloned populations of *T. parva* sporozoites produced by Morzaria *et al.* (1995) was generated from the same buffalo-derived isolate used in the experiments reported by Maritim *et al.* (1992). This cloned population was obtained by tick pick-up from an animal infected with a cloned derivative from a bovine cell line infected *in vitro* with the buffalo *T. parva* isolate. Although this clone is clearly tick transmissible, the level of infection produced in ticks is lower than that observed with clones of cattle-maintained *T. parva*.

Transmission of South African buffalo-derived *T. parva* from cattle has proved extremely difficult, and there are no reports of 'transformation' of parasite behaviour. Until recently, despite numerous attempts, there was only one report of experimental transmission, and that was from a splenectomized calf (Neitz, 1957). However, Latif *et al.* (2019) reported successful experimental transmission following tick feeding on one of four cattle that had recovered from natural infection with buffalo-derived *T. parva* during a disease outbreak in the KwaZulu-Natal province of South Africa.

The experimental studies discussed above clearly demonstrate that transformation of the behaviour of at least some buffalo-derived isolates of *T. parva* can be achieved following experimental tick transmission in cattle. If this were a frequent event in the field, the populations of *T. parva* in cattle and buffalo might be expected to become relatively homogeneous. However, as discussed below, this is clearly not the case. This discrepancy may relate to conditions used for experimental transmission, namely use of large numbers of heavily infected ticks for serial passage from the acute phase of infection with the same parasite isolate. Such circumstances are extremely unlikely to be replicated under field conditions. A potential mechanism underlying the experimental transformation of the parasite is discussed further in Section 5.10.

5.8 A Live ECF Vaccine Does Not Protect Cattle against Buffalo-Derived *T. parva*

As discussed elsewhere in this book (see Chapters 12 and13 of this volume), a live vaccine, involving infection of cattle with sporozoites from three *T. parva* isolates (the Muguga cocktail) and simultaneous treatment with long-acting oxytetracycline, has been developed for vaccinating cattle against ECF. The vaccine has been shown to provide robust protection against experimental challenge with different isolates of cattle *T. parva* (Radley *et al.*, 1975a, b; Leemans *et al.*, 1999b) and against field challenge, predominantly with cattle-maintained *T. parva* (Di Giulio *et al.*, 2009; Babo Martins *et al.*, 2010). However, a number of studies have shown that the vaccine does not protect against buffalo-derived *T. parva*. This was first demonstrated in a study using an experimental paddock that had been 'cleaned' of infection and then infected by introducing two infected buffalo along with clean ticks (Young *et al.*, 1977a). Animals vaccinated by infection and treatment introduced into the paddock were not protected. In another study in the same paddock (Young *et al.*, 1977b), cattle were immunized separately with three different parasite isolates from the buffaloes used to seed the paddock. Following introduction into the paddock, protection was observed with two of the isolates, which had been generated by pooling several tick feeds, whereas the third isolate derived from a single tick feed failed to give protection. The results of these experiments, in addition to showing that the ECF vaccine did not protect against buffalo-derived *T. parva*, provided evidence of antigenic heterogeneity in the buffalo *T. parva* parasites used to seed the paddock. The lack of protection against buffalo-derived parasites was confirmed in a further study, which involved experimental challenge with several buffalo-derived parasite isolates (Radley *et al.*, 1979).

Two more recent studies, in which groups of naïve or Muguga cocktail-vaccinated cattle were introduced into field sites grazed solely or predominantly by buffalo (Bishop *et al.*, 2015; Sitt *et al.*, 2015), revealed that the vaccinated cattle remained fully susceptible to natural challenge, clearly demonstrating antigenic disparity between buffalo-derived parasites and the parasites used in the vaccine.

5.9 Genotypic and Antigenic Diversity in *T. parva*

5.9.1 Early studies with monoclonal antibodies and molecular techniques

Early use of *T. parva*-specific monoclonal antibodies and DNA probes detected antigenic and molecular differences among *T. parva* isolates of both cattle and buffalo origin (Minami *et al.*, 1983; Conrad *et al.*, 1987a, b, 1989; Leemans *et al.*, 1999b). The restriction fragment length polymorphism (RFLP) profiles obtained with DNA probes and the reactivities of monoclonal antibodies with buffalo parasites often differed substantially from those obtained with cattle parasites, with considerably more parasite heterogeneity within buffalo cell lines and in *ex vivo* buffalo samples (Conrad *et al.*, 1989; Bishop *et al.*, 1993). Since most of the monoclonal antibodies used in these studies were specific for a single polymorphic parasite protein (the polymorphic immunodominant molecule – PIM; Toye *et al.*, 1991) and most studies employing DNA probes targeted a single repetitive DNA element (*Tpr* – *T. parva* repeat; see Chapter 9 of this volume for a further description of *Tpr*), these tools provided limited resolution at the genome level. In particular, they did not provide a means of clearly distinguishing buffalo-derived parasites from those from cattle.

Sequencing of the *T. parva* genome in 2005 (Gardner *et al.*, 2005) opened up opportunities to develop new molecular typing methods, allowing more detailed interrogation of the genetic composition of parasite populations. Use of satellite DNA markers distributed across the genome, identified from the genome sequence, demonstrated that different parasite isolates had unique molecular fingerprints. Typing of carrier cattle in the field with these tools revealed that most infections were genotypically mixed and that the genetic complexity of the parasites in the blood of infected cattle increased with the age of the animals (Oura *et al.*, 2003, 2005, Oura *et al.*, 2011b). Analyses of samples from buffalo revealed an even greater level of complexity, indicating the presence of at least nine different *T. parva* genotypes in single blood samples from some animals (Oura *et al.*, 2011a). These findings implied that cattle and buffalo acquire multiple infections over time, consistent with experimental findings in cattle that immunity against *T. parva*, which protects against clinical disease, does not prevent establishment of infection upon parasite challenge.

5.9.2 Greater diversity of antigen-encoding genes in buffalo parasites

The availability of a genome sequence for *T. parva* coupled with progress in identifying antigens recognized by antibodies and T cells from immune cattle allowed a detailed comparison of the genetic and antigenic diversity of buffalo- and cattle-derived parasite populations.

Evidence that CD8 T cell responses play a key role in immunity to the parasite (McKeever *et al.*, 1994; Taracha *et al.*, 1995) led to the identification of a number of antigens recognized by CD8 T cells from immune cattle (Graham *et al.*, 2006). Detailed studies of two of these antigens (Tp1 and Tp2) demonstrated that they displayed sequence polymorphism that resulted in differential recognition by CD8 T cells (MacHugh *et al.*, 2009; Connelley *et al.*, 2011). Using the genes encoding these antigens as genetic markers, Pelle *et al.* (2011) undertook an analysis of sequence polymorphism in a series of 79 cell lines infected with *T. parva*. They examined cell lines that had either been infected *in vitro* with laboratory-maintained strains of *T. parva* or were isolated from naturally infected cattle or buffalo in various field locations. The cattle isolates included parasites from cattle in buffalo-free areas or from sentinel cattle introduced into an area populated predominantly by buffalo. The Tp1 and Tp2 genes proved to be highly polymorphic, showing single nucleotide polymorphisms (SNPs) in 12 and 61% of residues, resulting in 30 and 41 protein variants, respectively, among the 79 isolates examined. However, the most striking finding was that the isolates from buffalo or from cattle exposed to buffalo-grazed pasture displayed much greater sequence diversity compared to those from cattle in buffalo-free areas (results summarized in Table 5.2).

Table 5.2. Sequence diversity in the genes[a] encoding the CD8 T cell antigens Tp1 and Tp2 and their predicted proteins in a series of cattle-derived and buffalo-derived *T. parva* isolates or infected cell lines From Pelle *et al.*, 2011.

	Cattle derived (*N* = 39)		Buffalo derived (*N* = 38)	
Antigen	Nucleotide	Protein	Nucleotide	Protein
Tp1	12	9	26	26
Tp2	4	4	38	36

[a]Nucleotide sequences were obtained from PCR amplicons of a 432 bp segment of the Tp1 gene and the full length of Tp2.

Table 5.3. Sequence diversity in gene segments of six antigen-encoding *T. parva* genes detected by high-throughput sequencing of PCR amplicons from the blood of 14 African buffalo. From Hemmink *et al.*, 2018.

Antigen	Sequences obtained from 14 buffalo			Sequences obtained from one buffalo
	Nucleotide[a]	% Polymorphism[b]	Protein[c]	Nucleotide[a]
Tp1	72	11	66	15
Tp2	72	70	62	19
Tp4	76	30	3	23
Tp5	46	9	1	19
Tp6	36	9	2	15
Tp10	42	11	2	10

[a]Number of distinct nucleotide sequences.
[b]Percentage of polymorphic residues in nucleotide sequences.
[c]Number of distinct predicted protein sequences.

Further evidence of extensive heterogeneity in buffalo *T. parva* was obtained in a study that performed high-throughput sequencing of PCR amplicons of segments of six T cell antigen-encoding genes (including Tp1 and Tp2) using DNA obtained directly from buffalo blood samples (Hemmink *et al.*, 2018; results summarized in Table 5.3).

Thus, as shown in Table 5.2, only nine of the 30 Tp1 antigenic variants and four of the 41 Tp2 variants were present in the cattle-maintained parasite population. However, the majority of these cattle variants were also found among the parasites from buffalo and buffalo-associated populations, indicating that they do not represent a completely divergent population. Based on these findings, the authors concluded that the cattle-maintained parasites represent a subset of the *T. parva* population and, coupled with other evidence, suggest that these parasites are most likely to have been selected for their ability to undergo tick transmission between cattle.

In addition to confirming a high level of allelic diversity of each gene at the population level, the results revealed extensive allelic diversity within individual buffalo. For example, between 11 and 24 nucleotide sequence variants were detected for each of the six genes in one buffalo sample. Given that the infection rate of ticks with *T. parva* in the field is usually < 2% and that many infected ticks have only one or two infected salivary gland cells (each derived from a single *T. parva* zygote), these results again clearly indicate that the parasites in these buffalo must have arisen from multiple infection events. The simultaneous presence of multiple parasite genotypes in buffalo blood further highlights the enormous potential for genetic recombination to occur in ticks feeding on infected buffalo.

A more recent study used long-read sequencing to examine the sequences of three antigen genes (Tp1, Tp4 and Tp16) in cattle and buffalo in a region adjacent to the Serengeti National Park in Tanzania, where the cattle were likely to come into contact with buffalo-fed ticks (Allan *et al.*, 2021). The majority of the cattle examined (as well as the buffalo) had carrier infections. Overall, the results revealed a larger number of allelic variants of the antigen genes from parasites in both host species than in the previous studies, which the authors suggested was due to the near full-length sequences obtained compared to the short segments examined previously. However, again the numbers of variants obtained from buffalo were much greater than those obtained from cattle.

The study reported by Hemmink *et al.* (2018) included a comparison of sequences obtained from buffalo in Kenya and South Africa. Samples from both regions showed similar levels of sequence diversity, both at the population level and within animals. Although there was evidence for differentiation of the Kenyan and South African sequences, analyses of molecular variance for each gene revealed that the majority of the underlying nucleotide sequence polymorphism was common to both areas. Moreover, a comparison of the sequences of known CD8 T cell epitopes within the two most polymorphic genes, Tp1 and Tp2, revealed a high level of similarity in epitope variants in the Kenyan and South African buffalo samples, including epitope sequences in the South African samples that were identical to those found in East African cattle-maintained *T. parva*. These findings indicated that much of the sequence variation in these genes pre-dates geographical separation of the parasites.

The p67 *T. parva* sporozoite surface protein is involved in the initial binding of sporozoites to bovine lymphocytes, leading to cell invasion (Dobbelaere *et al.*, 1984, 1985; Musoke *et al.*, 1984; Nene *et al.*, 1992), and has been investigated as an antigen for vaccination against *T. parva* (Musoke *et al.*, 1992; discussed in further detail in Chapter 11 of this volume). To date, no variation in the sequence of the gene encoding p67 has been found in cattle-maintained *T. parva*. However, a sequence variant, which differed by the presence of an insert of 43 amino acids, was detected in an East African buffalo-derived parasite (Nene *et al.*, 1996). A subsequent study in South Africa, which examined the sequences of p67 in buffalo-derived isolates, identified a further two sequence variants, in addition to the cattle and buffalo sequences reported in East Africa (Sibeko *et al.*, 2010). The observed polymorphism affected sites of antibody epitopes within the protein (Obara *et al.*, 2015), although the effect on recognition by the respective monoclonal antibodies was not examined. The possibility that the sequence of p67 influences the ability of buffalo-derived parasites to infect cattle was addressed in a study that examined p67 sequences of parasites infecting cattle introduced into an area previously only grazed by buffalo, compared with sequences from buffalo in the same location (Sitt *et al.*, 2019). Over 40 sequence variants of p67 were identified, most representing minor variants of the previously described alleles; many of the variants were found in both cattle and buffalo, and there was no significant difference in the level of sequence diversity in the two host species. Up to five different sequence variants were found in individual cattle, confirming multiplicity of infection. These findings failed to reveal any restriction in the ability of buffalo parasites expressing different alleles of p67 to infect cattle, and added to the evidence that *T. parva* transmitted to cattle from buffalo are much more genotypically diverse than cattle-maintained *T. parva*.

The similar diversity seen in buffalo *T. parva* and in cattle *T. parva* acquired from buffalo in this study appears inconsistent with an earlier study in Uganda, which observed distinct satellite DNA marker profiles in parasites from cattle and buffalo grazing in close proximity (Oura *et al.*, 2011b). However, this almost certainly is due to the fact that the latter study examined animals with carrier infections rather than the acute infections studied by Sitt *et al.* (2019); as discussed above, such carrier infections in cattle are likely to originate only from challenge with cattle-maintained *T. parva*.

5.9.3 Analyses of full-length genome sequences

The use of genome sequencing offers a greater opportunity to identify potentially relevant functional genotypic differences between *T. parva* maintained in cattle and in buffalo. Hayashida *et al.* (2013) reported genome sequences of nine parasite isolates from various locations in East Africa, which included two parasites of buffalo origin, and found much greater sequence diversity of the buffalo isolates, with respect to the reference Muguga genome, than the cattle isolates. Similar divergence of the genome sequences of 12 isolates from South African buffalo, compared to the reference cattle-derived sequence, was reported by Maboko *et al.* (2021).

5.10 Why Has Genotypic Restriction of *T. parva* in Cattle Been Maintained?

The demonstration that experimental tick transmission of buffalo *T. parva* in cattle can sometimes result in the selection of parasites adapted to transmission between cattle (Barnett and Brocklesby, 1966a; Young and Purnell, 1973; Maritim *et al.*, 1992), might suggest that such adaptation has occurred frequently in the field. However, the limited genetic diversity of cattle-maintained *T. parva* (compared to buffalo parasites) indicates that this is not the case. It seems unlikely that fully cattle-transmissible parasites are present in the buffalo parasite population (even at low frequency), as such parasites would be expected to be readily selected upon transmission to cattle. Since buffalo *T. parva* are expected to undergo frequent sexual recombination, the selected parasites would carry with them a diversity of genetic backgrounds that would add to genetic diversity of the cattle *T. parva* population. For similar reasons, transmissibility in cattle is unlikely to be determined by a single parasite gene.

Nevertheless, in the experimental studies that demonstrated 'behavioural transformation' of buffalo *T. parva* following passage in cattle, the parasites must have had some residual capacity to differentiate to the tick-infective piroplasm stage in cattle. However, in each of these studies, several passages of the same parasite isolate, employing large numbers of ticks fed on multiple cattle during the acute phase of infection, were required to generate the tick transmissible parasites. Infection was not always initially detected in all animals, and only some passage lineages yielded 'transformed' parasites, indicating heterogeneity within the starting parasite population. The pressure for selection of transmissibility in these experiments is unlikely to be replicated in field situations. The levels of infection in ticks in the field are much lower than under experimental conditions, and the parasites are likely to be transmitted together with cattle-adapted parasites, reducing the capacity for selection. Clearly, the buffalo parasites used in these 'transformation' experiments must have possessed a degree of transmissibility in cattle. Moreover, the capacity of the selected buffalo parasites to be maintained in cattle would also depend on their ability to establish a carrier state. While two of the reported transformed populations of *T. parva* were found to establish a carrier state in cattle (Barnett and Brocklesby, 1966a; Young and Purnell, 1973), it is unclear whether the earlier passages of these parasites had this capability.

We propose a possible model to explain these observations, based on the assumption that full transmission competence of *T. parva* in cattle is dependent on multiple parasite genes. In this case, the fully cattle-adapted genotypes are not present in the starting buffalo parasite population but their generation requires recombination during tick transmission, coupled with selection in cattle for transmission, to generate the genotype(s) that facilitate efficient tick transmission. As indicated above, some of the parasites in the starting parasite population must possess alleles that allow low-level transmission. Recombinant events during subsequent tick passages might then facilitate selection of the combination of alleles that provide efficient transmission. This may be achievable under experimental conditions with some buffalo isolates but rarely occurs in the field. Molecular and genetic tools are now available to investigate this issue.

As discussed earlier in this chapter, the ability of cattle parasites to establish infection in buffalo following tick transmission is not known. If cattle-adapted parasites are successfully transmitted to buffalo, recombination with buffalo parasites in the course of further tick passage would likely generate genotypically diverse parasites, some of which may be transmissible back to cattle. On the other hand, it is possible that adaptation of *T. parva* to cattle has resulted in parasites that are poorly adapted to establishing persistent infection and transmission in buffalo.

In recent years, epigenetic mechanisms of regulating gene expression that affect cell phenotypes have received increasing attention (Lowdon *et al.*, 2016). Studies of *Plasmodium* parasites have implicated epigenetic processes in regulating a number of biological activities, including expression of variable antigen genes and differentiation of the sexual stages of the parasites in erythrocytes (reviewed in Cortés and Deitsch, 2017). However, to date, these findings have only been documented across generations of asexually replicating parasites, and we are unaware of evidence of inheritance of epigenetically determined traits following completion of the sexual cycle.

In practical terms, elucidation of the genetic basis of transmissibility in cattle would provide markers to distinguish cattle- and buffalo-derived parasites in areas co-grazed by both species and to identify buffalo parasites that could potentially adapt to transmission in cattle.

5.11 The Basis of Resistance to Disease in the Buffalo

There are very few experimental studies of infection with *T. parva* in the buffalo, largely due to difficulty in obtaining animals that are not already infected with the parasite. Most studies have used animals captured as calves and then reared in captivity. However, such animals remain untamed and require heavy sedation to conduct experimental procedures. There is one well-documented study using a single captive buffalo experimentally infected with buffalo-derived *T. parva*. This buffalo was rigorously tested before infection to confirm that it was negative for *T. parva* (Grootenhuis *et al.*, 1987a). In this regard, the status of animals used in some previous studies was less certain. The buffalo and two susceptible cattle were inoculated with sporozoites from a cryopreserved stabilate, which had been prepared with ticks fed on a naturally infected buffalo, and monitored over a period of 888 days. The buffalo suffered a very mild clinical reaction, with transient enlargement of the regional lymph node and elevation of body temperature for 1 day. By contrast, the two cattle developed acute lethal disease. Only two infected lymphoblasts were detected on 1 day in the regional lymph node of the buffalo. Piroplasms were observed in blood on day 15 and subsequently also at irregular intervals throughout the observation period. Seven of 11 attempts to isolate the parasite by feeding ticks during this period were successful, and establishment of cultures of infected lymphoblasts from blood samples was successful on six of ten occasions. These results, along with other findings, clearly show that the buffalo is refractory to the pathogenic effects of *T. parva*.

Studies to compare the susceptibility of cattle and buffalo cells to infection *in vitro* with *T. parva* have indicated that the two species are similarly susceptible to infection by the parasite (Baldwin *et al.*, 1986). *T. parva* sporozoites (from both cattle and buffalo *T. parva* isolates) were found to bind to similar percentages of cells in cattle and buffalo peripheral blood mononuclear cells (PBM). Infection of cattle and buffalo PBM with cattle and buffalo *T. parva* isolates in limiting dilution cultures revealed some differences between the parasites in the percentage of cells that established transformed cell lines. Cattle *T. parva* transformed a greater percentage of cattle cells than buffalo cells, and the converse was the case for the buffalo parasites. However, overall, the findings demonstrated that infections with *T. parva* parasites originating from the respective host species exhibit similar capacities to infect and transform host lymphocytes, implying that the resistance of the buffalo to disease is due to the nature of the response of the buffalo to infection.

As discussed above, the increasing availability of African buffalo genomic reference resources and population genomic data (de Jager *et al.*, 2021; Quinn *et al.*, 2023; Talenti *et al.*, 2024) means that it is becoming possible to consider interrogating the buffalo genome, in order to assess whether genomic regions can be identified where selection by *T. parva* has resulted in the over-representation of haplotypes or alleles that contain genes that are responsible for conferring tolerance. This is not straightforward, as signatures of selection will inevitably derive from multiple environmental pressures (for example, see the difficulty in identifying signatures of selection associated with the devastating rinderpest epidemic of the 1890s that resulted in enormous mortality of buffalo; Simonsen *et al.*, 1998; Van Hooft *et al.*,

2000; Heller *et al.*, 2008; Quinn *et al.*, 2023; Talenti *et al.*, 2024), and as discussed above, we cannot rely on contemporary metadata (e.g. vector and pathogen distribution) to infer historical selection. However, given that the African buffalo is the primary host of *T. parva* with a very lengthy co-evolution, and the profound amelioration of clinical signs in buffalo compared to cattle, it is likely that selection by *T. parva* will have resulted in detectable signatures in the buffalo genome.

A recent study assessed selective sweeps in the buffalo genome using a dataset that comprised samples from across the extant range of buffalo ($n = 196$ genomes; Talenti *et al.*, 2024). Analysis (using two distinct but complementary approaches: P_R and XP-EHH) revealed that the sets of genes shown to be under selection in both methods were significantly enriched for genes with predicted function related to the immune response. Of note were multiple genes that had previously been implicated in the host response to apicomplexan protozoa. Among these was tyrosine-phosphatase non-receptor type substrate 1-like (SIRPA-like), which intriguingly has also been detected as being under significant selection in the Asian water buffalo *B. bubalis* (Dutta *et al.*, 2020). *B. bubalis* is the host for the related parasite *T. annulata*, and experimental studies to investigate relative resistance of Sahiwal (*Bos indicus*) compared to Holstein (*Bos taurus*) cattle to *T. annulata* revealed significant differences between the breeds in expression of SIRP genes in both uninfected and infected monocytes (Glass *et al.*, 2012).

Clearly, such data and observations are still preliminary, and it will require further, much more detailed investigation (in particular at the cellular level) to confidently identify and validate the association of buffalo genes with the *T. parva* tolerance phenotype. However, in combination with ongoing work on cattle genetic tolerance (see Chapter 7 of this volume), the definition of host genetic components that contribute to tolerance to *T. parva* infection may prove in the long term to be a useful future tool for combating the disease. This will also require the development of approaches that enable such genetic markers to be usefully deployed in the field in the settings in which *T. parva* causes disease.

5.12 Practical Implications for Disease Control

The data discussed in this chapter have highlighted the extent of antigenic diversity in the buffalo *T. parva* population and the failure of the Muguga cocktail vaccine to provide protection against challenge with buffalo parasites. Despite this diversity, vaccination with the Muguga cocktail has been effective in some areas where buffalo are present (Di Giulio *et al.*, 2009; Babo Martins *et al.*, 2010). As argued elsewhere (Morrison *et al.*, 2015), this may be due to a relatively low abundance of buffalo-fed versus cattle-fed ticks in these areas. However, vaccine-induced immunity is likely to be breached in situations where cattle are farmed alongside a high density of wildlife or in close proximity to game reserves with buffalo populations. More information on the *T. parva* populations carried by ticks in such situations is required to provide a better understanding of the nature of the parasite challenge in relation to the risk of vaccine breakthrough. Further improvement of vaccination by infection and treatment by incorporation of buffalo-derived parasites is problematic because of lack of tick transmissibility of most buffalo isolates in cattle, thus hampering production of parasites for vaccination. In addition, the enormous diversity among the buffalo parasites may hinder the selection of representative buffalo-derived isolates for inclusion in a vaccine. Hence, vaccination against these parasites may need to await development of alternative vaccines.

In South Africa, the disease threat is confined to challenge with buffalo-derived parasites, and the control strategy for many decades has been to prevent contact between infected buffalo and cattle by fencing and restriction of animal movement (Potgieter *et al.*, 1988; Lawrence, 1990). Detailed surveillance of livestock is conducted to ensure rapid identification of outbreaks in cattle, and measures are imposed on infected farms to prevent spread of infection. Testing of buffalo for *T. parva* prior to movement is required to avoid spread of infection. As discussed above, the likelihood of buffalo *T. parva* adapting to transmission and maintenance in cattle seems remote in South Africa. However, the potentially disastrous consequences of such a rare event fully justify the control measures currently being applied.

5.13 Concluding Remarks

The African buffalo is fully susceptible to infection with *T. parva*, and infection persists as a carrier state that facilitates efficient transmission of the parasite. The profoundly different outcome of infection, compared to the severe disease produced in cattle, is believed to be a consequence of the prolonged period of co-evolution of buffalo with *T. parva*, which has allowed acquisition of the ability to control the infection and avoid the pathogenic effects observed in cattle. By contrast, cattle were first introduced into Africa within the last 10,000 years and clearly have not acquired the ability to control the parasite. However, although cattle are susceptible to infection with the range of *T. parva* genotypes found in buffalo, only a subset of these genotypes are maintained in the cattle population by tick transmission. The buffalo-derived parasites and those maintained in cattle produce similar diseases in cattle, but infection with the former results in no or few infected erythrocytes. Available evidence indicates that the inability of most buffalo *T. parva* to maintain infections in cattle is due to a failure of the parasites to differentiate to the tick-transmissible stages. Although most experimental studies have confirmed the lack of tick transmission of buffalo *T. parva* isolates in cattle, in a few studies, transmission has been achieved using large numbers of experimentally infected ticks, and further tick passage of the parasites has resulted in selection of parasites that behave in a manner similar to that of cattle-maintained parasites. However, the restricted genetic diversity of cattle-maintained *T. parva* implies that such transformation is not a frequent event in the field. The mechanisms underlying this 'behavioural transformation' of the parasite and the factors that maintain the restricted genetic diversity of cattle-maintained *T. parva* in the field are not understood. Herein, we argue that it is unlikely to arise from the presence of fully cattle-transmissible parasites in the buffalo, but rather may be determined by several parasite genes that need to undergo recombination to generate a haplotype that results in transmission competence.

References

Allan, F.K., Jayaraman, S., Paxton, E., Sindoya, E., Kibona, T. *et al.* (2021) Antigenic diversity in *Theileria parva* populations from sympatric cattle and African buffalo analyzed using long read sequencing. *Frontiers in Genetics* 12, 684127. DOI: 10.3389/fgene.2021.684127.

Babo Martins, S., Di Giulio, G., Lynen, G., Peters, A. and Rushton, J. (2010) Assessing the impact of East Coast fever immunisation by the Infection and Treatment Method in Tanzanian pastoralist systems. *Preventive Veterinary Medicine* 97(3–4), 175–182. DOI: 10.1016/j.prevetmed.2010.09.018.

Baldwin, C.L., Malu, M.N., Kinuthia, S.W., Conrad, P.A. and Grootenhuis, J.G. (1986) Comparative analysis of infection and transformation of lymphocytes from African buffalo and Boran cattle with *Theileria parva* subsp. parva and *T. parva* subsp. lawrencei. *Infection and Immunity* 53(1), 186–191. DOI: 10.1128/iai.53.1.186-191.1986.

Barnett, S.F. and Brocklesby, D.W. (1966a) The passage of '*Theileria lawrencei* (Kenya)' through cattle. *British Veterinary Journal* 122, 396–409. DOI: 10.1016/S0007-1935(17)40406-4.

Barnett, S.F. and Brocklesby, D.W. (1966b) The susceptibility of the African buffalo (*Syncerus caffer*) to infection with *Theileria parva* (Theiler 1904). *British Veterinary Journal* 122, 379–386. DOI: 10.1016/S0007-1935(17)40404-0.

Beierkuhnlein, C. (2015) *Bos primigenius* in Ancient Egyptian art – historical evidence for the continuity of occurrence and ecology of an extinct key species. *Frontiers of Biogeography* 7(3), 21527. DOI: 10.21425/F5FBG21527.

Bishop, R.P., Sohanpal, B.K., Allsopp, B.A., Spooner, P.R., Dolan, T.T. *et al.* (1993) Detection of polymorphisms among *Theileria parva* stocks using repetitive, telomeric and ribosomal DNA probes and anti-schizont monoclonal antibodies. *Parasitology* 107(1), 19–31. DOI: 10.1017/S0031182000079361.

Bishop, R.P., Hemmink, J.D., Morrison, W.I., Weir, W., Toye, P.G. *et al.* (2015) The African buffalo parasite *Theileria*. sp. (buffalo) can infect and immortalize cattle leukocytes and encodes divergent orthologues of *Theileria parva* antigen genes. *International Journal for Parasitology: Parasites and Wildlife* 4(3), 333–342. DOI: 10.1016/j.ijppaw.2015.08.006.

Brocklesby, D.W. and Barnett, S.F. (1966) The isolation of *Theileria lawrencei* (Kenya) from a wild buffalo (*Syncerus caffer*) and its serial passage through captive buffaloes. *British Veterinary Journal* 122, 387–395.

Caron, A., Cornélis, D., Chardonnet, P. and Prins, H.H.T. (eds) (2023) *Ecology and Management of the African Buffalo*. Cambridge University Press, Cambridge, UK.

Connelley, T.K., MacHugh, N.D., Pelle, R., Weir, W. and Morrison, W.I. (2011) Escape from CD8+ T cell response by natural variants of an immunodominant epitope from *Theileria parva* is predominantly due to loss of TCR recognition. *The Journal of Immunology* 187(11), 5910–5920. DOI: 10.4049/jimmunol.1102009.

Conrad, P.A., Iams, K., Brown, W.C., Sohanpal, B. and ole-MoiYoi, O.K. (1987a) DNA probes detect genomic diversity in *Theileria parva* stocks. *Molecular and Biochemical Parasitology* 25(3), 213–226. DOI: 10.1016/0166-6851(87)90085-5.

Conrad, P.A., Stagg, D.A., Grootenhuis, J.G., Irvin, A.D., Newson, J. *et al.* (1987b) Isolation of *Theileria* parasites from African buffalo and characterisation with monoclonal antibodies. *Parasitology* 94, 413–423. DOI: 10.1017/S0031182000055761.

Conrad, P.A., ole-MoiYoi, O.K., Baldwin, C.L., Dolan, T.T., O'Callaghan, C.J. *et al.* (1989) Characterization of buffalo-derived theilerial parasites with monoclonal antibodies and DNA probes. *Parasitology* 98(2), 179–188. DOI: 10.1017/S0031182000062089.

Cook, E.A.J., Sitt, T., Poole, E.J., Ndambuki, G., Mwaura, S. *et al.* (2021) Clinical evaluation of Corridor disease in *Bos indicus* (Boran) cattle naturally infected with buffalo-derived *Theileria parva*. *Frontiers in Veterinary Science* 8, 731238. DOI: 10.3389/fvets.2021.731238.

Cornelis, D., Renaud, P.C., Melletti, M., Fonteyn, D., Bonhotal, H. *et al.* (2023) Conservation status of the African buffalo: A continent-wide assessment. In: Caron, E., Cornelis, D., Chardonnet, P. and Prins, H.H.T. (eds) *Ecology and Management of the African Buffalo*. Cambridge, UK: Cambridge University Press. DOI: 10.1017/9781009006828.007.

Cortés, A. and Deitsch, K.W. (2017) Malaria epigenetics. *Cold Spring Harbor Perspectives in Medicine* 7(7): a025528. DOI: 10.1101/cshperspect.a025528.

de Jager, D., Glanzmann, B., Möller, M., Hoal, E., Helden, P. *et al.* (2021) High diversity, inbreeding and a dynamic pleistocene demographic history revealed by African buffalo genomes. *Scientific Reports* 11(1), 4540. DOI: 10.1038/s41598-021-83823-8.

Di Giulio, G., Lynen, G., Morzaria, S., Oura, C. and Bishop, R. (2009) Live immunization against East Coast fever – current status. *Trends in Parasitology* 25(2), 85–92. DOI: 10.1016/j.pt.2008.11.007.

Dobbelaere, D.A.E., Spooner, P.R., Barry, W.C. and Irvin, A.D. (1984) Monoclonal antibody neutralizes the sporozoite stage of different *Theileria parva* stocks. *Parasite Immunology* 6(4), 361–370. DOI: 10.1111/j.1365-3024.1984.tb00808.x.

Dobbelaere, D.A.E., Shapiro, S.Z. and Webster, P. (1985) Identification of a surface antigen on *Theileria parva* sporozoites by monoclonal antibody. *Proceedings of the National Academy of Sciences* 82(6), 1771–1775. DOI: 10.1073/pnas.82.6.1771.

Dutta, P., Talenti, A., Young, R., Jayaraman, S., Callaby, R. *et al.* (2020) Whole genome analysis of water buffalo and global cattle breeds highlights convergent signatures of domestication. *Nature Communications* 11(1), 4739. DOI: 10.1038/s41467-020-18550-1.

Gardner, M.J., Bishop, R., Shah, T., Villiers, E.P., Carlton, J.M. *et al.* (2005) Genome sequence of *Theileria parva*, a bovine pathogen that transforms lymphocytes. *Science* 309(5731), 134–137. DOI: 10.1126/science.1110439.

Gifford-Gonzalez, D. and Hanotte, O. (2011) Domesticating animals in Africa: Implications of genetic and archaeological findings. *Journal of World Prehistory* 24(1), 1–23. DOI: 10.1007/s10963-010-9042-2.

Ginja, C., Guimarães, S., Fonseca, R.R., Rasteiro, R., Rodríguez-Varela, R. *et al.* (2023) Iron age genomic data from Althiburos – Tunisia renew the debate on the origins of African taurine cattle. *iScience* 26(7), 107196. DOI: 10.1016/j.isci.2023.107196.

Glass, E.J., Crutchley, S. and Jensen, K. (2012) Living with the enemy or uninvited guests: Functional genomics approaches to investigating host resistance or tolerance traits to a protozoan parasite. *Veterinary Immunology and Immunopathology* 148(1–2), 178–189. DOI: 10.1016/j.vetimm.2012.03.006.

Graham, S.P., Pellé, R., Honda, Y., Mwangi, D.M., Tonukari, N.J. *et al.* (2006) *Theileria parva* candidate vaccine antigens recognized by immune bovine cytotoxic T lymphocytes. *Proceedings of the National Academy of Sciences* 103(9), 3286–3291. DOI: 10.1073/pnas.0511273103.

Grootenhuis, J.G., Leitch, B.L., Stagg, D.A., Dolan, T.T. and Young, A.S. (1987a) Experimental induction of *Theileria parva* lawrencei carrier state in an African buffalo (*Syncerus caffer*). *Parasitology* 94(Pt 3), 425–431. DOI: 10.1017/s0031182000055773.

Grootenhuis, J.G., Young, A.S., Stagg, D.A., Leitch, B.L., Dolan, T.T. *et al.* (1987b) Infection of African buffalo (*Syncerus caffer*) and cattle with *Theileria parva* lawrencei after serial passage in cattle. *Research in Veterinary Science* 42(3), 326–330. DOI: 10.1016/S0034-5288(18)30712-4.

Hanotte, O., Bradley, D.G., Ochieng, J.W., Verjee, Y., Hill, E.W. *et al.* (2002) African pastoralism: Genetic imprints of origins and migrations. *Science* 296(5566), 336–339. DOI: 10.1126/science.1069878.

Hanotte, O., Ronin, Y., Agaba, M., Nilsson, P., Gelhaus, A. *et al.* (2003) Mapping of quantitative trait loci controlling trypanotolerance in a cross of tolerant West African N'Dama and susceptible East African Boran cattle. *Proceedings of the National Academy of Sciences* 100(13), 7443–7448. DOI: 10.1073/pnas.1232392100.

Hayashida, K., Abe, T., Weir, W., Nakao, R., Ito, K. *et al.* (2013) Whole-genome sequencing of *Theileria parva* strains provides insight into parasite migration and diversification in the African continent. *DNA Research* 20(3), 209–220. DOI: 10.1093/dnares/dst003.

Heller, R., Lorenzen, E.D., Okello, J.B.A., Masembe, C. and Siegismund, H.R. (2008) Mid-holocene decline in African buffalos inferred from Bayesian coalescent-based analyses of microsatellites and mitochondrial DNA. *Molecular Ecology* 17(22), 4845–4858. DOI: 10.1111/j.1365-294X.2008.03961.x.

Heller, R., Bruniche-Olsen, A. and Siegismund, H.R. (2012) Cape buffalo mitogenomics reveals a Holocene shift in the African human-megafauna dynamics. *Molecular Ecology* 21, 3947–3959.

Hemmink, J.D., Sitt, T., Pelle, R., de Klerk-Lorist, L.-M., Shiels, B. *et al.* (2018) Ancient diversity and geographical sub-structuring in African buffalo *Theileria parva* populations revealed through metagenetic analysis of antigen-encoding loci. *International Journal for Parasitology* 48(3–4), 287–296. DOI: 10.1016/j.ijpara.2017.10.006.

Irvin, A.D. and Mwamachi, D.M. (1983) Clinical and diagnostic features of East Coast fever (*Theileria parva*) infection of cattle. *The Veterinary Record* 113(9), 192–198. DOI: 10.1136/vr.113.9.192.

Jura, W.G.Z. and Losos, G.J. (1980) A comparative study of the diseases in cattle caused by *Theileria lawrencei* and *Theileria parva*. 1. Clinical signs and parasitological observations. *Veterinary Parasitology* 7(4), 275–286. DOI: 10.1016/0304-4017(80)90047-3.

Katzer, F., Lizundia, R., Ngugi, D., Blake, D. and McKeever, D. (2011) Construction of a genetic map for *Theileria parva*: Identification of hotspots of recombination. *International Journal for Parasitology* 41(6), 669–675. DOI: 10.1016/j.ijpara.2011.01.001.

Kim, K., Kwon, T., Dessie, T., Yoo, D., Mwai, O.A. *et al.* (2020) The mosaic genome of indigenous African cattle as a unique genetic resource for African pastoralism. *Nature Genetics* 52(10), 1099–1110. DOI: 10.1038/s41588-020-0694-2.

Kim, K., Kim, D., Hanotte, O., Lee, C., Kim, H. *et al.* (2023) Inference of admixture origins in indigenous African cattle. *Molecular Biology and Evolution* 40(12), msad257. DOI: 10.1093/molbev/msad257.

Kwon, T., Kim, K., Caetano-Anolles, K., Sung, S., Cho, S. *et al.* (2022) Mitonuclear incompatibility as a hidden driver behind the genome ancestry of African admixed cattle. *BMC Biology* 20(1), 20. DOI: 10.1186/s12915-021-01206-x.

Latif, A.A., Troskie, P.C., Peba, S.B., Maboko, B.B., Pienaar, R. *et al.* (2019) Corridor disease (buffalo-associated *Theileria parva*) outbreak in cattle introduced onto a game ranch and investigations into their carrier-state. *Veterinary Parasitology, Regional Studies and Reports* 18, 100331. DOI: 10.1016/j.vprsr.2019.100331.

Lawrence, D.A. (1935) *Report of the Director of Veterinary Research, Southern Rhodesia, for the Year 1934*. Salisbury: Rhodesia Printing and Publishing Co. Ltd.

Lawrence, D.A. (1937) *Report of the Director of Veterinary Research, Southern Rhodesia, for the Year 1936*. Salisbury: Rhodesia Printing and Publishing Co. Ltd.

Lawrence, J.A. (1990) Summing up of strategies for tick-borne disease control in Africa, especially East Africa. *Parasitologia* 32, 113–115.

Leemans, I., Brown, D., Hooshmand-Rad, P., Kirvar, E. and Uggla, A. (1999a) Infectivity and cross-immunity studies of *Theileria lestoquardi* and *Theileria annulata* in sheep and cattle: I. *In vivo* responses. *Veterinary Parasitology* 82(3), 179–192. DOI: 10.1016/S0304-4017(99)00013-8.

Leemans, I., Brown, D., Fossum, C., Hooshmand-Rad, P., Kirvar, E. *et al.* (1999b) Infectivity and cross-immunity studies of *Theileria lestoquardi* and *Theileria annulata* in sheep and cattle: II. *In vitro* studies. *Veterinary Parasitology* 82(3), 193–204. DOI: 10.1016/S0304-4017(99)00014-X.

Lewis, E.A. (1943) East Coast fever and the African buffalo, the eland and the bushbuck. *The East African Agricultural Journal* 9(2), 90–92.

Lowdon, R.F., Jang, H.S. and Wang, T. (2016) Evolution of epigenetic regulation in vertebrate genomes. *Trends in Genetics* 32(5), 269–283. DOI: 10.1016/j.tig.2016.03.001.

Maboko, B.B., Sibeko-Matjila, K.P., Pierneef, R., Chan, W.Y., Josemans, A. *et al.* (2021) South Arican buffalo-derived *Theileria parva* is distinct from other buffalo and cattle-derived *T. parva*. *Frontiers in Genetics* 12, 666096. DOI: 10.3389/fgene.2021.666096.

MacHugh, N.D., Connelley, T., Graham, S.P., Pelle, R., Formisano, P. *et al.* (2009) CD8+ T-cell responses to *Theileria parva* are preferentially directed to a single dominant antigen: Implications for parasite strain-specific immunity. *European Journal of Immunology* 39(9), 2459–2469. DOI: 10.1002/eji.200939227.

Maritim, A.C., Young, A.S., Lesan, A.C., Ndungu, S.G., Stagg, D.A. *et al.* (1992) Transformation of *Theileria parva* derived from African buffalo (*Syncerus caffer*) by tick passage in cattle and its use in infection and treatment immunization. *Veterinary Parasitology* 43(1–2), 1–14. DOI: 10.1016/0304-4017(92)90043-9.

McKeever, D.J., Taracha, E.L., Innes, E.L., MacHugh, N.D., Awino, E. *et al.* (1994) Adoptive transfer of immunity to *Theileria parva* in the CD8+ fraction of responding efferent lymph. *Proceedings of the National Academy of Sciences* 91(5), 1959–1963. DOI: 10.1073/pnas.91.5.1959.

Mehlhorn, H. and Schein, E. (1984) The piroplasms: Life cycle and sexual stages. *Advances in Parasitology* 23, 37–103. DOI: 10.1016/s0065-308x(08)60285-7.

Michaux, J., Smitz, N. and Hooft, P. (2023) Taxonomic status of the African buffalo. In: Caron, A., Cornelis, D., Chardonnet, P. and Prins, H.H.T. (eds) *Ecology and Management of the African Buffalo*. Cambridge, UK: Cambridge University Press, pp. 49–65.

Minami, T., Spooner, P.R., Irvin, A.D., Ocama, J.G.R., Dobbelaere, D.A.E. *et al.* (1983) Characterisation of stocks of *Theileria parva* by monoclonal antibody profiles. *Research in Veterinary Science* 35(3), 334–340. DOI: 10.1016/S0034-5288(18)32029-0.

Morrison, W.I., Connelley, T., Hemmink, J.D. and MacHugh, N.D. (2015) Understanding the basis of parasite strain-restricted immunity to *Theileria parva*. *Annual Review of Animal Biosciences* 3(1), 397–418. DOI: 10.1146/annurev-animal-022513-114152.

Morzaria, S.P., Dolan, T.T., Norval, R.A.I., Bishop, R.P. and Spooner, P.R. (1995) Generation and characterization of cloned *Theileria parva* parasites. *Parasitology* 111(Pt 1), 39–49. DOI: 10.1017/s0031182000064581.

Musoke, A., Morzaria, S., Nkonge, C., Jones, E. and Nene, V. (1992) A recombinant sporozoite surface antigen of *Theileria parva* induces protection in cattle. *Proceedings of the National Academy of Sciences* 89(2), 514–518. DOI: 10.1073/pnas.89.2.514.

Musoke, A.J., Nantulya, V.M., Buscher, G., Masake, R.A. and Otim, B. (1984) Bovine immune response to *Theileria parva*: Neutralizing antibodies to sporozoites. *Immunology* 45, 663–668.

Neitz, W.O. (1955) Corridor disease: A fatal form of bovine teileriosis encountered in Zululand. *Bulletin of Epizootic Diseases in Africa* 3, 121–123.

Neitz, W.O. (1957) Theileriosis, gonderiosis and cytauxzoonoses: A review. *Onderstepoort Journal of Veterinary Research* 27, 275–430.

Neitz, W.O., Canham, A.S. and Kluge, E. (1955) Corridor disease: A fatal form of bovine theileriosis encountered in Zululand. *Journal of the South African Veterinary Association* 26, 78–87.

Nene, V., Iams, K.P., Gobright, E. and Musoke, A.J. (1992) Characterisation of the gene encoding a candidate vaccine antigen of *Theileria parva* sporozoites. *Molecular and Biochemical Parasitology* 51(1), 17–27. DOI: 10.1016/0166-6851(92)90196-q.

Nene, V., Musoke, A.J., Gobright, E. and Morzaria, S. (1996) Conservation of sporozoite p67 vaccine antigen in cattle-derived *Theileria parva* stocks with different cross-immunity profiles. *Infection and Immunity* 64(6), 2056–2061. DOI: 10.1128/iai.64.6.2056-2061.1996.

Obara, I., Ulrike, S., Musoke, T., Spooner, P.R., Jabbar, A. *et al.* (2015) Molecular evolution of a central region containimng B cell epitopes in the gene encoding the p67 sporozoite antigen within a field population of *Theileria parva*. *Parasitology Research* 114(5), 1729–1737. DOI: 10.1007/s00436-015-4358-6.

Obara, I., Githaka, N., Nijhof, A., Krücken, J., Nanteza, A. *et al.* (2020) The *Rhipicephalus appendiculatus* tick vector of *Theileria parva* is absent from cape buffalo (*Syncerus caffer*) populations and associated ecosystems in Northern Uganda. *Parasitology Research* 119(7), 2363–2367. DOI: 10.1007/s00436-020-06728-x.

Oura, C.A.L., Odongo, D.O., Lubega, G.W., Spooner, P.R., Tait, A. *et al.* (2003) A panel of microsatellite and minisatellite markers for the characterisation of field isolates of *Theileria parva*. *International Journal for Parasitology* 33(14), 1641–1653. DOI: 10.1016/s0020-7519(03)00280-7.

Oura, C.A.L., Asiimwe, B.B., Weir, W., Lubega, G.W. and Tait, A. (2005) Population genetic analysis and sub-structuring of *Theileria parva* in Uganda. *Molecular and Biochemical Parasitology* 140(2), 229–239. DOI: 10.1016/j.molbiopara.2004.12.015.

Oura, C.A.L., Tait, A., Asiimwe, B., Lubega, G.W. and Weir, W. (2011a) Haemoparasite prevalence and *Theileria parva* strain diversity in Cape buffalo (*Syncerus caffer*) in Uganda. *Veterinary Parasitology* 175(3–4), 212–219. DOI: 10.1016/j.vetpar.2010.10.032.

Oura, C.A.L., Tait, A., Asiimwe, B., Lubega, G.W. and Weir, W. (2011b) *Theileria parva* genetic diversity and haemoparasite prevalence in cattle and wildlife in and around Lake Mburo National Park in Uganda. *Parasitology Research* 108(6), 1365–1374. DOI: 10.1007/s00436-010-2030-8.

Pelle, R., Graham, S.P., Njahira, M.N., Osaso, J., Saya, R.M. *et al.* (2011) Two *Theileria parva* CD8 T cell antigen genes are more variable in buffalo than cattle parasites, but differ in pattern of sequence diversity. *PLoS ONE* 6(4), e19015. DOI: 10.1371/journal.pone.0019015.

Pitt, D., Sevane, N., Nicolazzi, E.L., MacHugh, D.E., Park, S.D.E. *et al.* (2018) Domestication of cattle: Two or three events. *Evolutionary Applications* 12(1), 123–136. DOI: 10.1111/eva.12674.

Potgieter, F.T., Stoltsz, W.H., Blouin, E.F. and Roos, J.A. (1988) Corridor disease in South Africa: A review of the current status. *Journal of the South Africa Veterinary Association* 59, 155–160.

Prins, H.H.T., Jong, J.F. and Geraads, D. (2023) The evolutionary history of the African buffalo: Is it truly a bovine? In: Caron, A., Cornélis, D., Chardonnet, P. and Prins, H.H.T. (eds) *Ecology and Management of the African Buffalo. Ecology, Biodiversity and Conservation*. Cambridge, UK: Cambridge University Press, pp. 25–48.

Quinn, L., Garcia-Erill, G., Santander, C., Brüniche-Olsen, A., Liu, X. *et al.* (2023) Colonialism in South Africa leaves a lasting legacy of reduced genetic diversity in Cape buffalo. *Molecular Ecology* 32(8), 1860–1874. DOI: 10.1111/mec.16851.

Radley, D.E., Brown, C.G.D., Burridge, M.J., Cunningham, M.P., Kirimi, I.M. *et al.* (1975a) East Coast fever: 1. Chemoprophylactic immunization of cattle against *Theileria parva* (Muguga) and five theilerial strains. *Veterinary Parasitology* 1(1), 35–41. DOI: 10.1016/0304-4017(75)90005-9.

Radley, D.E., Brown, C.G.D., Cunningham, M.P., Kimber, C.D., Musisi, F.L. *et al.* (1975b) East Coast fever: 3. Chemoprophylactic immunization of cattle using oxytetracycline and a combination of theilerial strains. *Veterinary Parasitology* 1(1), 51–60. DOI: 10.1016/0304-4017(75)90007-2.

Radley, D.E., Young, A.S., Grootenhuis, J.G., Cunningham, M.P., Dolan, T.T. *et al.* (1979) Further studies on the immunization of cattle against *Theileria lawrencei* by infection and chemoprophylaxis. *Veterinary Parasitology* 5(2–3), 117–128. DOI: 10.1016/0304-4017(79)90003-7.

Schreuder, B.E., Uilenberg, G. and Tondeur, W. (1977) Studies on Theileriidae (Sporozoa) in Tanzania. VIII. Experiments with African buffalo (*Syncerus caffer*). *Tropenmed Parasitologie* 28, 367–371.

Sibeko, K.P., Geysen, D., Oosthuizen, M.C., Matthee, C.A., Troskie, M. *et al.* (2010) Four p67 alleles identified in South African *Theileria parva* field samples. *Veterinary Parasitology* 167(2–4), 244–254. DOI: 10.1016/j.vetpar.2009.09.026.

Simonsen, B.T., Siegismund, H.R. and Arctander, P. (1998) Population structure of African buffalo inferred from mtDNA sequences and microsatellite loci: High variation but low differentiation. *Molecular Ecology* 7(2), 225–237. DOI: 10.1046/j.1365-294x.1998.00343.x.

Sitt, T., Poole, E.J., Ndambuki, G., Mwaura, S., Njoroge, T. *et al.* (2015) Exposure of vaccinated and naive cattle to natural challenge from buffalo-derived *Theileria parva*. *International Journal for Parasitology* 4(2), 244–251. DOI: 10.1016/j.ijppaw.2015.04.006.

Sitt, T., Henson, S., Morrison, W.I. and Toye, P. (2019) Similar levels of diversity in the gene encoding the p67 sporozoite surface protein of *Theileria parva* are observed in blood samples from buffalo and cattle naturally infected from buffalo. *Veterinary Parasitology* 269, 21–27. DOI: 10.1016/j.vetpar.2019.04.006.

Smitz, N., Berthouly, C., Cornélis, D., Heller, R., Hooft, P. *et al.* (2013) Pan-African genetic structure in the African buffalo (*Syncerus caffer*): Investigating intraspecific divergence. *PLoS ONE* 8(2), e56235. DOI: 10.1371/journal.pone.0056235.

Smitz, N., Cornélis, D., Chardonnet, P., Caron, A., Garine-Wichatitsky, M. *et al.* (2014) Genetic structure of fragmented southern populations of African Cape buffalo (*Syncerus caffer* caffer). *BMC Evolutionary Biology* 14(1), 203. DOI: 10.1186/s12862-014-0203-2.

Talenti, A., Wilkinson, T., Cook, E.A., Hemmink, J.D., Paxton, E. *et al.* (2024) Continent-wide genomic analysis of the African buffalo (*Syncerus caffer*). *Communications Biology* 7(1), 792. DOI: 10.1038/s42003-024-06481-2.

Taracha, E.L., Goddeeris, B.M., Teale, A.J., Kemp, S.J. and Morrison, W.I. (1995) Parasite strain specificity of bovine cytotoxic T cell responses to *Theileria parva* is determined primarily by immunodominance. *The Journal of Immunology* 155(10), 4854–4860. DOI: 10.4049/jimmunol.155.10.4854.

Toye, P.G., Goddeeris, B.M., Iams, K., Musoke, A.J. and Morrison, W.I. (1991) Characterization of a polymorphic immunodominant molecule in sporozoites and schizonts of *Theileria parva*. *Parasite Immunology* 13(1), 49–62. DOI: 10.1111/j.1365-3024.1991.tb00262.x.

Van Hooft, W.F., Groen, A.F. and Prins, H.H. (2000) Microsatellite analysis of genetic diversity in African buffalo (*Syncerus caffer*) populations throughout Africa. *Molecular Ecology* 9(12), 2017–2025. DOI: 10.1046/j.1365-294x.2000.01101.x.

Wragg, D., Cook, E.A.J., Latre de Laté, P., Sitt, T., Hemmink, J.D. *et al.* (2022) A locus conferring tolerance to *Theileria* infection in African cattle. *PLoS Genetics* 18(4), e1010099. DOI: 10.1371/journal.pgen.1010099.

Young, A.S. and Purnell, R.E. (1973) Transmission of *Theileria lawrencei* (Serengeti) by the ixodid tick, *Rhipicephalus appendiculatus*. *Tropical Animal Health and Production* 5(3), 146–152. DOI: 10.1007/BF02251383.

Young, A.S., Brown, C.G.D., Burridge, M.J., Cunningham, M.P., Kirimi, I.M. *et al.* (1973) Observations on the cross-immunity between *Theileria lawrencei* (Serengeti) and *Theileria parva* (Muguga) in cattle. *International Journal for Parasitology* 3(6), 723–728. DOI: 10.1016/0020-7519(73)90063-5.

Young, A.S., Brown, C.G.D., Burridge, M.J., Cunningham, M.P., Payne, R.C. *et al.* (1977a) Establishment of an experimental field population of *Theileria lawrencei*-infected ticks maintained by African buffalo (*Syncerus caffer*). *The Journal of Parasitology* 63(5), 903–907.

Young, A.S., Radley, D.E., Cunningham, M.P., Musisi, F.L., Payne, R.C. *et al.* (1977b) Exposure of immunized cattle to prolonged natural challenge of *Theileria lawrencei* derived from African buffalo (*Syncerus caffer*). *Veterinary Parasitology* 3(4), 283–290. DOI: 10.1016/0304-4017(77)90015-2.

Young, A.S., Brown, C.G.D., Burridge, M.J., Grootenhuis, G.K., Kanhau, G.K. *et al.* (1978) The incidence of theilerial parasites in East African buffalo (*Syncerus caffer*). *Tropenmed Parasitologie* 29, 281–288.

6 Disease Caused by *Theileria parva* in Southern Africa

Boitumelo B. Maboko, Ronel Pienaar and Ben J. Mans*
Epidemiology, Parasites and Vectors, Agricultural Research Council-Onderstepoort Veterinary Research, Onderstepoort, South Africa

6.1 Introduction

The nature of the disease threat from *T. parva* in southern Africa differs substantially from that in eastern Africa. Classical East Coast fever (ECF) was introduced into southern Africa at the beginning of the 20th century but was eradicated from South Africa in the 1950s following prolonged application of rigorous disease control measures. However, a less virulent form of the cattle-transmitted parasite remains in Zimbabwe, where it causes January disease. In both countries, endemic infection of African buffalo causes sporadic outbreaks of a condition known as Corridor disease in cattle that come into contact with buffalo. This chapter deals primarily with the history of ECF in southern Africa, specifically South Africa and Zimbabwe. It covers the recognized introduction of the disease in 1902, the measures applied to achieve its subsequent eradication from South Africa and the current control methods applied to prevent its re-establishment. The chapter also discusses the diseases caused by *T. parva* currently present in southern Africa (CD and January disease) and how they differ from classical ECF. The seasonal variation in the activity of the tick vector in southern Africa is highlighted as a key factor that influenced the eradication of ECF and currently determines the seasonal occurrence of disease. Finally, hypotheses concerning the origin of the different types of *T. parva* found in southern Africa and the factors that enabled the eradication of ECF are discussed.

6.2 Recognition of the Diseases Caused by *T. parva* in Southern Africa

6.2.1 The introduction of ECF into southern Africa

The first report of ECF in southern Africa was in Southern Rhodesia (now Zimbabwe) in January 1902 (Gray and Robertson, 1903). Shortly thereafter (May 1902), the disease was observed at Komatipoort and Nelspruit in the north-eastern part of South Africa (Fig. 6.1A). At this time, cattle were being imported from several countries to replenish the stock following a devastating outbreak of rinderpest, and it is widely recognized that the outbreak of ECF in southern Africa was associated with the importation of infected cattle from Tanzania into Zimbabwe and South Africa, through Malawi and Mozambique, respectively. The disease spread rapidly in both countries, and in South Africa reached Pretoria in November 1902 (Theiler, 1904). Widespread dissemination

*Corresponding author: MansB@arc.agric.za

 East Coast Fever: The Disease, its Impact and Control (eds W.I. Morrison and P. Toye)
DOI: 10.1079/9781800626324.0006

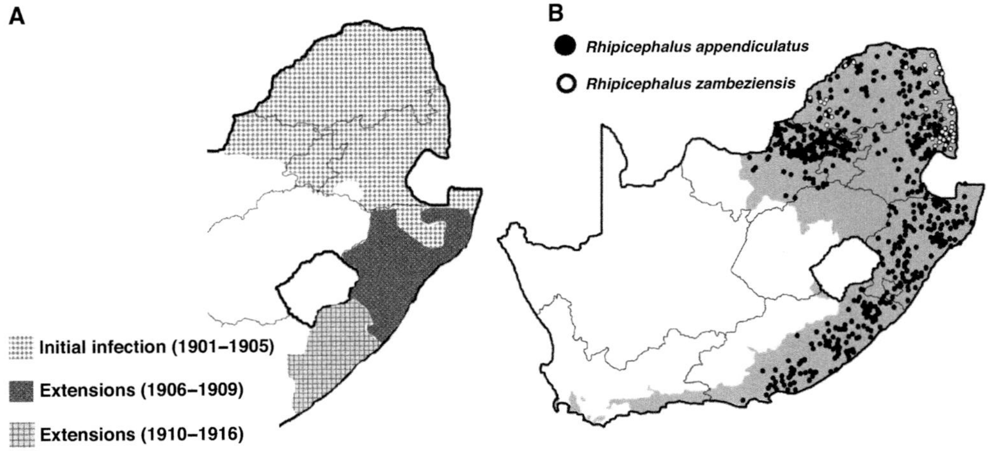

Fig. 6.1. The historic spread of ECF and the current distribution of the tick vectors in South Africa. A: The spread of ECF from 1901 to 1916. B: The shaded area shows the potential distribution for *R. appendiculatus* based on habitat suitability prediction (Norval *et al.*, 1982; Spickett, 2013). The circles represent locations of confirmed detection of *R. appendiculatus* and *R. zambeziensis* (another vector of *T. parva* – discussed in Section 6.4) (Horak *et al.*, 2018).

of the disease occurred within 7 months of its introduction, spanning autumn, winter and spring seasons. Despite extensive efforts to curtail it, by 1905 it had spread throughout the Transvaal and entered northern Natal via Swaziland, and by 1906 it had spread through north-eastern Natal (Diesel, 1948). By 1909, the disease was present throughout Natal, and in March 1910 it reached the Eastern Cape (Transkei) (Diesel, 1948). In 1912, ECF was established across most of the geographic distribution of the tick vector (Fig. 6.1A; Lawrence, 1991).

The main tick vector was identified as the brown ear tick, *Rhipicephalus appendiculatus* (Lounsbury, 1903). The geographic distribution of *R. appendiculatus* has changed very little in the past century (Fig. 6.1B; Horak *et al.*, 2018), a feature that will be considered for the period after the eradication of ECF. The identification of *T. parva* as the causative agent and its tick vector followed a period of intensive investigation of the disease, as discussed more fully in Chapter 1 of this volume.

6.2.2 Corridor disease

In 1934, a related disease caused by *Theileria* parasites was identified in Southern Rhodesia (now Zimbabwe) by Lawrence (1935) and subsequently recognized in South Africa (Neitz *et al.*, 1955). The disease showed similarities to ECF and, over the course of investigations, was shown to be caused by a parasite related to *T. parva*, derived from buffalo. The parasite was appropriately named *Theileria lawrencei* and the disease was named Corridor disease (CD), based on its occurrence in a land corridor that existed between the Hluhluwe and Imfolozi Game Parks in Natal at the time. The disease showed clinical differences from ECF relating to disease progression and time to death, and the levels of schizonts and piroplasms observed in lymph node aspirates and blood smears, respectively, were much lower than observed in ECF (Neitz *et al.*, 1955; Sitt *et al.*, 2015). Of particular significance was the observation that moving infected cattle from buffalo pastures to buffalo-free pastures known to be infested with ticks effectively halted the spread of the disease, indicating cessation of transmission of the parasite by ticks. By contrast, removal of cattle from infected pastures during the ECF epidemic had led to further spread of the disease. Neitz investigated transmission of infection from cattle infected with the CD parasite (Neitz, 1957, 1958) and was unable to demonstrate transmission by ticks fed on recovered cattle, although a brief period of transmission was found in a splenectomized calf and cattle treated with chemotherapeutics during infection (Neitz, 1958; Potgieter *et al.*, 1988). A later study of cattle infected with buffalo-derived *T. parva* in South Africa also failed to detect transmission of infection in recovered animals (Potgieter *et al.*, 1988). However, more recently, cattle that recovered from a CD outbreak were found to retain the infection for up to 3 months, as detected using the polymerase chain reaction (PCR) assay and tick transmission (Mbizeni *et al.*, 2013; Latif *et al.*, 2019).

6.2.3 January disease (Zimbabwe theileriosis)

In 1936, Lawrence reported another form of theileriosis in eastern Zimbabwe. Like CD, affected animals had fewer schizonts and piroplasms than observed in ECF, but it was not associated with buffalo (Lawrence, 1937). Neitz (1957) initially referred to the parasite causing Rhodesian/Zimbabwean theileriosis as *Gonderia bovis* but later referred to it as *Theileria bovis*. It was subsequently named *T. parva bovis* (Uilenberg, 1976). The disease is different from ECF in that it causes fewer fatalities (Matson, 1967). However, Norval *et al.* (1985) state that it is likely that the parasite associated with January disease originated from the parasites that cause ECF but is less virulent. The possibility that this strain can potentially revert to virulence has been considered (Uilenberg *et al.*, 1982).

6.3 Control of the Initial ECF Epidemic in Southern Africa

It is believed that 20–40% of the cattle population of southern Africa that survived the rinderpest epidemic were subsequently killed by ECF (Norval *et al.*, 1992). The initial efforts to control the disease were similar in South Africa and Zimbabwe, since scientists from both countries freely exchanged information and met at various conferences to design strategies for control of the disease (Lawrence, 1986). Control of the initial ECF epidemic involved dipping and spraying cattle for ticks at 10 day intervals and before movement from infected or suspected infected fields to new uninfected grazing areas. This method of control had limited success due to cattle owners not cooperating and the dipping interval not being short enough to control the vector (Lawrence, 1986).

In a meeting held in Bloemfontein in December 1903, the decision was taken to attempt eradication of the disease. This followed the realization that some animals could survive the infection and might become reservoirs for future outbreaks (Williams, 1904; Lawrence, 1986). Initial efforts involved quarantine and slaughter of infected animals, but it became costly, prompting a change in approach by the authorities involving the establishment of temperature camps. Animals that did not show any clinical symptoms were moved to clean grazing land and their temperatures monitored for about 3 months, depending on the circumstances. Those with elevated temperatures were slaughtered. The temperature camps had limited success and the practice was short-lived.

Short-interval dipping (in cycles 4, 5 and 5 days apart) was introduced in 1911 with the aim of replacing the practice of quarantine and slaughter of animals (Norval *et al.*, 1992). However, information presented at the November 1924 conference in Bulawayo (Anon, 1924) indicated that dipping suppressed the disease but did not eradicate it. The dipping strategy was briefly supplemented by the introduction of immunization based on the inoculation of naïve animals with 5 ml of blood from ECF-recovered animals. This approach was based on the observations of Koch (1903), who found that attempts to transmit infection from ECF cases with the blue tick (*Rhipicephalus (Boophilus)* spp.) resulted in infection of erythrocytes but no disease in recipient animals, which Koch erroneously interpreted as production of immunity. However, the transmitted parasites were subsequently believed to be a non-pathogenic species of *Theileria*. This control method was not well received, and during the Cape Town, May 1904 meeting it was noted that immunization was not effective and it was believed that it might help to sustain the outbreak (Anon, 1904; Lawrence, 1986). Additional vaccine strategies were attempted using tissues from ECF cases (Theiler, 1912; Spreull, 1914), but the vaccination protocols themselves resulted in fatalities and were abandoned once it became clear that dipping was more effective.

By 1928, it was realized that measures introduced to control the disease, namely short-interval dipping, quarantine and removal of cattle showing disease symptoms, were inadequate (du Toit and Viljoen, 1928). Therefore, a revised compulsory quarantine and slaughter policy was adopted in 1929, which incorporated extensive diagnostic testing of all suspect and clinical cases through microscopic slide examination to detect parasites and removing infected animals before the disease could spread further (Anon, 1929; Viljoen, 1929; Diesel, 1948; Diesel and Van Drimmelen, 1948; Anon, 1981). The diagnostic testing was laborious, but when properly executed, it was valuable in detecting the disease early before heavy mortalities and losses occurred. If an infection was missed at first, retracing was possible by examining smears and conducting follow-ups of farms that might have become infected due to cattle movement (Norval *et al.*, 1992). At one point, cattle were monitored monthly by veterinary authorities because movement permits were required when relocating cattle. The farmer had to account for any discrepancies.

This prolonged, concerted effort by the veterinary authorities eventually led to eradication of the disease in South Africa by 1955 (Diesel, 1948; Neitz, 1957). It was estimated that about 5.5 million cattle were lost at an approximate cost of 100 million rand in South Africa (Anon, 1981). Since 1955, no new cases of ECF have been reported.

6.4 Diapause and Seasonality of Tick Activity

The pronounced seasonality of tick activity in southern Africa is a major factor in determining differences in the epidemiology of infections with *T. parva*, compared to the situation in eastern Africa. Ambient temperature affects the speed of parasite development in the tick. Studies of infected ticks in an experimental paddock in Kenya showed that the minimum time required for transmission of infection acquired by nymphal ticks was 30 days during the warm season but 62 days during the cold season, where the mean temperature differed by 4°C (Young *et al.*, 1981). In contrast, in southern Africa, adult *R. appendiculatus* ticks have a seasonal diapausing behaviour, that is, ticks overwinter in a low metabolic state of suspended development (Randolph, 1997). Eastern African *R. appendiculatus* ticks do not exhibit diapause when exposed to a South African environment (Madder *et al.*, 2002). During diapause, adult ticks delay host-seeking and feeding. This delay is regulated primarily by photoperiod (i.e. daily length of daylight) but is also influenced by humidity and temperature (Short and Norval, 1981). The diapause period ranges from 3 to 7 months (Norval *et al.*, 1991; Randolph, 1997), largely in line with geographical latitude; ticks from Zambia exhibit a less pronounced diapause than those from South Africa and Zimbabwe (Madder *et al.*, 2002). Since ticks have been shown to be infective for at least 6 months after moulting (Neitz, 1957; Young *et al.*, 1981), an appreciable portion of ticks will retain infectivity after diapause. Diapause results in a degree of synchronization of the tick life cycle, influencing the seasonal prevalence of the different life-cycle stages of the tick. In South Africa, 90% of tick larvae are found between April and June, 90% of nymphs are found between May and November and 90% of adults are found between December and May (Rechav, 1981, 1982; Gallivan *et al.*, 2011; Spickett *et al.*, 2011). As a result of the climatic conditions and the diapause behaviour of the ticks, the resident ticks in southern Africa complete only one life cycle each year. By contrast, in countries close to the equator (e.g. Kenya), two or sometimes three life cycles can be completed annually, with no clear pattern of seasonal abundance of a life stage.

Rhipicephalus zambeziensis has also been shown to be a competent vector of *T. parva*. It can transmit the parasite experimentally (Lawrence *et al.*, 1983), although records of its role in *T. parva* outbreaks are scant. It is a non-diapausing tick (Berkvens *et al.*, 1995) whose contribution to the epidemiology of ECF is not clear, but its propensity for drier areas may impact disease prevalence in regions unsuitable for *R. appendiculatus*. *R. zambeziensis* is widespread in the northern and southern regions of Zimbabwe, while *R. appendiculatus* is found in the central and eastern regions. In South Africa, *R. zambeziensis* is found in the Northwest, Limpopo and Mpumalanga provinces (Norval *et al.*, 1982; Walker *et al.*, 2000; Norval and Horak, 2004). Blouin and Stoltsz (1989) experimentally showed that *R. zambeziensis* had higher *T. parva* infection rates than *R. appendiculatus*, indicating they may be better transmitters of the parasite. Its role in the original ECF outbreak was considered non-significant (Lawrence, 1991).

The conditions in South Africa result in a seasonal pattern of transmission of *T. parva* and occurrence of disease. As a consequence of diapause, CD outbreaks generally start from December or January, with a peak from March to May and some cases in June (Mbizeni *et al.*, 2013), while in Zimbabwe, January disease outbreaks are common from December to May. Tick nymphal stages are linked to occasional June and July outbreaks. The different seasonal patterns of abundance of the tick life-cycle stages also influence transmission of the parasite. During the period when adult ticks are abundant, there are very few larval and nymphal stages, which are required to transmit infection from acutely infected animals. Hence, it has been suggested that transmission is heavily dependent on ticks picking up infection from carrier animals (Norval *et al.*, 1991; discussed further below).

6.5 Potential Role of Non-diapausing Ticks in the ECF Epidemic

The presence of diapause in southern Africa raises the intriguing question of how the disease spread so quickly after introduction and through the colder months of the year. Norval *et al.* (1991) postulated that non-diapausing *R. appendiculatus* strains capable of transmitting virulent *T. parva* were imported into southern Africa during the original introduction of ECF and that persistence and spread of these ticks facilitated transmission of the parasite across seasons, hampering efforts to eradicate the disease. However, this hypothesis seems implausible, not least because imported non-diapausing ticks would not have been adapted to the seasonal fluctuations in climate that characterize South Africa and are unlikely to have been able to survive and spread throughout such a large area in competition with locally adapted ticks. Within 10 years of introduction of the disease into South Africa, it had spread rapidly through the total natural geographic range of the tick vector, and thereafter it took about 40 years to achieve eradication. Spread of the disease was obviously not hindered by the annual life cycle of *R. appendiculatus* in southern Africa. Disease was observed across the seasons, although the incidence was lower in the winter compared to autumn and summer months, associated with lower numbers of ticks (Neitz, 1957). The less pronounced seasonal occurrence of disease in the early outbreak may have been due to the much higher levels of parasites in the numerous cases of acute ECF, compared to transmission of CD from buffalo, allowing more efficient transmission across different seasons. The possible significance of the seasonal pattern of the disease in the early years of the epidemic was not discussed in early publications (Koch, 1903; Theiler, 1904; Diesel, 1948; Neitz, 1957).

Rather than involving an unlikely role for introduced non-diapausing ticks in contributing to the prolonged period required to eradicate ECF from South Africa, as mentioned above, persistence of the disease during the early years could be attributed to the inability to control the disease with dipping practices (du Toit and Viljoen, 1928). Indeed, right up to 1945, the tick vector remained extensively distributed across its range in South Africa (Lawrence, 1991). Implementation of a number of additional control measures by the South African government in 1929, involving an extensive system of diagnostic testing of all suspect animals and the quarantine and slaughter of such suspected animals (Anon, 1929), appears to have been instrumental in the eventual eradication of ECF. Nevertheless, the seasonal pattern of the disease in southern Africa may well have helped in achieving eradication.

6.6 The Importance of the Carrier State in the Rapid Spread of ECF in South Africa

Infection with *T. parva* is not detected microscopically in lymphocytes and erythrocytes in cattle that have recovered from ECF, and early studies by Theiler and Lounsbury failed to transmit infection with ticks fed on ECF-recovered cattle, leading to the belief that infection does not persist beyond the acute phase of the disease. Indeed, it had been argued that eradication by natural means could be achieved as no carrier state for ECF could be demonstrated in South Africa, and diapause would impair survival of the parasite across the winter seasons (du Toit, 1928; Neitz, 1948). However, observations that ECF recurred in areas of a previous outbreak after a period of 18 months suggested that persistence of infection in carrier animals may have occurred in some recovered cattle (Diesel and Van Drimmelen, 1948). This was based on earlier studies indicating that ticks may survive for up to 15 months under optimal temperature and humidity conditions (Lounsbury, 1905), indicating that pasture needs to lie fallow for at least 15–18 months to clear infection (Theiler, 1904; Diesel and Van Drimmelen, 1948). However, survival of ticks can vary depending on local environmental conditions, as indicated by the finding of Young *et al.* (1981) of one example of ticks surviving for 21 months in an experimental paddock in Kenya. Nevertheless, later studies in eastern Africa involving feeding of ticks on recovered cattle clearly showed that a potentially lifelong carrier state in cattle existed for *T. parva*, enabling infection to be maintained by tick-mediated cattle-to-cattle transmission (Young *et al.*, 1986; Kariuki *et al.*, 1995). Moreover, mathematical modelling has indicated that transmission from carrier animals plays an important role in maintaining infection in ECF-endemic areas (Medley *et al.*, 1993).

Mortality during the South African ECF epidemic is estimated to have varied from 78% to 100% (Neitz, 1957), indicating that significant numbers of cattle survived the disease. Current knowledge of the carrier state supports the perspective that the existence of persistent carrier infections in at least some of the recovered cattle during the original ECF epidemic in South Africa could have sustained the infection over the diapausing period each year to allow pick-up and transmission of infection in the subsequent season of tick activity. Moreover, as argued by Norval *et al.* (1992) and discussed above, the differences in the seasonal timing of different developmental stages of the tick in southern Africa implies that transmission of *T. parva* in this region is heavily dependent on tick pick-up of infection from carrier animals.

The ability of infected ticks to diapause allows parasite survival over the winter periods. The presence of carrier animals means year-round sources of parasites that can be picked up by different life stages of the vector tick, resulting in year-round outbreaks.

6.7 Was CD Introduced at the Time of the ECF Outbreak?

The fact that CD in cattle appears not to have been recognized before the ECF outbreak led to the proposal that the parasite that causes CD was introduced into African buffalo from the parasites that caused the ECF outbreak (Lawrence, 1986; Norval *et al.*, 1991, 1992). However, extensive research strongly refutes this hypothesis.

Firstly, buffalo-derived *T. parva* usually fails to produce a piroplasmic or carrier state in cattle and thus it is not transmitted from infected animals. As such, it is highly unlikely that buffalo-type parasites could have been transmitted from cattle imported from eastern Africa.

Secondly, if the parasites introduced at the time of the ECF outbreak were the only source of infections in buffalo, subsequently causing CD in cattle, it would be expected that all *T. parva* circulating in South African buffalo would show limited genetic diversity. Genome-wide genetic evidence for cattle-adapted *T. parva* from diverse countries, including Kenya, Rwanda, Tanzania, Uganda and Zambia, has indicated that the cattle-adapted parasites show limited genetic diversity compared to buffalo-adapted parasites (reviewed in Chapter 4 of this volume). As current evidence indicates that ECF was introduced into southern Africa once, or at most only a few times (J. Lawrence, 2016, unpublished observations), it is likely that the *T. parva* population introduced into southern Africa represented only a small subset of the cattle-adapted *T. parva* population. Unfortunately, only one laboratory isolate of the parasites that caused ECF in South Africa, the Schoonspruit strain, currently exists as a parasitized lymphoid cell line. It shows 99–100% sequence identity in the p67, p104 and PIM genes with those of the Muguga genome reference strain of *T. parva*. By contrast, genotypic analyses have revealed that South African buffalo parasites show extensive genotypic diversity, similar to that found in eastern African buffalo. A study in which the genes encoding p67, p104 and PIM were sequenced detected a very large amount of sequence diversity within the population of *T. parva* circulating among buffalo and cases associated with CD in South Africa (Sibeko *et al.*, 2010, 2011). Similar diversity in p67 was also observed in eastern Africa in cattle that developed CD when grazed on buffalo pasture, whereas only a single variant of p67 has been detected in cattle with ECF (Sitt *et al.*, 2019). In a further study in which the genes encoding two highly polymorphic T cell antigens (Tp1 and Tp2) in small samples of eastern African and South African buffalo also revealed similarly extensive sequence diversity in both populations (Hemmink *et al.*, 2018), which was much greater than had been observed in cattle *T. parva* isolates (Pelle *et al.*, 2011). More recently, analysis of single nucleotide polymorphisms from whole genome sequences has shown that, on a genome-wide scale, buffalo-derived *T. parva* from South Africa shows a level of genetic diversity as large as, if not surpassing, that of buffalo isolates from other countries (Maboko *et al.*, 2021a, b). A number of isolates in these studies were derived from cattle, but these were cattle infected with parasites of buffalo origin. Phylogenetic analysis also indicated that eastern African cattle-derived strains of *T. parva* diverged significantly from both South African and eastern African buffalo-derived strains (Fig. 6.2; Maboko *et al.*, 2021b). The implications of this are clear, namely that such large genetic diversity does not fit with the introduction of a genetically restricted population of parasites but rather indicates that *T. parva* has been circulating in South African buffalo for many thousands of years. In the unlikely event that the parasites which currently infect buffalo were introduced with cattle during the ECF epidemic, reversion to cattle–cattle transmissible parasites would have been highly likely in the buffalo parasite population. This has clearly not been the case.

Finally, it has been estimated that Cape buffalo migrated from central and eastern Africa into southern Africa between 83,000 and 29,000 years ago and that this introduction may have occurred several times (Smitz *et al.*, 2013; see also Chapter 4 of this volume). Since buffalo are considered lifelong carriers of *T. parva* (Norval *et al.*, 1992), it is likely that this natural migration introduced *T. parva* strains into southern Africa and may also have introduced the tick vector, given the low level of genetic diversity observed in *R. appendiculatus* in southern Africa (Amzati *et al.*, 2018). These issues have been discussed recently (Mans, 2020; Morrison *et al.*, 2020), with the conclusion that *T. parva* was present in buffalo in southern Africa well before the introduction of ECF.

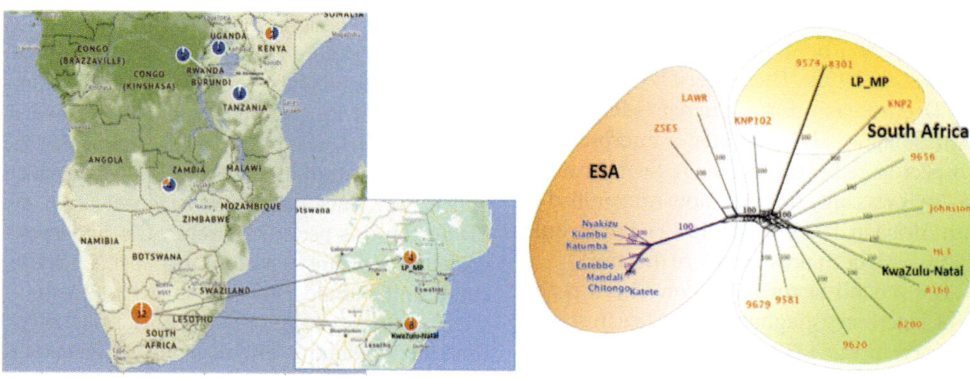

Fig. 6.2. Genome-wide SNP analysis of *Theileria parva* from various geographic regions and host origins. Cattle-derived strains are indicated with a blue font and buffalo-derived strains with an orange font. LP, MP and ESA represent Limpopo, Mpumalanga and eastern and southern Africa, respectively. Maximum likelihood analysis was performed using PAUP* with 1000 bootstrap replicates to assess nodal support. The scale bar indicates 0.01 nucleotide substitutions. Samples 9574, 9656, Johnston, 8200 and 9620 were collected from cattle. From Maboko *et al.* (2021b).

6.8 Why Was CD Not Recognized Before the ECF Epidemic?

If *T. parva* was present in buffalo in southern Africa before introduction of ECF, then why was CD not recognized in cattle, particularly given the acute and fatal nature of the disease? To answer this question, a number of factors can be considered.

The first relates to the rudimentary knowledge of tick-borne diseases in the period prior to the introduction of ECF into southern Africa. As discussed in Chapter 1 of this volume, the first blood-borne piroplasms to be identified as pathogens were the causal agents of redwater in cattle, by Babes (1888) and Smith and Kilborne (1893). The organisms were subsequently named *Babesia bovis* and *Babesia bigemina*, transmitted by the tick species *Boophilus bovis* and *Rhipicephalus annulatus*, respectively. *Babesia bigemina* and the alternative vector *Rhipicephalus decoloratus* were known to occur in South Africa by the time of the introduction of ECF and to have caused Texas redwater, known locally as South African redwater (Hutcheon, 1898; Koch, 1898; Theiler, 1904, 1905). Indeed, ECF was at first misdiagnosed as a form of redwater, and it was subsequently recognized that co-infections with the parasites that cause ECF and redwater occurred (Koch, 1903; Theiler, 1904). Although Theiler (1905) suggested that redwater may have been introduced into South Africa around 1870, others have argued that it was endemic in South Africa well before this date (Norval *et al.*, 1992). Therefore, it is possible that any CD outbreaks that occurred before 1902 were misdiagnosed as redwater or interpreted in retrospect as redwater. Asiatic redwater caused by *B. bovis* was only unambiguously identified in South Africa in 1941 (Neitz, 1941), but it could possibly have been present before this time.

The second factor to be considered is the lack of veterinary diagnostic expertise in southern Africa in the 1800s. The first veterinarian to be appointed in South Africa was in 1874 (Bothma, 1987), and therefore the recognition of CD before this period may have been limited by the absence of diagnostic expertise, as well as being confounded by the presence of other diseases. Any outbreak due to CD after 1902 would probably have been ascribed to the ECF epidemic. The transient nature of CD outbreaks, where removal of animals from infected pastures effectively stops the disease, could also have confounded its identification.

A third consideration is the presence of trypanosomiasis in the same cattle populations. Bruce (1895), working in northern KwaZulu-Natal, demonstrated that the tsetse was the vector for the causative agent of nagana or animal trypanosomiasis and later identified *Trypanosoma brucei* (Baker, 1995). Four major tsetse species are vectors for nagana, namely *Glossina morsitans morsitans*, which occurred in the northern areas of South Africa (including the Kruger National Park), and *G. austeni*, *G. brevipalpis* and *G. pallidipes*, which occurred in northern KwaZulu-Natal (Kappmeier *et al.*, 1998). These areas correspond closely with the current distribution of *R. appendiculatus* (Fig. 6.1A). Trypanosomiasis made these regions uninhabitable for cattle. Tsetse flies are considered to be associated with wildlife (buffalo act as a host for both tsetse flies and the trypanosome parasites), and a commonly held belief was that the tsetse fly and nagana only occur where wildlife are present (Bruce, 1895). It is possible that the occurrence of CD and nagana in cattle that came in contact with buffalo pasture may have hindered recognition of CD as a unique disease. Disappearance of nagana from regions where wildlife was actively hunted out, to be replaced by cattle (Kappmeier *et al.*, 1998), would also have coincided with disappearance of CD in these regions.

Finally, it should also be considered that the rinderpest outbreak in South Africa lasted from 1896 to 1899 (Vogel and Heyne, 1996). Theiler (1904) remarked on superficial similarities in clinical presentation of ECF and rinderpest, which may have confounded identification of CD during this period. However, the rinderpest epidemic had a more profound impact, since the cattle and buffalo populations were so extensively reduced (estimated 80–90% mortality) that the remaining buffalo could not sustain the tsetse fly (Vogel and Heyne, 1996). *Glossina m. morsitans* disappeared from South Africa, while *G. pallidipes* was eradicated in 1954. *G. austeni* and *G. brevipalpis* retracted to very small pockets, notably the Hluhluwe and Umfolozi reserves proclaimed as Game Reserves in 1897 by the British Government (Kappmeier *et al.*,

1998). Most probably, the only regions where buffalo extensively occurred after the rinderpest epidemic were the Kruger National Park (established 1898) and the Hluhluwe-Umfolozi Game Reserves. The substantial reduction in buffalo after the rinderpest epidemic is likely to have limited cattle and buffalo contact to an extent that would have reduced the incidence of CD outbreaks.

In conclusion, a number of confounding factors may have prevented the recognition of CD as a distinct disease in South Africa before its discovery in 1934 in Zimbabwe and 1955 in South Africa.

6.9 The Disease Situation Following Eradication of ECF

6.9.1 Recognition of *T. parva* as the cause of ECF, CD and January disease

A key factor in understanding the disease situation in southern Africa was the recognition that the three diseases, despite different clinical presentations, are caused by the same parasite species. A close relationship of the parasites causing ECF and CD was indicated following reports from eastern Africa that repeated experimental tick passage of some buffalo-derived *T. parva* isolates in cattle could transform the parasites to cause a disease similar to ECF, casting doubt on the validity of different species for *T. parva* and *T. lawrencei* (discussed in Section 6.9.3). An antigenic relationship between *T. parva* and *T. lawrencei* was also inferred based on partial cross-protection between some isolates (Neitz, 1957) and serological cross-reactivity in the immunofluorescent antibody test (Löhr and Ross, 1969; Schindler *et al.*, 1969; Lawrence, 1977). These findings led to the proposal that *T. parva* is composed of a complex of subtypes, namely *T. parva parva* causing ECF, *T. parva lawrencei* causing CD and *T. parva bovis* causing January disease (Uilenberg, 1976; Lawrence, 1979). The trinomial system was replaced in 1989 by referring to the parasites as buffalo-derived *T. parva* (*T. p. lawrencei*) or cattle-derived *T. parva* (*T. p. parva* and *T. p. bovis*) (Anon, 1989), to acknowledge the understanding that different subsets of the same parasite species are responsible for the different disease manifestations. This history of changes in the nomenclature of *T. parva* is described by Perry and Young (1993).

6.9.2 The current situation

In South Africa, theileriosis continues to be a problem only where CD outbreaks occur when cattle graze on pastures infested with ticks that fed on buffalo (Mbizeni *et al.*, 2013; Latif *et al.*, 2019). The CD area comprises part of the eastern side of South Africa including the Kruger National Park in Limpopo and Mpumalanga, extending down to the Hluhluwe-Imfolozi Game Park in KwaZulu-Natal (Mbizeni *et al.*, 2013). As discussed earlier, the peak of CD outbreaks is between March and May (Mbizeni *et al.*, 2013) and correlates with activity of adult ticks (Rechav, 1981, 1982; Spickett *et al.*, 2011). As discussed elsewhere, the outbreaks are curtailed when cattle are moved away from buffalo grazing areas. Sampling and testing of cattle outside the CD area, but within the *R. appendiculatus*-infested area, indicate no signs of infection with *T. parva* (Mans *et al.*, 2011, 2016).

In the case of Zimbabwe, the only diseases thought to remain are CD and January disease (Lawrence, 1986). A relatively low incidence of theileriosis outbreaks occurred from 1995 to 2011 (992 cases), but subsequently increased from 2012, continuing with more than 6000 theileriosis cases reported annually from 2012 to 2018 (Manyenyeka *et al.*, 2022). The new outbreaks have been linked with climate change and possible increase of *R. zambeziensis* in the drier areas during recent droughts (Manyenyeka *et al.*, 2022). However, the increase in cases has not abated, and it has been estimated that more than 500,000 cattle have died since 2021 (Muvhuringi *et al.*, 2022; Dube-Matutu, 2024). It is unclear whether this outbreak is due to farmers not adhering to recommended control measures due to the high cost of acaricides, tick resistance, an increase in the incidence of January disease or whether ECF has reappeared due either to reversion to virulence of the January disease parasites or to the reintroduction of ECF parasites from elsewhere.

6.9.3 Transformation of CD parasites to resemble those causing ECF

Although infections of cattle with the buffalo-derived parasites that cause CD generally are not tick-transmissible, it is possible that this situation may change and ECF will reappear in South Africa. As discussed elsewhere in this book, experimental studies in eastern Africa have demonstrated tick transmission of some buffalo *T. parva* isolates, which upon repeated passage produced disease similar to ECF (Barnett and Brocklesby, 1966a). This phenomenon, referred to as 'transformation', demonstrated the potential of buffalo-type *T. parva* to adapt to transmission in cattle. However, studies in South Africa could not demonstrate transformation of buffalo-type *T. parva* to resemble ECF strains (Potgieter *et al.*, 1988). Transmission from cattle infected with buffalo parasites could only be achieved on one occasion using a splenectomized calf. It is important to note that this 'transformation' has only been reported on three occasions in eastern Africa by feeding of large numbers of ticks on cattle infected experimentally with buffalo-derived parasites (Barnett and Brocklesby, 1966a; Young and Purnell, 1973; Maritim *et al.*, 1992). Hence, it is unclear how frequently (if at all) it occurs under natural conditions. The seasonality observed in tick activity and the abundance of different tick life-cycle stages in southern Africa (Mbizeni *et al.*, 2013) further decreases the likelihood of parasites acquired from buffalo going through several cattle passages that would allow transformation as described in eastern Africa. Nevertheless, the South African veterinary authorities do treat the potential reappearance of ECF in South Africa as a serious threat and ensure that CD is strictly controlled to reduce the risk of buffalo-adapted *T. parva* transforming to cattle-adapted forms (Potgieter *et al.*, 1988). The transformation process, which may involve adaptive changes in the parasite or selection of rare genotypes with the ability to undergo tick transmission in cattle, is discussed in further detail in Chapter 4 of this volume.

6.9.4 The origin of January disease in Zimbabwe

The seasonality of the occurrence of disease associated with *T. parva* and its presentation changed in Southern Rhodesia (Zimbabwe) over the course of the 50 or so years it took to eradicate ECF. Prior to eradication of ECF, disease during the early stages of the ECF epidemic occurred across the year, with peaks in January–February and May–July. This gradually changed until a disease peak was largely confined to January–March. The disease also changed from a virulent form that had a mortality of 95% to a much less virulent form. This less virulent form was first observed in the eastern regions of the country in 1936 and differed from ECF in displaying a shorter duration of clinical signs, absence of lesions associated with ECF, low schizont and piroplasm parasitemia and providing no consistent cross-protection against experimental challenge with more virulent strains (Lawrence, 1937). The disease was named January disease and it was effectively controlled by short-interval dipping of cattle with acaricides. More stringent control for typical ECF and less stringent control for the new disease resulted in this latter disease becoming the dominant form of theileriosis in Zimbabwe (Norval *et al.*, 1992). One of the outcomes of a less virulent isolate was the development of the *T. parva* (Boleni) live vaccine that could be used without concomitant chemotherapy (Irvin *et al.*, 1989; Latif and Hove, 2011).

The epidemiology of this disease suggests that the parasite was a subpopulation of the original ECF stock, which was selected as a less virulent form. It is known that within the *T. parva* population that causes ECF, strains that differ in virulence exist (Barnett and Brocklesby, 1966b; Mbogo *et al.*, 1996; Musisi *et al.*, 1996; Tindih *et al.*, 2010). The relaxed control methods towards this disease, coupled with the strict control of virulent ECF, probably allowed it to establish in the country. Whether the emergence of this form of the parasite was due to selection of a better adapted strain (a 'bottleneck' effect) in the eastern regions of the country or mutation in a population is difficult to ascertain to date. The relatively low cattle numbers at the start of the ECF epidemic due to the rinderpest epidemic and the further decimation by ECF itself (Norval *et al.*, 1992) may have resulted in favourable conditions for a bottleneck effect, since a small host population would restrict the parasite population and may have favoured emergence of a subpopulation (Papkou *et al.*, 2016). Monoclonal antibody profiles indicated that *T. parva* (Boleni) shows similar patterns of reactivity to ECF isolates from other countries, with the exception that one monoclonal antibody (MAb 7) does not react with the Zimbabwean isolates (Koch *et al.*, 1988). The only genetic data currently generated for *T. parva* from Zimbabwe come from a restriction fragment length polymorphism (RFLP)-based study that analysed both cattle-derived and buffalo-derived parasites (Bishop *et al.*, 1994). This study showed that all cattle-derived isolates, including the well characterized *T. parva* (Boleni) (Koch *et al.*, 1988), showed a homogeneous *Tpr* allele profile, while buffalo-derived isolates gave a large diversity of alleles. This may support the idea that a bottleneck effect resulted in selection of a subpopulation of parasites exhibiting reduced virulence. Microsatellite analysis indicated that *T. parva* (Boleni) groups with other ECF isolates from Kenya, Uganda and Zambia, to the exclusion of buffalo-derived isolates (Oura *et al.*, 2003), consistent with the view that it was derived by selection from the original ECF stock. However, better resolution would be obtained if full genome sequencing could be performed on the Zimbabwean isolates and compared using, for example, single nucleotide polymorphism (SNP) analysis (Maboko *et al.*, 2021b).

6.10 Current Control Measures in Southern Africa

In South Africa, CD and ECF are listed as controlled diseases (Animal Diseases Act, 1984). Any suspected cases or outbreaks need to be reported to the authorities for investigation and diagnostic testing performed. Positive cases are reported to the Department of Animal Health. All buffalo that are moved need to be tested, and all movements need to be approved by the State Veterinary Offices. The immunofluorescence antibody assay test (IFAT) and Hybrid II real-time PCR test are used (see Chapter 8 of this volume). Testing for the parasite that causes CD is regarded as a herd test, such that if one or more buffalo in a herd show a positive test reaction, the whole herd (i.e. all buffalo on the whole property) must be regarded as infected or potentially infected with the parasite. Government protocol dictates that positive results must be reported to the Department of Animal Health immediately. As the disease is transmitted by ticks that can be carried by a variety of animal species and may infest pastures for at least 18 months, the whole land on which the infected herd was present has to be quarantined for 2 years after the officially confirmed removal of all buffalo. Alternatively, with the written approval of the Department of Animal Health, the buffalo may be translocated tick-free to land registered for the keeping of infected buffalo. The destruction or translocation must happen as soon as possible, and care should be taken to ensure that every buffalo is accounted for (Department of Agriculture, Forestry and Fisheries, 2017).

In Zimbabwe, January disease is a notifiable disease according to the Animal Health (Theileriosis) Regulations of 1976. This entails short interval dipping (5:5:4) and quarantine for 28 days in the event of disease outbreak (Chifamba, 2024; Zimbabwe Agricultural Growth Programme, 2024).

6.10.1 Control of cattle importation

Cattle importation is allowed in South Africa provided the animals are disease-free, as required by the legislation (Animal Diseases Act 35 of 1984 and Animal Improvement Act 62 of 1998), demonstrated by testing using the IFAT and Hybrid II real-time PCR test. Zimbabwe requires that a country where animals are sourced should be ECF-free for 3 years before animal importation (Statutory Instrument 57 of 1989).

6.10.2 Vaccination and chemotherapy

Currently, vaccination against *T. parva* and chemotherapy of infected animals with theilericidal compounds are both prohibited in South Africa, in order to avoid the risk of establishing carrier infections, which could be a source of future transmission of infection (Kariuki *et al.*, 1995). In contrast to South Africa, where treatment is prohibited, treatment in Zimbabwe using drugs like buparvaquone is recommended with antipyretics and antihistaminics, oxytetracycline, haematinics, ruminotorics and liver tonics used as supportive treatment options (Chifamba, 2024; Zimbabwe Agricultural Growth Programme, 2024).

A vaccine using the Boleni strain of *T. parva*, registered as Bolvac, a mild version of the parasite that causes January disease, is used in Zimbabwe. It was first produced in 1989 by the Zimbabwean Central Veterinary laboratory, but production was stopped due to lack of skilled personnel and financial constraints in the 1990s. Vaccine production was resumed in 2021. Vaccination does not require the administration of oxytetracycline, making it very cost-effective (Kanhai *et al.*, 1997). It is effective against January disease, but not against buffalo-type *T. parva* (Latif *et al.*, 2001; Perry, 2016).

6.10.3 Regulations restricting movement of buffalo, especially in relation to game ranching

T. parva-infected buffalo are considered permanent carriers of the parasite and are allowed only on land registered for the keeping of buffalo within the CD-controlled areas of KwaZulu-Natal, Mpumalanga and Limpopo provinces. Buffalo must be individually identified with a microchip and with an ear tag or other externally visible identification number or mark; this is essential for record keeping of test results and movements of animals.

The South African government regulation dictates that anyone who wishes to have a buffalo farm needs to register the land on which the buffalo are going to be kept. The land must be fenced with double game-proof electrified fences (the inner and outer fences at least 5 m apart) to prevent contact with stray buffalo, and at least 100 m away from international borders such as Mozambique and Zimbabwe. Contact between cattle and buffalo should be prevented and thus no buffalo may be moved onto the same land where cattle are being kept, and vice versa. Non-compliance may lead to loss of land registration and buffalo not being allowed to be kept on the land.

Should a suspected outbreak or positive cases of CD be identified, the farm and animals are quarantined by the responsible State Veterinarian. In this case, no contact or potential contact between the positive cases and any other susceptible animals is allowed, including on grazing land and at water points, stables, pens, camps, dip tanks or crush facilities.

6.10.4 Veterinary movement permits/ Red Cross permit

Veterinary movement permits, whose purpose is to monitor and control movements that pose or have potential animal health risks, are issued by State Veterinarians or by a veterinary official delegated in writing by a State Veterinarian. They are required for all movements of live buffalo in the whole of South Africa. In addition to the movement permit, Red Cross permits are required for all movements of live buffalo. A Red Cross permit should have information including the tag/microchip number of the buffalo, origin and destination of the buffalo being moved and the information of the owner at origin and destination farms.

This also applies during auctions, which are considered to be a high biosecurity risk, due to the mixing of animals of potentially different health status. Care should be taken that there is no possible contact between buffalo from different groups, no possible contact with other species and that the land at destination is registered for buffalo of the appropriate health status.

All buffalo being moved to an auction facility must have a Red Cross permit, negative results in the real-time PCR (Hybrid II assay) (Pienaar *et al.*, 2011) and IFAT (Burridge and Kimber, 1972) from an accredited (ISO17025), government-approved laboratory, before the movement. In the case of South Africa, it is the Agricultural Research Council-Onderstepoort Veterinary Research (ARC-OVR). Following the auction and within 90 days of the blood collection date for disease status tests, the buffalo may be moved back to the land of origin, or to land registered for the keeping of buffalo as stated in the Red Cross permit (Department of Agriculture, Forestry and Fisheries, 2017).

6.11 Conclusions

The introduction of ECF and its subsequent eradication occurred over the same timescale in South Africa and Zimbabwe. However, differences in disease control strategies led to different outcomes. For South Africa, there was complete eradication of cattle-derived *T. parva*, while in Zimbabwe, a milder form of disease remains, namely January disease. It took over 50 years to eradicate ECF by a concerted effort of the veterinary authorities in both countries. This effort included early attempts at quarantine and dipping, but the final solution was a protracted campaign of ruthless quarantine and slaughter supported by extensive diagnostic monitoring. As discussed earlier, the seasonal variation in the activity of the tick vector in southern Africa is highlighted as a key factor that determines the seasonal incidence of disease caused by *T. parva* and almost certainly influenced the eradication of ECF. Since eradication, ECF has not resurfaced, and South Africa and Zimbabwe are two countries where the parasite and its tick vector occur yet are free of this scourge and where it is not considered the tick-borne disease with the highest economic impact.

Towards the end of the eradication campaign, a disease in cattle known as Corridor disease, caused by buffalo-derived *T. parva*, was identified. *T. parva* was circulating in buffalo in southern Africa long before the ECF epidemic, as attested to by the extensive genetic diversity found in the buffalo-associated *T. parva* population. Various factors contributed to its not being detected before 1955, including the lack of veterinary expertise, masking by co-morbid diseases such as nagana and redwater, decimation of the buffalo population by hunting and rinderpest and effective sequestering of buffalo in the Kruger National Park, the Hluhluwe and Umfolozi Game Reserves and other wildlife reserves and the ECF epidemic itself.

The greatest risk of reoccurrence of ECF in southern Africa would be the non-observance of biosecurity measures and illegal introduction of infected cattle or ticks. Surveillance of theileriosis and adherence to control measures have so far proven effective against the reintroduction of ECF and, in the case of Zimbabwe, the parasites that cause January disease. A prime example of this relates to the establishment in 2002 of the Great Limpopo Transfrontier Park encompassing contiguous parts of Mozambique, South Africa and Zimbabwe, which allows free movement of wildlife and the diseases and ticks they carry. Despite this, neither January disease nor ECF have been reported in South Africa. It is clear that the potentially devastating effects of reintroducing the ECF parasite on the cattle industry in southern Africa fully justify the strict control measures currently in place. Further investigations into the recurring Zimbabwe theileriosis might shed light on whether ECF has reappeared due either to reversion to virulence of the January disease parasites or to the reintroduction of ECF parasites from elsewhere.

In conclusion, the various aspects of the history of *T. parva* in southern Africa, encompassing the interplay among the parasite, vectors and hosts, the various clinical manifestations caused by different strains of the parasite and the sustained and monumental effort to remove ECF from South Africa, combine to create an important and fascinating narrative.

References

Amzati, G.S., Pelle, R., Muhigwa, J.-B.B., Kanduma, E.G., Djikeng, A. *et al.* (2018) Mitochondrial phylogeography and population structure of the cattle tick *Rhipicephalus appendiculatus* in the African Great Lakes region. *Parasites & Vectors* 11(1), 329. DOI: 10.1186/s13071-018-2904-7.

Anon (1904) *Report of Proceedings at Inter-colonial Veterinary Conference on "Animals" Diseases in South Africa Held at Cape Town on 25th, 26th, 27th, 28th, 30th and 31st May, 1904.* Cape Times Ltd, Government Printers. Cape Town, South Africa.

Anon (1924) *Report of Veterinary Conference Held at Bulawayo on 4th, 5th and 6th November, 1924*. Argus Publishing and Printing Co. Ltd, Salisbury, Southern Rhodesia, p. 44.

Anon (1929) *Report of Proceedings: Pan-African Agricultural and Veterinary Conference, Pretoria, 1-17 August, 1929*. Government Printer. Pretoria, South Africa.

Anon (1981) The eradication of East Coast Fever in South Africa. *Journal of the South African Veterinary Association* 52, 71–73.

Anon (1989) Classification of *Theileria parva* reactions in cattle. In: Dolan, T.T. (ed.) *Theileriosis in Eastern, Central and Southern Africa. Proceedings of a Workshop on East Coast Fever Immunization*, International Laboratory for Research on Animal Diseases, Nairobi, Kenya, pp. 187–188.

Babes, V. (1888) Sur l'hémoglobinurie bactérienne du boeuf. *Comptes Rendus de l'Académie Des Sciences* 107, 692–694.

Baker, J.R. (1995) The subspecific taxonomy of *Trypanosoma brucei*. *Parasite* 2(1), 3–12. DOI: 10.1051/parasite/1995021003.

Barnett, S.F. and Brocklesby, D.W. (1966a) The passage of "*Theileria lawrencei* (Kenya)" through cattle. *British Veterinary Journal* 122, 396–409. DOI: 10.1016/S0007-1935(17)40406-4.

Barnett, S.F. and Brocklesby, D.W. (1966b) Recent investigations into theileridae of cattle and buffalo in Africa: A mild form of East Coast Fever (*Theileria parva*) with persistence of infection. *British Veterinary Journal* 122, 361–370. DOI: 10.1016/S0007-1935(17)40402-7.

Berkvens, D.L., Pegram, R.G. and Brandt, J.R.A. (1995) A study of the diapausing behaviour of *Rhipicephalus appendiculatus* and *R. zambeziensis* under quasi-natural conditions in Zambia. *Medical and Veterinary Entomology* 9(3), 307–315. DOI: 10.1111/j.1365-2915.1995.tb00139.x.

Bishop, R.P., Spooner, P.R., Kanhai, G.K., Kiarie, J., Latif, A.A. *et al.* (1994) Molecular characterization of *Theileria* parasites: Application to the epidemiology of theileriosis in Zimbabwe. *Parasitology* 109(Pt 5), 573–581. DOI: 10.1017/s0031182000076459.

Blouin, E.F. and Stoltsz, W.H. (1989) Comparative infection rates of *Theileria parva lawrencei* in salivary glands of *Rhipicephalus appendiculatus* and *Rhipicephalus zambeziensis*. *The Onderstepoort Journal of Veterinary Research* 56(3), 211–213.

Bothma, J.D.P. (1987) The veterinarian as biologist. *Journal of the South African Veterinary Association* 58(4), 213–217.

Bruce, D. (1895) *Preliminary Report on the Tsetse Fly Disease or Nagana, in Zululand*. South Africa, Bennett and Davis, Durban.

Burridge, M.J. and Kimber, C.D. (1972) The indirect fluorescent test for experimental East Coast Fever (*Theileria parva* infection in cattle). *Research in Veterinary Science* 13(5), 451–456. DOI: 10.1016/S0034-5288(18)33992-4.

Chifamba, O. (2024) Farmers warned as january disease peaks. *The Herald*. 2 January 2024. Available at: https://www.herald.co.zw/farmers-warned-as-january-disease-peaks (accessed 2 January 2025).

Department of Agriculture, Forestry and Fisheries (2017) Veterinary procedural notice for buffalo disease risk management in South Africa. Department of Agriculture, Forestry and Fisheries, Directorate Animal Health. Available at: https://www.elsenburg.com/wp-content/uploads/2022/02/Buffalo-Disease-Risk-Management-VPN_Signed-2017-02-17.pdf (accessed 2 January 2025).

Diesel, A.M. (1948) The campaign against East Coast Fever in South Africa. *Onderstepoort Journal of Veterinary Science* 23, 19–31.

Diesel, A.M. and Van Drimmelen, G.C. (1948) The diagnosis of East Coast Fever in South Africa: A review. *Journal of the South African Veterinary Medical Association* 19, 81–92.

Dube-Matutu, S. (2024) January disease under control, farmers urged to dip cattle regularly. *The Chronicle*. 1 February 2024. Available at: www.chronicle.co.zw/january-disease-under-control-farmers-urged-to-dip-cattle-regularly/ (accessed 2 January 2025).

du Toit, P.J. (1928) Observations on immunity in East Coast fever. *South African Journal of Science* 25, 282–287.

du Toit, P.J. and Viljoen, P.R. (1928) *Dipping as Method of Eradicating East Coast Fever*. 15th Annual Report of the Director of Veterinary Services and Animal Industry. Union of South Africa, Pretoria.

Gallivan, G.J., Spickett, A., Heyne, H., Spickett, A.M. and Horak, I.G. (2011) The dynamics of questing ticks collected for 164 consecutive months off the vegetation of two landscape zones in the Kruger National Park (1988-2002). Part II. *Rhipicephalus appendiculatus* and *Rhipicephalus zambeziensis*. *Onderstepoort Journal of Veterinary Research* 78(1), 233. DOI: 10.4102/ojvr.v78i1.41.

Gray, C.E. and Robertson, W. (1903) *Report upon Texas Fever or Redwater in Rhodesia*. Argus Printing & Publishing, Cape Town, South Africa.

Hemmink, J.D., Sitt, T., Pelle, R., Klerk-Lorist, L.-M., Shiels, B. *et al.* (2018) Ancient diversity and geographical sub-structuring in African buffalo *Theileria parva* populations revealed through metagenetic analysis of antigen-encoding loci. *International Journal for Parasitology* 48(3–4), 287–296. DOI: 10.1016/j.ijpara.2017.10.006.

Horak, I.G., Heyne, H., Williams, R., Gallivan, G.J., Spickett, A.M. *et al.* (2018) *The Ixodid Ticks (Acari: Ixodidae) of Southern Africa*. Springer International Publishing, Cham, Switzerland.

Hutcheon, D. (1898) Redwater and its history. *Agricultural Journal of the Cape Colony* 17, 331–339.

Irvin, A.D., Morzaria, S.P., Munatswa, F.C. and Norval, R.A.I. (1989) Immunization of cattle with a *Theileria parva* bovis stock from Zimbabwe protects against challenge with virulent *T.p. parva* and *T.p. lawrencei* stocks from Kenya. *Veterinary Parasitology* 32(4), 271–278. DOI: 10.1016/0304-4017(89)90037-X.

Kanhai, G.K., Pegram, R.G., Hargreaves, S.K., Hove, T. and Dolan, T.T. (1997) Immunisation of cattle in Zimbabwe using *Theileria parva* (Boleni) without concurrent tetracycline therapy. *Tropical Animal Health and Production* 29(2), 92–98. DOI: 10.1007/BF02632324.

Kappmeier, K., Nevill, E.M. and Bagnall, R.J. (1998) Review of tsetse flies and trypanosomosis in South Africa. *The Onderstepoort Journal of Veterinary Research* 65(3), 195–203.

Kariuki, D.P., Young, A.S., Morzaria, S.P., Lesan, A.C., Mining, S.K. *et al.* (1995) *Theileria parva* carrier state in naturally infected and artificially immunised cattle. *Tropical Animal Health and Production* 27(1), 15–25. DOI: 10.1007/BF02236328.

Koch, R. (1898) *Reise-Berichte über Rinderpest, Bubonenpest in Indien und Afrika, Ttetse- oder Surrahkrankheit, Texasfieber, tropische Malaria, Schwarzwasserfieber*. Springer, Berlin, Germany. DOI: 10.1007/978-3-662-39506-6.

Koch, R. (1903) Interim report on Rhodesian redwater or African Coast Fever. *Journal of Comparative Pathology and Therapeutics* 16, 273–280. DOI: 10.1016/S0368-1742(03)80079-6.

Koch, H.T., Ocama, J.G.R., Munatswa, F.C., Byrom, B., Norval, R.A.I. *et al.* (1988) Isolation and characterization of bovine Theileria parasites in Zimbabwe. *Veterinary Parasitology* 28(1–2), 19–32. DOI: 10.1016/0304-4017(88)90015-5.

Latif, A.A. and Hove, T. (2011) History and critical review of *Theileria parva* (Boleni), the vaccine stock against Zimbabwean cattle theileriosis. *Ticks and Tick-Borne Diseases* 2(3), 163–167. DOI: 10.1016/j.ttbdis.2011.06.002.

Latif, A.A., Hove, T., Kanhai, G.K. and Masaka, S. (2001) Exposure of cattle immunized with different stocks of *Theileria parva* to buffalo-associated Theileria challenge on two game parks in Zimbabwe. *Onderstepoort Journal of Veterinary Research* 68, 197–201.

Latif, A.A., Troskie, P.C., Peba, S.B., Maboko, B.B., Pienaar, R. *et al.* (2019) Corridor disease (buffalo-associated *Theileria parva*) outbreak in cattle introduced onto a game ranch and investigations into their carrier-state. *Veterinary Parasitology* 18, 100331. DOI: 10.1016/j.vprsr.2019.100331.

Lawrence, D.A. (1935) *Theileriosis. South Rhodesia Report to the Director of Veterinary Research for the Year 1934*. Rhodesia Printing and Publishing Co. Ltd, Salisbury.

Lawrence, D.A. (1937) *Report of the Director of Veterinary Research for the Year 1936*. Rhodesia Printing and Publishing Co. Ltd, Salisbury, p. 12.

Lawrence, J.A. (1977) The serological relationship between *Theileria parva* (Muguga) and *Theileria lawrencei* from Rhodesia. *Veterinary Record* 100(22), 470–471. DOI: 10.1136/vr.100.22.470.

Lawrence, J.A. (1979) The differential diagnosis of the bovine Theilerias of Southern Africa. *Journal of the South African Veterinary Medical Association* 50, 311–313.

Lawrence, J.A. (1986) *East Coast Fever in Southern Africa 1901-1960*. Faculty of Veterinary Science, University of Zimbabwe.

Lawrence, J.A. (1991) Retrospective observations on the geographical relationship between *Rhipicephalus appendiculatus* and East Coast Fever in Southern Africa. *Veterinary Record* 128(8), 180–183. DOI: 10.1136/vr.128.8.180.

Lawrence, J.A., Norval, R.A.I. and Uilenberg, G. (1983) *Rhipicephalus zambeziensis* as a vector of bovine Theileriae. *Tropical Animal Health and Production* 15(1), 39–42. DOI: 10.1007/BF02250760.

Löhr, K.-F. and Ross, J.P.J. (1969) Serological response in cattle to East Coast Fever (*Theileria parva* infection) as measured by the indirect fluorescent antibody test. *Research in Veterinary Science* 10(5), 453–461. DOI: 10.1016/S0034-5288(18)34412-6.

Lounsbury, C.P. (1903) Ticks and African Coast Fever. *Transvaal Agricultural Journal* 2, 4–13.

Lounsbury, C.P. (1905) Habits and peculiarities of some South African ticks. *South African Journal of Science* 3, 13–26.

Maboko, B.B., Featherston, J., Sibeko-Matjila, K.P. and Mans, B.J. (2021a) Whole genome sequencing of *Theileria parva* using target capture. *Genomics* 113(2), 429–438. DOI: 10.1016/j.ygeno.2020.12.033.

Maboko, B.B., Sibeko-Matjila, K.P., Pierneef, R., Chan, W.Y., Josemans, A. *et al.* (2021b) South african buffalo-derived *Theileria parva* is distinct from other buffalo and cattle-derived *T. parva*. *Frontiers in Genetics* 12, 666096. DOI: 10.3389/fgene.2021.666096.

Madder, M., Speybroeck, N., Brandt, J., Tirry, L., Hodek, I. *et al.* (2002) Geographic variation in diapause response of adult *Rhipicephalus appendiculatus* ticks. *Experimental & Applied Acarology* 27(3), 209–221. DOI: 10.1023/A:1021694207456.

Mans, B.J. (2020) The history of East Coast Fever in Southern Africa. In: *Proceedings of the 44th International Congress of the World Association for the History of Veterinary Medicine*, Pretoria, South Africa, pp. 52–54.

Manyenyeka, M., Tagwireyi, W.M., Marufu, M.C., Spargo, R.M. and Etter, E. (2022) Spatio-temporal clustering and risk factor analysis of bovine Theileriosis (*Theileria parva*) in Zimbabwe from 1995 to 2018. *Transboundary and Emerging Diseases* 69(3), 1186–1196. DOI: 10.1111/tbed.14081.

Mans, B.J., Pienaar, R., Latif, A.A. and Potgieter, F.T. (2011) Diversity in the 18S SSU rRNA V4 hyper-variable region of *Theileria* spp. in cape buffalo (*Syncerus caffer*) and cattle from Southern Africa. *Parasitology* 138(6), 766–779. DOI: 10.1017/S0031182011000187.

Mans, B.J., Pienaar, R., Ratabane, J., Pule, B. and Latif, A.A. (2016) Investigating the diversity of the 18S SSU rRNA hyper-variable region of *Theileria* in cattle and cape buffalo (*Syncerus caffer*) from Southern Africa using a next generation sequencing approach. *Ticks and Tick-Borne Diseases* 7(5), 869–879. DOI: 10.1016/j.ttbdis.2016.04.005.

Maritim, A.C., Young, A.S., Lesan, A.C., Ndungu, S.G., Stagg, D.A. *et al.* (1992) Transformation of *Theileria parva* derived from African buffalo (*Syncerus caffer*) by tick passage in cattle and its use in infection and treatment immunization. *Veterinary Parasitology* 43(1–2), 1–14. DOI: 10.1016/0304-4017(92)90043-9.

Matson, B.A. (1967) Theileriosis in Rhodesia: A study of diagnostic specimens over two seasons. *Journal of South African Veterinary Association* 38, 93–102.

Mbizeni, S., Potgieter, F.T., Troskie, C., Mans, B.J., Penzhorn, B.L. *et al.* (2013) Field and laboratory studies on corridor disease (*Theileria parva* infection) in cattle population at the livestock/game interface of Uphongolo-Mkuze area, South Africa. *Ticks and Tick-Borne Diseases* 4(3), 227–234. DOI: 10.1016/j.ttbdis.2012.11.005.

Mbogo, S.K., Kariuki, D.P., Ngumi, P.N. and McHardy, N. (1996) A mild *Theileria parva* parasite with potential for immunisation against East Coast Fever. *Veterinary Parasitology* 61, 41–47.

Medley, G.F., Perry, B.D. and Young, A.S. (1993) Preliminary analysis of the transmission dynamics of *Theileria parva* in Eastern Africa. *Parasitology* 106(3), 251–264. DOI: 10.1017/S0031182000075077.

Morrison, W.I., Hemmink, J.D. and Toye, P.G. (2020) *Theileria parva*: A parasite of African buffalo, which has adapted to infect and undergo transmission in cattle. *International Journal for Parasitology* 50(5), 403–412. DOI: 10.1016/j.ijpara.2019.12.006.

Musisi, F.L., Quiroga, J.C., Kanhai, G.K., Kamwendo, S.P., Mzoma, F.J. *et al.* (1996) *Theileria parva* (Kasoba): Isolation and challenge of cattle recovered from infection with other *Theileria parva* stocks. *Revue d'elevage et de Medecine Veterinaire Des Pays Tropicaux* 49(1), 42–45.

Muvhuringi, P.B., Murisa, R., Sylvester, D., Chigede, N. and Mafunga, K. (2022) Factors worsening tick borne diseases occurrence in rural communities. A case of Bindura district, Zimbabwe. *Cogent Food & Agriculture* 8(1), 2082058. DOI: 10.1080/23311932.2022.2082058.

Neitz, W.O. (1941) The occurrence of *Babesia bovis* in South Africa. *Journal of the South African Veterinary Association* 12, 62–66.

Neitz, W.O. (1948) Studies in East Coast Fever. *South African Journal of Science* 1, 133–135.

Neitz, W.O. (1957) Theileriosis, gonderiosis and cytauxzoonoses: A review. *Onderstepoort Journal of Veterinary Research* 27, 275–430.

Neitz, W.O. (1958) Can corridor disease-recovered cattle serve as reservoirs of *Gonderia lawrencei? Bulletin of Epizootic Diseases of Africa* 6, 151–154.

Neitz, W.O., Canham, A.S. and Kluge, E. (1955) Corridor disease: A fatal form of bovine theileriosis encountered in Zululand. *Journal of the South African Veterinary Association* 26, 78–87.

Norval, R.A., Fivaz, B.H., Lawrence, J.A. and Brown, A.F. (1985) Epidemiology of tick-borne diseases of cattle in Zimbabwe. III. *Theileria Parva* Group. *Tropical Animal Health and Production* 17(1), 19–28. DOI: 10.1007/BF02356128.

Norval, R.A., Perry, B.D. and Young, A.S. (1992) *The Epidemiology of Theileriosis in Africa*. Academic Press, London, pp. 136–154.

Norval, R.A.I. and Horak, I.G. (2004) Vectors: Ticks. In: Coetzer, J.A.W. and Tustin, R.C. (eds) *Infectious Diseases of Livestock*, 2nd edn. Oxford University Press, Cape Town, South Africa, pp. 3–42.

Norval, R.A.I., Walker, J.B. and Colborne, J. (1982) The ecology of *Rhipicephalus zambeziensis* and *Rhipicephalus appendiculatus* (Acarina, Ixodidae) with particular reference to Zimbabwe. *Onderstepoort Journal of Veterinary Research* 49, 181–190.

Norval, R.A.I., Lawrence, J.A., Young, A.S., Perry, B.D., Dolan, T.T. *et al*. (1991) *Theileria parva*: Influence of vector, parasite and host relationships on the epidemiology of theileriosis in Southern Africa. *Parasitology* 102(3), 347–356. DOI: 10.1017/S0031182000064295.

Oura, C.A.L., Odongo, D.O., Lubega, G.W., Spooner, P.R., Tait, A. *et al*. (2003) A panel of microsatellite and minisatellite markers for the characterisation of field isolates of *Theileria parva*. *International Journal for Parasitology* 33(14), 1641–1653. DOI: 10.1016/S0020-7519(03)00280-7.

Papkou, A., Gokhale, C.S., Traulsen, A. and Schulenburg, H. (2016) Host-parasite coevolution: Why changing population size matters. *Zoology* 119(4), 330–338. DOI: 10.1016/j.zool.2016.02.001.

Pelle, R., Graham, S.P., Njahira, M.N., Osaso, J., Saya, R.M. *et al*. (2011) Two *Theileria parva* CD8 T cell antigen genes are more variable in buffalo than cattle parasites, but differ in pattern of sequence diversity. *PLoS ONE* 6(4), e19015. DOI: 10.1371/journal.pone.0019015.

Perry, B.D. and Young, A.S. (1993) The naming game: The changing fortunes of East Coast Fever and *Theileria parva*. *Veterinary Record* 133, 613–616.

Perry, B.D. (2016) The control of East Coast Fever of cattle by live parasite vaccination: A science-to-impact narrative. *One Health* 2, 103–114. DOI: 10.1016/j.onehlt.2016.07.002.

Pienaar, R., Potgieter, F.T., Latif, A.A., Thekisoe, O.M.M. and Mans, B.J. (2011) The hybrid II assay: A sensitive and specific real-time hybridization assay for the diagnosis of *Theileria parva* infection in Cape buffalo (*Syncerus caffer*) and cattle. *Parasitology* 138(14), 1935–1944. DOI: 10.1017/S0031182011001454.

Potgieter, F.T., Stoltsz, W.H., Blouin, E.F. and Roos, J.A. (1988) Corridor disease in South Africa: A review of the current status. *Journal of the South African Veterinary Association* 59, 155–160.

Randolph, S.E. (1997) Abiotic and biotic determinants of the seasonal dynamics of the tick *Rhipicephalus appendiculatus* in South Africa. *Medical and Veterinary Entomology* 11, 25–37. DOI: 10.1111/j.1365-2915.1997.tb00286.x.

Rechav, Y. (1981) Ecological factors affecting the seasonal activity of the brown ear tick *Rhipicephalus appendiculatus*. In: Whitehead, G.B. and Gibson, J.D. (eds) *Tick Biology and Control*. Tick Research Unit, Rhodes University, Makhanda, South Africa, pp. 187–191.

Rechav, Y. (1982) Dynamics of tick populations (Acari: Ixodoidea) in the Eastern Cape province of South Africa. *Journal of Medical Entomology* 19, 679–700. DOI: 10.1093/jmedent/19.6.679.

Schindler, R., Mehlitz, D. and Matson, B.A. (1969) Serologische und immunologische untersuchungen bei der *Theileria lawrencei* - Infektion des Rindes. *Zeitschrift Für Tropenmedizin Und Parasitologie* 20, 162–183.

Short, N.J. and Norval, R.A.I. (1981) Regulation of seasonal occurrence in the tick *Rhipicephalus appendiculatus* Neumann, 1901. *Tropical Animal Health and Production* 13(1), 19–26. DOI: 10.1007/BF02237881.

Sibeko, K.P., Geysen, D., Oosthuizen, M.C., Matthee, C.A., Troskie, M. *et al*. (2010) Four p67 alleles identified in South African *Theileria parva* field samples. *Veterinary Parasitology* 167, 244–254. DOI: 10.1016/j.vetpar.2009.09.026.

Sibeko, K.P., Collins, N.E., Oosthuizen, M.C., Troskie, M., Potgieter, F.T. *et al*. (2011) Analyses of genes encoding *Theileria parva* p104 and polymorphic immunodominant molecule (PIM) reveal evidence of the presence of cattle-type alleles in the South African *T. parva* population. *Veterinary Parasitology* 181(2–4), 120–130. DOI: 10.1016/j.vetpar.2011.04.035.

Sitt, T., Poole, E.J., Ndambuki, G., Mwaura, S., Njoroge, T. *et al*. (2015) Exposure of vaccinated and naive cattle to natural challenge from buffalo-derived *Theileria parva*. *International Journal for Parasitology* 4(2), 244–251. DOI: 10.1016/j.ijppaw.2015.04.006.

Sitt, T., Henson, S., Morrison, W.I. and Toye, P. (2019) Similar levels of diversity in the gene encoding the p67 sporozoite surface protein of *Theileria parva* are observed in blood samples from buffalo and cattle naturally infected from buffalo. *Veterinary Parasitology* 269, 21–27. DOI: 10.1016/j.vetpar.2019.04.006.

Smith, T. and Kilborne, F.L. (1893) *Investigations into the Nature, Causation, and Prevention of Texas or Southern Cattle Fever*. (Bulletin, No. 1). Department of Agriculture, Bureau of Animal Industry, Washington, DC, p. 133.

Smitz, N., Berthouly, C., Cornélis, D., Heller, R., Hooft, P. *et al.* (2013) Pan-African genetic structure in the African buffalo (*Syncerus caffer*): Investigating intraspecific divergence. *PLoS ONE* 8(2), e56235. DOI: 10.1371/journal.pone.0056235.

Spickett, A.M. (2013) Ixodid ticks of major economic importance and their distribution in South Africa. In: Oberem, P. (ed.) *Ticks and Tick-Borne Diseases, Monograph 1*, 1st edn. Agri Connect (Pty) Ltd, Pretoria, South Africa, pp. 1–79.

Spickett, A.M., Gallivan, G.J. and Horak, I.G. (2011) The dynamics of questing ticks collected for 164 consecutive months off the vegetation of two landscape zones in the Kruger National Park (1988-2002). Part II. *Rhipicephalus appendiculatus* and *Rhipicephalus zambeziensis*. *Onderstepoort Journal of Veterinary Research* 78(1), 233.

Spreull, J. (1914) East Coast Fever inoculations in the Transkeian territories, South Africa. *Journal of Comparative Pathology and Therapeutics* 27, 299–304. DOI: 10.1016/S0368-1742(14)80052-0.

Theiler, A. (1904) Rhodesian tick fever. *Transvaal Agricultural Journal* 2, 421–438.

Theiler, A. (1905) Redwater. *Transvaal Agricultural Journal* 3, 476–496.

Theiler, A. (1912) The Immunisation of Cattle against East Coast Fever. *Second Report of the Director of Veterinary Research, Union of South Africa, Department of Agriculture*. Cape Times Limited, Government Printer, Cape Town, pp. 266–314.

Tindih, H.S., Marcotty, T., Naessens, J., Goddeeris, B.M. and Geysen, D. (2010) Demonstration of differences in virulence between two *Theileria parva* isolates. *Veterinary Parasitology* 168(3–4), 223–230. DOI: 10.1016/j.vetpar.2009.11.006.

Uilenberg, G. (1976) Tick-borne livestock diseases and their vectors, 2. Epizootiology of tick-borne diseases. *World Animal Review* 17, 8–15.

Uilenberg, G., Perié, N.M., Lawrence, J.A., de Vos, A.J., Paling, R.W. *et al.* (1982) Causal agents of bovine theileriosis in Southern Africa. *Tropical Animal Health and Production* 14(3), 127–140. DOI: 10.1007/BF02242143.

Viljoen, P.R. (1929) The East Coast fever Problem in the union. Paper no.15. Veterinary Section: Pan-African Agricultural and Veterinary Conference, Pretoria, 1–17 August 1929. Government Printer, Pretoria, South Africa.

Vogel, S.W. and Heyne, H. (1996) Rinderpest in South Africa – 100 years ago. *Journal of the South African Veterinary Association* 67(4), 164–170.

Walker, J.B., Keirans, J.E. and Horak, I. (2000) *The Genus Rhipicephalus (Acari, Ixododae)*. Cambridge University Press, Cambridge, UK.

Williams, G. (1904) *Report of the Proceedings of the Conference on Diseases amongst Cattle and Other Animals in South Africa. Held on 3rd, 4th and 5th December 1903*. Argus Printing and Publishing Co. Ltd, Bloemfontein, p. 62.

Young, A.S. and Purnell, R.E. (1973) Transmission of *Theileria lawrencei* (Serengeti) by the ixodid tick, *Rhipicephalus appendiculatus*. *Tropical Animal Health and Production* 5(3), 146–152. DOI: 10.1007/BF02251383.

Young, A.S., Leitch, B.L. and Newson, R.M. (1981) The occurrence of a *Theileria parva* carrier state in cattle from an East Coast Fever endemic area of Kenya. In: Irvin, A.D., Cunningham, M.P. and Young, A.S. (eds) *Advances in the Control of Theileriosis. Current Topics in Veterinary Medicine and Animal Science*. Springer, Dordrecht, The Netherlands, pp. 60–62.

Young, A.S., Leitch, B.L., Newson, R.M. and Cunningham, M.P. (1986) The occurrence of a *Theileria parva* carrier state in cattle from an East Coast Fever endemic area of Kenya. *Parasitology* 93, 9–16.

Zimbabwe Agricultural Growth Programme (2024) Theileriosis (January disease) in cattle. Department of Veterinary Services. Available at: https://zagp.org.zw/Content/recource_center_files/891cafe5-0928-4599-b343-d36f4c5b7b6d.pdf (accessed 2 January 2025).

7 Heritable Resistance to Disease Caused by *Theileria parva*

Philip Toye*
International Livestock Research Institute, Nairobi, Kenya

7.1 Introduction

The clinical outcome of infection with a pathogen can vary greatly among individuals of the same host species. Although many factors may contribute to this variability, the genetic background of the individual is an important determinant of susceptibility to infectious disease, to the extent that infectious diseases are a major contributor to the genomic evolution of host species (Lederberg, 1999). An early example where a genetic basis for resistance to human disease was identified is that of the sickle cell trait and malaria (Allison, 1954). More recently, Fumagalli *et al.* (2011) correlated mutation frequencies in distinct human populations with a set of environmental factors and concluded that pathogens have exerted predominant selective pressure on human evolution. Similarly for livestock, genetic differences in susceptibility to several diseases are well known, e.g. ticks, trypanosomes and helminths, and in some cases, these have strongly influenced the breeds of animals used in endemic regions. However, the precise mechanisms underlying resistance to these diseases are seldom fully understood.

The recent advent of powerful genomics tools, such as high-throughput sequencing coupled with refined statistical analyses, has spurred research aimed at identifying the genes mediating disease resistance and the cellular mechanisms involved. As well as underpinning traditional breeding programmes and those based on marker-assisted selection, a potential application of the findings from such studies is use of genomic manipulation to disseminate the beneficial alleles more rapidly through target populations (Jenko *et al.*, 2015). It is also possible that this research will lead to the identification of new preventative and therapeutic agents to combat such diseases.

There are several aspects of *Theileria parva* infection that promote natural selection for genetic resistance to the disease it causes in cattle, East Coast fever (ECF). The disease is highly fatal in susceptible populations, with mortality rates approaching 100%. Calves of a pre-reproductive age are not spared the lethal outcome of infection, allowing the disease to exert an extremely strong selective pressure. There is a high infection pressure in endemic areas, which can be constant in the equatorial regions. The presence of African buffalo, which

*Corresponding author: pgtoye@gmail.com

DOI: 10.1079/9781800626324.0007

Box 7.1. Resistance or tolerance?

The phenomenon that is the subject of this chapter has been referred to as both 'resistance' and 'tolerance'. A commonly held distinction between the two is that resistance refers to a trait which prevents a pathogen from infecting or proliferating within the host, whereas tolerance reduces the consequences of infection without affecting the pathogen (Roy and Kirchner, 2000). Assigning one or the other to a disease situation necessarily requires a detailed knowledge of the infection dynamics and pathogenesis. The situation with ECF is not yet clear. Although there are indications, discussed in the chapter, which suggest that less severe disease occurs through limiting the proliferation of the parasite, this is yet to be conclusively established. In this review chapter, the terms are used somewhat interchangeably but usually consistent with the publication being described.

are susceptible to infection with *T. parva* but do not suffer disease, represents a highly potent reservoir for infection of cattle. Finally, it is estimated that *Bos taurus* cattle were brought into Africa from the Middle East about 8000 years ago and *Bos indicus* cattle arrived in eastern Africa from Asia about 3000–4000 years ago, followed by a major arrival about 1400 years ago (Hanotte, 2019; Chapter 5 of this volume). This would provide ample time for inherited resistance to have arisen or been selected for. As an example from infectious diseases of humans, which have a longer generation time than cattle, a recent study to identify mutations selected by the European plague pandemic showed significant enrichment of mutations in regions of the genome containing immune-related genes in post-pandemic samples (AD1350–1539) compared to pre-pandemic ones (AD1000–1250) (Klunk *et al.*, 2022).

This chapter will review the early field observations that indicated that an inherited resistance to ECF has arisen and more recent experimental studies that have yielded some initial insights into how this resistance is mediated.

7.2 Early Observations of ECF Resistance in Cattle

Since evidence of genetic resistance to *T. parva* is poorly documented in contemporary Theileria literature, a detailed discussion is provided here of the findings in historical literature that have provided clear evidence of resistance. In 1936, Mettam and Carmichael published a survey of ECF in Uganda, in which they noted that ECF is a 'very fatal disease to imported or grade cattle, and even to native cattle from clean areas, but is of lower pathogenicity for indigenous animals' (Mettam and Carmichael, 1936, p.256). They reported mortality rates of about 20% in indigenous herds, compared to up to 90% in susceptible populations, and ascribed the lower mortality rates in indigenous cattle to a resistance resulting from 'centuries' of exposure to infected ticks. The possibility that it was due to a loss of pathogenicity in local strains of the parasite was dismissed in the light of the 'appalling' losses that occurred when susceptible animals were introduced into endemic regions.

7.2.1 Studies in western Kenya on East African zebu

One of the earliest detailed field studies describing the innate resistance of indigenous cattle in an endemic area was reported by Barnett and Bailey (1955a). The study was located in western Kenya, where 1169 calves were monitored for up to 1 year at two sites. The overall mortality rate due to ECF in the study areas was calculated to be 8.0% (Barnett, 1957). That the calves had been exposed to a virulent field challenge was shown by the high mortality rates observed in a limited number of susceptible 'high-grade' animals introduced into the areas. In addition, a sample of older indigenous animals (about 1 year of age) survived an otherwise lethal experimental infection. The authors concluded that most animals in the area survived and developed an immunity to infection by 1 year of age without having shown any clinical signs of ECF. This contrasted emphatically with the fate of zebu-Sahiwal cross-bred animals that had been sent into the area to improve productivity. The area was regarded as 'one of the worst areas for the dreaded disease East Coast Fever and all the other tick-borne diseases that went with it' and 'almost all the animals that went out eventually succumbed to one of these diseases' (described by Conelly, 1998, p. 1742).

Interestingly, a large epidemiology study of 548 calves undertaken more than 50 years later (2007–2009) in the same area of western Kenya estimated the ECF-related mortality rate in indigenous calves to be about 3.6%, despite a *T. parva* infection rate of 83% (Bronsvoort *et al.*, 2013; Woolhouse *et al.*, 2015). This study, the Infectious Diseases of East African Livestock (IDEAL), involved only indigenous zebu cattle, which were monitored for up to 12 months and maintained in the absence of any animal health interventions.

Following their field observations, Barnett and Bailey undertook experimental studies to identify how indigenous cattle survived infection (Barnett and Bailey, 1955b). Four factors were considered: maternal immunity, a genetic basis, age of exposure and the level of challenge. The experiments focused on the susceptibility of progeny of zebu animals from endemic areas to a controlled tick challenge. To avoid the possibility of early infection in the experimental animals, cows and bulls were transported from the endemic area of western Kenya to a disease-free facility at Muguga, near Nairobi in central Kenya, and the progeny calves were recruited into the experimental cohort (called 'calves from immune dams' by the authors). There was a 'control' group ('calves from susceptible dams') born to animals that had never been maintained in endemic areas or were three generations removed from animals from endemic areas. The latter introduces some uncertainty in interpretation when testing for an inherited factor, which was compounded by the lack of information provided by the authors on relative numbers within the mixed group.

In the key experiment, groups of calves of different ages were challenged with a single infected tick from a batch of ticks fed on an experimentally infected animal (Table 7.1).

The overall survival rate in the calves born to dams from the endemic area was 89% (63 out of 71), compared to 35% (18/51) for those from non-endemic areas and 4% (1/25) in a third group comprising 'high grade steers' (i.e. European *B. taurus* animals). The mortality rate of 11% in the 'endemic' group of calves was similar to that obtained from the field observations (8%), as described above.

The authors discounted a role for maternal immunity by recalling that large amounts of ECF convalescent sera fail to protect animals, a finding later supported by Muhammed *et al.* (1975) and Cunningham *et al.* (1989).

The clear difference in results between the three groups immediately pointed to a genetic basis for the resistance. There also appeared to be a modest decrease in the resistance with age, which is discussed later in this chapter (see Section 7.5). The observation that the resistance was discernible after successful feeding of a single infected tick suggested that the inherited resistance was not due to tick resistance, that is, differences in the percentage of ticks which can successfully attach.

To examine the effect of the level of challenge, increasing numbers of ticks were applied to additional calves born to cows from the endemic and non-endemic areas. Increasing mortality rates were observed as the number of applied ticks increased in both groups, especially

Table 7.1. Percentage recovery in zebu cattle infested with a single *T. parva*-infected tick. Adapted from Barnett, 1957, Table I.

Average age of calf group	Calves from immune dams[a]	Calves from susceptible dams[a]	1–2 year-old high-grade steers[b]
1 month	100% (20)[c]	20% (20)	0% (9)
4 months	100% (20)	46% (24)	9% (11)
14 months	80% (20)	43% (7)	0% (3)
27 months	64% (11)	–	0% (2)

[a]'Calves from immune dams' were born to dams from an endemic area of Kenya, whereas 'calves from susceptible dams' were born to dams from non-endemic areas.
[b]This group was included as a control for virulence of the challenge infection.
[c]The figures in brackets represent the number of animals in each group.

Table 7.2. Percentage recovery in zebu cattle infested with different numbers of *T. parva*-infected ticks. Adapted from Barnett, 1957, Table II.

Tick infestation	Calves from immune dams[a]	Calves from susceptible dams[a]
1 adult	100% (20)[b]	46% (24)
7 adults	73% (26)	40% (30)
20 adults	63% (19)	25% (20)
50 adults	36% (22)	–

[a]Calves were 3–4 months old.
[b]The figures in brackets represent the number of animals in each group.

the endemic group, where the mortality rate rose from 0% with one infected adult tick to 64% with 50 infected adult ticks (Table 7.2).

This was the first clear demonstration that the genetic resistance in indigenous cattle was not absolute but could be 'broken though' under heavy challenge. A similar comparison with 'high-grade' steers could not be performed as challenge with a single tick killed 95% of calves and adults alike.

The authors concluded that 'it would be reasonable to suppose that some genetic resistance to E.C.F. exists among the cattle of the enzootic areas' (Barnett and Bailey, 1955b). The results also suggested that the resistance trait is not entirely absent but only less common in the zebu calves from non-endemic areas, a not unexpected result.

7.2.2 Nganda cattle in Uganda

Shortly after this, an investigation was undertaken in Uganda to assess the possibility of exploiting the inherited resistance of indigenous cattle to establish 'an E.C.F. resistant type of dairy cattle' (Guilbride and Opwata, 1963, p. 289). The specific aims were to estimate the survival rate of cross-bred cattle, to determine whether there was any genetic factor connected with resistance and whether such a factor could be exploited by cross-breeding with more productive breeds. The authors noted that it was an 'incomplete experiment' that was terminated prematurely, possibly due to the untimely death of one of the principal investigators. Nevertheless, some valid conclusions can be gathered from the data that were collected.

The study animals were progeny of local Nganda dams and Jersey bulls, produced by artificial insemination. The Nganda is a stable breed of zebu-sanga ancestry. When challenged by application of 10 infected ticks, 44% (19/43) of the cross-bred animals survived. In contrast, 92% (11/12) 'pure' Nganda control animals survived, and all five Guernsey control animals died.

This experimental study was followed by a field study in which similar animals were placed on pasture in a known endemic area. The groups comprised seven Nganda–Jersey crosses, ten Nganda and seven Guernseys. The challenge appears to have been very severe, as all animals died. However, it was observed that the mean survival time for the Nganda animals was much longer (65.6 days) than that of the Guernsey control animals (22.6 days), whereas the survival time of the naïve Nganda–Jersey crosses was intermediate (41 days). Although the numbers are small, the results support the concept that the indigenous Nganda carry a heritable resistance to ECF, which can be broached by a severe challenge.

Guilbride and Opwata (1963) also recorded the maximum body temperatures for the different breeds following challenge and made the general observation that the maximum temperatures in the Nganda group were less than those in the other two groups. A retrospective analysis (presented here and converted to Celsius from the original Fahrenheit) shows that the mean maximum temperature of the Nganda was 40.6°C, compared to 41.1°C and 41.4°C for the cross-bred and Jersey animals, respectively. Within the cross-bred animals, which was the only group with substantial numbers of both susceptible and recovered animals, the mean maximum temperature of the survivors (40.7°C) was significantly less (logistic regression $p = 0.019$) than that of those that died (41.3°C). These results suggested that the resistant animals experienced a less severe pyrexia in response to *T. parva* infection, a finding confirmed in more recent, detailed studies (see Section 7.4.1).

7.2.3 Boran-zebu cross-bred animals in Uganda

A similar investigation was undertaken, again in Uganda, in which the response to field exposure to *T. parva* was compared among 'pure' Boran animals, local small East African zebu and cross-bred animals (Stobbs, 1966). The pure Boran were progeny of heifers, brought in from three Kenyan farms free of ECF and mated to local Boran bulls, and the cross-breds were from the local zebu, also mated to Boran bulls. Stobbs considered the Boran to be susceptible to ECF when introduced into an endemic area, as did Barnett (1968). In all, 398 calves were monitored (93 Boran, 74 crosses and 231 local zebu). The survival rate for the pure Boran calves was 23% (21/93), compared to 57% (42/74) for the Boran–zebu crosses and 77% (178/231) for the local zebu.

A minor drawback of the study was that ECF could not be fully established as the cause of death in a minority of cases. However, 86% of cases where ECF was suspected were supported by laboratory examination of blood and lymph node smears, and very few other tick-borne diseases had been positively recorded on the farm where the cattle were raised. In line with the previous studies, the results strongly suggested the presence of inherited resistance to ECF in indigenous zebu from endemic areas. It is not clear whether the survival of some of the Boran calves was due to a low infection pressure or to a degree of genetic resistance in some of the animals.

Stobbs (1966) also noted that the time between initial signs of ECF and death was shorter in the Boran animals (reported as 7 ± 4 days) compared to the zebu (12 ± 5 days), with the Boran–zebu crosses showing an intermediate interval (9 ± 5 days), although it was not made clear what the '±' range indicated. In addition, the mean maximum temperatures followed the trend observed in the Guilbride and Opwata study, in that the resistant zebu recorded a mean maximum temperature of 39.9°C ± 0.17, compared to the 'susceptible' Boran (40.4°C ± 0.5) and cross-bred animals (40.3°C ± 0.5). Overall, the results provided an early indication that there was a slower development of the disease in the animals that carried the resistance trait even if the animals eventually succumbed.

7.2.4 Resistance in Ankole cattle

Resistance in a different breed of cattle was reported by Paling *et al.* (1991). The Ankole is classified as a sanga type, a series of breeds which have descended from a mixture of indicine and African taurine cattle (Mwai *et al.*, 2015). In a series of experiments, the survival rate of Ankole cattle was compared to that of cross-bred animals (Ankole–Jersey or Ankole–Sahiwal) following challenge with infected ticks, subcutaneous inoculation of various *T. parva* stabilates or field exposure. The cattle came from two farms that were considered free of ECF. When taken together, the results showed a significantly ($p < 0.01$) greater level of survival in the Ankole (68% or 49/72) compared to the cross-bred animals (36% or 12/33). In those experiments where a direct comparison could be made between the breeds (same method and level of exposure), the survival rates were also significantly different ($p < 0.01$), being 64% (16/25) and 32% (6/19) for Ankole and cross-breds, respectively. In the field study, although all animals including the Ankole eventually succumbed, the time to death in the Ankole (23–67 days) was considerably longer than for the cross-breds (17–23 days).

An additional result from these experiments was the confirmation that the resistance to ECF cannot be due solely to tick resistance, as clear differences in survival were observed in experiments where needle inoculation with infected tick homogenate was used to challenge the animals. This was reinforced by a later study (Dolan *et al.*, 1982) investigating the comparative susceptibility of taurine (Friesian) and indicine (Boran) cattle that were infected by administration of infected lymphocyte cell lines, one of which was derived from a taurine donor and one from an indicine donor. Irrespective of origin of the cell line, fewer Boran cattle died or suffered severe reactions than the Friesian ones.

Two key insights into the mechanism of resistance were revealed by laboratory analyses undertaken during the Paling study. First, the researchers examined the intensity of the parasitosis by estimating the macroschizont index (MSI), being the number of macroschizonts, both free and intracellular, per 100 lymphocytes in smears of lymph node aspirates. The mean maximum MSI of Ankole cattle was estimated to be 5.24%, which was almost three times less than that of the cross-bred animals (15.55%, $p < 0.001$). A slightly different analysis revealed that the mean maximum MSI in the animals that survived the stabilate challenge was 1.58%, compared to 13.72% for the susceptible ones. The results suggested that the resistant animals avoided severe disease by controlling the proliferation of macroschizonts.

7.2.5 Small African zebu cattle in southern Kenya

In the 1980s, Moll and co-workers published epidemiological observations of theileriosis in indigenous calves in the southern Transmara region of Kenya, which is endemic for ECF. The cattle under study were from Maasai pastoralist herds and were classified as small African zebu. The authors concluded that 'The calf population was highly resistant to theileriosis since they had a 100% morbidity, but only 2.6% mortality' (Moll *et al.*, 1984, pp. 801–802). Some caution needs to be observed with this conclusion, as there were several confounding factors, which illustrate the challenges with field observations under normal, 'uncontrolled' conditions. Foremost among these was the application of acaricide every 10–20 days, which may have reduced the parasite challenge to a sub-lethal level. Antibiotic use was widespread, including the use of oxytetracycline to treat suspected cases of ECF, which may have led to an underestimate of potential deaths due to ECF. The authors also reported the presence of other pathogens, including *Theileria mutans*, which complicates the identification of the precise cause of mortality and morbidity. Finally, and importantly when attempting to establish a heritable trait, there was no control group available for study. The nearest the researchers came to this was to note that ticks removed from the study area were invariably fatal when applied to European cattle away from the study site. Nevertheless, the study does provide reasonably strong grounds for believing that resistance was observed and that it was remarkable enough for the authors to consider that it derived from '... an important gene pool from which *Theileria* resistant cattle of improved productivity could be developed' (Moll *et al.*, 1984, p. 829).

7.2.6 Resistance observed in experimental infections

A detailed clinical and parasitological comparison of the susceptibility of taurine and indicine cattle to experimental infection was reported by Ndungu *et al.* (2005). Four groups of cattle comprising Friesian, Boran and zebus, with the last group comprising animals from non-endemic and from endemic regions were examined. The animals in the last group were born to dams that had been removed from the endemic area prior to calving. The parasites were delivered by needle inoculation with an infected tick stabilate at an estimated 50% lethal dose (LD_{50}). Although the numbers of animals were small (ten per group), there was a significantly higher survival rate in the endemic zebus compared to the other three groups, in which there was no significant difference in mortality rate. If the numbers of animals that either died or developed a severe reaction are combined, it is seen that only three of the endemic zebu were in this category, compared to all ten of the Boran, eight of the Friesian and seven of the non-endemic zebu. Apart from supporting earlier observations that indigenous cattle from endemic areas are more resistant to ECF, the results also indicated that indigenous cattle from non-endemic areas are as susceptible as non-indigenous ones. It must be stressed that the numbers are small and insufficient to allow extrapolation of the conclusions to the general population.

These early field and experimental observations (summarized in Fig. 7.1) strongly indicated that cattle from endemic areas have been selected for a degree of resistance to ECF. Until recently, there was no concerted effort to identify the genetic elements responsible for this resistance for use in marker-assisted breeding programmes. This is due to the lack of the powerful genetic tools required for such analyses, which, as presented below, has now changed.

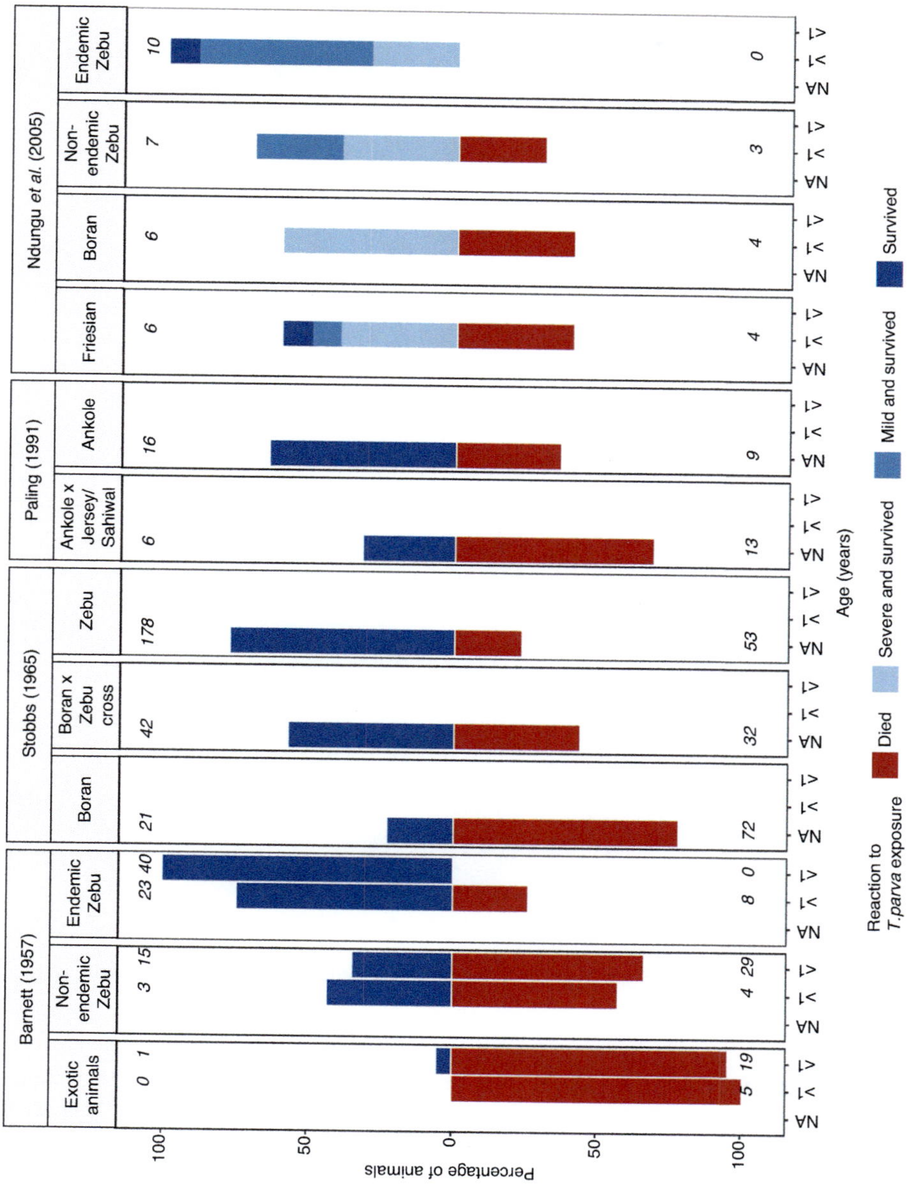

Fig. 7.1. Summarized results of early observations indicating the presence of a genetic resistance to disease caused by *T. parva* in cattle. (Kindly provided by James Prendergast.)

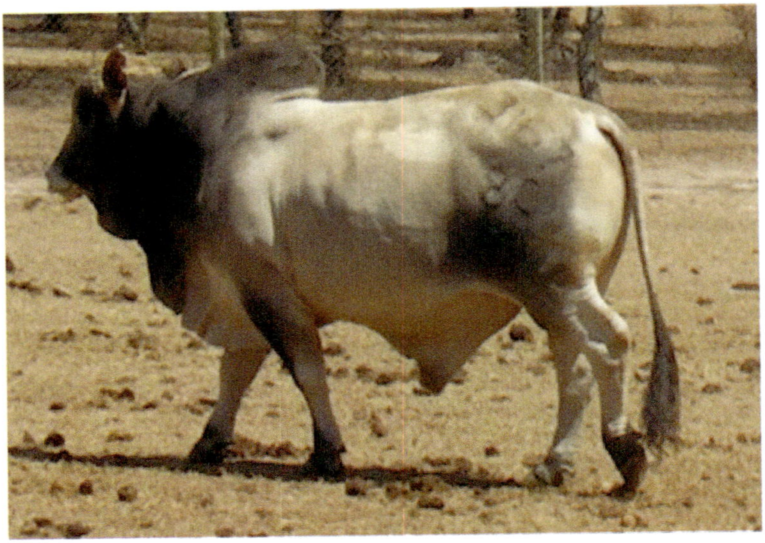

Fig. 7.2. Bull 3167. (Photograph taken at Kapiti Plains Estate (ILRI) and kindly provided by Liam Morrison.)

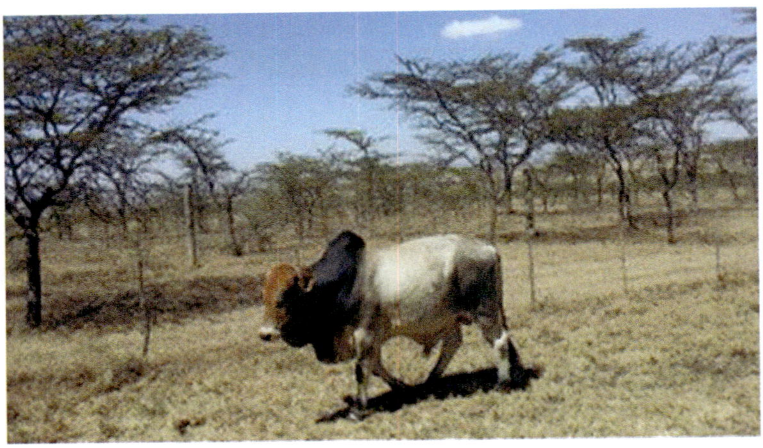

Fig. 7.3. First-generation offspring of bull 3167. (Photograph taken at Ol Pejeta Conservancy by Philip Toye.)

7.3 The Ol Pejeta Field Studies

7.3.1 Resistance observed in a single lineage of Boran animals

Substantial insights into the nature of the resistance in indicine cattle have come from a series of field studies conducted at Ol Pejeta, a conservancy in central Kenya with a high *T. parva* challenge derived from a resident buffalo population. The studies were prompted, quite unexpectedly, by the outcome of a field trial examining the efficacy of the Muguga cocktail version of the Infection and Treatment Method (ITM) vaccine against buffalo-derived challenge (Sitt *et al.*, 2015). Vaccinated and unvaccinated *B. indicus* (Boran) cattle (12 animals per group) from the International Livestock Research Institute's facility at Kapiti, which is considered free of ECF, were transported to the Ol Pejeta

Conservancy and maintained in an area grazed only by buffalo. The study demonstrated that the vaccine offered no protection against this challenge, as nine cattle died from *T. parva* infection in both the vaccinated and unvaccinated groups. However, Dr Tatjana Sitt, a postdoctoral fellow attached to the project, noted that all three surviving unvaccinated cattle were from the same sire, a Boran bull known as '3167' (Fig. 7.2). The only other experimental animal from this bull was in the vaccinated group and it also survived. The result was the more remarkable as Boran were previously believed to be a susceptible breed (Stobbs, 1966; Barnett, 1968; Ndungu *et al.*, 2005).

As the number of animals from the bull was very small, a second field study was undertaken to explore the possibility that the offspring had inherited a resistance trait from 3167. The bull had died of unknown causes at about the time of the study, but there were several first-generation offspring available at Kapiti (Fig. 7.3).

Breeding records were used to select a group of 12 offspring of the bull together with a second group of 12 age-matched but apparently unrelated animals. (The details of all field studies in this series conducted at Ol Pejeta have been published by Latré de Laté *et al.*, 2021; Wragg *et al.*, 2022). All animals were unvaccinated and serologically negative for *T. parva* antibodies. Genome analysis undertaken after the study confirmed the relatedness of the animals, apart from two of the 'offspring', which were shown not to be related to the bull and were reassigned to the unrelated group. Following exposure at Ol Pejeta, four of the offspring survived the field challenge, as did one of the unrelated animals. There was no statistically significant difference in survival rates between the groups, most likely due to the small number of survivors. There were, however, two interesting aspects of the survival time (time from field exposure to death, euthanasia or treatment *in extremis*) in the study animals. Firstly, the mean survival time for the unrelated animals was 16.2 days, compared to 21.4 days in the first study (Table 7.3). These short durations indicated that the calves in the second study were exposed to an exceptionally high level of challenge. The second aspect was that the mean survival time of the offspring was significantly longer (22.3 days) compared to that of the unrelated animals (16.2 days). These results were considered sufficiently promising to justify a further field study.

The third study comprised 15 progeny of bull 3167 and ten unrelated animals, initially selected on pedigree records and then reallocated

Table 7.3. Survival rates and survival times of animals in the Ol Pejeta field studies.

		Survived	Succumbed[a]	Total	Survival rate	Survival time[b]
2013	First generation	3[c]	0	3	100%	n/a
	Unrelated	0	9	9	0%	21.4
2014	First generation	4	6	10	40%	22.3
	Unrelated	1	13	14	7%	16.2
2015	First generation	12	3	15	80%	23.7
	Unrelated	0	10	10	0%	18.9
	Third degree	2	3	5	40%	19.0
2017	Second generation	17	7	24	71%	20.0
	Unrelated	1	6	7	14%	17.3
2018	Second generation	7	16	23	30%	20.8
	Unrelated	2	4	6	33%	18.8

[a]'Succumbed' refers to animals which developed severe clinical signs and died or were euthanazed or treated.
[b]'Survival time' is the time in days between when the animals were introduced to the field site and when they succumbed (death from *T. parva* infection, euthanasia or treatment *in extremis*).
[c]Although there were four progeny of 3167 in this trial, one animal had been vaccinated and is not included in the analysis.

following genomic analysis to confirm their pedigree. In this study, the difference in survival rate between the two groups was highly significant. All ten unrelated animals succumbed to the *T. parva* challenge compared to only three of the 15 progeny. The mean survival times of animals that succumbed to infection were also different (18.9 days and 23.7 days, respectively).

With clear evidence that the progeny of 3167 possessed a significant degree of resistance to *T. parva*, two more studies were undertaken with second-generation progeny of 3167, for two reasons. The first was to determine if the resistance trait was 'strong' enough to be passed on by the direct offspring of the bull. The second was to obtain, in the absence of suitable first-generation animals, more DNA samples from phenotypically characterized animals to facilitate the localization of genomic regions responsible for the resistance trait and to increase the number of recombination events to reduce the linkage interval. Due to constraints imposed by the availability of animals and the limit on the number of animals that can be rigorously monitored and sampled in the field, two separate studies were undertaken. The two studies together comprised 47 progeny of five first-generation bulls from 3167, and 13 unrelated calves. The respective survival rates were 51% (24/47) and 23% (3/13). Among the progeny group, there was no bias in survival with respect to sire.

Apart from the 121 study animals that were included in the five studies above, five additional calves were included as unrelated animals and underwent field challenge but were later excluded from the survival analysis following genomic analysis undertaken after the trials. Four of these were estimated to be related (third-degree relatives) to the first-generation progeny and the fifth was a second-generation descendant of 3167 through its dam. Two of the four relatives of the first-generation animals survived the field exposure. Despite being censored from the survival analysis, the animals and their samples and metadata were included in the subsequent analyses to identify the genomic region responsible for tolerance (Section 7.3.2).

Collectively, the five field studies took place over a period of about 5 years (June 2013–July 2018), due in part to the need to have progeny animals reach a suitable (post-weaning) age. The combined results demonstrated the inherited nature of the resistance phenotype, which was reflected in both a significantly greater survival rate of progeny (mean survival rate of 68% (19/28) and 51% (24/47) for first- and second-generation animals, respectively, compared to 8.7% (4/46) for unrelated cattle) and a significantly longer mean survival time for those animals which did succumb (24.1, 20.4 and 18.7 days, respectively). The survival rates and survival times for the different groups of calves are shown in Table 7.3 and illustrated in Fig. 7.4. The data provided an estimated heritability (h^2) of the tolerance phenotype of 0.67 (s.e. = 0.57) (Wragg *et al.*, 2022).

The Ol Pejeta site provided a rigorous system for detecting the resistance phenotype under field conditions. Across the five studies, the animals were exposed to a constant, high level of parasite challenge, which ensured rapid infection of all animals. Thus, with one exception, parasites were detected in the draining lymph nodes of all animals within 17 days of arrival on the field site. (The exception died on day 16, and parasites were detected in organ impression smears taken at the post-mortem examination.) The highly lethal nature of the challenge was reflected in the mortality rate of 91.3% (42/46) in the unrelated control animals, almost all of which (95% or 40/42) succumbed within 21 days of arrival at the field site.

In summary, the Ol Pejeta studies clearly demonstrated differences in susceptibility to disease caused by *T. parva* between the descendants of a single *B. indicus* (Boran) animal and unrelated animals of the same breed and provided strong evidence to support the earlier observations by several researchers in different countries and with different *B. indicus* breeds.

7.3.2 Identification of a genomic region associated with resistance

The availability of pedigree information, biological samples and parasitological and clinical data from the animals in the Ol Pejeta field studies prompted a search for the genomic region controlling the resistance phenotype (Wragg *et al.*, 2022). As mentioned above,

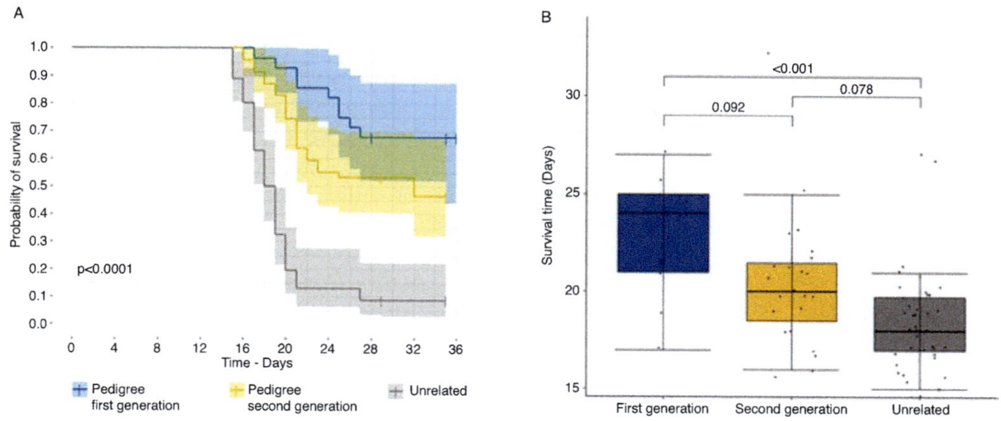

Fig. 7.4. Survival outcomes for calves in the five Ol Pejeta field studies. (A) shows the survival curves of first- (blue) and second- (orange) generation offspring of sire 3167 vesus unrelated (grey) animals. Shaded areas correspond to 95% confidence intervals. (B) shows the comparison of survival time (or time to death) of animals that succumbed to infection for first- (blue) and second- (orange) generation offspring of sire 3167 and unrelated (grey) animals. The *p* values for the specific paired comparisons from the linear regression (adjusted for multiple comparisons using Tukey) are shown above the boxplot. (Reproduced with permission from Latré de Laté *et al.*, 2021.)

the sire, 3167, died as the first field study was completed and no tissue samples were recovered from him. Thus, the initial task was to infer the bull's genotypes from those of his offspring used in the field studies. Whole-genome sequences were obtained for 43 animals, including all 28 first-generation animals, together with array data from a further 78 animals. The genotypes of the first-generation offspring were then used in simulation analyses to impute the genotypes of the sire. Haplotype analysis was undertaken by calculating the Hamming distance of 1 Mbp regions of each animal's genome with the corresponding paternal and maternal regions. The four distances were used to determine the strength of association between survival and haplotypes derived from or similar to those of 3167, so as not to exclude the possibility of resistance being inherited down the maternal line. This resulted in the identification of a segment at chromosome 15, 49–50 Mb, which is highly associated with the resistance trait ($p = 4.12 \times 10^{-07}$). This segment plus flanking regions (chromosome 15, 45–51 Mb) underwent further analysis to identify candidate single nucleotide variants (SNVs) that could generate the resistance phenotype using the assumption that the relevant candidate SNVs affect either the level of expression or the coding regions of genes whose protein products are involved in tolerance.

Variants affecting gene expression levels were identified by sequencing mRNA in leucocytes obtained from animals at various time points before or during the fifth field study. Although nominal associations were found between 720 variants and the expression of genes within or near the target segment, and a further 587 variants were tagged as response expression quantitative trait loci, no significant associations were found after applying a false discovery correction.

The SNVs were then assessed for impact on coding regions, which resulted in the identification of 58,066 high-quality SNVs. After excluding variants over-represented in European cattle (alternative allele frequency > 0.1) that are highly susceptible to ECF, and variants under-represented in the tolerant progeny of 3167 (alternative allele frequency < 0.5), 52 SNVs remained. Four of these were predicted to have high impact. Two were located in olfactory receptor genes, one in a paralogue of the haemoglobin subunit beta receptor, while the fourth results in a stop codon within a paralogue of the FAS-associated factor 1 (FAF1). Currently, there is no clearly established role for any of these proteins in the pathogenesis of *T. parva* infection. However, FAS has been shown to induce apoptosis, and *T. parva*-infected lymphocytes circumvent apoptotic pathways (Küenzi *et al.*, 2003). It was due to this association that the FAF1 paralogue was examined further.

The paralogue, which has been named FAF1B, is located on chromosome 15, whereas the authentic FAF1 gene is found on chromosome 3. The nucleotide sequence of FAF1B shows 96.8% identity with 68.77% of the authentic FAF1 gene (Wragg *et al.*, 2022). The variant in FAF1B is a C:T mutation at position 15:50823230, which is predicted to convert an arginine codon (cga) to a stop codon (tga), resulting in a truncated protein. This variant has not been observed in the authentic FAF1 gene.

The association of the FAF1B variant with survival in the field trials was analysed more deeply. As the variant is not present on the array used to genotype some of the calves in the haplotype analysis, these and a further 22 animals were genotyped at the locus by PCR and sequencing (Wragg *et al.*, 2022). As expected, the analysis revealed a highly significant association between the presence of the allele and both survival rate and survival time. It was noted that seven of the eight (88%) offspring homozygous for the derived T allele survived the field challenge, as did 62% (36/58) of heterozygotes. In contrast, only 12% (4/34) of cattle homozygous for the ancestral C allele survived. (When the genotypes were subsequently available for all 126 animals in the field study, these figures were revised to 88% (7/8), 57% (37/65) and 9% (5/53), respectively [P. Toye, Nairobi, personal communication]). The analysis also revealed that the mean survival time for the animals that succumbed was longer ($p = 0.00073$; Mann Whitney U test) for the CT heterozygotes (21.27 ± 2.25 days) than for the CC homozygotes (18.55 ± 1.7 days). These results are illustrated in Fig. 7.5.

As noted above, only four unrelated animals survived the field exposure. Genotyping revealed that three of these were CT heterozygotes and the fourth was a TT homozygote. They had presumably inherited the protective allele outside the 3167-descendant lineage. It was also noted that two of the five animals regarded as third-degree relatives to the 3167 first-generation progeny survived. Both were CT heterozygotes, while the three that succumbed were CC homozygotes.

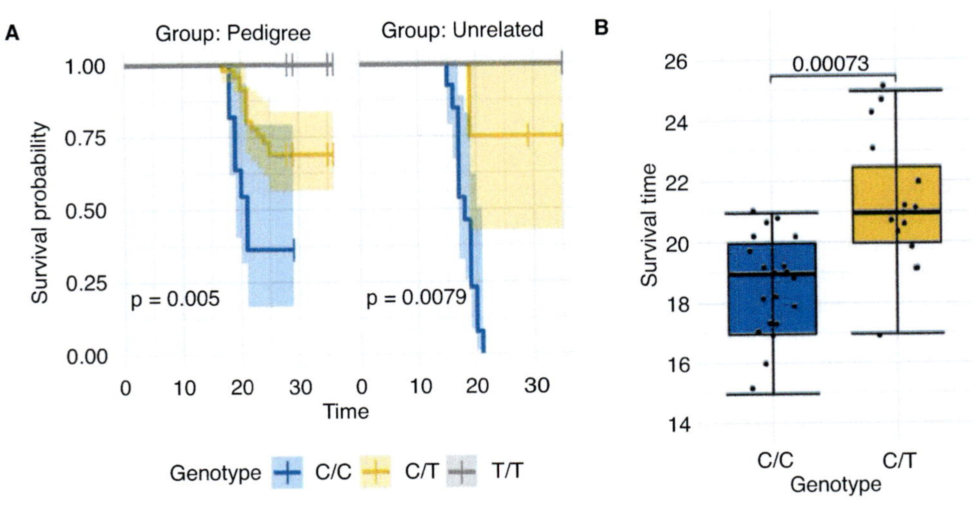

Fig. 7.5. Survival curves (A) and survival times (B) vs variant genotype for first- and second-generation and unrelated animals from the Ol Pejeta field studies. Log-rank *p* values (A) and a Mann-Whitney U test *p* value is reported (B). (Reproduced with permission from Wragg *et al.*, 2022.)

Table 7.4. Genotypes of the IDEAL calf cohort. Miyunga *et al.*, 2026.

Genotype	Total	Survived	Succumbed	
			ECF	Non-ECF
CC	265 (48.4%)	224 (84.5%)	16 (6.0%)	25 (9.4%)
CT	227 (41.4%)	187 (82.4%)	16 (7.0%)	24 (10.6%)
TT	56 (10.2%)	49 (87.5%)	0 (0%)	7 (12.5%)
Total	548	460	32	56

The percentages in brackets are based on the total number of animals in the corresponding rows, except for the 'Total' column, which is based on the total number of animals.

7.3.3 Evidence for an association of the variant with survival from a cattle-derived challenge

As the Ol Pejeta experiments involved a buffalo-derived challenge, it was important to analyse cattle from an area endemic for cattle-derived infection. Advantage was taken of the availability of clinical data and DNA samples from the calves in the IDEAL study conducted in western Kenya between 2007 and 2009, as mentioned above (Section 7.2.1). All 548 animals in the IDEAL cohort were genotyped for the FAF1B C:T mutation by PCR and sequencing or by a real-time PCR hybridization assay (Wragg *et al.*, 2022; Miyunga *et al.*, 2026).

The cohort included 56 TT homozygous animals, but none of these animals were among the 32 animals that died from ECF in the study, although seven died from causes other than ECF (Table 7.4). There was a significant difference in the genotype frequencies of the animals that died of ECF compared both to the rest of the population (likelihood ratio test, $p = 0.026$) and specifically to the animals that died of causes other than ECF ($p = 0.035$). On the other hand, the genotype frequencies of the animals that died of causes other than ECF were not significantly different from those of the surviving population ($p = 0.69$). As there were equal numbers of the CC or CT genotypes in the animals that died of ECF, no effect of a single copy of the T haplotype on survival was discerned, although the numbers of animals involved are small. Nevertheless, this retrospective analysis did detect an association of the T haplotype when present in homozygous form with survival from ECF in a farming system where the mortality rate from ECF was calculated to be only 7% in the calves that were known to have been exposed to *T. parva* (Woolhouse *et al.*, 2015).

This result is important as it demonstrates the association of the resistance haplotype with survival following a cattle-derived challenge in animals of a different breed in a different farming system to that of the Ol Pejeta studies. It is also clear that, with only a 7% fatality rate from ECF and a calculated exposure rate to *T. parva* of 83% in the total population (Woolhouse *et al.*, 2015), most of the CC animals were resistant. As historical reports state that the challenge to non-indigenous cattle in this region was invariably fatal (Barnett, 1957; Conelly, 1998), the survival of the CC animals in the IDEAL study suggests that, in addition to the genetic region associated with the FAF1B mutation, other genes can confer resistance to *T. parva* infection.

Currently, there is no evidence available to confirm that FAF1B is involved in mediating resistance to ECF. Indeed, examination of RNA from infected and uninfected blood leukocytes has failed to show any expression of the gene (Wragg *et al.*, 2022). Consistent with these observations, a recent update of the Ensembl database has indicated that the FAF1B sequence is no longer classified as a gene (Dyer *et al.*, 2025). Thus, the FAF1B sequence variant is unlikely to be responsible for resistance, but rather the C:T mutation in the DNA is closely linked to a causal allele yet to be identified. Further experimentation, including analysis of the indicine genome, is required to elucidate the precise genetic basis of the resistance to ECF.

In summary, the data and samples derived from the Ol Pejeta studies allowed the identification of a region of the bovine genome strongly associated with the tolerance phenotype and

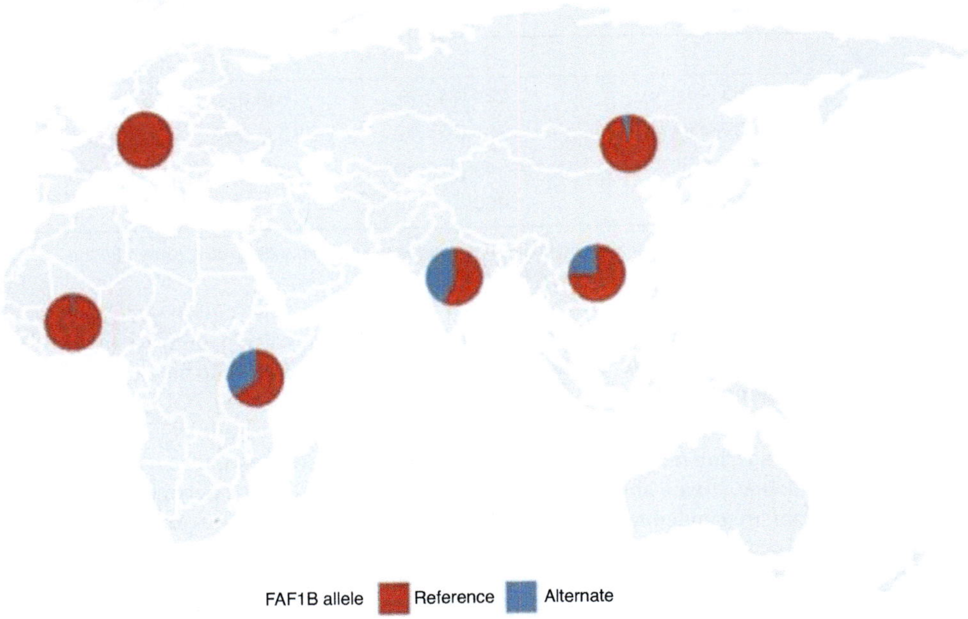

Fig. 7.6. Frequency of the T haplotype in cattle from different geographic areas. (Kindly provided by James Prendergast.)

provides the basis for further work to identify the causal allele(s) and mechanisms mediating resistance to ECF.

7.3.4 The variant is found in other *B. indicus* populations

Wragg *et al.* (2022) also determined the frequency of FAF1B mutation in various cattle populations across the globe. The samples were obtained from 436 cattle and comprised 145 European taurine, 44 East Asian taurine, 35 African taurine, 112 African indicine, 64 Chinese indicine and 36 Indian indicine animals. The results are presented graphically in Fig. 7.6. The mutation was found at a frequency of < 4% in the European taurine, which is not a surprising result given that a selection filter of an alternative allele frequency of < 10% in European taurine had been applied in identifying the allele. There was a similarly low frequency (< 9%) in African taurine animals, almost all of which were from West Africa, where *T. parva* does not occur. There were relatively high frequencies of 22–54% in both African and Asian indicine cattle. As the African indicine breeds were introduced from Asia, the results suggest that the mutation is likely to have arisen there.

7.4 Parasitological and Clinical Parameters Associated with Resistance

7.4.1 Clinical and parasitological results from the Ol Pejeta studies

Analysis of the clinical and parasitological data obtained in the Ol Pejeta field studies showed that both first- and second-generation survivors of the field exposure experienced a delayed and less severe parasitosis compared to unrelated susceptible animals (Latré de Laté *et al.*, 2021). For example, the time to first detection of parasites in either the parotid or prescapular lymph nodes in the first- and second-generation surviving progeny and the unrelated susceptible animals was 13.0, 12.9 and 11.6 days, respectively (least square means, $p < 0.001$), and the maximum Infection Index (mean percentage of infected lymphocytes in parotid and prescapular lymph nodes) was estimated to be 1.01 in the surviving progeny, compared to 4.00 in the susceptible unrelated animals (least square means, $p < 0.001$). The susceptible progeny showed a parasitological response intermediate between these two groups. In addition, the time from initial parasitosis to death was 11.3, 8.1 and 7.0 days in susceptible first-generation, second-generation and unrelated animals, respectively (least square means, $p < 0.001$), indicating a slower progression of the pathogenic response in the progeny.

The pyrexic response followed a similar pattern. The time to detection of fever (> 39.4°C) was 15.2, 15.5 and 12.9 days (least square means, $p = 0.003$), and the mean maximum temperature was 40.8°C, 40.6°C and 41.5°C (least square means, $p < 0.001$) in the three groups as above, respectively. In addition, the pyrexia intensity (the mean increase above 39.4°C on the days on which an elevated temperature was recorded) was 0.81, 0.73 and 1.19, respectively (least square means, $p < 0.001$).

When the clinical and parasitological data were re-analysed following the identification of a strong association of the C:T mutation with survival, a similar trend was observed. Animals homozygous for the protective T allele showed a delayed and less severe parasitological and pyrexic response compared to those homozygous for the C allele, with heterozygotes exhibiting an intermediate reaction (Fig. 7.7).

7.4.2 *In vitro* studies from the Ol Pejeta field studies

The previous results showed that tolerance to ECF is due to fewer infected lymphocytes in animals possessing the inherited resistance genotype. The availability of lymphocytes that had been collected and cryopreserved before the animals were exposed in the fifth Ol Pejeta field study in 2018 provided an opportunity to obtain supporting data from *in vitro* experiments (Latré de Laté *et al.*, 2021). When the lymphocytes were infected and cultivated *in vitro*, it was clear that the increase in infected cell numbers from the resistant animals progressed much more slowly on average than those from susceptible cattle (Fig. 7.8). A similar difference in numbers of infected cells was also observed in animals of the TT genotype compared to CC animals in cells harvested from additional cattle not involved in the field study (Fig. 7.9). In both experiments, the presence of proliferating uninfected cells in the cultures does not allow a conclusion to be drawn as to whether the reduced numbers of infected cells in cultures from resistant animals

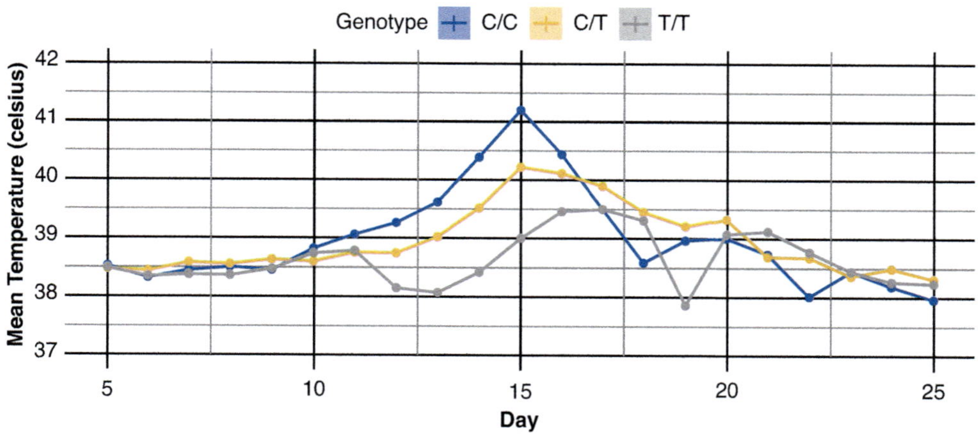

Fig. 7.7. Mean daily temperature for all animals in the Ol Pejeta field studies grouped by genotype. (Adapted with permission from Wragg *et al.*, 2022.)

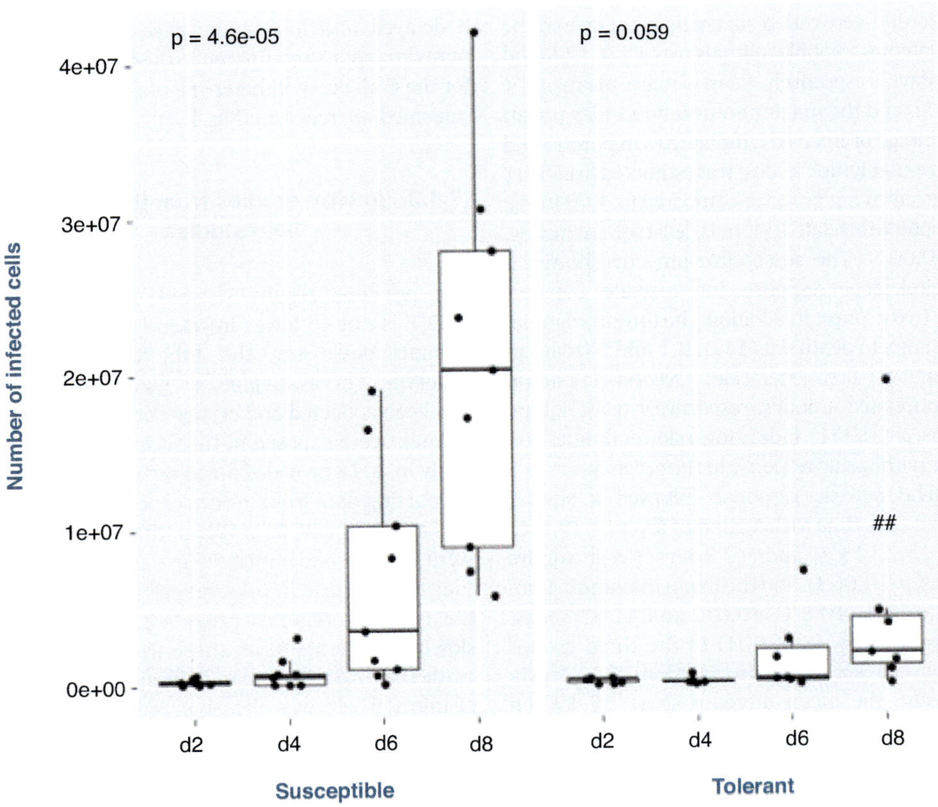

Fig. 7.8. Increase in numbers of infected cells from tolerant and susceptible animals during *in vitro* culture. The *p* values represent the probability of a difference in the values at different days within each group (Kruskal–Wallis test). The probability of a difference in values on the same day between susceptible and tolerant populations is shown as ## $p < 0.01$. (Adapted with permission from Latré de Laté *et al.*, 2021.)

is due to an intrinsic impairment of proliferation of the infected cells or to a unique population of effector cells present in resistant animals that suppress the proliferation of infected lymphocytes. It is also not yet clear whether the reduction in the numbers of infected lymphocytes occurs in all lymphocytes or in specific lineages.

In summary, it appears that animals carrying the C:T mutation in FAF1B limit the multiplication of infected lymphocytes, which results in delayed and less severe pathogenic consequences. This in turn allows the animals to resolve the infection, most likely by the induction of a protective T cell-mediated immune response (see Chapter 11 of this volume).

7.5 Is the Inherited Resistance to *T. parva* Related to Age?

It is known that young cattle infected with other haemoparasites such as *Babesia bovis* display less severe clinical signs than older animals (reviewed by Brown *et al.*, 2006). The concept that young calves are more resistant to ECF

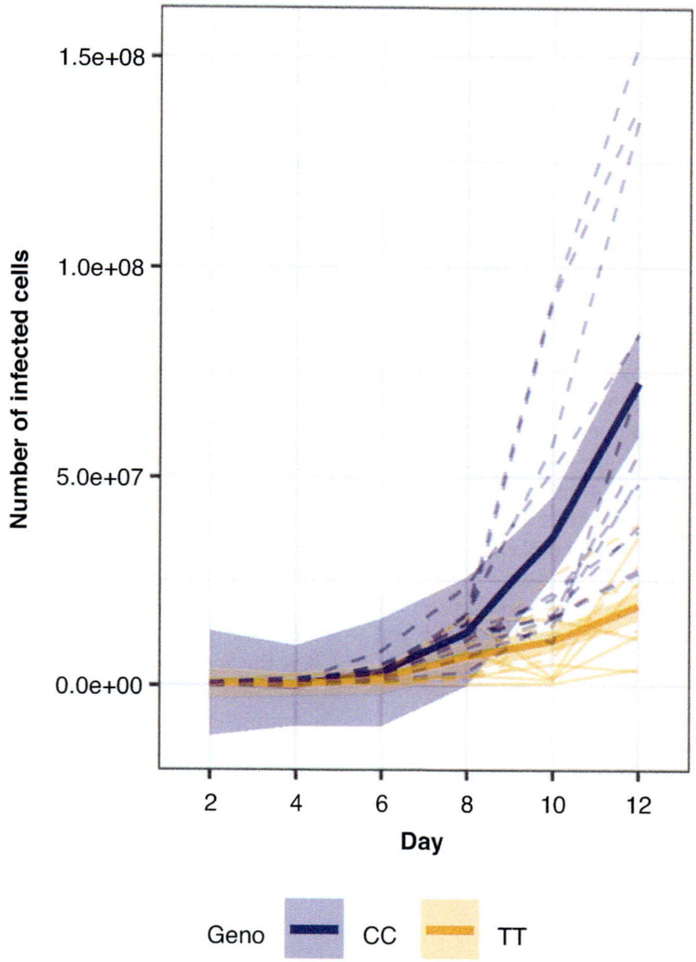

Fig. 7.9. *In vitro* cultures of cells from TT homozygous animals contain significantly fewer infected cells than those from CC animals (F-test p = 7.56 x 10^{-09}). The blue and orange ribbons and thick blue and orange lines indicate the 95% confidence interval around the mean for the corresponding genotypes, respectively. Thin dashed lines represent results from unrelated animals while thin solid lines represent results from animals from the ECF-resistant pedigree. (Adapted with permission from Wragg *et al.*, 2022).

than older animals has also been promoted. Hornby (1934, cited by Wilson, 1950) observed that 50% of calves in endemic areas recovered from infection, and he considered age as a possible factor in the resistance shown by calves in endemic areas. Wilson (1950) infected calves of various ages (5–35 months), but there was no conclusive evidence of an age-related resistance. As mentioned earlier (Section 7.2.1), Barnett and Bailey (1955b) investigated age as one of the possible factors associated with resistance. They infected calves of various ages by application of a single infected tick. Although an apparent decline in resistance with age was observed in calves from endemic areas, the opposite was observed in calves from non-endemic areas (Table 7.1). Thus, the study suggested that any age-related resistance was restricted to calves from the 'endemic' group. Given the small numbers of animals in each age group, it is very difficult to apply any solid conclusions regarding a purely age-related resistance to the general population.

Koch *et al.* (1990) attempted to explain why field reports in Zimbabwe showed a lower ECF case incidence in calves under 7 months of age (relative incidence 0.18) compared to those aged between 7 and 18 months (2.17) or older than 18 months (2.04). When groups of seven Holstein-Friesian calves of 1, 4, 7, 10 and 13 months were challenged with an LD_{40} of the local *T. parva* (*bovis*) tick stabilate, the highest mortality rates and disease severity were seen in the 4- and 13-month age groups and the lowest in the calves of 1 month of age. The authors concluded that there was no evidence for an age-related resistance in young calves, apart from those at a very young age, and that the apparent resistance in the field was the result of a lower tick challenge.

In summary, there appears to be no conclusive evidence for an age-related resistance to *T. parva* comparable to that seen with *Babesia* and *Anaplasma* species.

7.6 The Role of Inherited Resistance in Endemic Stability

Endemic stability is the epidemiological situation that occurs when there is a high prevalence of infection with a pathogen but limited clinical disease. Mahoney (1977) applied the concept to a parasitic disease in describing the epidemiology of *Babesia bovis*, where endemic stability is attained in areas where calves are exposed to a low but persistent parasite challenge. They are protected from severe disease by increased resistance of calves compared to adults and the presence of colostral antibody (Young, 1981). This allows a non-fatal infection and the development of protective immunity against challenge in later life.

Endemic stability has also been used to describe the low ECF-related mortality in calves of indigenous cattle residing in endemic areas (Young, 1981; Norval *et al.*, 1992). Although these authors suggested that age-related resistance of calves contributed to this endemic stability, current evidence indicates that there is no significant age-related resistance to *T. parva*. Hence, genetic resistance coupled with sustained low infection levels in ticks appear to be the key factors in maintaining endemic stability and, as discussed below, they are interdependent.

Previous studies have shown that the inherited resistance to *T. parva* can be overcome by high levels of challenge. Barnett (1957) noted that the 100% survival rate seen with a one-tick challenge was reduced to 36% when the challenge was increased to 50 ticks (Table 7.2). Similarly, Wilson (1950) reported that attachment of three or four infected ticks led to a fatal ECF episode, whereas one or two ticks resulted in an asymptomatic infection. An interpretation of the results of the second field trial at Ol Pejeta, in which there was a higher mortality rate due to ECF among the first-generation 3167 offspring compared to the first and third trials, is that these animals were exposed to a much heavier parasite challenge that 'broke through' the resistance phenotype.

Given that the inherited resistance can be overcome with a sufficiently high dose of sporozoites, the level of initial challenge encountered in the field is an important consideration in explaining endemic stability, but one that is difficult to quantify. Barnett (1957) reported that seven infected ticks led to death in 27% (7/26) of indigenous calves but considered that 'a challenge dose of 10 adult ticks is greater than that likely to be encountered in the field' (Barnett, 1957, p. 352). These studies used experimentally infected ticks, which have high levels of infection. In endemic regions of Kenya, it has been estimated that the tick infection rate is < 3%. Although most infected ticks have one or two infected salivary gland cells, or acini, a few ticks can have over 30 infected acini (Leitch and Young, 1981; Moll *et al.*, 1986). Thus, field challenge will result in a dose of parasites that, although lethal for fully susceptible breeds of calves, is likely to be sub-lethal for most calves of indigenous breeds. However, the inherited resistance may be overcome in the field if calves encounter a tick carrying an above average number of sporozoites. This may account for the small proportion of indigenous animals that do succumb in endemic areas. The fact that there are relatively few instances of severe disease with high parasite burdens in indigenous animals may be an important factor in ensuring that feeding ticks usually do not acquire high levels of infection.

Thus, it could be argued that the inherited resistance in indigenous cattle has evolved in such a way as to enable the survival of the great majority of animals under the low levels of parasite challenge that prevail in endemic areas, while at the same time, the low level of challenge is maintained by the low parasitaemia encountered by feeding ticks in the surviving carrier animals. The balanced interdependence between these two factors is possibly the strongest, and perhaps only, driver for maintaining endemic stability. Despite the presence of endemic stability, annual mortality rates of up to 10–20% have been recorded, which represents a considerable loss, especially among smallholder farmers, and which necessitates expensive control measures.

7.7 Inherited Resistance in Infections with *T. annulata*

As mentioned above, analysis of whole genome sequences from several cattle populations showed that the T allele identified in the Ol Pejeta studies is present in other indicine cattle populations, including those from Asia where the related parasite *T. annulata* is endemic and causes the disease tropical theileriosis. As the eastern African cattle populations originated from the Indian subcontinent several thousand years ago (see Chapter 5 of this volume), it is possible that the causal mutation arose in response to *T. annulata*. Although the host cell type differs for *T. annulata* (B lymphocytes and macrophages/monocytes), the pathogenesis of the diseases caused by the parasites is similar (reviewed by Nene and Morrison, 2016).

There is a general acceptance that *B. indicus* cattle are more resistant to *T. annulata* than *B. taurus* animals. For example, Bakheit and Latif (2002) showed that Kenana cattle from an endemic region of Sudan were resistant to *T. annulata* infection delivered by stabilate inoculation. They observed a significantly ($p < 0.05$) lower mean MSI in the tolerant Kenana cattle. Similarly, Glass *et al.* (2005) showed that Sahiwal cattle, an indicine breed from the Punjab, were more resistant to disease following inoculation of *T. annulata* sporozoites than were European taurine (Holstein) cattle. However, there is currently no evidence that demonstrates an association between the CT variant in the FAF1 gene paralogue and resistance to disease caused by *T. annulata*.

7.8 Conclusions

It is puzzling why the innate resistance to ECF has not been more fully and formally exploited, as had been suggested by several early workers (Mettam and Carmichael, 1936; Barnett and Bailey, 1955a, b; Moll *et al.*, 1984; Ndungu *et al.*, 2005). Indigenous cattle, despite their low productivity, are still used by many smallholders and pastoralists in ECF endemic areas due to their resistance to ECF, and attempts to introduce more productive breeds into these areas have been unsuccessful due to their susceptibility to the disease. At the same time, the poor productivity of these indigenous animals limits their attraction as a starting point for genetic improvement in traditional breeding programmes. The identification of genes that confer resistance would enhance marker-assisted selection in breeding programmes to incorporate the causal allele(s) into the genetic backgrounds of more productive animals by cross-breeding. Alternatively, precise identification of the causal allele(s) could ultimately facilitate the use of genome-edited animals to achieve this outcome and reduce the impact of ECF in affected regions. Future studies of the resistance are required in two areas:

1. The underlying genetic basis and mechanism of resistance.
    - More precisely identify the causal allele and the associated molecular/cellular phenotype.
    - Determine whether impaired multiplication of infected cells from resistant cattle *in vitro* is due to a direct effect on the infected cells or to involvement of another cell type that acts on the infected cells.

   Addressing these issues would provide a more direct genetic marker of the resistance and potentially facilitate development of an *in vitro* biological assay for predicting the resistance status of animals.

2. Issues that need to be addressed to determine the feasibility of commercial exploitation of the resistance.
    - Obtain further evidence in other farming systems that animals with the resistance genotype survive infection with cattle-maintained *T. parva*.
    - Estimate the financial benefit to livestock owners of using resistant cattle through reduced mortality and morbidity and decreased use of acaricides. This would include an assessment of any negative production consequences associated with the resistance phenotype.

Addressing these issues will provide further impetus for the selection and use of resistant cattle at a time when better control methods for disease caused by *T. parva* are urgently required.

Acknowledgements

The series of field experiments at Ol Pejeta were only possible with the permission and extensive assistance of the Ol Pejeta management and staff, under the astute management of Giles Prettejohn. I should also like to acknowledge James Prendergast, who led the genetic analyses of the Ol Pejeta animals, and read the drafts of this chapter and provided critical insights.

References

Allison, A.C. (1954) Protection afforded by sickle-cell trait against subtertian malarial infection. *British Medical Journal* 1(4857), 290–294. DOI: 10.1136/bmj.1.4857.290.

Bakheit, M.A. and Latif, A.A. (2002) The innate resistance of Kenana cattle to tropical theileriosis (*Theileria annulata* infection) in the Sudan. *Annals of the New York Academy of Sciences* 969, 159–163. DOI: 10.1111/j.1749-6632.2002.tb04370.x.

Barnett, S.F. (1957) Theileriasis control. *Bulletin of Epizootic Diseases of Africa* 5, 343–357.

Barnett, S.F. and Bailey, K.P. (1955a) *A Field Survey of East Coast fever and calf mortality in an enzootic E.C.F. area*. East African Veterinary Research Organization Annual Report 1954-1955 incorporating Annual Reports 1952 & 1953. Nairobi: East Africa High Commission.

Barnett, S.F. and Bailey, K.P. (1955b) *The Susceptibility of zebu Calves to East Coast Fever under Experimental Conditions at Muguga*. East African Veterinary Research Organization Annual Report 1954-1955 incorporating Annual Reports 1952 & 1953. Nairobi: East Africa High Commission.

Barnett, S.F. (1968) Theileriasis. In: Weinman, D. and Ristic, M. (eds) *Infectious Blood Diseases of Man and Animals. Diseases Caused by Protista. Volume II. The Pathogens, the Infections, and the Consequences*. London: Academic Press, pp. 307–328.

Bronsvoort, B.M. de C., Thumbi, S.M., Poole, E.J., Kiara, H., Auguet, O.T. *et al.* (2013) Design and descriptive epidemiology of the Infectious Diseases of East African Livestock (IDEAL) project, a longitudinal calf cohort study in western Kenya. *BMC Veterinary Research* 9(1), 171. DOI: 10.1186/1746-6148-9-171.

Brown, W.C., Norimine, J., Knowles, D.P. and Goff, W.L. (2006) Immune control of *Babesia bovis* infection. *Veterinary Parasitology* 138(1–2), 75–87. DOI: 10.1016/j.vetpar.2006.01.041.

Conelly, W.T. (1998) Colonial era livestock development policy: Introduction of improved dairy cattle in high-potential farming areas of Kenya. *World Development* 26, 1733–1748.

Cunningham, M.P., Brown, C.G.D., Burridge, M.J., Morzaria, S.P. and Urquhart, G.M. (1989) *Theileria parva*: The immune status of calves born of dams immunised against East Coast fever. *Research in Veterinary Science* 46(1), 90–94. DOI: 10.1016/S0034-5288(18)31124-X.

Dolan, T.T., Njuguna, L.N. and Stagg, D.A. (1982) The response of *Bos taurus* and *Bos indicus* cattle types to inoculation of lymphoblastoid cell lines infected with *Theileria parva* schizonts. *Tropenmedizin Und Parasitologie* 33(1), 57–62.

Dyer, S.C., Austine-Orimoloye, O., Azov, A.G., Barba, M., Barnes, I. *et al.* (2025) Ensembl 2025. *Nucleic Acids Research* 53(D1), D948–D957. Available at: https://www.ensembl.org/Bos_taurus/Gene/Idhistory?g=ENSBTAG00000040380

Fumagalli, M., Sironi, M., Pozzoli, U., Ferrer-Admetlla, A., Pattini, L. *et al.* (2011) Signatures of environmental genetic adaptation pinpoint pathogens as the main selective pressure through human evolution. *PLoS Genetics* 7(11), e1002355. DOI: 10.1371/journal.pgen.1002355.

Glass, E.J., Preston, P.M., Springbett, A., Craigmile, S., Kirvar, E. *et al.* (2005) *Bos taurus* and *Bos indicus* (Sahiwal) calves respond differently to infection with *Theileria annulata* and produce markedly different levels of acute phase proteins. *International Journal for Parasitology* 35(3), 337–347. DOI: 10.1016/j.ijpara.2004.12.006.

Guilbride, P.D.L. and Opwata, B. (1963) Observations on the resistance of Jersey/Nganda calves to East Coast fever (*Theileria parva*). *Bulletin of Epizootic Diseases of Africa* 11, 289–298.

Hanotte, O. (2019) Why cattle matter: An enduring and essential bond. In: Dessie, T. and Mwai, O. (eds) *International Livestock Research Institute, the Rural Development Administration of the Republic of Korea and the African Union-InterAfrican Bureau for Animal Resources,* Nairobi. pp. 6–11.

Jenko, J., Gorjanc, G., Cleveland, M.A., Varshney, R.K., Whitelaw, C.B.A. *et al.* (2015) Potential of promotion of alleles by genome editing to improve quantitative traits in livestock breeding programs. *Genetics, Selection, Evolution* 47(1), 55. DOI: 10.1186/s12711-015-0135-3.

Klunk, J., Vilgalys, T.P., Demeure, C.E., Cheng, X., Shiratori, M. *et al.* (2022) Evolution of immune genes is associated with the black death. *Nature* 611(7935), 312–319. DOI: 10.1038/s41586-022-05349-x.

Koch, H.T., Kambeva, L., Norval, R.A., Ocama, J.G., Masaka, S. *et al.* (1990) Age resistance to *Theileria parva* bovis infection in calves. *Veterinary Parasitology* 37(3–4), 197–206. DOI: 10.1016/0304-4017(90)90003-t.

Küenzi, P., Schneider, P. and Dobbelaere, D.A.E. (2003) *Theileria parva*-transformed T cells show enhanced resistance to Fas/Fas ligand-induced apoptosis. *Journal of Immunology* 171(3), 1224–1231. DOI: 10.4049/jimmunol.171.3.1224.

Latré de Laté, P., Cook, E.A.J., Wragg, D., Poole, E.J., Ndambuki, G. *et al.* (2021) Inherited tolerance in cattle to the apicomplexan protozoan *Theileria parva* is associated with decreased proliferation of parasite-infected lymphocytes. *Frontiers in Cellular and Infection Microbiology* 11, 751671. DOI: 10.3389/fcimb.2021.751671.

Lederberg, J. (1999) J. B. S. Haldane (1949) on infectious disease and evolution. *Genetics* 153(1), 1–3. DOI: 10.1093/genetics/153.1.1.

Leitch, B.L. and Young, A.S. (1981) Theileria infections in *Rhipcephalus appendiculatus* ticks collected in the field. In: Irvin, A.D., Cunningham, M.P. and Young, A.S. (eds) *Current Topics in Veterinary Medicine and Animal Sciences. Advances in the Control of Theileriosis*, Vol. 14. The Netherlands: Martinus Nijhoff, The Hague, pp. 63–65.

Mahoney, D.F. (1977) Babesia of domestic animals. In: Kreier, J.P. (ed.) *Parasitic Protozoa*. Academic Press, New York, pp. 1–52.

Mettam, R.W.M. and Carmichael, J. (1936) Turning sickness, a protozoan encephalitis of cattle in Uganda: Its relationship with East Coast Fever. *Parasitology* 28(2), 254–283. DOI: 10.1017/S0031182000022447.

Miyunga, A.A., Karani, B.E., Njeru, R., Nangekhe, G., Cook, E.A.J. *et al.* (2026) Genotyping of an intensively monitored cohort of *Bos indicus* cattle in western Kenya for the FAF1B allele associated with resistance to East Coast fever (*Theileria parva* infection) with a real-time PCR assay. *Veterinary Parasitology: Regional Studies and Reports* 69, 101439.

Moll, G., Lohding, A. and Young, A.S. (1984) Epidemiology of theilerioses in the Trans-Mara Division, Kenya: Husbandry and disease background and preliminary investigations on theilerioses in calves. *Preventive Veterinary Medicine* 2(6), 801–831. DOI: 10.1016/0167-5877(84)90035-7.

Moll, G., Lohding, A., Young, A.S. and Leitch, B.L. (1986) Epidemiology of theileriosis in calves in an endemic area of Kenya. *Veterinary Parasitology* 19(3–4), 255–273. DOI: 10.1016/0304-4017(86)90073-7.

Muhammed, S.I., Lauerman, L.H. and Johnson, L.W. (1975) Effect of humoral antibodies on the course of *Theileria parva* infection (East Coast fever) of cattle. *American Journal of Veterinary Research* 36(4), 399–402.

Mwai, O., Hanotte, O., Kwon, Y.-J. and Cho, S. (2015) African indigenous cattle: Unique genetic resources in a rapidly changing world. *Asian-Australasian Journal of Animal Sciences* 28(7), 911–921. DOI: 10.5713/ajas.15.0002R.

Ndungu, S.G., Brown, C.G.D. and Dolan, T.T. (2005) *In vivo* comparison of susceptibility between *Bos indicus* and *Bos taurus* cattle types to *Theileria parva* infection. *The Onderstepoort Journal of Veterinary Research* 72(1), 13–22. DOI: 10.4102/ojvr.v72i1.220.

Nene, V. and Morrison, W.I. (2016) Approaches to vaccination against *Theileria parva* and *Theileria annulata*. *Parasite Immunology* 38(12), 724–734. DOI: 10.1111/pim.12388.

Norval, R.A.I., Perry, B.D. and Young, A.S. (1992) *The Epidemiology of Theileriosis in Africa*. Academic Press, London.

Paling, R.W., Mpangala, C., Luttikhuizen, B. and Sibomana, G. (1991) Exposure of Ankole and cross-bred cattle to theileriosis in Rwanda. *Tropical Animal Health and Production* 23(4), 203–214. DOI: 10.1007/BF02357101.

Roy, B.A. and Kirchner, J.W. (2000) Evolutionary dynamics of pathogen resistance and tolerance. *Evolution; International Journal of Organic Evolution* 54(1), 51–63. DOI: 10.1111/j.0014-3820.2000.tb00007.x.

Sitt, T., Poole, E.J., Ndambuki, G., Mwaura, S., Njoroge, T. *et al*. (2015) Exposure of vaccinated and naive cattle to natural challenge from buffalo-derived *Theileria parva*. *International Journal for Parasitology: Parasites and Wildlife* 4(2), 244–251. DOI: 10.1016/j.ijppaw.2015.04.006.

Stobbs, T.H. (1966) The introduction of Boran cattle into an E.C.F. endemic area. *East African Agricultural and Forestry Journal* 31(3), 298–304. DOI: 10.1080/00128325.1966.11662057.

Wilson, S.G. (1950) An experimental study of East Coast fever in Uganda. I. A study of the type of East Coast fever reactions produced when the number of infected ticks is controlled. *Parasitology* 40(3–4), 195–209. DOI: 10.1017/s0031182000018059.

Woolhouse, M.E.J., Thumbi, S.M., Jennings, A., Chase-Topping, M., Callaby, R. *et al*. (2015) Co-infections determine patterns of mortality in a population exposed to parasite infection. *Science Advances* 1(2), e1400026. DOI: 10.1126/sciadv.1400026.

Wragg, D., Cook, E.A.J., Latré de Laté, P., Sitt, T., Hemmink, J.D. *et al*. (2022) A locus conferring tolerance to *Theileria* infection in African cattle. *PLoS Genetics* 18(4), e1010099. DOI: 10.1371/journal.pgen.1010099.

Young, A.S. (1981) The epidemiology of theileriosis in east Africa. In: Irvin, A.D., Cunningham, M.P. and Young, A.S. (eds) *Advances in the Control of Theileriosis*. The Netherlands: Martinius Nijhoff, The Hague, pp. 38–55.

8 *Theileria* Diagnostics and Species Definition

Ronel Pienaar, Boitumelo B. Maboko and Ben J. Mans*
Epidemiology, Parasites and Vectors, Agricultural Research Council-Onderstepoort Veterinary Research, Onderstepoort, South Africa

8.1 Introduction

Diagnostics refers to the activities used to determine the cause of ill-health in animals or plants, and as a discipline has probably existed since the first diseases were recognized by mankind. Since then, ever more complicated and intricate means to diagnose diseases have been developed. Accurate diagnosis of a disease and its causative agents is essential for disease control and management. As such, diagnostics remain the bedrock of global disease management, and for veterinary diseases, general test procedures are prescribed by the World Organisation for Animal Health (WOAH), formerly known as the Office International des Epizooties (OIE) (WOAH, 2023b).

Diagnostic tests are used both for diagnosing infection or disease in individual animals and for surveying herds to determine the distribution and prevalence of infection at the population level. Different levels of sensitivity and specificity of individual assays are required, depending on the purpose of the diagnosis.

This chapter reviews the development and application of diagnostic assays to detect infection with *T. parva*. Diagnosis of disease caused by *T. parva* is an excellent example of diagnostic assay development because, from the initial identification of *T. parva* as the causal agent in 1902, the methods used to diagnose the disease include most of the trends in diagnostics development since the turn of the last century (Fig. 8.1).

The first section of this chapter deals with clinical diagnosis, that is, determining the cause of illness in individual animals or of outbreaks affecting a herd to facilitate management of the disease. The second section comprises a description of methods used predominantly in epidemiological studies, which are used mainly as research and policy tools. The final section examines attempts to define theilerial species and characterize strains within species, and to develop species-specific assays. This is of particular concern for theilerial infections as the bovid hosts can be infected concurrently with pathogenic as well as benign species of *Theileria* that cause no clinical signs. The current understanding of speciation of *Theileria*, including some of the conundrums with discovered/described species in the *Theileria* genus, is discussed.

8.2 Clinical Diagnosis

As discussed elsewhere (see Chapters 5 and 6 of this volume), infection of cattle with *T. parva* can present as three main clinical entities:

*Corresponding author: MansB@arc.agric.za

DOI: 10.1079/9781800626324.0008

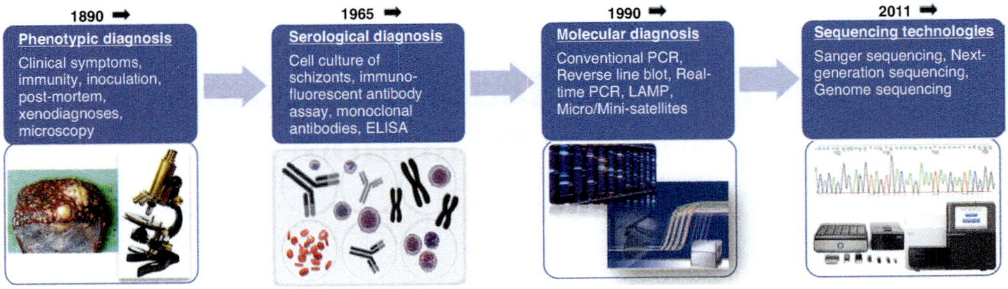

Fig. 8.1. General trends in diagnostics since the formal recognition of East Coast fever in 1902. The major phases of diagnostic methodology and their corresponding dates of origin are shown.

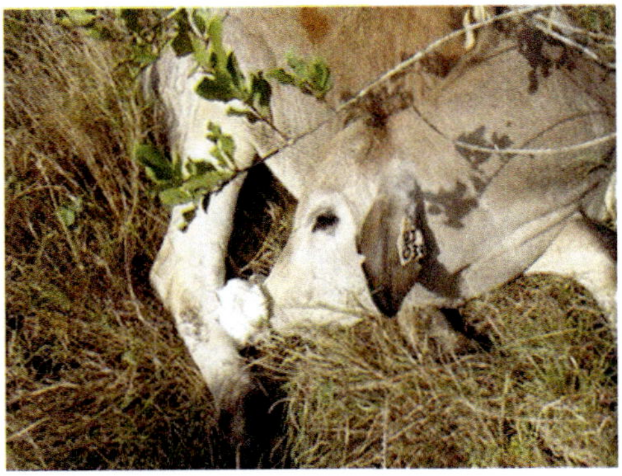

Fig. 8.2. Frothy exudate observed in a calf succumbing to *T. parva* infection. (Photo credit P. Toye.)

- classical East Coast fever (ECF) caused by *T. parva* transmitted from other cattle;
- Corridor disease (CD) caused by infection with *T. parva* transmitted from buffalo; and
- January disease, a mild form of ECF found predominantly in Zimbabwe.

8.2.1 Field observations and post-mortem signs

The initial confusion and delay in recognizing ECF as a distinct disease at the time of the southern African epidemic (see Chapters 1 and 6 of this volume) was a consequence of some of the signs associated with ECF being shared with other diseases. These have been described at length in other places (e.g. Irvin and Mwamachi, 1983). Here we summarize only the commonly occurring key signs that are most particular to *T. parva* infection that can aid specific diagnosis, noting that a history of the disease in the area will underpin diagnosis.

The initial sign is enlargement of the parotid and prescapular lymph nodes, which drain the preferred site of tick attachment in the ear. Development of fever, which occurs concurrently, can be quite marked compared to other diseases and often exceeds 41°C. Several days later, affected animals develop an increased respiratory rate, leading to a phase of respiratory distress, with nasal discharge in the later stages of the disease. A reversible, corneal opacity due to invasion of infected lymphocytes may also be observed in CD. In the terminal stages, body temperature can drop rapidly and a severe pan-leukopenia is observed.

A telling sign observed immediately after death is the presence of a frothy, sometimes bloody, exudate issuing from the nostrils. A marked example of this is shown in Fig. 8.2. Upon dissection, the pleural cavity contains straw-coloured fluid, and the lungs contain copious oedema fluid. The draining lymph nodes appear enlarged, haemorrhagic and oedematous.

The signs mentioned above are those most indicative of ECF and CD. The reader is referred elsewhere for a more complete account of the clinical signs associated with *T. parva* infection (Irvin and Mwamachi, 1983).

8.2.2 Light microscopy

The first laboratory tool employed to aid in the diagnosis of *T. parva* infection was light

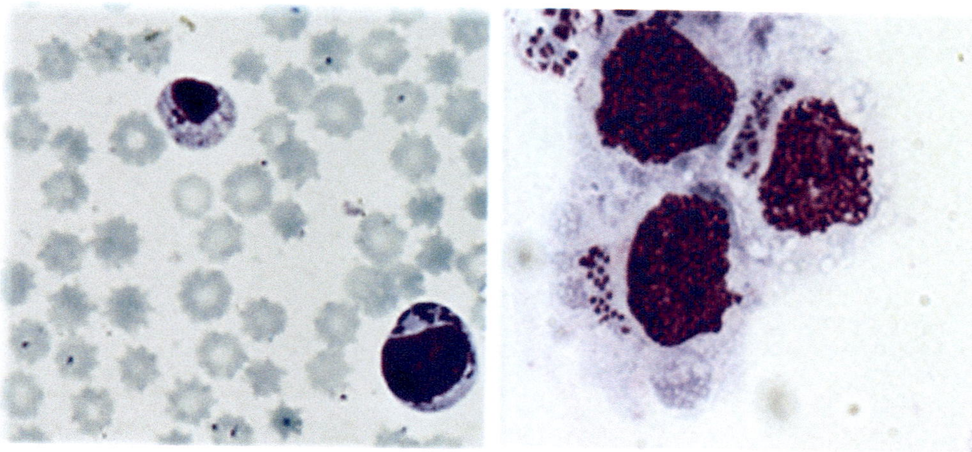

Fig. 8.3. Schizonts in lymphocytes on a blood smear (left) and in tissue culture (right). (Photo credit ARC slide archive.)

microscopy. By 1902, the use of blood smears and light microscopy was an accepted practice to confirm disease diagnosis (Gray and Robertson, 1902). Following the observation of intracellular blue bodies in lymphoid tissues (schizonts) by Koch in 1903 (Fig. 8.3; Chapter 1 of this volume), microscopic examination of smears of lymph node cells was used to confirm diagnosis. It is unlikely that Giemsa stain (azure-methylene blue; Giemsa, 1902) was implemented before this time, but both Koch (1903) and Theiler (1904) report the use of Giemsa stain in the early stages of the southern African epidemic.

Light microscopy is routinely used to detect either the macroschizont stage, usually in lymph node needle aspirates or post-mortem impression smears, or the piroplasm in thin blood smears (Diesel and Van Drimmelen, 1948). Apart from *T. velifera* piroplasms, it is impossible to distinguish among the cattle-borne *Theileria* species by morphology alone. An additional drawback of microscopy is that piroplasms are usually not detectable in clinically normal carrier animals. Thus, the chief uses of light microscopy currently are: (i) as a relatively quick and economic way to support a diagnosis of ECF/CD based on clinical and field observations or post-mortem findings; (ii) as a means of distinguishing *Theileria* infections from other haemoprotozoan diseases (Fig. 8.4); and (iii) as a research tool in experimental studies to determine the kinetics of infection in relation to the development of disease or establishment of immunity (e.g. Latré de Laté *et al.*, 2021).

8.3 Assays Used in Epidemiological Studies

8.3.1 Serology

The development of antibody-detection methods ushered in a new era for *T. parva* diagnostics. The major application of serology is to monitor ongoing outbreaks and incursions into non-endemic regions, as well as in vaccination exercises, where it can be used to avoid immunization of already exposed animals and to assess seroconversion rates following vaccination. It is also a valuable experimental tool in efforts to prevent the inclusion of previously exposed animals in vaccination and other trials. Unfortunately, serological assays have limited use in detecting acute clinical cases as animals undergoing a fatal infection usually lack antibodies (Sitt *et al.*, 2015). This is due to the time required for antibodies to appear and the disruption of architecture of lymphoid tissues that occurs during severe infection.

Two serological methods, the immunofluorescent antibody test (IFAT) and enzyme-linked immunosorbent assay (ELISA), are widely used. The IFAT is currently recommended by WOAH as

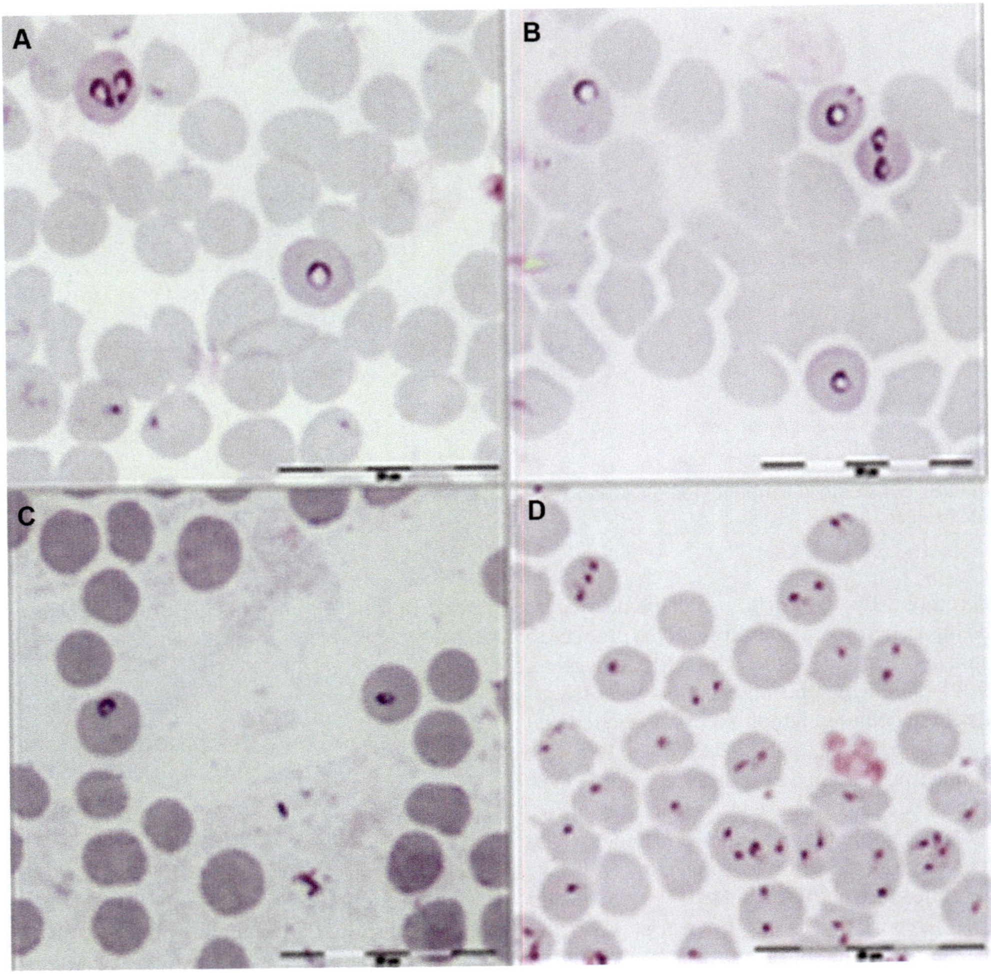

Fig. 8.4. Giemsa-stained blood smears of A: African redwater; B: Asiatic redwater; C: theileriosis caused by *Babesia bigemina*, *B. bovis* and *Theileria* parasites, respectively. As opposed to the larger paired and singular pear-shaped pyrosoma seen in babesiosis, ECF displays smaller parasites of different shapes (D). Scale 20 μm.

the gold standard diagnostic assay for detection of *T. parva* exposure in animals (WOAH, 2023a).

8.3.1.1 Immunofluorescent antibody test (IFAT)

The most commonly used format for the *T. parva* IFAT is an indirect Coon's method in which fluorescently labelled secondary antibodies detect primary host antibodies bound to piroplasms or schizonts fixed to slides (Fig. 8.5; Schindler and Mehlitz, 1965, 1969; Löhr and Ross, 1969; Burridge, 1971).

During its development, the IFAT was shown to be more sensitive than blood smear analysis to detect animals that had been infected with *T. parva* (Burridge, 1971), and schizont preparations were found to be better than piroplasms. A major advance that facilitated the use of IFAT was the ability to culture infected lymphocytes *in vitro* as continuously growing cell lines (Moulton *et al.*, 1971; Brown *et al.*, 1973; Malmquist and Brown, 1974). This provided a means of obtaining antigen easily and consistently for use in the IFAT.

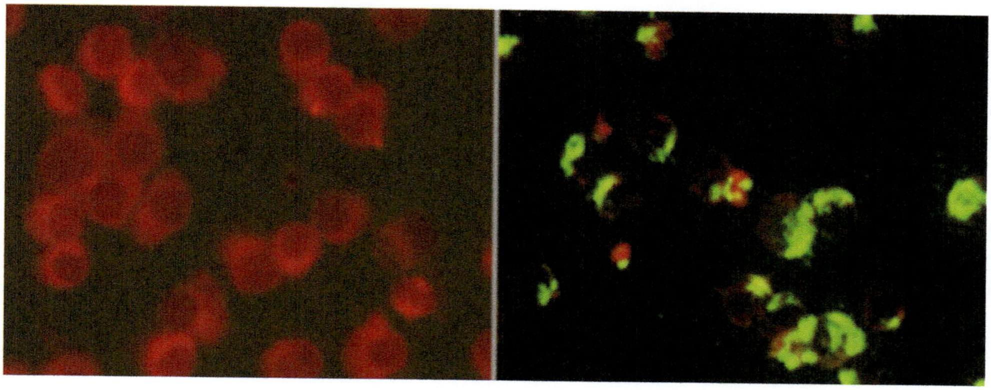

Fig. 8.5. A negative (left) and positive (right) reaction on the IFAT using *T. parva*-infected lymphocytes from *in vitro* culture. The positive reaction has strong fluorescence localized to the parasite schizonts in cultured cells.

In the early studies on IFAT, no difference in serological titres was observed between sera from animals exposed to cattle-derived and buffalo-derived parasites (Löhr and Ross, 1969), and a serological response was detected for 12–73 weeks (mean 29 weeks) after infection (Burridge and Kimber, 1973). However, the IFAT possesses inherent drawbacks. It displays significant cross-reactivity with closely related species, for example between *T. parva* and *T. taurotragi* and *T. parva* and *T.* sp. (buffalo) (De Vos and Roos, 1981a; Jongejan *et al.*, 1986; Conrad *et al.*, 1987; Pienaar *et al.*, 2014). As it is operator dependent with subjective interpretation of a fluorescent result, it is difficult to standardize and is a laborious process (Katende *et al.*, 1998). Nevertheless, IFAT is an economical and simple assay for use in epidemiological studies or, in the absence of species-specific molecular tests, to support clinical diagnosis (Thompson *et al.*, 2008; Mans *et al.*, 2011; Mbizeni *et al.*, 2013).

8.3.1.2 Enzyme-linked immunosorbent assay (ELISA)

Monoclonal antibodies generated against different stages of the parasite allowed the detection of specific antigens in sporozoite and schizont stages and were used to identify the genes coding for these proteins in recombinant expression libraries. These included the sporozoite antigen p67 (Musoke *et al.*, 1984; Nene *et al.*, 1992) and the sporozoite and schizont antigens p104 (Iams *et al.*, 1990; Huber *et al.*, 2018), the polymorphic immunodominant molecule (PIM; Shapiro *et al.*, 1987; Toye *et al.*, 1991, 1995b) and p150 (Skilton *et al.*, 1998). Analysis of 160 field sera from immune cattle indicated that these four proteins were the most immunogenic in *T. parva* and they were investigated for their potential for use in ELISA for diagnostic use (Katende *et al.*, 1998). The most immunogenic antigens in sporozoites were p67 and p104, while PIM was the most immunogenic in schizonts. PIM was shown to be recognized by all anti-schizont monoclonal antibodies for which the corresponding antigen was identified (Toye *et al.*, 1991). Antibodies to the PIM antigen were detected in 92% of 160 field samples tested, while responses to p150, p104 and p67 were detected in only 70%, 80 and 83%, respectively. PIM elicited a longer lasting immune response in experimentally infected cattle, being detectable 215 days after infection, compared to 60, 90 and 120 days for p67, p150 and p104, respectively. In addition, the PIM ELISA was compared to the gold standard schizont IFAT and shown to be more sensitive and able to detect a wide array of *T. parva* strains. Antibody responses to PIM were also shown to persist for at least 9 months within an endemic setting (Katende *et al.*, 1998). Analytical sensitivity, determined using 12 experimentally infected animals, was reported to be > 99%. However, based on current WOAH standards (WOAH, 2023a), this number of animals is too low to derive accurate estimates for sensitivity and specificity.

Diagnostic specificity was determined using 721 sera from a non-endemic region where animals were exposed to *Anaplasma marginale*, *Babesia bigemina* and *T. taurotragi*, and resulted in a specificity of 98%. In addition, sera of animals known to be infected with *B. bigemina*, *B. bovis*, *T. buffeli*, *T. annulata*, *T. mutans*, *T. taurotragi*, *Trypanosoma brucei*, *T. congolense* and *T. vivax* did not give titres above the cutoff (Katende *et al.*, 1998). As mentioned above, antibody responses to PIM are rarely detected in animals that die of ECF or CD (Kiara *et al.*, 2014; Sitt *et al.*, 2015), and the current serological assays are of no value in establishing *T. parva* as a cause of death.

The PIM ELISA was subsequently made available as a diagnostic ELISA kit using a monoclonal antibody raised against cattle IgG as secondary conjugate. Due to the failure of this antibody to recognize buffalo immunoglobulins, the test did not work for African buffalo. It was modified using a polyclonal anti-cattle IgG, which cross-reacts with buffalo Ig (B.J. Mans, South Africa, personal observation). The commercial test kits have been discontinued due primarily to lack of demand, given the unsuitability of serology to detect clinical cases (P. Toye, Nairobi, personal communication), and a perceived incomplete specificity (OIE, 2014). Despite the discontinuation of the commercial kit, it remains a widely used method to detect seropositivity for *T. parva* (Gitau *et al.*, 2000; Kivaria *et al.*, 2004, 2012; Rubaire-Akiiki *et al.*, 2006; Swai *et al.*, 2007; Bazarusanga *et al.*, 2008; Salih *et al.*, 2008, 2010; Gachohi *et al.*, 2010, 2011; Marcellino *et al.*, 2012, 2017; Wesonga *et al.*, 2015; Kimaro *et al.*, 2017; Silatsa *et al.*, 2020).

With regard to specificity of the PIM ELISA, there has been no published study documenting the low specificity. It is not clear how widespread the problem is nor which organisms affect the specificity of the ELISA, although *T. sp.* (buffalo) is a candidate. Cross-reactivity of monoclonal antibodies raised against *T. parva* PIM with *T.* sp. (buffalo) has been shown to occur due to the similarity with a PIM orthologue in the latter parasite (Bishop *et al.*, 2015; Kanduma *et al.*, 2016; B.J. Mans, South Africa, personal observation). Infection of cattle with *T.* sp. (buffalo) sometimes occurs in *T. parva*-endemic regions where cattle come into contact with buffalo, although this usually occurs as co-infection with buffalo *T. parva* (Bishop *et al.*, 2015; Pienaar *et al.*, 2020b). Nevertheless, exposure to *T.* sp. (buffalo) alone could result in false seropositivity for *T. parva*. Since PIM is the major immunodominant antigen in schizonts, it implies that the schizont IFAT would present similar drawbacks in specificity.

Assays based on the PIM antigen possess a major advantage in being able to detect a wide array of field strains, but there is the potential of a small number of false positive results. PIM possesses a central polymorphic region flanked by conserved regions and shows variation in size and antibody epitope expression due to the hypervariability of the central region (Toye *et al.*, 1991, 1995b, 1996). It has been suggested that the conserved flanking regions are responsible for the high sensitivity of the ELISA (Katende *et al.*, 1998). However, the central region is of low complexity, rich in repeats, especially of glutamic acid, glutamine and proline (Toye *et al.*, 1995b; Geysen *et al.*, 2004). Given this low complexity, it is likely that this region induces antibodies that cross-react with other organisms, resulting in the incomplete specificity of the ELISA. For example, the two monoclonal antibodies (numbers 10 and 12) that cross-react with *T. sp.* (buffalo) target epitopes in this central region (Bishop *et al.*, 2015).

Given the dominance of antibody responses to the four major *T. parva* antigens discussed above, it is unlikely that a new antigen will be identified that surpasses their sensitivity. Further investigation to determine conclusively the extent and nature of potential cross-reactivity of antibodies reactive with these four antigens is required to explore how the diagnostic assays can be improved. In the case of the PIM antigen, further research is required to determine the presence and extent of cross-reactivity with other *Theileria* species and to define the antigenic regions responsible for cross-reactivity. One potential approach might be to use components of more than one antigen to improve the sensitivity of the assay.

8.3.2 DNA-based assays

The introduction of molecular technologies in the early 1990s presented new opportunities in *T. parva* diagnostics through the targeting of nucleic acid sequences using a large array of techniques and approaches, almost all of which are based on the polymerase chain reaction (PCR). An in-depth discussion on molecular diagnostics, specifically related to the Piroplasmida, has been given elsewhere (Mans, 2022), but some of the methodologies and target genes employed for *T. parva* will be highlighted here.

8.3.2.1 PCR assays for the Tpr1, *p67 and p104 genes*

Initial attempts to develop PCR assays for diagnostic purposes focused on genes for which full-length nucleotide sequences were available at the time, namely *Tpr1*, p67 and p104. The *Tpr1* gene is present within a repetitive region (Tpr) in the genome (Conrad *et al.*, 1987; Allsopp and Allsopp, 1988), which comprises a tandemly repeated array of open reading frames, the encoded products of which are of unknown function (Baylis *et al.*, 1991). The p67 antigen is a sporozoite surface protein involved in attachment to and invasion of host lymphocytes by the sporozoite stage of the parasite (Musoke *et al.*, 1984). The p104 protein was initially identified as an antigen in sporozoites recognized by antibodies (Iams *et al.*, 1990) and subsequently also shown to be expressed in schizonts (Huber *et al.*, 2018). PCR assays were developed for *Tpr1* and p67 (Bishop *et al.*, 1992) and shown to detect carrier animals with low parasitaemia, as well as those undergoing acute infections. However, the *Tpr1* assay failed to detect all strains (Bishop *et al.*, 1992; Pienaar *et al.*, 2011b; Pienaar *et al.*, 2013), most likely because of sequence polymorphism.

A conventional PCR test was developed using p104 to investigate the carrier state in immune animals (Skilton *et al.*, 2002). Specificity was assessed using DNA from *T. annulata*, *T. buffeli*, *T. lestoquardi*, *T. mutans* and *T. taurotragi*. Sensitivity was shown to be ~1–2 parasites/μl of infected blood. To improve sensitivity, Odongo *et al.* (2010) developed a nested PCR and compared it to the original conventional p104 PCR and the reverse line blot (see below). The analytical sensitivities were shown to be 9.2×10^{-6}%, 2.8×10^{-5}% and 8.3×10^{-5}%, respectively. In a field population of carrier animals, the conventional PCR detected a prevalence of 37.7%, while the prevalence using the nested PCR was 42.3%, effectively four extra animals out of 151 sampled. The attractiveness of the p104 gene lies in its low level of polymorphism in *T. parva* (Morrison *et al.*, 2021) and its relatively low level of sequence identity with orthologues in other *Theileria* species (e.g. 42% with *T. annulata*; Huber *et al.*, 2018).

In a subsequent comparison of real-time PCR assays based on the three genes, the *Tpr1* assay detected the fewest positives (87%) compared to assays with p67N (N-terminus primer) (95%), p67C (C-terminus primer) (92%) and p104 (98%) (Pienaar *et al.*, 2013).

8.3.2.2 Real-time PCR assays for the 18S ribosomal RNA gene

The 18S ribosomal RNA gene is considered to be highly conserved among members of the same species but distinct between species (Eickbush and Eickbush, 2007). In the case of *T. parva*, two identical copies exist in the genome (Gardner *et al.*, 2005). Two real-time PCR assays that target the 18S ribosomal RNA gene of *T. parva* have been developed (Sibeko *et al.*, 2008; Papli *et al.*, 2011). The first test was a hybridization assay that used a *T. parva*-specific forward primer and a *Theileria* genus-specific reverse primer to amplify a 167 bp product (Sibeko *et al.*, 2008). The assay employed two hybridization probe pairs, one targeting the V4 hypervariable region with anchor and sensor probes specific for *T. parva* (detected at an emission wavelength of 640 nm), while the other anchor and sensor probe pair targeted the conserved region for the *Theileria* genus (detected at an emission wavelength of 705 nm). For *T. parva* positive samples, this resulted in two amplification and melting curves, one for *T. parva* at 640 nm and one for the *Theileria* genus at 705 nm. Both melting peaks gave an optimum melting temperature (Tm) of about 63°C (Fig. 8.6). The detection limit of the test at 80% sensitivity was 3.87 parasites or a parasitaemia of 9×10^{-6}%, comparing well with the p104 PCR assay (Odongo *et al.*, 2009).

The second test was a Taqman assay that used universal *Theileria* primers for amplification and a *T. parva*-specific probe (Papli *et al.*, 2011). The sensitivity at 100% detection limit was 3.5 parasites or 2×10^{-6}% parasitaemia.

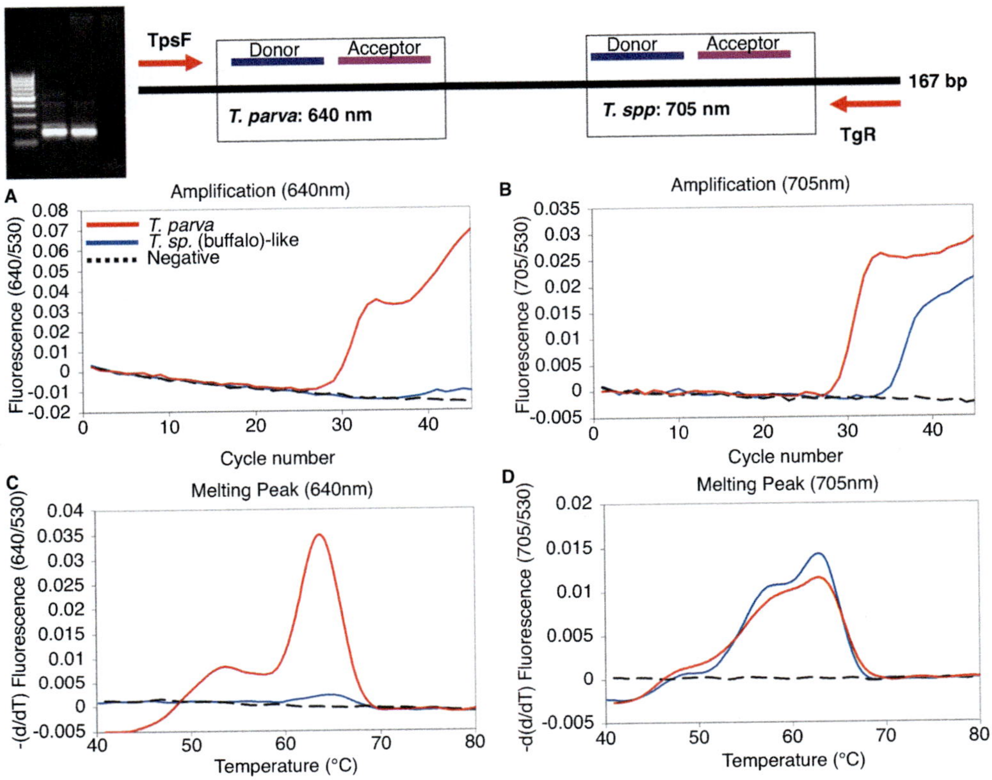

Fig. 8.6. The real-time hybridization assay for *Theileria parva*. Indicated is an insert of an agarose gel of the PCR products obtained using the real-time assay. Samples on the gel include a *T. parva* (Tp) positive sample, a *T. sp.* (buffalo) (TspB)-positive sample and a negative control. Also indicated is a diagrammatic representation of the PCR with *T. parva*-specific forward (TpsF) and *Theileria* genus-specific reverse (TgR) primers indicated, as well as the probe acceptor pairs for the *T. parva*-specific probe (640 nm) and the *Theileria* genus-specific probe (705 nm). At the bottom, typical PCR results are indicated with amplification curves for the 640 nm probe in panel A, amplification curves for the 705 nm probe in panel B, melting curves for the 640 nm probe in panel C and melting curves for the 705 nm probe in panel D.

During the validation phase of the hybridization assay, it was determined that the primers also amplified *T.* sp. (buffalo) and *T.* sp. (bougasvlei) (Sibeko *et al.*, 2008; Pienaar *et al.*, 2011b). This resulted in samples that were negative for *T. parva* but positive for either of these genotypes, and produced an amplification curve and melting peak at 705 nm but low amplification and a small melting hump at 640 nm. It was also shown that, in the case of mixed infections of *T. parva* and *T.* sp. (buffalo), the latter may suppress the 640 nm amplification and melting peak signal when present at higher parasitaemia, due to PCR template competition (Pienaar *et al.*, 2011b). Suppression of PCR signal due to template competition was also observed for the Taqman PCR since it used universal *Theileria* primers (R. Pienaar, South Africa, personal communication). This made interpretation of field samples quite difficult for both assays and led to the development of a new test based on the 18S ribosomal RNA gene, called the Hybrid II assay (Pienaar *et al.*, 2011a). The Hybrid II assay uses a *Theileria* genus-specific forward primer and a *T. parva*-specific reverse primer with the same 640 nm anchor and sensor probe pair used in the hybridization assay. This primer combination allows specific amplification of a 145 bp *T. parva* template in the presence of an excess *T.* sp. (buffalo)

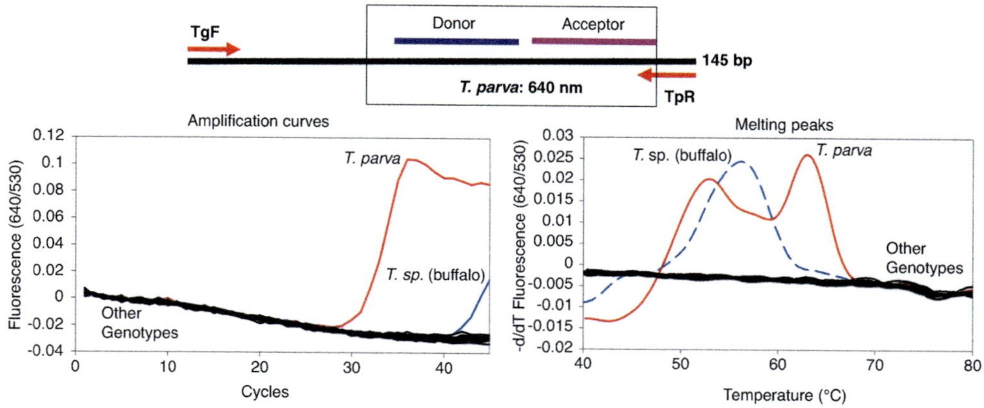

Fig. 8.7. The real-time Hybrid II assay for *Theileria parva* (in red). Indicated is a diagrammatic representation of the PCR with the *Theileria* genus-specific forward (TgF) and *T. parva*-specific reverse (*TpR*) primers indicated, as well as the probe acceptor pairs for the *T. parva*-specific probe (640 nm). At bottom left, amplification curves for the 640 nm probe, and at bottom right, melting curves for the 640 nm probe. Note that samples containing *T.* sp. (buffalo) (in blue), even at high parasitaemia as observed in the field, are not amplified below 40 cycles due to inefficiency of the PCR.

template without compromising sensitivity or signal strength, making the interpretation of the assay much simpler and reducing potential false negatives (Fig. 8.7). The sensitivity of the test is similar to the hybridization assay at 2×10^{-6}% parasitaemia. In a comparison with the assays targeting genes encoding the p67N, p67C, p104 and *Tpr1* proteins, the Hybrid II assay was more sensitive (Pienaar *et al.*, 2013) and remains the test of choice when screening African buffalo for *T. parva* infection. The Hybrid II assay is the current gold standard accredited assay used for *T. parva* diagnostics in South Africa.

8.3.2.3 LAMP assays for the PIM and p150 genes

Loop-mediated isothermal amplification (LAMP) is a PCR technique that was developed to amplify DNA under isothermal conditions. The resultant product can be detected using a variety of methods, such as colorimetry, fluorescence and turbidity, allowing its use under field conditions (Notomi *et al.*, 2000). For *T. parva*, the PIM and p150 genes were targeted for development of LAMP assays (Thekisoe *et al.*, 2010). The assays could detect *T. parva* in as little as 100 fg schizont-infected lymphocyte genomic DNA. The assays showed 100% sensitivity in detecting *T. parva* in 90 carrier buffaloes. While the study reported targeting of the p150 gene, it actually targeted the adjacent S5 ribosomal gene and not the reported p150 gene (B.J. Mans, South Africa, personal communication). Benchmarking studies of 210 gold standard positive *T. parva* samples showed that the PIM and p150 LAMP assays only detected 40–50% of positives compared to the real-time hybridization assays (R. Pienaar, South Africa, personal communication). The low performance was probably due to sequence variation. Only two LAMP assays have been developed for the detection of *T. parva* DNA to date.

8.3.3 DNA-based assays used to detect multiple *Theileria* species

8.3.3.1 Reverse line blot (RLB)

Sequencing of the 18S ribosomal RNA gene from various *Theileria spp.* indicated that, while large portions of the gene are conserved between species, specific regions, such as the V4 hypervariable region, show interspecies differences (Allsopp *et al.*, 1993). These differences were exploited to develop the reverse line blot (RLB) method to simultaneously detect up to nine species within one assay (Gubbels *et al.*,

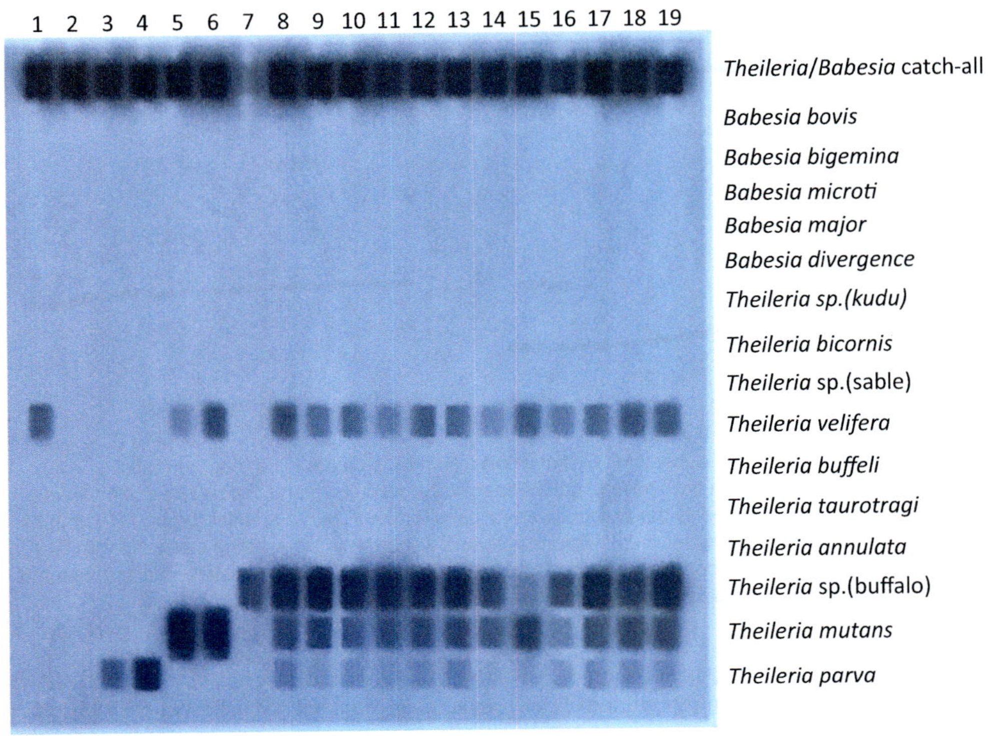

Fig. 8.8. An example of an RLB result after exposure of the membrane to radiographic film. Indicated at the top are samples 1–20 and, on the right, the various probes that were used in the blot. In this case, the blot represented buffalo sampled from the Kruger National Park, with the assays revealing preponderance of *T. mutans*, *T. parva*, *T. sp.* (buffalo) and *T. velifera*.

1999). The number of species that can be tested for has subsequently expanded over the years to include up to 28 species of *Theileria* and *Babesia* (Brothers *et al.*, 2011).

The RLB uses universal primers conserved within both *Babesia* and *Theileria* to amplify the V4 hypervariable region. PCR products are transferred onto a nitrocellulose membrane in a perpendicular array and biotinylated probes specific to the V4 hypervariable region of each species are hybridized. Visualization of a positive reaction is completed using streptavidin-labelled peroxidase and a suitable substrate that produces a chemiluminescent reaction detectable by radiographic film. Stringent washes in between steps ensure specificity. This results in an array of spots if the sample is positive for more than one species. A positive *Babesia* and *Theileria* probe that targets a conserved region is also included to enable detection of novel genotypes when none of the probes in the array hybridize with a sample (Fig. 8.8).

Detection of novel genotypes worked particularly well when vertebrates with unique piroplasm species were screened. Novel species were detected in giraffe, grey duiker, kudu, rhinoceros, and sable antelope (Nijhof *et al.*, 2003, 2005; Matjila *et al.*, 2008; Oosthuizen *et al.*, 2008, 2009; Bosman *et al.*, 2010). When animals possess mixed infections, detection of novel genotypes may be masked by the existing genotypes. As sequence diversity increased, it also became apparent that some of the probes were not genotype specific (Mans *et al.*, 2011). Comparison of the RLB with other single-gene PCR methods for *T. parva* indicated that it performed worse with regard to sensitivity (Odongo *et al.*, 2010; Pienaar *et al.*, 2011b, 2013; Silatsa *et al.*, 2020). This is mostly due to the use of universal primers that result in PCR template competition between genotypes. In a mixed infection, genotypes with higher parasitaemia can outcompete genotypes with lower parasitaemia. It became apparent that members of the *T. mutans*, *T. velifera* and *T. buffeli* clades were present at much higher parasitaemia than *T. parva* (Mans *et al.*, 2016). Prevalence of *T. parva* is, therefore, mostly underestimated when using RLB. The same argument may also hold for other genotypes, making the RLB a qualitative test that detects those genotypes with the highest parasitaemia in a sample. Even so, RLB has been used extensively to study the prevalence of *T. parva* and other *Theileria* in cattle and buffalo (Oura *et al.*, 2004; Salih *et al.*, 2007; Salih *et al.*, 2010; Yusufmia *et al.*, 2010; Chaisi *et al.*, 2011; Eygelaar *et al.*, 2015; Njiiri *et al.*, 2015; Tembo *et al.*, 2018; Silatsa *et al.*, 2020; Byaruhanga *et al.*, 2021).

8.3.3.2 Real-time PCR assay for the Cox III gene

A real-time PCR test that targets the Cox III gene was developed with the aim of differentiating all known bovine *Theileria* using universal primers, a conserved anchor probe and a sensor probe for which the probe region varies among different *Theileria* species (Chaisi *et al.*, 2013b). The variation in the sensor probe region resulted in unique Tm values. While this test had an interesting design, it will suffer the same limitations as the RLB due to the use of universal primers. In addition, the presence of mixed infections would likely make the number of melting peaks that can be attained so complex that interpretation of the data would not be trivial. Indeed, correlation between the Cox III and RLB assays was poor.

8.3.4 Assays to examine genotypic and antigenic diversity

8.3.4.1 Restriction fragment length polymorphisms (RFLP)

Early work aimed at identifying differences in *T. parva* isolates used non-specific approaches to detect differences in DNA sequences between parasite isolates. The RFLP assay involved restriction enzyme digestion of genomic DNA and detection of DNA fragments of the repetitive *Tpr* region in agarose electrophoresis gels by hybridization with a DNA probe (Conrad *et al.*, 1987; Allsopp and Allsopp, 1988). The repetitive *Tpr* restriction fragments were initially cloned, sequenced and used to design the probes used in the RFLP assays. Studies using the RFLP assay confirmed that there were genetic differences between strains that can be used to differentiate subpopulations within the *T. parva* population (Conrad *et al.*, 1987; Allsopp and Allsopp, 1988; Allsopp *et al.*, 1989).

Another assay, known as pulsed field gel electrophoresis (Morzaria *et al.*, 1990), aims to examine restriction fragment polymorphism of whole parasite DNA digested with different restriction enzymes. However, this assay is not suitable for routine diagnostic use and has been used principally as a specialist research tool. The results obtained indicated that the *T. parva* genome is composed of four chromosomes and confirmed that significant polymorphism exists between field strains of *T. parva* across all chromosomes.

8.3.4.2 Microsatellite and minisatellite polymorphisms

A shortcoming of the RFLP assay focused on *Tpr* is that it is restricted to analysis of a small region of the parasite genome. Satellite DNAs are short tandemly repeated segments (minisatellites 8–100 bp; microsatellites 2–6 bp) of DNA distributed throughout the genome, which show polymorphism in copy number and in nucleotide sequences. Two minisatellites were initially identified by Bishop *et al.* (1998), and subsequently Oura *et al.* (2003) identified a panel of minisatellites and microsatellites from the then recently completed *T. parva* genome sequence (Bishop *et al.*, 1998; Oura *et al.*, 2003). Oura and colleagues analysed laboratory isolates of *T. parva* and field populations of the parasite in Uganda, which provided information on genotypic diversity of *T. parva* and sub-structuring in parasite populations at local and larger scales (Oura *et al.*, 2005, Oura *et al.*, 2011a, 2011b; Asiimwe *et al.*, 2013). Their analyses also indicated that parasites at a local level are likely to undergo frequent genetic exchange (Oura *et al.*, 2005). The satellite panels have been used extensively in further studies to investigate diversity and sub-structuring in *T. parva* at local and larger-scale levels and include studies in Burundi (Atuhaire *et al.*, 2021), Kenya (Odongo *et al.*, 2006), Malawi (Chatanga *et al.*, 2020), Mozambique and South Africa (Lubembe *et al.*, 2020), Sudan (Salih *et al.*, 2018), Tanzania (Elisa *et al.*, 2015; Rukambile *et al.*, 2016), Uganda (Muwanika *et al.*, 2016) and Zambia (Muleya *et al.*, 2012). The majority of these studies indicate geographic sub-structuring of populations with limited gene flow between populations.

The satellite DNAs along with other markers have been used to construct a genetic map of *T. parva* in order to investigate sexual recombination during co-transmission of genotypically distinct strains of the parasite (Katzer *et al.*, 2007). Minisatellies and microsatellites were also used to examine genotypic diversity within the Muguga cocktail used for Infection and Treatment Method (ITM) vaccination (Patel *et al.*, 2011; Hemmink *et al.*, 2016). The data showed that, although there were several genotypes in the vaccine stabilates, there was relatively little allelic diversity (see Chapter 12 of this volume).

8.3.4.3 Monoclonal antibodies

Early studies to examine diversity in *T. parva* used monoclonal antibodies generated against schizont antigens. These antibodies frequently showed differential recognition of parasite isolates, which allowed differentiation among laboratory isolates, including those used in the ITM vaccine, and in some cases different clones of the same isolate (Pinder and Hewett, 1980; Minami *et al.*, 1983). More recent studies showed that many of these antibodies recognize the PIM antigen (Toye *et al.*, 1991). This line of work eventually resulted in comparison of cattle- and buffalo-derived strains using panels of the monoclonal antibodies, which revealed cross-reactivity of some of the antibodies, but differences in monoclonal antibody profiles between cattle- and buffalo-derived strains (Conrad *et al.*, 1986). It also confirmed that diverse *T. parva* populations exist within carrier animals (Morzaria *et al.*, 1995). A fuller account of the development and use of anti-*T. parva* monoclonal antibodies can be found in Toye *et al.* (2020). More recently, use of monoclonal antibodies has been superseded by antigen gene sequencing to investigate antigenic diversity.

8.3.4.4 Sequencing to examine antigenic diversity

Sequencing of genes encoding a number of antigens recognized by antibody- or T cell-mediated immune responses has been used to study genetic diversity in *T. parva* and as a means of identifying the antigenic differences that determine lack of cross-protection between some parasite strains. Sequencing of the PIM gene revealed extensive diversity in its central low complexity region, with variable indels in both sympatric and allopatric populations (Toye *et al.*, 1995a, b; Geysen *et al.*, 2004; Sibeko *et al.*, 2011). Sequencing of the p67 antigen gene, which has been explored for inducing immunity against the sporozoite stage of the parasite, has shown that the sequence of this gene is conserved in cattle-derived *T. parva* but shows variability in buffalo-derived isolates, with numerous alleles characterized to date (Sibeko *et al.*, 2010; Sitt *et al.*, 2019). The latter study examined parasites from cattle grazed on pasture that previously had only been grazed by buffalo and therefore the parasites were of buffalo origin. A series of antigens recognized by CD8 T cells from immune cattle have been identified (Graham *et al.*, 2006; Hemmink *et al.*, 2016). Sequencing of a subset of these antigens (Tp1, Tp2, Tp4, Tp5, Tp7, Tp8, Tp9, Tp10) in a small panel of parasites revealed that three of the antigen genes (Tp1, Tp2 and Tp9) show a particularly high level of polymorphism. CD8 T cells specific for these three antigens exhibit parasite strain specificity. Sequencing of the Tp1 and Tp2 genes in a series of parasites confirmed that the genes are highly polymorphic, but that only a small proportion of the alleles detected in buffalo are present in the cattle-derived isolates (Pelle *et al.*, 2011). This is consistent with other evidence that cattle *T. parva* comprise a subset of the buffalo population, which have adapted to cattle. A further study employed high-throughput sequencing to obtain sequences of PCR amplicons of six antigen-encoding genes (Tp1, Tp2, Tp4, Tp5, Tp6 and Tp10) from blood samples collected from small groups of buffalo in Kenya and South Africa (Hemmink *et al.*, 2018). The results revealed diversity in most of the antigen genes in both the Kenyan and the South African populations, with the Tp1 and Tp2 genes again exhibiting greatest diversity. Multiple alleles of the genes (up to 24) were detected in individual buffalo in both populations. Sequencing of these genes has been of value not only for studying the role of the antigens in immunity, but also in understanding the structure of *T. parva* populations. The Tp1, Tp2 and Tp9 genes are among the most polymorphic genes in the *T. parva* genome, and analysis of their sequences provides a rapid means of assessing genotypic diversity in a parasite population.

8.3.4.5 *Sequencing to examine species and genotypic diversity*

8.3.4.5.1 SEQUENCING THE 18S RIBOSOMAL RNA GENE. Sequencing of the 18S ribosomal RNA gene may be the most direct and unbiased way to gain insight into the genotypic diversity of the *Theileria* (Allsopp *et al.*, 1993) and has been used in a number of studies (Allsopp *et al.*, 1994; Chae *et al.*, 1999b; Chansiri *et al.*, 1999; Criado-Fornelio *et al.*, 2004; Reichard *et al.*, 2005; Criado *et al.*, 2006; Altay *et al.*, 2007; Bhoora *et al.*, 2009). However, most of these studies aimed to genotype specific isolates and did not address diversity in field samples. A systematic study using Sanger sequencing to uncover *Theileria* diversity targeted 111 buffalo and cattle samples, from which an 18S ribosomal RNA gene fragment was amplified and cloned and ten randomly selected clones from each sample were sequenced, generating about 1000 sequences (Mans *et al.*, 2011). This study uncovered single nucleotide polymorphisms (SNPs) in the V4 hypervariable region for *T. parva* that were confirmed by differences in the melting peak of the real-time PCR hybridization assay. The study showed that the cattle and buffalo harboured mixed infections and confirmed the major genotypes present in cattle and buffalo.

This work was followed up by a study employing, for the first time, next-generation sequencing to uncover *Theileria* diversity in southern Africa (Mans *et al.*, 2016). The study used Roche 454 technology to screen 1152 samples from buffalo and cattle, generating 825,711 sequences that could be assigned to genotypes. Roche 454 technology allowed amplification and sequencing of the 1100 bp fragment that covers the V4 hypervariable region. No new genotypes were uncovered, indicating that Sanger sequencing of about 10 clones may be enough to find the major genotypes within a sample. The study highlighted the promising prospect of incorporating high-throughput sequencing into routine diagnostic protocols. A subsequent study with amplicon sequencing using Illumina MiSeq technologies enabled the generation of millions of reads for analysis (Chaudhry *et al.*, 2019; Glidden *et al.*, 2020). RLB primers were used to amplify the V4 hypervariable region, after which a second round of PCR was performed to barcode the samples. Following validation of the assay using samples from Asiatic buffalo, cattle and sheep (Chaudhry *et al.*, 2019), it was used to examine samples collected from 66 African buffalo over a period of 16 months (Glidden *et al.*, 2020). Sequencing of 443 samples collected every 2–3 months yielded an estimated 69,407 reads per sample. The species composition and relative abundance of each genotype was very similar to that obtained previously for African buffalo (Mans *et al.*, 2011, 2016). The only differences were two unique genotypes grouping in the *T. mutans* and *T. velifera* clades. These were present at very low relative frequency in one or two of the animals sampled. Several other studies using high-throughput sequencing to examine *Theileria* diversity in wildlife and cattle have been published (Ghafar *et al.*, 2020; Pienaar *et al.*, 2020a; Squarre *et al.*, 2020), indicating that such approaches are likely to be applied more widely in the future.

8.3.4.5.2 WHOLE-GENOME SEQUENCING. The use of whole-genome sequencing for diagnostic purposes has not been implemented on a large scale. However, advances in this field promise to change the way that *T. parva* may be analysed in future, specifically to differentiate between strains and lineages within the species. The first *T. parva* genome to be published was the cattle-derived strain Muguga, which remains the reference genome (Gardner *et al.*, 2005). The next genomes for *T. parva* included the Marikebuni and Uganda strains and two offspring of these crossed with the Muguga strain obtained following tick pick-up of parasites from animals co-infected with two cloned parasites (Henson et al., 2012). This study confirmed recombination between the strains, with extensive crossovers in the genome. These genomes were all sequenced by extracting genomic material from piroplasms purified from blood, facilitated by the high piroplasm parasitaemia attainable by ECF strains. The next study, which used DNA prepared from schizonts purified from *T. parva*-infected cell lines, involved sequencing of nine *T. parva* strains, seven cattle-derived (Chitongo – Zambia, Katete – Zambia, Kiambu – Kenya, Mandali – Zambia, Entebbe – Uganda, Nyakizu – Rwanda and Katumba – Tanzania) and two buffalo-derived (LAWR – Kenya, Z5E5 –Zambia) (Hayashida *et al.*, 2013). The ECF strains were sourced over a large geographic region representing the natural distribution of *T. parva*. One of the main conclusions was that cattle-adapted ECF strains showed lower numbers of SNPs with respect to the Muguga reference strain (40,501 ± 7136) than buffalo-derived strains (112,713 ± 12,491). The implication is that buffalo strains show more genetic variation, fitting with an ancestral population, while cattle strains show less diversity due to adaptation of a subpopulation to cattle. This was supported by neighbour-net analysis that showed that ECF strains grouped into a tight clade. The next studies focused on the characterization of strains that comprise the Muguga cocktail version of the ITM vaccine (buffalo-derived Serengeti and cattle-derived Muguga and Kiambu) and showed that Serengeti and Muguga only show 420 SNPs, while Muguga and Kiambu show about 40,000 SNPs (the expected variation between ECF strains) (Norling *et al.*, 2015). The possibility that the Serengeti stock was contaminated in the past with Muguga was considered the most likely explanation for the high similarity between Serengeti and Muguga.

New developments in genome sequencing tried to circumvent the difficult process of purifying enough genomic material from schizonts for sequencing in the absence of contaminating host DNA. For this, bait capture methods were developed to allow specific pulldown of *T. parva* DNA from preparations of lysed *T. parva*-infected cells prior to Illumina sequencing (Palmateer *et al.*, 2020; Maboko *et al.*, 2021a). This approach allows sequencing of parasite genomic material directly extracted from infected cells without prior purification. Direct sampling from blood may also be possible with better advances in technology, which would enable routine sequencing of parasites directly from the field (Maboko *et al.*, 2021b). Although previous studies had provided evidence that buffalo *T. parva* in South Africa exhibit similar genotypic diversity to those in eastern Africa (Hemmink *et al.*, 2018), implying that *T. parva* was endemic in South African buffalo prior to the introduction of ECF in 1902, confirmatory evidence that this is the case was provided by a study involving genome sequencing of South African *T. parva* (Maboko *et al.*, 2021b). In this study, 12 buffalo-derived strains were sequenced; none grouped within the ECF clade but they showed an average SNP variation of 135,611 ± 43,377 compared to the Muguga reference strain. It may be noted that the estimated number of total SNPs is much higher than that of Hayashida *et al.* (2013). The study re-analysed the Hayashida dataset, and the numbers of SNPs obtained for ECF strains (14,093 ± 3121) and buffalo strains (41,350 ± 6407) were lower than in the original study, suggesting that *T. parva* in South African buffalo may contain greater diversity. The implication of this study and others is that future genome sequencing will allow the identification of genetic elements that clearly differentiate buffalo- and cattle-adapted strains and which can be incorporated into more routine laboratory assays. This approach may become a standard way of distinguishing strains in the future and may also allow differentiation of the parasites causing classic ECF and January disease.

8.4 *Theileria* Species that Infect Cattle and Buffalo

In addition to *T. parva*, several other *Theileria* species are known to infect cattle and/or African buffalo. Although the species that are present in Africa (apart from *T. parva*) do not usually cause clinical disease in cattle, their presence requires diagnostic assays that can distinguish them from *T. parva*. The discovery of the different *Theileria* species is discussed briefly in Chapter 1 of this volume. Since the different species are difficult to distinguish morphologically, assignment to species in early studies was based largely on biological properties of the parasites, including their mammalian host range, their tick vector species and their pathogenicity. Moreover, serological assays were not always reliable in distinguishing closely related species. The advent of molecular techniques has helped to clarify the relationship between the species and to correct earlier erroneous species assignments.

Phylogenetic analyses of the species that infect cattle and African buffalo, based on sequences of their 18S ribosomal RNA genes, distinguish four main clades, namely, *T. buffeli/orientalis*, *T. mutans*, *T. taurotragi* and *T. velifera* (Fig. 8.9; Mans *et al.*, 2011). The *T. taurotragi* clade includes *T. parva*, *T. annulata*, *T. lestoquardi* and *T. taurotragi*, as well as genotypes not yet assigned to a definitive species, namely *T.* sp. (buffalo) and *T.* sp. (bougasvlei). Parasites within the remaining three clades are currently each assigned to a single species, although each clade contains numerous distinct genotypes (Bishop *et al.*, 2004); further studies may eventually result in the identification of distinct species within these clades (discussed further below). It is evident that these clades do not share a monophyletic origin but share closer sister relationships with clades from other ruminants. Indeed, colonization of domestic animals by clade members may have occurred at different times in the past (Pienaar *et al.*, 2018).

8.4.1 The *T. taurotragi* clade

The parasites within this clade have been characterized in greater detail than those within the other clades, largely due to the strategic importance of *T. parva* and *T. annulata* as pathogens and consequently the much greater research effort they have received. The distribution of *T. parva* and its vectors are discussed in detail in Chapter 15 of this volume. *T. annulata* causes tropical theileriosis in cattle in countries around the Mediterranean, in the Middle East and in Asia. In Africa, its distribution extends into Sudan, which is the only country where the distribution of *T. parva* and *T. annulata* overlap. *T. lestoquardi*, which is genetically closely related to *T. annulata*, causes malignant ovine theileriosis in small ruminants, roughly in the same geographic region (Brown *et al.*, 1998). Both species are vectored by *Hyalomma* species of ticks. *T. taurotragi* causes bovine cerebral theileriosis (turning sickness) and, like *T. parva*, is transmitted by *R. appendiculatus* (De Vos and Roos, 1981a). While *T. parva* infects cattle and buffalo, *T. taurotragi* infects cattle and antelope species (Pienaar *et al.*, 2018). *T.* sp. (buffalo) and *T.* sp. (bougasvlei) have been shown to be genetically closely related to but distinct from *T. parva* and infect buffalo (Pienaar *et al.*, 2014). Their tick vectors have not been identified. No specific disease syndrome has been associated with these parasites, although co-infections with *T. parva* and *T.* sp. (buffalo) have been detected in cattle infected by transmission from buffalo (Bishop *et al.*, 2015). In common with other species within this clade, *T.* sp. (buffalo) has been shown to transform bovine lymphocytes *in vitro* (Zweygarth *et al.*, 2009; Bishop *et al.*, 2015).

8.4.2 The *T. buffeli/orientalis* clade

The parasites in this clade were initially assigned to a number of different species, including *Theileria buffeli* (Neveu-Lemaire, 1912), *Theileria orientalis* (Yakimoff and Soudatschenkoff, 1931), *Theileria sergenti* (Yakimoff and Dekhtereff, 1930) and *Theileria sinensis* (Bai *et al.*, 2002). However, based on morphology, pathology, serological cross-reactivity and transmission by *Haemaphysalis* species of ticks, this group was synonymized to one species, with *Theileria orientalis* initially designated as the species name (Uilenberg *et al.*, 1985), but other groups preferring *Theileria buffeli* (Stewart *et al.*, 1996; Gubbels *et al.*, 2000). Currently, about 13 genotypes are recognized in this clade (Mans *et al.*, 2015) based on the 18S ribosomal RNA gene sequences. Differences between genotypes range from 3 to 22 bp in the V4 hypervariable region of the gene (Mans *et al.*, 2016).

Most of these parasites are considered benign and are found across the globe. Some have been found to be restricted to cattle and some restricted to Asian or African buffalo (Mans *et al.*, 2016). So at least for some members in this clade there seems to be evidence of host specificity. Parasites of at least one genotype within this group are recognized as being pathogenic to cattle, namely the Ikeda genotype originally

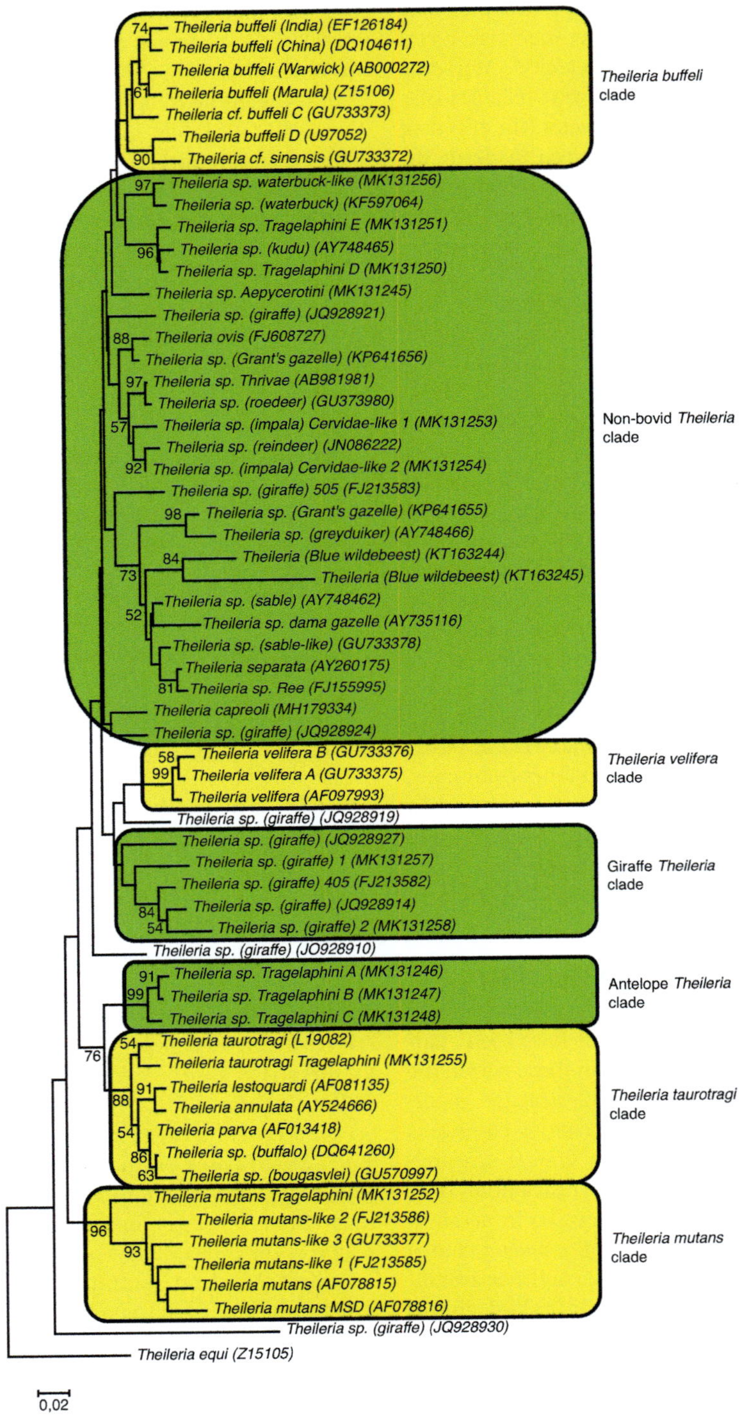

Fig. 8.9. A phylogenetic tree of the *Theileria*, based on 18S rRNA gene sequences. The major clades found in cattle and buffalo are boxed in yellow, while clades found in other ruminants are shaded in green.

isolated from Japan, when it was described as *T. sergenti* (Yakimoff and Dekhtereff, 1930). This genotype has caused considerable concern since it and its tick vector, *Haemaphysalis longicornis*, have been introduced to a number of countries where the parasite causes outbreaks of disease, including Australia (Izzo *et al.*, 2010), New Zealand (McFadden *et al.*, 2011, 2016), Pakistan, Vietnam (Gebrekidan *et al.*, 2017) and the USA (Beard *et al.*, 2018; Oakes *et al.*, 2019).

8.4.3 The *T. mutans* clade

The original description of *T. mutans* was that of a small piroplasm that can be transmitted by transfer of blood (Theiler, 1906). Although *T. mutans* has been reported in various countries, such as the UK (Brocklesby and Barnett, 1972; Morzaria *et al.*, 1974), Australia (Oteng, 1972) and Germany (Liebisch *et al.*, 1976), follow-up studies based on serological cross-reactivity indicated that these parasites are from the *T. orientalis*/*T. buffeli* group (Morzaria *et al.*, 1977; Uilenberg *et al.*, 1977; Joyner *et al.*, 1979) and that *T. mutans* is confined to Africa. Sequencing of the small-subunit ribosomal RNA gene confirmed that this was the case (Chae *et al.*, 1999a). *T. mutans* is transmitted by *Amblyomma hebraeum* and *A. variegatum* (Young *et al.*, 1978; De Vos and Roos, 1981b). Other reports that implicate *R. appendiculatus* and *R. evertsi* as vectors (Theiler, 1906) were shown to relate to transmission of *T. taurotragi* (De Vos and Roos, 1981a).

The *T. mutans* clade currently has six genotypes (Pienaar *et al.*, 2020b). Two genotypes have been found in cattle, *T. mutans* and *T. mutans* MSD (Theiler, 1906; De Vos and Roos, 1981b), while another three genotypes (mutans-1, mutans-2 and mutans-3) are limited to African buffalo (Mans *et al.*, 2011; Chaisi *et al.*, 2013a; Mans *et al.*, 2016) and a further genotype has been exclusively found in various African antelope species (Pienaar *et al.*, 2020b). Sequence differences between genotypes range from 9 to 20 bp in the V4 hypervariable region of the 18S ribosomal RNA gene (Mans *et al.*, 2016). Studies involving sequencing of the 18S ribosomal RNA gene and the use of *T. mutans* (Intona)-specific probes in the RLB (Gubbels *et al.*, 1999) have detected *T. mutans* in Angola (Sili *et al.*, 2021), Benin and Burkina Faso (Ouedraogo *et al.*, 2021), Botswana (Eygelaar *et al.*, 2015), Ethiopia (Hailemariam *et al.*, 2017), Kenya (Njiiri *et al.*, 2015), Mozambique (Martins *et al.*, 2010), South Africa (Yusufmia *et al.*, 2010), Southern Sudan (Salih *et al.*, 2007), Uganda (Oura *et al.*, 2004) and Zambia (Tembo *et al.*, 2018), indicating that at least some *T. mutans* genotypes probably occur over the distribution range of *A. variegatum* and *A. hebraeum*.

8.4.4 The *T. velifera* clade

Theileria velifera was differentiated from other *Theileria* by the presence of a veil associated with the piroplasm (Uilenberg, 1964). It was first described in cattle and buffalo (Uilenberg, 1964, 1970) but was recently also found in dogs (Salim *et al.*, 2019). It is transmitted by *Amblyomma* spp. (Uilenberg and Schreuder, 1976). To date, three genotypes have been described in this clade, namely *T. velifera*, *T. velifera* A and *T. velifera* B (Pienaar *et al.*, 2020b). Sequence differences between genotypes range from 3 to 9 bp in the V4 hypervariable region of the 18S ribosomal RNA gene (Mans *et al.*, 2016). Reverse line blot indicates the presence of this clade in Angola (Sili *et al.*, 2021), Benin and Burkina Faso (Ouedraogo *et al.*, 2021), Botswana (Eygelaar *et al.*, 2015), Ethiopia (Hailemariam *et al.*, 2017), Kenya (Njiiri *et al.*, 2015), Mozambique (Martins *et al.*, 2010), South Africa (Yusufmia *et al.*, 2010), Southern Sudan (Salih *et al.*, 2007), Uganda (Oura *et al.*, 2004) and Zambia (Tembo *et al.*, 2018).

8.4.5 Differentiation of *Theileria* species

As discussed above, differences in serological cross-reactivity and virulence are not always reliable parameters to define different species of *Theileria*. While the highly virulent nature of *T. parva* and *T. annulata* is a characteristic feature of these species, many other pathogens exhibit variation in virulence among strains. The definition of species has recently relied largely on genomic similarities and has focused on sequences of the18S ribosomal RNA gene as the most reliable marker. The sequences of the V4 variable region of this gene in buffalo and cattle *T. parva* and in the parasites that cause January disease are 100% identical (Allsopp *et al.*, 1993; Mans *et al.*, 2011). In addition, whole-genome comparisons of isolates from cattle and buffalo indicate that the overall sequence identity across the genomes is greater than 98% (Maboko *et al.*, 2021a). These properties indicate that these isolates all belong to the same species. Thus, there is no compelling reason to raise these entities to species level. However, it should be acknowledged that sub-structuring of species based on different biological properties, such as tick transmissibility of *T. parva* in cattle, may be appropriate.

By contrast, the genotypes within the *T. buffali/orientalis*, *T. mutans* and *T. velifera* clades exhibit significant differences in their ribosomal RNA gene sequences. The observed differences in the V4 hypervariable region of the gene among genotypes of the *T. orientalis*, *T.mutans* and *T. velifera* clades (3–22 bp, 9–20 bp, 3–9 bp, respectively) are comparable to some of the species differences (1–19 bp) observed in the *T. taurotragi* clade parasites. Moreover, available evidence indicates that some of the genotypes of *T. orientalis* and T. *mutans* infect different mammalian hosts. These features clearly suggest the existence of distinct species within these clades.

A key feature of apicomplexan parasites that defines species identity is their ability to undergo sexual recombination, which occurs for *Theileria* parasites during development in the tick vector. Recombination between genotypically distinct parasites clearly depends on the parasites infecting the same mammalian host and being transmissible by the same tick species. The parasites also need to possess a similar genome structure and synteny in gene order and content to facilitate genetic alignment that will allow recombination. Use of genome sequencing should help to clarify the existence of distinct species within the *T. buffeli/orientalis*, *T.mutans* and *T. velifera* clades. Following publication of the first *T. orientalis* genome sequence in 2012 (Hayashida *et al.*, 2012), comparison of genome sequence data was now possible for single isolates of three *T. orientalis* genotypes (Ikeda, Chitose and Buffeli), which revealed pairwise genetic identities ranging from 81.7 to 85.4% (Bogema *et al.*, 2018; Yam *et al.*, 2022). This compares with 79% pairwise identity observed between *T. annulata* and *T. parva*. These and other findings led Bogema *et al.* (2018) to suggest that the parasites represent distinct species. More extensive application of genome sequencing will be required to confirm these findings and to examine other genotypes within these clades. In the meantime, the current species names applied to these clades can continue to be used until distinct species can be identified unambiguously. In relation to diagnosis, current knowledge of the parasites and available technologies allow these other species of *Theileria* to be distinguished from *T. parva*.

8.5 Conclusions

Diagnosing *Theileria parva*, the causative agent of East Coast fever and Corridor disease in cattle, is crucial for both individual animal health and population-level disease management. Different diagnostic assays are recommended for different intended purposes, such as confirmation of clinical cases, investigation of suspected outbreaks, population freedom from infection, individual animal freedom from infection prior to movement, prevalence of infection (surveillance) or subpopulation examination. For most purposes, obtaining baseline data on prevalence of disease and the carrier state in both endemic and non-endemic regions is essential if proper disease control and diagnosis are to be managed. Passive surveillance programmes are essential to obtain this information to assess the likelihood of future outbreaks of disease. Such baseline data will assist in determining the suitability of various diagnostic techniques for the specific purposes.

8.5.1 Confirmation of clinical cases

In suspected cases of disease and in animals that have died, clinical signs or post-mortem pathology, respectively, are important for differential diagnosis. Microscopic examination of blood smears or organ impression smears will detect high levels of schizonts in lymph node cells and piroplasms in blood characteristic of East Coast fever; animals that die also usually show severe pulmonary oedema. In the case of Corridor disease, much lower levels of schizonts are observed, and usually there is no detectable piroplasm parasitaemia; such results may be confounded by *T. taurotragi* infection.

Serological tests are of no value for confirming diagnosis, as animals do not produce antibodies during the acute phase of infection. Such tests are valuable for estimating the prevalence of infection within a population over time. Molecular tests can be used, but positive results are not definitive, as animals in endemic areas suffering other diseases may also harbour *T. parva* carrier infections. Microscopic examination of smears of infected cells by immunofluorescence or immunocytochemistry using *T. parva*-specific antibody can be used to confirm diagnosis.

8.5.2 Population freedom from infection

Population freedom from infection depends on screening of sufficient numbers of animals to be certain in demonstrating absence of infection. Numbers depend on estimated disease prevalence in a region, population size and the desired level of confidence, as well as test sensitivity and specificity (WOAH, 2023b). Generally, multiple herds need to be screened over a period of time using tests with high sensitivity and specificity to support the claim of freedom from infection. Clearly, the absence of any previous cases of disease is essential. Microscopic examination of lymph node cells and blood for the presence of carrier infections is of limited use for this purpose due to poor sensitivity. Molecular and serological tests are more useful since they allow for carrier state detection as well as historical exposure to infection. Tests for population freedom require high sensitivity, while lower specificity would make the declaration of freedom much more stringent. Tests suitable for this would include the IFAT or PIM ELISA for serology since these are sensitive, while lower specificity would not compromise the declaration of freedom from infection. For molecular testing, the real-time Hybrid II PCR assay (Pienaar *et al.*, 2011a) or the nested p104 PCR assay (Odongo *et al.*, 2010) would be considered suitable since both present high sensitivity and specificity.

8.5.3 Individual animal freedom from infection prior to movement

To declare individual animals free of infection for movement purposes requires sensitive and specific diagnostic tests. Clinical signs and microscopic tests are of limited use for this purpose due to low sensitivity and specificity. Molecular tests are very sensitive and specific and allow for carrier state detection at low parasitaemia, even if antibody titres have waned. Serological tests are useful since they may indicate prior exposure even if the parasitaemia is below the detection limits of molecular tests. A combination of molecular and serological tests is preferred to cover various states of infection. The movement history of the animal, its origin and association with disease animals or regions are also important considerations, and any diagnostic test result should assess these factors before movement. Depending on country-specific regulations, animals may be placed under quarantine and monitored over time before being declared free of disease. Tests currently in use for individual freedom include the IFAT for serology and the real-time Hybrid II PCR assay (Pienaar *et al.*, 2011a) for molecular analysis.

8.5.4 Prevalence of infection

Surveillance of disease prevalence provides important baseline information to assess disease risk and support different intended purposes of testing. Sensitive and specific diagnostic methods are important for accurate estimation of prevalence. As such, molecular and serological methods will be preferred and, used in combination, can provide accurate estimates of prevalence and also serve to give insight into epidemiology of disease. Tests suitable for prevalence would include the IFAT or PIM ELISA for serology, or for molecular testing, the real-time Hybrid II PCR assay (Pienaar *et al.*, 2011a) or the nested p104 PCR assay (Odongo *et al.*, 2010).

8.5.5 Parasite subpopulation analysis

Differentiation of subpopulations can be important to track introduction of new disease strains into regions or understand the flow and distribution of parasites across a region. Methods that allow differentiation may not necessarily be useful for routine diagnostics but should be able to differentiate genetics at individual, population or regional level. As such, antibody panels can identify differences in antigenic profiles between populations. Microsatellites can differentiate alleles unique to individuals or populations. Whole-genome sequencing and SNP analysis may be able to differentiate individuals or populations.

Overall, a combination of diagnostic methods tailored to the specific situation and objectives is recommended for effective management and control of *Theileria parva* infection in cattle and buffalo populations. This approach ensures accurate diagnosis, timely intervention and informed decision making for disease control and prevention.

References

Allsopp, B.A. and Allsopp, M.T.E.P. (1988) *Theileria parva*: Genomic DNA studies reveal intraspecific sequence diversity. *Molecular and Biochemical Parasitology* 28(1), 77–83. DOI: 10.1016/0166-6851(88)90183-1.

Allsopp, B.A., Baylis, H.A., Allsopp, M.T., Cavalier-Smith, T., Bishop, R.P. *et al.* (1993) Discrimination between six species of *Theileria* using oligonucleotide probes which detect small subunit ribosomal RNA sequences. *Parasitology* 107(2), 157–165. DOI: 10.1017/s0031182000067263.

Allsopp, B., Carrington, M., Baylis, H., Sohal, S., Dolan, T. *et al.* (1989) Improved characterization of *Theileria parva* isolates using the polymerase chain reaction and oligonucleotide probes. *Molecular and Biochemical Parasitology* 35(2), 137–147. DOI: 10.1016/0166-6851(89)90116-3.

Allsopp, M.T., Cavalier-Smith, T., Waal, D.T. and Allsopp, B.A. (1994) Phylogeny and evolution of the piroplasms. *Parasitology* 108(2), 147–152. DOI: 10.1017/s0031182000068232.

Altay, K., Dumanli, N. and Aktas, M. (2007) Molecular identification, genetic diversity and distribution of *Theileria* and *Babesia* species infecting small ruminants. *Veterinary Parasitology* 147(1–2), 161–165. DOI: 10.1016/j.vetpar.2007.04.001.

Asiimwe, B.B., Weir, W., Tait, A., Lubega, G.W. and Oura, C.A.L. (2013) Haemoparasite infection kinetics and the population structure of *Theileria parva* on a single farm in Uganda. *Veterinary Parasitology* 193(1–3), 8–14. DOI: 10.1016/j.vetpar.2012.12.017.

Atuhaire, D.K., Muleya, W., Mbao, V., Niyongabo, J., Nyabongo, L. *et al.* (2021) Molecular characterization and population genetics of *Theileria parva* in Burundi's unvaccinated cattle: Towards the introduction of East Coast fever vaccine. *PloS One* 16(5), e0251500. DOI: 10.1371/journal.pone.0251500.

Bai, Q., Liu, G., Yin, H., Zhao, Q., Liu, D. *et al.* (2002) *Theileria sinensis* sp nov: A new species of bovine *Theileria*-classical taxonomic studies. *Acta Veterinaria et Zootechnica Sinica* 33, 73–77.

Baylis, H.A., Sohal, S.K., Carrington, M., Bishop, R.P. and Allsopp, B.A. (1991) An unusual repetitive gene family in *Theileria parva* which is stage-specifically transcribed. *Molecular and Biochemical Parasitology* 49(1), 133–142. DOI: 10.1016/0166-6851(91)90136-t.

Bazarusanga, T., Geysen, D., Vercruysse, J. and Marcotty, T. (2008) The sensitivity of PCR and serology in different *Theileria parva* epidemiological situations in Rwanda. *Veterinary Parasitology* 154(1–2), 21–31. DOI: 10.1016/j.vetpar.2008.02.017.

Beard, C.B., Occi, J., Bonilla, D.L., Egizi, A.M., Fonseca, D.M. *et al.* (2018) Multistate infestation with the exotic disease-vector tick *Haemaphysalis longicornis* – United States, August 2017–September 2018. *Morbidity and Mortality Weekly Report* 67(47), 1310–1313. DOI: 10.15585/mmwr.mm6747a3.

Bhoora, R., Franssen, L., Oosthuizen, M.C., Guthrie, A.J., Zweygarth, E. *et al.* (2009) Sequence heterogeneity in the 18S rRNA gene within *Theileria equi* and *Babesia caballi* from horses in South Africa. *Veterinary Parasitology* 159(2), 112–120. DOI: 10.1016/j.vetpar.2008.10.004.

Bishop, R., Sohanpal, B., Kariuki, D.P., Young, A.S., Nene, V. *et al.* (1992) Detection of a carrier state in *Theileria parva*-infected cattle by the polymerase chain reaction. *Parasitology* 104(Pt 2), 215–232. DOI: 10.1017/s0031182000061655.

Bishop, R., Morzaria, S. and Gobright, E. (1998) Linkage of two distinct AT-rich minisatellites AT multiple loci in the genome of *Theileria parva*. *Gene* 216, 245–254. DOI: 10.1016/s0378-1119(98)00336-9.

Bishop, R., Musoke, A., Morzaria, S., Gardner, M. and Nene, V. (2004) *Theileria*: Intracellular protozoan parasites of wild and domestic ruminants transmitted by ixodid ticks. *Parasitology* 129(S1), S271–S283. DOI: 10.1017/s0031182003004748.

Bishop, R.P., Hemmink, J.D., Morrison, W.I., Weir, W., Toye, P.G. *et al.* (2015) The African buffalo parasite *Theileria*. sp. (buffalo) can infect and immortalize cattle leukocytes and encodes divergent orthologues of *Theileria parva* antigen genes. *International Journal for Parasitology: Parasites and Wildlife* 4(3), 333–342. DOI: 10.1016/j.ijppaw.2015.08.006.

Bogema, D.R., Micallef, M.L., Liu, M., Padula, M.P., Djordjevic, S.P. *et al.* (2018) Analysis of *Theileria orientalis* draft genome sequences reveals potential species-level divergence of the Ikeda, Chitose and Buffeli genotypes. *BMC Genomics* 19(1), 298. DOI: 10.1186/s12864-018-4701-2.

Bosman, A.M., Oosthuizen, M.C., Peirce, M.A., Venter, E.H. and Penzhorn, B.L. (2010) *Babesia lengau* sp. nov., a novel *Babesia* species in cheetah (*Acinonyx jubatus*, Schreber, 1775) populations in South Africa. *Journal of Clinical Microbiology* 48(8), 2703–2708. DOI: 10.1128/JCM.02266-09.

Brocklesby, D.W. and Barnett, S.F. (1972) The tick *Haemaphysalis punctata*, shown to be a vector of *Theileria mutans* in Britain. *The Veterinary Record* 90(18), 512–513. DOI: 10.1136/vr.90.18.512.

Brothers, P.S., Collins, N.E., Oosthuizen, M.C., Bhoora, R., Troskie, M. *et al.* (2011) Occurrence of blood-borne tick-transmitted parasites in common tsessebe (*Damaliscus lunatus*) antelope in Northern Cape Province, South Africa. *Veterinary Parasitology* 183(1–2), 160–165. DOI: 10.1016/j.vetpar.2011.06.015.

Brown, C.G.D., Stagg, D.A., Purnell, R.E., Kanhai, G.K. and Payne, R.C. (1973) Infection and transformation of bovine lymphoid cells *in vitro* by infective particles of *Theileria parva*. *Nature* 245(5420), 101–103. DOI: 10.1038/245101a0.

Brown, C.G.D., Ilhan, T., Kirvar, E., Thomas, M., Wilkie, G. *et al.* (1998) *Theileria lestoquardi* and *T. annulata* in cattle, sheep, and goats. In: *In Vitro and in Vivo Studies. Annals of the New York Academy of Sciences*, Vol. 849. pp. 44–51. DOI: 10.1111/j.1749-6632.1998.tb11032.x.

Burridge, M.J. (1971) Application of the indirect fluorescent antibody test in experimental East Coast fever (*Theileria parva* infection of cattle). *Research in Veterinary Science* 12(4), 338–341. DOI: 10.1016/S0034-5288(18)34160-2.

Burridge, M.J. and Kimber, C.D. (1973) Duration of serological response to the indirect fluorescent antibody test of cattle recovered from *Theileria parva* infection. *Research in Veterinary Science* 14(2), 270–271. DOI: 10.1016/S0034-5288(18)33929-8.

Byaruhanga, C., Akure, P.C., Lubembe, D.M., Sibeko-Matjila, K., Troskie, M. *et al.* (2021) Molecular detection and characterisation of protozoan and rickettsial pathogens in ticks from cattle in the pastoral area of Karamoja, Uganda. *Ticks and Tick-Borne Diseases* 12(4), 101709. DOI: 10.1016/j.ttbdis.2021.101709.

Chae, J.S., Allsopp, B.A., Waghela, S.D., Park, J.H., Kakuda, T. *et al.* (1999a) A study of the systematics of *Theileria* spp. based upon small-subunit ribosomal RNA gene sequences. *Parasitology Research* 85(11), 877–883. DOI: 10.1007/s004360050651.

Chae, J.S., Waghela, S.D., Craig, T.M., Kocan, A.A., Wagner, G.G. *et al.* (1999b) Two *Theileria* cervi SSU rRNA gene sequence types found in isolates from white-tailed deer and elk in North America. *Journal of Wildlife Diseases* 35(3), 458–465. DOI: 10.7589/0090-3558-35.3.458.

Chaisi, M.E., Sibeko, K.P., Collins, N.E., Potgieter, F.T. and Oosthuizen, M.C. (2011) Identification of *Theileria parva* and *Theileria* sp. (buffalo) 18S rRNA gene sequence variants in the African buffalo (*Syncerus caffer*) in southern Africa. *Veterinary Parasitology* 182(2–4), 150–162. DOI: 10.1016/j.vetpar.2011.05.041.

Chaisi, M.E., Janssens, M.E., Vermeiren, L., Oosthuizen, M.C., Collins, N.E. *et al.* (2013a) Evaluation of a real-time PCR test for the detection and discrimination of *Theileria* species in the African buffalo (*Syncerus caffer*). *PloS ONE* 8(10), e75827. DOI: 10.1371/journal.pone.0075827.

Chaisi, M.E., Collins, N.E., Potgieter, F.T. and Oosthuizen, M.C. (2013b) Sequence variation identified in the 18S rRNA gene of *Theileria mutans* and *Theileria velifera* from the African buffalo (*Syncerus caffer*). *Veterinary Parasitology* 191(1–2), 132–137. DOI: 10.1016/j.vetpar.2012.08.005.

Chansiri, K., Kawazu, S., Kamio, T., Terada, Y., Fujisaki, K. *et al.* (1999) Molecular phylogenetic studies on *Theileria* parasites based on small subunit ribosomal RNA gene sequences. *Veterinary Parasitology* 83(2), 99–105. DOI: 10.1016/s0304-4017(99)00052-7.

Chatanga, E., Hayashida, K., Muleya, W., Kusakisako, K., Moustafa, M.A.M. *et al.* (2020) Genetic diversity and sequence polymorphism of two genes encoding *Theileria parva* antigens recognized by CD8+ T cells among vaccinated and unvaccinated cattle in Malawi. *Pathogens* 9(5), 334. DOI: 10.3390/pathogens9050334.

Chaudhry, U., Ali, Q., Rashid, I., Shabbir, M.Z., Ijaz, M. *et al.* (2019) Development of a deep amplicon sequencing method to determine the species composition of piroplasm haemoprotozoa. *Ticks and Tick-Borne Diseases* 10(6), 101276. DOI: 10.1016/j.ttbdis.2019.101276.

Conrad, P.A., Denham, D. and Brown, C.G.D. (1986) Intraerythrocytic multiplication of *Theileria parva in vitro*: An ultrastructural study. *International Journal for Parasitology* 16(3), 223–229. DOI: 10.1016/0020-7519(86)90047-0.

Conrad, P.A., Stagg, D.A., Grootenhuis, J.G., Irvin, A.D., Newson, J. *et al.* (1987) Isolation of *Theileria parasites* from African buffalo (*Syncerus caffer*) and characterization with anti-schizont monoclonal antibodies. *Parasitology* 94(3), 413–423. DOI: 10.1017/s0031182000055761.

Criado, A., Martinez, J., Buling, A., Barba, J.C., Merino, S. *et al.* (2006) New data on epizootiology and genetics of piroplasms based on sequences of small ribosomal subunit and cytochrome *b* genes. *Veterinary Parasitology* 142(3–4), 238–247. DOI: 10.1016/j.vetpar.2006.07.004.

Criado-Fornelio, A., Gónzalez-del-Río, M.A., Buling-Saraña, A. and Barba-Carretero, J.C. (2004) The "expanding universe" of piroplasms. *Veterinary Parasitology* 119(4), 337–345. DOI: 10.1016/j.vetpar.2003.11.015.

De Vos, A.J. and Roos, J.A. (1981a) The isolation of *Theileria*? *taurotragi* in South Africa. *The Onderstepoort Journal of Veterinary Research* 48(3), 149–153.

De Vos, A.J. and Roos, J.A. (1981b) Observations on the transmission of *Theileria mutans* in South Africa. *The Onderstepoort Journal of Veterinary Research* 48(1), 1–6.

Diesel, A.M. and Van Drimmelen, G.C. (1948) The diagnosis of East Coast fever in South Africa: A review. *Journal of the South African Veterinary Association* 19, 81–92.

Eickbush, T.H. and Eickbush, D.G. (2007) Finely orchestrated movements: Evolution of the ribosomal RNA genes. *Genetics* 175(2), 477–485. DOI: 10.1534/genetics.107.071399.

Elisa, M., Hasan, S.D., Moses, N., Elpidius, R., Skilton, R. *et al.* (2015) Genetic and antigenic diversity of *Theileria parva* in cattle in Eastern and Southern zones of Tanzania. A study to support control of East Coast fever. *Parasitology* 142(5), 698–705. DOI: 10.1017/S0031182014001784.

Eygelaar, D., Jori, F., Mokopasetso, M., Sibeko, K.P., Collins, N.E. *et al.* (2015) Tick-borne haemoparasites in African buffalo (*Syncerus caffer*) from two wildlife areas in Northern Botswana. *Parasites & Vectors* 8(1), 26. DOI: 10.1186/s13071-014-0627-y.

Gachohi, J.M., Ngumi, P.N., Kitala, P.M. and Skilton, R.A. (2010) Estimating seroprevalence and variation to four tick-borne infections and determination of associated risk factors in cattle under traditional mixed farming system in Mbeere District, Kenya. *Preventive Veterinary Medicine* 95(3–4), 208–223. DOI: 10.1016/j.prevetmed.2010.03.015.

Gachohi, J.M., Kitala, P.M., Ngumi, P.N. and Skilton, R.A. (2011) Environment and farm factors associated with exposure to *Theileria parva* infection in cattle under traditional mixed farming system in Mbeere District, Kenya. *Tropical Animal Health and Production* 43(1), 271–277. DOI: 10.1007/s11250-010-9688-x.

Gardner, M.J., Bishop, R., Shah, T., Villiers, E.P., Carlton, J.M. *et al.* (2005) Genome sequence of *Theileria parva*, a bovine pathogen that transforms lymphocytes. *Science* 309(5731), 134–137. DOI: 10.1126/science.1110439.

Gebrekidan, H., Nelson, L., Smith, G., Gasser, R.B. and Jabbar, A. (2017) An outbreak of oriental theileriosis in dairy cattle imported to Vietnam from Australia. *Parasitology* 144(6), 738–746. DOI: 10.1017/S0031182016002328.

Geysen, D., Bazarusanga, T., Brandt, J. and Dolan, T.T. (2004) An unusual mosaic structure of the PIM gene of *Theileria parva* and its relationship to allelic diversity. *Molecular and Biochemical Parasitology* 133(2), 163–173. DOI: 10.1016/j.molbiopara.2003.10.004.

Ghafar, A., Koehler, A.V., Hall, R.S., Gauci, C.G., Gasser, R.B. *et al.* (2020) Targeted next-generation sequencing and informatics as an effective tool to establish the composition of bovine piroplasm populations in endemic regions. *Microorganisms* 9(1), 21. DOI: 10.3390/microorganisms9010021.

Giemsa, G. (1902) Färbemethoden für malariaparasiten Zentralblatt für Bakteriologie, I. Abteilung. *Abteilung Originale* 307–313.

Gitau, G.K., McDermott, J.J., Katende, J.M., O'Callaghan, C.J., Brown, R.N. *et al.* (2000) Differences in the epidemiology of theileriosis on smallholder dairy farms in contrasting agro-ecological and grazing strata of highland Kenya. *Epidemiology and Infection* 124(2), 325–335. DOI: 10.1017/s0950268800003526.

Glidden, C.K., Koehler, A.V., Hall, R.S., Saeed, M.A., Coppo, M. *et al.* (2020) Elucidating cryptic dynamics of *Theileria* communities in African buffalo using a high-throughput sequencing informatics approach. *Ecology and Evolution* 10(1), 70–80. DOI: 10.1002/ece3.5758.

Graham, S.P., Pellé, R., Honda, Y., Mwangi, D.M., Tonukari, N.J. *et al.* (2006) *Theileria parva* candidate vaccine antigens recognized by immune bovine cytotoxic T-lymphocytes. *Proceedings of the National Academy of Sciences* 103(9), 3286–3291. DOI: 10.1073/pnas.0511273103.

Gray, C.E. and Robertson, W. (1902) *Report upon Texas Fever or Redwater in Rhodesia.* Cape Town, South Africa: Argus Printing & Publishing.

Gubbels, J.M., Vos, A.P., van der Weide, M., Viseras, J., Schouls, L.M. *et al.* (1999) Simultaneous detection of bovine *Theileria* and *Babesia* species by reverse line blot hybridization. *Journal of Clinical Microbiology* 37(6), 1782–1789. DOI: 10.1128/JCM.37.6.1782-1789.1999.

Gubbels, M.J., Hong, Y., Weide, M., Qi, B., Nijman, I.J. *et al.* (2000) Molecular characterisation of the *Theileria buffeli/orientalis*-group. *International Journal for Parasitology* 30(8), 943–952. DOI: 10.1016/s0020-7519(00)00074-6.

Hailemariam, Z., Krücken, J., Baumann, M., Ahmed, J.S., Clausen, P.-H. *et al.* (2017) Molecular detection of tick-borne pathogens in cattle from Southwestern Ethiopia. *PLoS ONE* 12(11), e0188248. DOI: 10.1371/journal.pone.0188248.

Hayashida, K., Hara, Y., Abe, T., Yamasaki, C., Toyoda, A. *et al.* (2012) Comparative genome analysis of three eukaryotic parasites with differing abilities to transform leukocytes reveals key mediators of *Theileria*-induced leukocyte transformation. *mBio* 3(5), e00204-12. DOI: 10.1128/mBio.00204-12.

Hayashida, K., Abe, T., Weir, W., Nakao, R., Ito, K. *et al.* (2013) Whole-genome sequencing of *Theileria parva* strains provides insight into parasite migration and diversification in the African continent. *DNA Research* 20(3), 209–220. DOI: 10.1093/dnares/dst003.

Hemmink, J.D., Weir, W., MacHugh, N.D., Graham, S.P., Patel, E. *et al.* (2016) Limited genetic and antigenic diversity within parasite isolates used in a live vaccine against *Theileria parva*. *International Journal for Parasitology* 46(8), 495–506. DOI: 10.1016/j.ijpara.2016.02.007.

Hemmink, J.D., Sitt, T., Pelle, R., Klerk-Lorist, L.-M., Shiels, B. *et al.* (2018) Ancient diversity and geographical sub-structuring in African buffalo *Theileria parva* populations revealed through metagenetic analysis of antigen-encoding loci. *International Journal for Parasitology* 48(3–4), 287–296. DOI: 10.1016/j.ijpara.2017.10.006.

Henson, S., Bishop, R.P., Morzaria, S., Spooner, P.R., Pelle, R. *et al.* (2012) High-resolution genotyping and mapping of recombination and gene conversion in the protozoan *Theileria parva* using whole genome sequencing. *BMC Genomics* 13, 503. DOI: 10.1186/1471-2164-13-503.

Huber, S., Karagenc, T., Ritler, D., Rottenberg, S. and Woods, K. (2018) Identification and characterisation of a *Theileria annulata* proline-rich microtubule and SH3 domain-interacting protein (TaMISHIP) that forms a complex with CLASP1, EB1, and CD2AP at the schizont surface. *Cellular Microbiology* 20(7), e12838. DOI: 10.1111/cmi.12838.

Iams, K.P., Young, J.R., Nene, V., Desai, J., Webster, P. *et al.* (1990) Characterisation of the gene encoding a 104-kilodalton microneme-rhoptry protein of *Theileria parva*. *Molecular and Biochemical Parasitology* 39(1), 47–60. DOI: 10.1016/0166-6851(90)90007-9.

Irvin, A.D. and Mwamachi, D.M. (1983) Clinical and diagnostic features of East Coast fever (*Theileria parva*) infection of cattle. *The Veterinary Record* 113(9), 192–198. DOI: 10.1136/vr.113.9.192.

Izzo, M.M., Poe, I., Horadagoda, N., De Vos, A.J. and House, J.K. (2010) Haemolytic anaemia in cattle in NSW associated with *Theileria* infections. *Australian Veterinary Journal* 88(1–2), 45–51. DOI: 10.1111/j.1751-0813.2009.00540.x.

Jongejan, F., Musisi, F.L., Moorhouse, P.D., Snacken, M. and Uilenberg, G. (1986) *Theileria taurotragi* in Zambia. *The Veterinary Quarterly* 8(3), 261–263. DOI: 10.1080/01652176.1986.9694051.

Joyner, L.P., Payne, R.C., Takahashi, K., Brocklesby, D.W. and Irvin, A.D. (1979) Serological comparison of British *Theileria mutans* and Japanese *T. sergenti*. *Research in Veterinary Science* 26(3), 387–388. DOI: 10.1016/S0034-5288(18)32901-1.

Kanduma, E.G., Mwacharo, J.M., Mwaura, S., Njuguna, J.N., Nzuki, I. *et al.* (2016) Multi-locus genotyping reveals absence of genetic structure in field populations of the brown ear tick (*Rhipicephalus appendiculatus*) in Kenya. *Ticks and Tick-Borne Diseases* 7(1), 26–35. DOI: 10.1016/j.ttbdis.2015.08.001.

Katende, J., Morzaria, S., Toye, P., Skilton, R., Nene, V. *et al.* (1998) An enzyme-linked immunosorbent assay for detection of *Theileria parva* antibodies in cattle using a recombinant polymorphic immunodominant molecule. *Parasitology Research* 84(5), 408–416. DOI: 10.1007/s004360050419.

Katzer, F., Ngugi, D., Schnier, C., Walker, A.R. and McKeever, D.J. (2007) Influence of host immunity on parasite diversity in *Theileria parva*. *Infection and Immunity* 75(10), 4909–4916. DOI: 10.1128/IAI.00710-07.

Kiara, H., Jennings, A., Bronsvoort, B.M.D.C., Handel, I.G., Mwangi, S.T. *et al.* (2014) A longitudinal assessment of the serological response to *Theileria parva* and other tick-borne parasites from birth to one year in a cohort of indigenous calves in western Kenya. *Parasitology* 141(10), 1289–1298. DOI: 10.1017/S003118201400050X.

Kimaro, E.G., Mor, S.M., Gwakisa, P. and Toribio, J.A. (2017) Seasonal occurrence of *Theileria parva* infection and management practices amongst Maasai pastoralist communities in Monduli District, Northern Tanzania. *Veterinary Parasitology* 246, 43–52. DOI: 10.1016/j.vetpar.2017.08.023.

Kivaria, F.M., Heuer, C., Jongejan, F., Okello-Onen, J., Rutagwenda, T. *et al.* (2004) Endemic stability for *Theileria parva* infections in Ankole calves of the Ankole ranching scheme, Uganda. *The Onderstepoort Journal of Veterinary Research* 71(3), 189–195. DOI: 10.4102/ojvr.v71i3.259.

Kivaria, F.M., Kapaga, A.M., Mbassa, G.K., Mtui, P.F. and Wani, R.J. (2012) Epidemiological perspectives of ticks and tick-borne diseases in South Sudan: Cross-sectional survey results. *The Onderstepoort Journal of Veterinary Research* 79(1), E1–E10. DOI: 10.4102/ojvr.v79i1.400.

Koch, R. (1903) Interim report on Rhodesian redwater or African Coast fever. *Journal of Comparative Pathology and Therapeutics* 16, 273–280. DOI: 10.1016/S0368-1742(03)80079-6.

Latré de Laté, P., Cook, E.A.J., Wragg, D., Poole, E.J., Ndambuki, G. *et al.* (2021) Inherited tolerance in cattle to the apicomplexan protozoan *Theileria parva* is associated with decreased proliferation of parasite-infected lymphocytes. *Frontiers in Cellular and Infection Microbiology* 11, 751671. DOI: 10.3389/fcimb.2021.751671.

Liebisch, A., Rahman, M.S. and Melfsen, J. (1976) Isolation of *Theileria mutans* (Theiler, 1906) from the blood of cattle in northern Germany (shor communication). *Deutsche Tierarztliche Wochenschrift* 83, 433.

Löhr, K.F. and Ross, J.P. (1969) Serological response in cattle to East Coast fever (*Theileria parva* infection) as measured by the indirect fluorescent antibody test. *Research in Veterinary Science* 10(5), 453–460.

Lubembe, D.M., Odongo, D.O., Salih, D.A. and Sibeko-Matjila, K.P. (2020) Microsatellite and minisatellite genotyping of *Theileria parva* population from southern Africa reveal possible discriminatory allele profiles with parasites from eastern Africa. *Ticks and Tick-Borne Diseases* 11(6), 101539. DOI: 10.1016/j.ttbdis.2020.101539.

Maboko, B.B., Featherston, J., Sibeko-Matjila, K.P. and Mans, B.J. (2021a) Whole genome sequencing of *Theileria parva* using target capture. *Genomics* 113(2), 429–438. DOI: 10.1016/j.ygeno.2020.12.033.

Maboko, B.B., Sibeko-Matjila, K.P., Pierneef, R., Chan, W.Y., Josemans, A. *et al.* (2021b) South African buffalo-derived *Theileria parva* is distinct from other buffalo and cattle-derived *T. parva*. *Frontiers in Genetics* 12, 666096. DOI: 10.3389/fgene.2021.666096.

Malmquist, W.A. and Brown, C.G.D. (1974) Establishment of *Theileria parva*-infected lymphoblastoid cell lines using homologous feeder layers. *Research in Veterinary Science* 16(1), 134–135. DOI: 10.1016/S0034-5288(18)33795-0.

Mans, B.J. (2022) The basis of molecular diagnostics for piroplasmids: Do the sequences lie? *Ticks and Tick-Borne Diseases* 13(2), 101907. DOI: 10.1016/j.ttbdis.2022.101907.

Mans, B.J., Pienaar, R., Latif, A.A. and Potgieter, F.T. (2011) Diversity in the 18S SSU rRNA V4 hyper-variable region of *Theileria* spp. in Cape buffalo (*Syncerus caffer*) and cattle from southern Africa. *Parasitology* 138(6), 766–779. DOI: 10.1017/S0031182011000187.

Mans, B.J., Pienaar, R. and Latif, A.A. (2015) A review of *Theileria* diagnostics and epidemiology. *International Journal for Parasitology: Parasites and Wildlife* 4(1), 104–118. DOI: 10.1016/j.ijppaw.2014.12.006.

Mans, B.J., Pienaar, R., Ratabane, J., Pule, B. and Latif, A.A. (2016) Investigating the diversity of the 18S SSU rRNA hyper-variable region of *Theileria* in cattle and Cape buffalo (*Syncerus caffer*) from southern Africa using a next generation sequencing approach. *Ticks and Tick-Borne Diseases* 7(5), 869–879. DOI: 10.1016/j.ttbdis.2016.04.005.

Marcellino, W.L., Salih, D.A., Julla, I.I. and El Hussein, A.R.M. (2012) Seroprevalence of East Coast fever in Central Equatoria State, South Sudan. *Veterinaria Italiana* 48(4), 379–385.

Marcellino, W.L., Salih, D.A., Njahira, M.N., Ndiwa, N., Araba, A. *et al.* (2017) The emergence of *Theileria parva* in Jonglei State, South Sudan: Confirmation using molecular and serological diagnostic tools. *Transboundary and Emerging Diseases* 64(4), 1229–1235. DOI: 10.1111/tbed.12495.

Martins, T.M., Neves, L., Pedro, O.C., Fafetine, J.M., Do Rosário, V.E. *et al.* (2010) Molecular detection of *Babesia* spp. and other haemoparasitic infections of cattle in Maputo Province, Mozambique. *Parasitology* 137(6), 939–946. DOI: 10.1017/S003118200999196X.

Matjila, P.T., Leisewitz, A.L., Oosthuizen, M.C., Jongejan, F. and Penzhorn, B.L. (2008) Detection of a *Theileria* species in dogs in South Africa. *Veterinary Parasitology* 157(1–2), 34–40. DOI: 10.1016/j.vetpar.2008.06.025.

Mbizeni, S., Potgieter, F.T., Troskie, C., Mans, B.J., Penzhorn, B.L. *et al.* (2013) Field and laboratory studies on Corridor disease (*Theileria parva* infection) in cattle population at the livestock/game interface of uPhongolo-Mkuze area, South Africa. *Ticks and Tick-Borne Diseases* 4(3), 227–234. DOI: 10.1016/j.ttbdis.2012.11.005.

McFadden, A.M.J., Rawdon, T.G., Meyer, J., Makin, J., Morley, C.M. *et al.* (2011) An outbreak of haemolytic anaemia associated with infection of *Theileria orientalis* in naive cattle. *New Zealand Veterinary Journal* 59(2), 79–85. DOI: 10.1080/00480169.2011.552857.

McFadden, A.M.J., Gias, E., Heuer, C., Stevens McFadden, F.J. and Pulford, D.J. (2016) Prevalence and spatial distribution of cattle herds infected with *Theileria orientalis* in New Zealand between 2012 and 2013. *New Zealand Veterinary Journal* 64(1), 55–59. DOI: 10.1080/00480169.2015.1090891.

Minami, T., Spooner, P.R., Irvin, A.D., Ocama, J.G., Dobbelaere, D.A. *et al.* (1983) Characterisation of stocks of *Theileria parva* by monoclonal antibody profiles. *Research in Veterinary Science* 35(3), 334–340.

Morrison, W.I., Aguado, A., Sheldrake, T.A., Palmateer, N.C., Ifeonu, O.O. *et al.* (2021) CD4 T-cell responses to *Theileria parva* in immune cattle recognize a diverse set of parasite antigens presented on the surface of infected lymphoblasts. *Journal of Immunology* 207(8), 1965–1977. DOI: 10.4049/jimmunol.2100331.

Morzaria, S.P., Barnett, S.F. and Brocklesby, D.W. (1974) Isolation of *Theileria mutans* from cattle in Essex. *The Veterinary Record* 94(12), 256. DOI: 10.1136/vr.94.12.256.

Morzaria, S.P., Young, A.S., Kimber, C.D. and Brocklesby, D.W. (1977) The serological relationship of a British *Theileria* with other *Theileria* species using the indirect fluorescent antibody test. *Research in Veterinary Science* 22(3), 330–333. DOI: 10.1016/S0034-5288(18)33257-0.

Morzaria, S.P., Spooner, P.R., Bishop, R.P., Musoke, A.J. and Young, J.R. (1990) *Sfi*I and *Not*I polymorphisms in *Theileria* stocks detected by pulsed field gel electrophoresis. *Molecular and Biochemical Parasitology* 40(2), 203–211. DOI: 10.1016/0166-6851(90)90042-k.

Morzaria, S.P., Dolan, T.T., Norval, R.A., Bishop, R.P. and Spooner, P.R. (1995) Generation and characterization of cloned *Theileria parva* parasites. *Parasitology* 111(Pt 1), 39–49. DOI: 10.1017/s0031182000064581.

Moulton, J.E., Krauss, H.H. and Malmquist, W.A. (1971) Growth characteristics of *Theileria parva*-infected bovine lymphoblast cultures. *American Journal of Veterinary Research* 32(9), 1365–1370. DOI: 10.2460/ajvr.1971.32.09.1365.

Muleya, W., Namangala, B., Simuunza, M., Nakao, R., Inoue, N. *et al.* (2012) Population genetic analysis and sub-structuring of *Theileria parva* in the northern and eastern parts of Zambia. *Parasites & Vectors* 5, 255. DOI: 10.1186/1756-3305-5-255.

Musoke, A.J., Nantulya, V.M., Rurangirwa, F.R. and Buscher, G. (1984) Evidence for a common protective antigenic determinant on sporozoites of several *Theileria parva* strains. *Immunology* 52(2), 231–238.

Muwanika, V., Kabi, F. and Masembe, C. (2016) Population genetic structure of *Theileria parva* field isolates from indigenous cattle populations of Uganda. *Ticks and Tick-Borne Diseases* 7(2), 291–297. DOI: 10.1016/j.ttbdis.2015.11.004.

Nene, V., Iams, K.P., Gobright, E. and Musoke, A.J. (1992) Characterisation of the gene encoding a candidate vaccine antigen of *Theileria parva* sporozoites. *Molecular and Biochemical Parasitology* 51(1), 17–27. DOI: 10.1016/0166-6851(92)90196-q.

Neveu-Lemaire, M. (1912) *Parasitologie des animaux domestiques: Maladies parasitaires non bactériennes*. Paris: J. Lamarre et Cie.

Nijhof, A.M., Penzhorn, B.L., Lynen, G., Mollel, J.O., Morkel, P. *et al.* (2003) *Babesia bicornis* sp. nov. and *Theileria bicornis* sp. nov.: Tick-borne parasites associated with mortality in the black rhinoceros (*Diceros bicornis*). *Journal of Clinical Microbiology* 41(5), 2249–2254. DOI: 10.1128/JCM.41.5.2249-2254.2003.

Nijhof, A.M., Pillay, V., Steyl, J., Prozesky, L., Stoltsz, W.H. *et al.* (2005) Molecular characterization of *Theileria* species associated with mortality in four species of African antelopes. *Journal of Clinical Microbiology* 43(12), 5907–5911. DOI: 10.1128/JCM.43.12.5907-5911.2005.

Njiiri, N.E., Bronsvoort, B.M. deC, Collins, N.E., Steyn, H.C., Troskie, M. *et al.* (2015) The epidemiology of tick-borne haemoparasites as determined by the reverse line blot hybridization assay in an intensively studied cohort of calves in western Kenya. *Veterinary Parasitology* 210(1–2), 69–76. DOI: 10.1016/j.vetpar.2015.02.020.

Norling, M., Bishop, R.P., Pelle, R., Qi, W., Henson, S. *et al.* (2015) The genomes of three stocks comprising the most widely utilized live sporozoite *Theileria parva* vaccine exhibit very different degrees and patterns of sequence divergence. *BMC Genomics* 16, 729. DOI: 10.1186/s12864-015-1910-9.

Notomi, T., Okayama, H., Masubuchi, H., Yonekawa, T., Watanabe, K. *et al.* (2000) Loop-mediated isothermal amplification of DNA. *Nucleic Acids Research* 28(12), e63–e63. DOI: 10.1093/nar/28.12.e63.

Oakes, V.J., Yabsley, M.J., Schwartz, D., LeRoith, T., Bissett, C. *et al.* (2019) *Theileria orientalis* Ikeda genotype in cattle, Virginia. *Emerging Infectious Diseases* 25(9), 1653–1659. DOI: 10.3201/eid2509.190088.

Odongo, D.O., Oura, C.A.L., Spooner, P.R., Kiara, H., Mburu, D. *et al.* (2006) Linkage disequilibrium between alleles at highly polymorphic mini- and micro-satellite loci of *Theileria parva* isolated from cattle in three regions of Kenya. *International Journal for Parasitology* 36(8), 937–946. DOI: 10.1016/j.ijpara.2006.01.008.

Odongo, D.O., Ueti, M.W., Mwaura, S.N., Knowles, D.P., Bishop, R.P. *et al.* (2009) Quantification of *Theileria parva* in *Rhipicephalus appendiculatus* (Acari: Ixodidae) confirms differences in infection between selected tick strains. *Journal of Medical Entomology* 46(4), 888–894. DOI: 10.1603/033.046.0422.

Odongo, D.O., Sunter, J.D., Kiara, H.K., Skilton, R.A. and Bishop, R.P. (2010) A nested PCR assay exhibits enhanced sensitivity for detection of *Theileria parva* infections in bovine blood samples from carrier animals. *Parasitology Research* 106(2), 357–365. DOI: 10.1007/s00436-009-1670-z.

OIE (Office International des Epizooties) (2014) *Manual of Diagnostic Tests and Vaccines for Terrestrial Animals*, 7th edn., Vol. 1–2. Paris, France: Office International des Epizooties.

Oosthuizen, M.C., Zweygarth, E., Collins, N.E., Troskie, M. and Penzhorn, B.L. (2008) Identification of a novel *Babesia* sp. from a sable antelope (*Hippotragus niger* Harris, 1838). *Journal of Clinical Microbiology* 46(7), 2247–2251. DOI: 10.1128/JCM.00167-08.

Oosthuizen, M.C., Allsopp, B.A., Troskie, M., Collins, N.E. and Penzhorn, B.L. (2009) Identification of novel *Babesia* and *Theileria* species in South African giraffe (*Giraffa camelopardalis*, Linnaeus, 1758) and roan antelope (*Hippotragus equinus*, Desmarest 1804). *Veterinary Parasitology* 163(1–2), 39–46. DOI: 10.1016/j.vetpar.2009.03.045.

Oteng, A.K. (1972) Development of schizonts directly from the blood piroplasms of the Australian *Theileria mutans*. *The British Veterinary Journal* 128(6), 23–25.

Ouedraogo, A.S., Zannou, O.M., Biguezoton, A.S., Kouassi, P.Y., Belem, A. *et al.* (2021) Cattle ticks and associated tick-borne pathogens in Burkina Faso and Benin: Apparent northern spread of *Rhipicephalus microplus* in Benin and first evidence of *Theileria velifera* and *Theileria annulata*. *Ticks and Tick-Borne Diseases* 12(4), 101733. DOI: 10.1016/j.ttbdis.2021.101733.

Oura, C.A.L., Odongo, D.O., Lubega, G.W., Spooner, P.R., Tait, A. *et al.* (2003) A panel of microsatellite and minisatellite markers for the characterisation of field isolates of *Theileria parva*. *International Journal for Parasitology* 33(14), 1641–1653. DOI: 10.1016/s0020-7519(03)00280-7.

Oura, C.A.L., Bishop, R., Wampande, E.M., Lubega, G.W. and Tait, A. (2004) The persistence of component *Theileria parva* stocks in cattle immunized with the 'Muguga cocktail' live vaccine against East Coast fever in Uganda. *Parasitology* 129(Pt 1), 27–42. DOI: 10.1017/s003118200400513x.

Oura, C.A.L., Asiimwe, B.B., Weir, W., Lubega, G.W. and Tait, A. (2005) Population genetic analysis and sub-structuring of *Theileria parva* in Uganda. *Molecular and Biochemical Parasitology* 140(2), 229–239. DOI: 10.1016/j.molbiopara.2004.12.015.

Oura, C.A.L., Tait, A., Asiimwe, B., Lubega, G.W. and Weir, W. (2011a) Haemoparasite prevalence and *Theileria parva* strain diversity in Cape buffalo (*Syncerus caffer*) in Uganda. *Veterinary Parasitology* 175(3–4), 212–219. DOI: 10.1016/j.vetpar.2010.10.032.

Oura, C.A.L., Tait, A., Asiimwe, B., Lubega, G.W. and Weir, W. (2011b) *Theileria parva* genetic diversity and haemoparasite prevalence in cattle and wildlife in and around Lake Mburo National Park in Uganda. *Parasitology Research* 108(6), 1365–1374. DOI: 10.1007/s00436-010-2030-8.

Palmateer, N.C., Tretina, K., Orvis, J., Ifeonu, O.O., Crabtree, J. *et al.* (2020) Capture-based enrichment of *Theileria parva* DNA enables full genome assembly of first buffalo-derived strain and reveals exceptional intra-specific genetic diversity. *PLoS Neglected Tropical Diseases* 14(10), e0008781. DOI: 10.1371/journal.pntd.0008781.

Papli, N., Landt, O., Fleischer, C., Koekemoer, J.O., Mans, B.J. *et al.* (2011) Evaluation of a TaqMan real-time PCR for the detection of *Theileria parva* in buffalo and cattle. *Veterinary Parasitology* 175(3–4), 356–359. DOI: 10.1016/j.vetpar.2010.10.038.

Patel, E.H., Lubembe, D.M., Gachanja, J., Mwaura, S., Spooner, P. *et al.* (2011) Molecular characterization of live *Theileria parva* sporozoite vaccine stabilates reveals extensive genotypic diversity. *Veterinary Parasitology* 179(1–3), 62–68. DOI: 10.1016/j.vetpar.2011.01.057.

Pelle, R., Graham, S.P., Njahira, M.N., Osaso, J., Saya, R.M. *et al.* (2011) Two *Theileria parva* CD8 T-cell antigen genes are more variable in buffalo than cattle parasites, but differ in pattern of sequence diversity. *PloS ONE* 6(4), e19015. DOI: 10.1371/journal.pone.0019015.

Pienaar, R., Potgieter, F.T., Latif, A.A., Thekisoe, O.M.M. and Mans, B.J. (2011a) The Hybrid II assay: A sensitive and specific real-time hybridization assay for the diagnosis of *Theileria parva* infection in Cape buffalo (*Syncerus caffer*) and cattle. *Parasitology* 138(14), 1935–1944. DOI: 10.1017/S0031182011001454.

Pienaar, R., Potgieter, F.T., Latif, A.A., Thekisoe, O.M.M. and Mans, B.J. (2011b) Mixed *Theileria* infections in free-ranging buffalo herds: Implications for diagnosing *Theileria parva* infections in Cape buffalo (*Syncerus caffer*). *Parasitology* 138(7), 884–895. DOI: 10.1017/S0031182011000503.

Pienaar, R., Latif, A.A., Mans, B.J. and Thekisoe, O. (2013) Protein gene candidates for the qualitative molecular detection of *Theileria parva* in African buffalo (*Syncerus caffer*) using the real-time SYBR green polymerase chain reaction. In: Howarth, G.S. (ed.) *Annual International Conference on Advances in Veterinary Science Research, Global Science and Technology (GSTF)*, pp. 41–46. DOI: 10.5176/2382-5685_VETSCI13.20.

Pienaar, R., Latif, A.A., Thekisoe, O.M.M. and Mans, B.J. (2014) Geographic distribution of *Theileria* sp. (buffalo) and *Theileria* sp. (bougasvlei) in Cape buffalo (*Syncerus caffer*) in southern Africa: Implications for speciation. *Parasitology* 141, 411–424. DOI: 10.1017/S0031182013001728.

Pienaar, R., Latif, A.A. and Mans, B.J. (2018) Investigations into the host specificity of *Theileria taurotragi*. *Veterinary Parasitology* 254, 30–35. DOI: 10.1016/j.vetpar.2018.03.003.

Pienaar, R., Josemans, A., Latif, A.A. and Mans, B.J. (2020a) The host-specificity of *Theileria* sp. (sable) and *Theileria* sp. (sable-like) in African Bovidae and detection of novel *Theileria* in antelope and giraffe. sable, *Parasitology* 147, 213–224. DOI: 10.1017/S003118201900132X.

Pienaar, R., Troskie, P.C., Josemans, A.I., Potgieter, F.T., Maboko, B.B. *et al.* (2020b) Investigations into the carrier-state of *Theileria* sp. (buffalo) in cattle. *International Journal for Parasitology* 11, 136–142. DOI: 10.1016/j.ijppaw.2020.01.009.

Pinder, M. and Hewett, R.S. (1980) Monoclonal antibodies detect antigenic diversity in *Theileria parva* parasite. *Journal of Immunology* 124(2), 1000–1001.

Reichard, M.V., Den Bussche, R.A., Meinkoth, J.H., Hoover, J.P. and Kocan, A.A. (2005) A new species of Cytauxzoon from Pallas' cats caught in Mongolia and comments on the systematics and taxonomy of piroplasmids. *The Journal of Parasitology* 91(2), 420–426. DOI: 10.1645/GE-384R.

Rubaire-Akiiki, C.M., Okello-Onen, J., Musunga, D., Kabagambe, E.K., Vaarst, M. *et al.* (2006) Effect of agro-ecological zone and grazing system on incidence of East Coast fever in calves in Mbale and Sironko Districts of Eastern Uganda. *Preventive Veterinary Medicine* 75(3–4), 251–266. DOI: 10.1016/j.prevetmed.2006.04.015.

Rukambile, E., Machuka, E., Njahira, M., Kyalo, M., Skilton, R. *et al.* (2016) Population genetic analysis of *Theileria parva* isolated in cattle and buffaloes in Tanzania using minisatellite and microsatellite markers. *Veterinary Parasitology* 224, 20–26. DOI: 10.1016/j.vetpar.2016.04.038.

Salih, D.A., El Hussein, A.M., Seitzer, U. and Ahmed, J.S. (2007) Epidemiological studies on tick-borne diseases of cattle in Central Equatoria State, Southern Sudan. *Parasitology Research* 101(4), 1035–1044. DOI: 10.1007/s00436-007-0583-y.

Salih, D.A., Liu, Z., Bakheit, M.A., Ali, A.M., El Hussein, A.M. *et al.* (2008) Development and evaluation of a loop-mediated isothermal amplification method for diagnosis of tropical theileriosis. *Transboundary and Emerging Diseases* 55(5–6), 238–243. DOI: 10.1111/j.1865-1682.2008.01033.x.

Salih, D.A., El Hussein, A.R.M., Ahmed, J. and Seitzer, U. (2010) Comparison between reverse line blot and enzyme-linked immunosorbent assay in diagnosis of major tick-borne diseases of cattle in Southern Sudan. *Transboundary and Emerging Diseases* 57(1–2), 61–62. DOI: 10.1111/j.1865-1682.2010.01103.x.

Salih, D.A., Mwacharo, J.M., Pelle, R., Njahira, M.N., Odongo, D.O. *et al.* (2018) Genetic diversity and population structure of *Theileria parva* in South Sudan. *Ticks and Tick-Borne Diseases* 9(4), 806–813. DOI: 10.1016/j.ttbdis.2018.03.002.

Salim, B., Alanazi, A.D., Omori, R., Alyousif, M.S., Alanazi, I.O. *et al.* (2019) Potential role of dogs as sentinels and reservoirs for piroplasms infecting equine and cattle in Riyadh City, Saudi Arabia. *Acta Tropica* 193, 78–83. DOI: 10.1016/j.actatropica.2019.02.029.

Schindler, R. and Mehlitz, D. (1965) Versuche zur differenzierung der *Theilerien* spezies des rindes durch serologische untersuchungen. *Tropical Medicine and Parasitology* 16, 85–87.

Schindler, R. and Mehlitz, D. (1969) Serologic studies on *Theileria mutans* infection in cattle. *Zeitschrift Für Tropenmedizin Und Parasitologie* 20(4), 459–473.

Shapiro, S.Z., Fujisaki, K., Morzaria, S.P., Webster, P., Fujinaga, T. *et al.* (1987) A life-cycle stage-specific antigen of *Theileria parva* recognized by anti-macroschizont monoclonal antibodies. *Parasitology* 94(1), 29–37. DOI: 10.1017/s0031182000053427.

Sibeko, K.P., Oosthuizen, M.C., Collins, N.E., Geysen, D., Rambritch, N.E. *et al.* (2008) Development and evaluation of a real-time polymerase chain reaction test for the detection of *Theileria parva* infections in Cape buffalo (*Syncerus caffer*) and cattle. *Veterinary Parasitology* 155(1–2), 37–48. DOI: 10.1016/j.vetpar.2008.03.033.

Sibeko, K.P., Geysen, D., Oosthuizen, M.C., Matthee, C.A., Troskie, M. *et al.* (2010) Four p67 alleles identified in South African *Theileria parva* field samples. *Veterinary Parasitology* 167(2–4), 244–254. DOI: 10.1016/j.vetpar.2009.09.026.

Sibeko, K.P., Collins, N.E., Oosthuizen, M.C., Troskie, M., Potgieter, F.T. *et al.* (2011) Analyses of genes encoding *Theileria parva* p104 and polymorphic immunodominant molecule (PIM) reveal evidence of the presence of cattle-type alleles in the South African *T. parva* population. *Veterinary Parasitology* 181(2–4), 120–130. DOI: 10.1016/j.vetpar.2011.04.035.

Silatsa, B.A., Simo, G., Githaka, N., Kamga, R., Oumarou, F. *et al.* (2020) First detection of *Theileria parva* in cattle from Cameroon in the absence of the main tick vector *Rhipicephalus appendiculatus*. *Transboundary and Emerging Diseases* 67, 68–78. DOI: 10.1111/tbed.13425.

Sili, G., Byaruhanga, C., Horak, I., Steyn, H., Chaisi, M. *et al.* (2021) Ticks and tick-borne pathogens infecting livestock and dogs in Tchicala-Tcholoanga, Huambo Province, Angola. *Parasitology Research* 120(3), 1097–1102. DOI: 10.1007/s00436-020-07009-3.

Sitt, T., Poole, E.J., Ndambuki, G., Mwaura, S., Njoroge, T. *et al.* (2015) Exposure of vaccinated and naive cattle to natural challenge from buffalo-derived *Theileria parva*. *International Journal for Parasitology* 4(2), 244–251. DOI: 10.1016/j.ijppaw.2015.04.006.

Sitt, T., Henson, S., Morrison, W.I. and Toye, P. (2019) Similar levels of diversity in the gene encoding the p67 sporozoite surface protein of *Theileria parva* are observed in blood samples from buffalo and cattle naturally infected from buffalo. *Veterinary Parasitology* 269, 21–27. DOI: 10.1016/j.vetpar.2019.04.006.

Skilton, R.A., Bishop, R.P., Wells, C.W., Spooner, P.R., Gobright, E. *et al.* (1998) Cloning and characterization of a 150 kDa microsphere antigen of *Theileria parva* that is immunologically cross-reactive with the polymorphic immunodominant molecule (PIM). *Parasitology* 117(4), 321–330. DOI: 10.1017/s0031182098003163.

Skilton, R.A., Bishop, R.P., Katende, J.M., Mwaura, S. and Morzaria, S.P. (2002) The persistence of *Theileria parva* infection in cattle immunized using two stocks which differ in their ability to induce a carrier state: Analysis using a novel blood spot PCR assay. *Parasitology* 124(Pt 3), 265–276. DOI: 10.1017/s0031182001001196.

Squarre, D., Nakamura, Y., Hayashida, K., Kawai, N., Chambaro, H. *et al.* (2020) Investigation of the piroplasm diversity circulating in wildlife and cattle of the greater Kafue ecosystem, Zambia. *Parasites & Vectors* 13(1), 599. DOI: 10.1186/s13071-020-04475-7.

Stewart, N.P., Uilenberg, G. and Vos, A.J. (1996) Review of Australian species of *Theileria*, with special reference to *Theileria buffeli* of cattle. *Tropical Animal Health and Production* 28(1), 81–90. DOI: 10.1007/BF02250731.

Swai, E.S., Karimuribo, E.D., Kambarage, D.M., Moshy, W.E. and Mbise, A.N. (2007) A comparison of seroprevalence and risk factors for *Theileria parva* and *T. mutans* in smallholder dairy cattle in the Tanga and Iringa regions of Tanzania. *Veterinary Journal* 174(2), 390–396. DOI: 10.1016/j.tvjl.2006.08.004.

Tembo, S., Collins, N.E., Sibeko-Matjila, K.P., Troskie, M., Vorster, I. *et al.* (2018) Occurrence of tick-borne haemoparasites in cattle in the Mungwi District, Northern Province, Zambia. *Ticks and Tick-Borne Diseases* 9(3), 707–717. DOI: 10.1016/j.ttbdis.2018.02.004.

Theiler, A. (1904) Rhodesian tick fever. *Transvaal Agricultural Journal* 2, 421–437.

Theiler, A. (1906) Piroplasma mutans (n. spec.) of South African cattle. *Journal of Comparative Pathology and Therapeutics* 19, 292–300. DOI: 10.1016/S0368-1742(06)80073-1.

Thekisoe, O.M.M., Rambritch, N.E., Nakao, R., Bazie, R.S., Mbati, P. *et al.* (2010) Loop-mediated isothermal amplification (LAMP) assays for detection of *Theileria parva* infections targeting the PIM and p150 genes. *International Journal for Parasitology* 40(1), 55–61. DOI: 10.1016/j.ijpara.2009.07.004.

Thompson, B.E., Latif, A.A., Oosthuizen, M.C., Troskie, M. and Penzhorn, B.L. (2008) Occurrence of *Theileria parva* infection in cattle on a farm in the Ladysmith district, KwaZulu-Natal, South Africa. *Journal of the South African Veterinary Association* 79(1), 31–35. DOI: 10.4102/jsava.v79i1.237.

Toye, P.G., Goddeeris, B.M., Iams, K., Musoke, A.J. and Morrison, W.I. (1991) Characterization of a polymorphic immunodominant molecule in sporozoites and schizonts of *Theileria parva*. *Parasite Immunology* 13(1), 49–62. DOI: 10.1111/j.1365-3024.1991.tb00262.x.

Toye, P., Gobright, E., Nyanjui, J., Nene, V. and Bishop, R. (1995a) Structure and sequence variation of the genes encoding the polymorphic, immunodominant molecule (PIM), an antigen of *Theileria parva* recognized by inhibitory monoclonal antibodies. *Molecular and Biochemical Parasitology* 73(1–2), 165–177. DOI: 10.1016/0166-6851(95)00110-m.

Toye, P.G., Metzelaar, M.J., Wijngaard, P.L., Nene, V., Iams, K. *et al.* (1995b) Characterization of the gene encoding the polymorphic immunodominant molecule, a neutralizing antigen of *Theileria parva*. *Journal of Immunology* 155(3), 1370–1381. DOI: 10.4049/jimmunol.155.3.1370.

Toye, P., Nyanjui, J., Goddeeris, B. and Musoke, A.J. (1996) Identification of neutralization and diagnostic epitopes on PIM, the polymorphic immunodominant molecule of *Theileria parva*. *Infection and Immunity* 64(5), 1832–1838. DOI: 10.1128/iai.64.5.1832-1838.1996.

Toye, P., Kiara, H., Ole-Moiyoi, O., Enahoro, D. and Rich, K.M. (2020) The management and economics of East Coast fever. In: McIntyre, J. and Grace, D. (eds) *The Impact of the International Livestock Research Institute*. Wallingford, UK: CAB International, pp. 239–273.

Uilenberg, G. (1964) *Haematoxenus veliferus*, n.g., n.sp., parasite incertae sedis du sang de bovins à Madagascar. *Revue d'élevage et de Médecine Vétérinaire Des Pays Tropicaux* 17(4), 655. DOI: 10.19182/remvt.7306.

Uilenberg, G. (1970) Existence of *Haematoxenus veliferus* (Sporozoa, *Theileriidae*) in Central Africa. Presence of *Haematoxenus* sp. in the African buffalo. *Revue d'élevage et de Médecine Vétérinaire Des Pays Tropicaux* 23(4), 455. DOI: 10.19182/remvt.7674.

Uilenberg, G. and Schreuder, B.E.C. (1976) Studies on *Theileriidae* (Sporozoa) in Tanzania. I. Tick transmission of *Haematoxenus veliferus*. *Tropenmedizin Und Parasitologie* 27(1), 106–111.

Uilenberg, G., Mpangala, C., McGregor, W. and Callow, L.L. (1977) Biological differences between African *Theileria mutans* (Theiler 1906) and two benign species of *Theileria* of cattle in Australia and Britain. *Australian Veterinary Journal* 53(6), 271–273. DOI: 10.1111/j.1751-0813.1977.tb00214.x.

Uilenberg, G., Perié, N.M., Spanjer, A.A.M. and Franssen, F.F.J. (1985) *Theileria orientalis*, a cosmopolitan blood parasite of cattle: Demonstration of the schizont stage. *Research in Veterinary Science* 38(3), 352–360. DOI: 10.1016/S0034-5288(18)31808-3.

Wesonga, F.D., Gachohi, J.M., Kitala, P.M., Gathuma, J.M. and Njenga, M.J. (2015) *Theileria parva* infection seroprevalence and associated risk factors in cattle in Machakos County, Kenya. *Tropical Animal Health and Production* 47(1), 93–101. DOI: 10.1007/s11250-014-0690-6.

WOAH (2023a) Chapter 1.1.6. validation of diagnostic assays for infectious diseases of terrestrial animals. In: *Manual of Diagnostic Tests and Vaccines for Terrestrial Animals*, 12th edn. pp. 1–27.

WOAH (2023b) *Terrestrial Animal Health Code* [Online]. Paris: OIE. Available at: https://www.woah.org/en/what-we-do/standards/codes-and-manuals/terrestrial-code-online-access/ (accessed 20 April 2024).

Yakimoff, W.L. and Dekhtereff, N.A. (1930) Zur frage fiber die theileriose in Ostsibirien. *Archiv Für Protistenkunde* 72, 179–189.

Yakimoff, W.L. and Soudatschenkoff, W.W. (1931) Zur frage der piroplasmiden der rinder in ost-sibirien. *Archiv Für Protistenkunde* 75, 179–190.

Yam, J., Bogema, D.R., Micallef, M.L., Djordjevic, S.P. and Jenkins, C. (2022) Complete genomes of *Theileria orientalis* Chitose and Buffeli genotypes reveal within species translocations and differences in ABC transporter content. *Pathogens* 11(7), 801. DOI: 10.3390/pathogens11070801.

Young, A.S., Purnell, R.E., Payne, R.C., Brown, C.G. and Kanhai, G.K. (1978) Studies on the transmission and course of infection of a Kenyan strain of *Theileria mutans*. *Parasitology* 76(1), 99–115. DOI: 10.1017/s0031182000047430.

Yusufmia, S.B.A.S., Collins, N.E., Nkuna, R., Troskie, M., Bossche, P. *et al.* (2010) Occurrence of *Theileria parva* and other haemoprotozoa in cattle at the edge of Hluhluwe-iMfolozi Park, KwaZulu-Natal, South Africa. *Journal of the South African Veterinary Association* 81(1), 45–49. DOI: 10.4102/jsava.v81i1.95.

Zweygarth, E., Koekemoer, O., Josemans, A.I., Rambritch, N., Pienaar, R. *et al.* (2009) *Theileria*-infected cell line from an African buffalo (*Syncerus caffer*). *Parasitology Research* 105(2), 579–581. DOI: 10.1007/s00436-009-1467-0.

9 The *Theileria parva* Genome

Joana C. Silva[1]* and Richard P. Bishop[2]
[1]*School of Medicine, The University of Maryland, Baltimore, USA;* [2]*Department of Veterinary Microbiology and Pathology, Washington State University, Pullman, USA*

9.1 Introduction

The era of genomics has ushered in unparalleled insights into the biology and evolution of living organisms, including tick-transmitted pathogen species (Seehausen *et al.*, 2014; Ashley, 2021; Wong *et al.*, 2021). Many pathogens, including parasites, have relatively small genomes, facilitating the comprehensive characterization of their gene complement and respective gene products, from which gene losses and gains and detailed metabolic pathways can be inferred (Harb *et al.*, 2016). Resequencing projects, in turn, by providing additional genomes for each species, allow estimation of the degree of conservation of specific genes or genomic features within and between pathogen populations, and the contribution of genetic variation to various phenotypes of interest (IGVF Consortium, 2024). All this information can then be interrogated by infectious disease researchers to identify potential vulnerabilities in pathogens, such as traits that can be exploited to develop rationally designed drugs and identify genes encoding candidate vaccine antigens (Sadiq *et al.*, 2018; Su *et al.*, 2019; Howden *et al.*, 2023). Examples include the presence of conserved, taxon-specific genes, which can be targeted without the risk of cross-reactions with host proteins, or the absence of specific metabolic pathways that render pathogens vulnerable to compounds they cannot metabolize or secrete.

Theileria parva, a eukaryotic pathogen, is a tick-transmitted apicomplexan protozoan parasite of bovids in Eastern and Southern Africa, including cattle (*Bos indicus* and *Bos taurus*) and African Cape buffalo (*Syncerus caffer*). *T. parva* infection in cattle causes East Coast fever (ECF), resulting in substantial financial losses to smallholder farmers and the dairy industry in eastern and southern Africa (see Chapter 2 of this volume). The species is thought to have evolved as a parasite of the buffalo, which tolerates the parasite without apparent clinical symptoms, but infection in domesticated cattle with strains transmitted by ticks, either from cattle or buffalo, is rapidly lethal (see Chapters 4 and 5 of this volume). However, some indigenous breeds of cattle residing in tick-infested areas exhibit a degree of resistance and suffer lower levels of mortality. Three major drivers of genomics research in *T. parva* are: (i) the desire to understand the molecular basis of the biology of the species, which is unusual among eukaryote species in its ability to transform the host leukocytes, allowing the parasitized cells to be established as immortalized cell lines *in vitro* (see Chapter 3 of this volume); (ii) the quest to develop an effective subunit vaccine against the parasite (see Chapter 11 of this volume), and ascertain how genetic variation in the species might impact vaccine efficacy; and (iii) the question of whether the *T. parva* strains of buffalo

*Corresponding author: jcsilva@som.umaryland.edu

 East Coast Fever: The Disease, its Impact and Control (eds W.I. Morrison and P. Toye)
DOI: 10.1079/9781800626324.0009

origin and those of cattle origin represent the same or different taxonomic units, with implications for vaccine design.

In this chapter, we present a summary of the main features of the *T. parva* genome and discuss aspects of the biology of the parasite and its ability to cause disease that require further genome sequencing and analyses.

9.2 The *T. parva* Genome

The first sequence of a *T. parva* genome was published by Gardner *et al.* in 2005 and was the result of a collaboration led by The Institute for Genomic Research and the International Livestock Research Institute (Gardner *et al.*, 2005). The sequence was derived from DNA isolated from piroplasms of the *T. parva* Muguga isolate and it covered the complete genome apart from small gaps in chromosomes 3 and 4. Sequences for the mitochondrial and apicoplast genomes were also revealed. A subsequent study in which the same parasite sequence was subjected to a more thorough annotation process was published by Tretina *et al.* 15 years later (Tretina *et al.*, 2020). This analysis was based on an extensive schizont RNA-seq dataset and corrected errors in the annotation of over 50% of the genes. At about the same time, the group used parasite DNA captured from bovine lymphocytes infected *in vitro* to produce genome assemblies of two additional cattle-derived isolates (*T. parva* Marikebuni and *T. parva* Uganda) and a buffalo-derived isolate (Palmateer *et al.*, 2020).

9.2.1 The reference *T. parva* strain

The reference genome of *T. parva* is based on an extensively laboratory-passaged parasite strain, *T. parva* Muguga. This strain was isolated in Kenya in the early 1960s and was subsequently maintained in the laboratory by regular passage through ticks and cattle until methods to cryopreserve the infective stages of the parasite were established in the 1970s (see Chapter 12 of this volume). *T. parva* Muguga is thought to have lost the ability to sustain long term tick-transmissible infections, known as the 'carrier state' (Skilton *et al.*, 2002), a key factor in the transmission biology and epidemiology of the parasite. The Muguga stock was chosen for genome sequencing because of the availability of a large body of background information on the properties of the Muguga isolate derived from experimental studies carried out with the parasite. It was also known to generate high levels of infected erythrocytes, allowing production of purified piroplasm DNA following infection of cattle. This was essential when the first *T. parva* genome sequence was generated in 2005, since it enabled the isolation of sufficiently large amounts of high molecular weight parasite DNA to build high-quality genomic libraries for the Sanger sequencing platform. The reference *T. parva* Muguga genome was completed using conventional Sanger dideoxy technology and published in 2005 (Gardner *et al.*, 2005), simultaneously with that of the closely related species *Theileria annulata* (Pain *et al.*, 2005).

9.2.2 Genome features

9.2.2.1 Genome size and protein-coding genes

At 8.31 Mbp in length, the *T. parva* genome is small (Gardner *et al.*, 2005), even among the haemosporidia. *Plasmodium falciparum*, the most studied of the haemosporidia and the cause of cerebral malaria in humans, has a 23.3 Mb genome (Gardner *et al.*, 2002). The *T. parva* nuclear genome is encoded on four chromosomes, substantially fewer than the 14 chromosomes found in *P. falciparum*. The original genome annotation of *T. parva* included 4035 predicted genes as compared to 3995 genes in *T. annulata* (Pain *et al.*, 2005) and 5268 in *P. falciparum* (Gardner *et al.*, 2002). The updated annotation of Tretina *et al.* (2020) included the addition of 128 genes and significant modifications in hundreds of genes, such as gene merges or gene splitting, and alterations to intron–exon boundaries. The re-annotation process resulted in 157 gene models being split, and 38 genes being replaced by new genes encoded in the reverse orientation. In addition, exon boundaries were corrected in over a thousand genes. Overall, 83% of all nuclear genes in the original annotation were modified, most significantly by the addition of untranslated region (UTR) coordinates to most genes. The re-annotation led to significant changes to the predicted proteome, with 53% of the nuclear proteins in the original annotation predicted to have altered amino acid sequences and an increase in the average coding sequence (CDS) length by about 50 bp. An additional 200,000 bp (corresponding to 2.4% of the genome), previously classified as intergenic/UTR or intronic sequences, were reassigned to the proteome.

Palmateer *et al.* (2020) used a capture DNA approach to selectively enrich the DNA pool for parasite DNA prior to sequencing, enabling them to construct *de novo* genome assemblies. The authors estimated the genome of an isolate of buffalo origin to be at least 20 kbp longer than the reference *T. parva* Muguga isolate. The additional DNA was predicted to contain 25 genes, 19 of which were additional copies of genes present elsewhere in the *T. parva* genome and which encode mostly hypothetical proteins. The remaining six were most similar to genes found in other *Theileria* species (*T. annulata* and *Theileria orientalis*).

9.2.2.2 A gene-dense genome

The annotation of the original genome sequence produced by Gardner *et al.* in 2005 predicted 4035 protein-encoding genes. This was increased to 4055 in the subsequent re-annotation by Tretina *et al.* in 2020. These results indicate that the *T. parva* genome is very gene-dense, with CDSs making up 71% of the nuclear genome (Fig. 9.1; Tretina *et al.*, 2020). This is similar to the *T. annulata* genome (73%; summarized in Kappmeyer *et al.*, 2012) but much more compact than the genome of *P. falciparum*, where CDSs make up only about 53% of the genome (Gardner *et al.*, 2002; Alvarez-Jarreta *et al.*, 2024). The observation that the length of regions between CDSs (consisting of intergenic regions and UTRs) increases with the number of promoters in those regions (zero, one or two, depending on the orientation of the flanking genes) led the authors to postulate that the compact genome is the result of selection against excess (non-functional) DNA (Guo and Silva, 2008; Tretina *et al.*, 2016).

The high gene density found in the *T. parva* genome is reflected in several features of the non-coding DNA. In addition to the increase in the length of non-coding sequences (NCSs) between CDSs with transcription regulation-associated functions, these NCSs in *T. parva* are short, with an average distance of 405 bp between CDSs, a fourth of the length in *P. falciparum* (Gardner *et al.*, 2005). In addition, RNA-seq data revealed overlap between transcripts of ~1300 consecutive genes pairs, which can be extensive (mean overlap >100 bp, with a maximum of >1 kb), and which involves mostly UTRs but also the overlap of predicted CDSs in a few dozen cases (Tretina *et al.*, 2020). Introns are also short, although there are more introns per gene and more genes with introns than are found in *Plasmodium* (Gardner *et al.*, 2005).

Consistent with the small genome size, there is an absence of extensive tracts of non-coding repetitive DNA in the genome, even though AT-rich minisatellites were reported early in the study of this genome (Bishop *et al.*, 1998). Unlike *P. falciparum*, long tracts of telomere-associated non-coding repetitive DNA that were thought to facilitate recombination between non-homologous telomeres are also absent (Sohanpal *et al.*, 1995; Bishop *et al.*, 2000). A short conserved sequence, approximately 140 bp in length, that is present proximal to the telomeric repeats (Sohanpal *et al.*, 2000), may however be sufficient to contribute to ectopic recombination between the termini of non-homologous chromosomes (Fig. 9.2).

9.2.2.3 Ribosomal DNA

Ribosomal DNA (rDNA) loci are essential to cell function, by encoding rRNA molecules required for translation and by contributing to assemblage of the nucleolus, an organelle central to genome stability, cell cycle regulation and many other vital cellular processes (Cerqueira and Lemos, 2019; Potapova and Gerton, 2019). Most eukaryotes, from the single celled *Saccharomyces cerevisiae* to plants and mammals, have >100 to a few thousand copies of the rDNA unit, each consisting of 18S, 5.8S and 28S subunits, often tandemly arrayed, and which can differ in sequence (Alvarez-Jarreta *et al.*, 2024; D'Alfonso *et al.*, 2024; Rodriguez-Algarra *et al.*, 2025). In *T. parva*, there are only

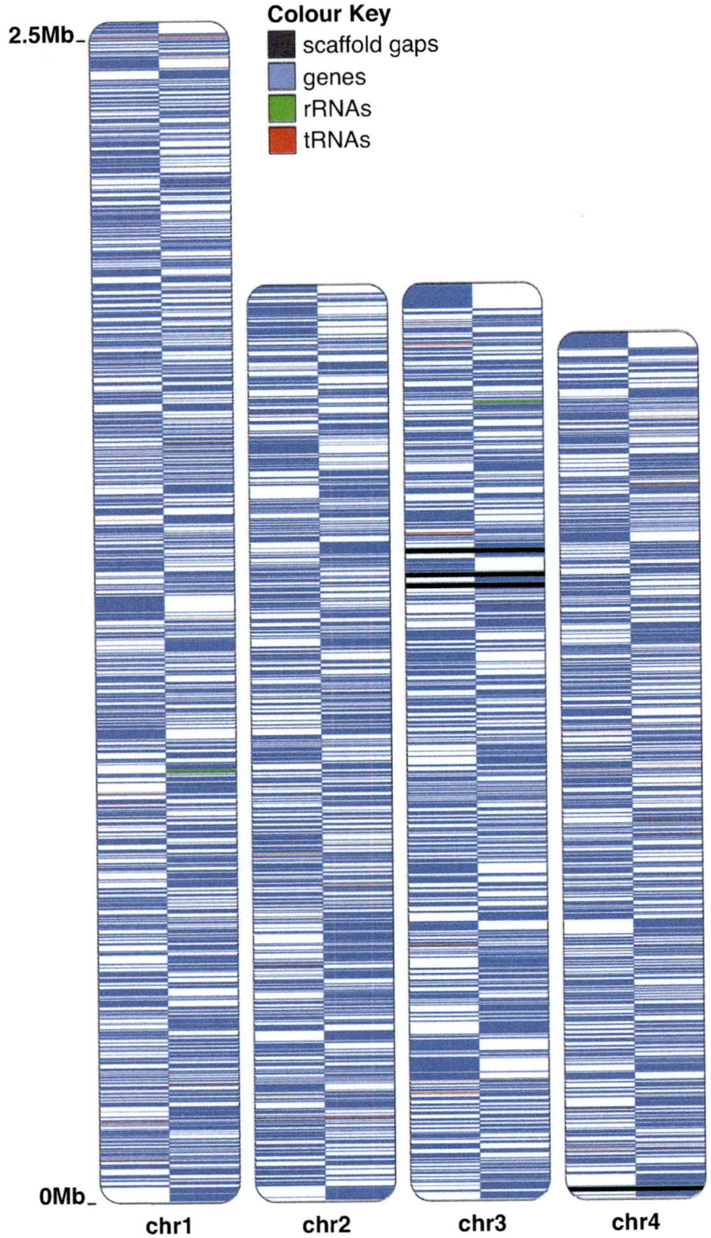

Fig. 9.1. Schematic of the nuclear genome assembly of the *T. parva* Muguga reference strain. Depiction of each of the four linear nuclear chromosomes, with the location of each protein-coding locus (blue) and loci encoding rRNAs (green) and tRNAs (purple). Location of loci in the forward (left, in each chromosome) and reverse (right) strands is shown. The four physical gaps present in the reference assembly are shown (black). Chromosome orientation is arbitrary and here it refers to the published structural annotation in Tretina *et al.* (2020). (Figure kindly provided by Jonathan Crabtree.)

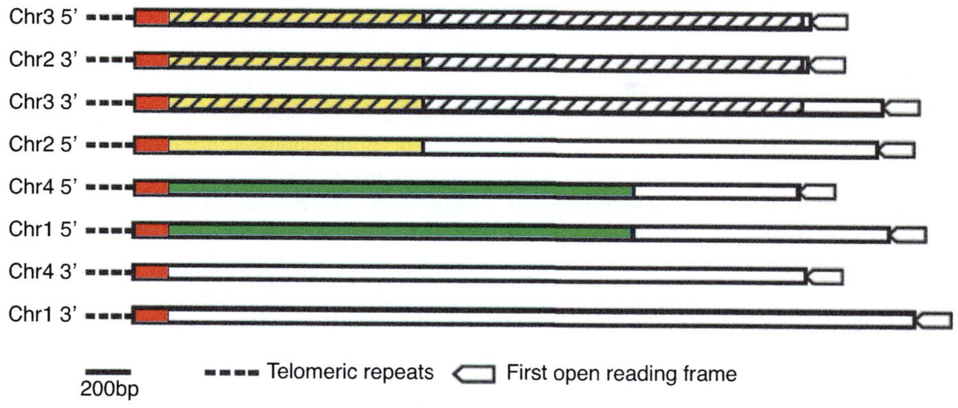

Fig. 9.2. Organization of *T. parva* subtelomeric repeat regions based on Clustal W alignment of nucleotides. Coloured and hatched areas indicate a level of sequence identity, with red highlighting the 100% conserved 140 followed by chromosomal 5' or 3' end as defined in the 2005 annotation of the genome. The repeats differ between chromosomal ends and vary between unit sizes of 153 and 579 bp. (Reproduced and adapted with permission from Gardner *et al*., 2005, supplementary data.)

two rDNA units, encoded by genes located one each on chromosomes 1 and 3 (Kibe *et al.*, 1994; Gardner *et al.*, 2005). The two small subunit ribosomal units are identical, and there is no evidence that they are differentially transcribed between life-cycle stages, as is the case in other parasitic protozoa including *P. falciparum* (McCutchan *et al.*, 1995), through mechanisms still being elucidated (Sharma *et al.*, 2023). There is micro-heterogeneity between the long subunits (Sohanpal *et al.*, 2000). This represents one of the smallest numbers of rDNA coding units in eukaryotes and further highlights the streamlined nature of the genome of *T. parva*.

9.2.3 Transcriptomics

9.2.3.1 Regulation of gene expression

In eukaryotic cells, transcription regulatory elements (i.e. DNA sequences that control the timing, level and duration of transcription) are predominantly found in the NCSs between CDSs, and especially in the DNA upstream of the protein-coding region (i.e. between the 5' UTR and the intergenic sequence directly upstream of it). Guo and Silva (2008) suggested that the small size of these NCSs in the theilerial genome have resulted in unusual transcriptional initiation signals. In line with this, no classical eukaryotic elements were found in *Theileria* (Gardner *et al.*, 2005). Identification of transcription control regions in *Theileria* is a step towards elucidating the biology of this parasite.

Guo and Silva (2008) attempted to find such regions by seeking location-constrained sequence motifs enriched in *Theileria* NCSs, particularly in NCSs containing 5' UTRs and, upstream of them, promoter regions. Since, at the time, the start and end coordinates of most genes were unknown (few UTRs were annotated), CDS coordinates were used to define the boundaries of NCSs. Then, they classified NCSs according to the three possible orientations of the CDSs that flank them: 5'–5' NCSs, those flanked by genes encoded in opposite DNA strands and transcribed away from each other (genes said to be in head-to-head orientation); 5'–3' or 3'–5' NCSs, those flanked by consecutive genes encoded in the same DNA strand, and therefore in head-to-tail or tail-to-head orientation; and, finally, 3'–3' NCSs, flanked by genes in opposite strands and transcribed towards each other (and said to be in tail-to-tail orientation). They observed that 5'–5' NCSs tend to be longer (median length: 493 bp) and slightly more AT-rich than 3'–3' NCSs (median length: 154 bp), and 5'–3' or 3'–5' NCSs are of intermediate length (median length: 309 bp) and

AT composition. Tretina *et al.* (2020) extended this observation to three other *Theileria* species. When accounting for the length taken by UTRs, these results suggest extremely short intergenic regions, composed mostly of regulatory motifs. In a compact genome, intergenic space comes at a cost and the correlation between their length and the number of flanking 5' regions suggests that there is increased functionality in the 5' region due to cis-acting elements controlling transcription.

Using NCRs between pairs of orthologues in *T. parva* and *T. annulata*, Guo and Silva (2008) identified three over-represented sequence motifs with conserved positions relative to transcriptional start sites. In 2016, Tretina *et al.* (2016) validated those findings and characterized the presence of these and other motifs across additional *Theileria* and *Babesia* species. These studies found that the most abundant and taxonomically widespread motif, with several hundred to over 1000 copies per genome, was the Spe2 motif, which has a completely conserved core of three thymines and two guanines (AA**TGTGT**AA) and is thought to be recognized by a family of transcription factors involved in the progression across blood stages of the life cycle (Pieszko *et al.*, 2015). Another motif, with roughly 300 copies in the *T. parva* genome, has consensus sequence ATGGGG, is similar to the G-box motif in *Plasmodium* and is over-represented upstream of secreted proteins in *T. parva* as well as in *T. annulata* and *T. orientalis* (Tretina *et al.*, 2016). The third most abundant motif found in *T. parva* promoter regions was GATTCC, and is similar to a motif recognized by NF-κB in mammals. In addition, Tretina and colleagues (2016) also identified a degenerate motif, with sequence T(C/T)A(C/T)(A/T)(A/T)(A/T) and previously identified in *Babesia bovis* (Yamagishi *et al.*, 2014), over-represented at transcription start sites.

Finally, Tretina *et al.* (2016) identified a motif present more frequently than expected by chance in *Theileria* 3'−3' NCSs, with consensus sequence TAGTATATTATA. Its preponderance in 3'−3' NCS, lower frequency in CDSs, introns, UTRs and 5'−5' NCSs, absence near transcription start sites, peak abundance near transcription termination sites and potential to form hairpin structure, led the authors to speculate that this motif may play a structural role in transcription termination.

Antisense transcription appears to be widespread in *Theileria*. Bishop *et al.* (2005) estimated that 13.8% of the transcripts in their massively parallel signature sequencing (MPSS) data were antisense to the predicted open reading frames in the original genome annotation. These results were supported by RNA-seq data on a genome-wide level, which revealed antisense transcription to be widespread throughout all four nuclear chromosomes (Tretina *et al.*, 2020). Tretina *et al.* (2016) suggested that this may be a form of transcription control, for example by collision of RNA polymerases on opposite strands, although it is not yet known if nearby regions of both strands are transcribed in the same cell at the same time.

9.2.3.2 *Life cycle stage-specific transcription*

Despite its small genome, *Theileria* parasites must cope with an intimate association with several types of cells in the vertebrate and arthropod hosts, which, it is assumed, will require differential expression of the proteome.

An early attempt to assess transcription in *T. parva* involved MPSS in which 20 bp signature sequences were generated from a schizont cDNA library (Bishop *et al.*, 2005). The signatures were mapped against the genome sequence published by Gardner *et al.* in 2005. The schizonts were isolated from a cell line derived from the lymph node of an animal infected with a clone of the *T. parva* Muguga isolate and cultured *in vitro*. Transcripts were reliably detected for 73% of the genes predicted from the *T. parva* genome. Overall, this early study suggested that the schizont stage of the parasite expressed a substantial proportion of the genes predicted from the *T. parva* genome.

The almost universal expression of genes comprising the theilerial nuclear genome by the schizont stage was confirmed by Tonui and colleagues (2018). More remarkably, the RNA-seq data analysis of Tretina *et al.* (2020) in re-annotation of the *T. parva* Muguga genome predicted that 98% of all protein-coding sequences were transcribed by the schizont, with transcripts detected for all but 43 of the 4054 protein-coding genes.

Tonui *et al.* (2018) and, later, Atchou and colleagues (2020) compared gene expression during different life-cycle stages of *T. parva*. Atchou *et al.* compared transcripts in schizonts from infected lymphocytes cultured *in vitro* and piroplasms from infected erythrocytes harvested from an infected calf. Differential expression levels were detected in 3279 genes, with about half of these being upregulated in the schizont relative to the piroplasm stages and the other half down-regulated (51% and 49%, respectively). Only 200 genes were considered to be stage-specific. After combining the results from both studies, the authors concluded that each stage from sporoblast to piroplasm expressed most of the predicted genes, with the sporoblast showing the fewest differentially transcribed genes (Tonui *et al.*, 2018), but that genes were expressed at widely varying levels in the different stages.

The overall picture that has emerged is one where transcripts of almost all *T. parva* genes are present during most life-cycle states, with only a very limited number that are stage-specific, suggesting that relative transcript amounts, more so than the presence/absence of gene expression, define life-cycle stage. However, these studies were conducted primarily without the availability of synchronized cultures, extensive biological replicates or biospecimens from diverse environmental conditions. It is also possible that qualitative aspects of the transcripts, such as base modifications or alternative splicing, may regulate translation. It should be noted that there are as yet no studies for the tick gut-associated life-cycle stages, including the kinetes, due to the difficulty of obtaining relevant samples of these stages.

9.2.4 The apicoplast

In addition to the nuclear and mitochondrial genomes found in mammalian and other eukaryotic cells, most apicomplexans contain a third genome in an organelle called the apicoplast. Apicoplasts, which are found in all apicomplexan parasites except *Cryptosporidium*, have been incorporated into the apicomplexan cell through the secondary endosymbiosis of a red alga (reviewed by van Dooren and Striepen, 2013; McFadden and Yeh, 2017). The apicoplast undertakes basic metabolic functions in apicomplexans, including pathways required for the synthesis of heme, short chain isoprenoids and type II fatty acids, and is essential for the parasite to establish infection (Fleige *et al.*, 2010; Lim and McFadden, 2010; Besteiro, 2017; Akkerman *et al.*, 2025). The different evolutionary history of the apicoplast and its indispensable relationship with the host cells has attracted the interest of researchers aiming to develop novel therapeutic agents for the diseases caused by apicomplexans, especially malaria but also for theileriosis (McFadden and Roos, 1999; Wiesner and Seeber, 2005; Lizundia *et al.*, 2009; Chen *et al.*, 2024).

The initial sequence of the *T. parva* apicoplast was published by Gardner *et al.* (2005). This 39.5 kb organellar genome differs from that of *P. falciparum* in several ways, including that all genes are encoded in the same strand and some genes differ in copy number and structure (Gardner *et al.*, 2005). Slightly more than half of the *T. parva* apicoplast protein-coding genes have orthologues in the *P. falciparum* apicoplast, albeit with a wide range of sequence similarity (27–61%; Gardner *et al.*, 2005). The function of the apicoplast relies heavily on proteins that are encoded by nuclear genes and imported into the organelle. Of the 345 proteins predicted to be imported (fewer than the 555 predicted in *P. falciparum*), only about 100 were common to both species, suggesting that some apicoplast functions might differ. It is possible that, of the functions previously associated with the apicoplast, both *T. parva* and *T. annulata* have only retained isoprenoid biosynthesis since, unlike *Plasmodium*, they reside in the host cell's cytoplasm instead of within a parasitophorous vacuole.

In the capture DNA approach described above (Palmateer *et al.*, 2020), the probes were designed to overlap and capture both nuclear DNA and 64 of the predicted 70 genes of the apicoplast. Alignment of the sequence reads from the two additional cattle-derived isolates and the one from buffalo resulted in coverage of at least 68 apicoplast genes in each isolate. Analysis of the synonymous and non-synonymous mutations indicated that the apicoplast genome is evolving more slowly than the nuclear genome, which supports the observation that the genes encode proteins involved in functions critical for the parasite.

The apicoplast genes are conserved across several apicomplexan species.

9.3 Multigene Families in *Theileria*

Multigene, or multicopy gene, families are groups of paralogous genes thought to have arisen through one or more duplication and unequal crossing-over events, and which can share a wide range of sequence similarity, from identical to <50% sequence identity. They can occupy a non-trivial proportion of genome space, especially in gene-dense genomes such as *Theileria*'s, and are of high evolutionary significance. They can improve the fitness of an organism by allowing duplicated but slightly different proteins to perform an altered function without losing the function of the original gene product. Prime examples of multigene families are found in components of the immune system of vertebrates, such as the immunoglobulin genes and those encoding the major histocompatibility complex. They also provide redundancy in complex and vital cellular functions.

Despite the low amount of non-protein encoding repetitive DNA in the *T. parva* genome, several protein-encoding multigene families have been identified. The original genome annotation identified 384 protein families containing a combined total of 1063 paralogues (Gardner *et al.*, 2005), more than a quarter of all protein-coding genes. Despite the high abundance of multigene families in *T. parva*, relatively little is known about their function. However, by analogy with other species of parasitic protozoa, it is likely that some of these predicted proteins are involved in parasite–host or parasite–vector interactions (Wahlgren *et al.*, 2017; Goo, 2022; Singh *et al.*, 2024; Hakimi *et al.*, 2025; Zhan *et al.*, 2025).

Although the functions of multigene families in *T. parva* are yet to be fully established, their underlying importance justifies further research to uncover targets for immunological or therapeutic intervention. We describe here some of the most studied multigene families in *T. parva* (Fig. 9.3).

9.3.1 *Theileria parva* repeat (*Tpr*) genes

The most dynamic multigene family in *T. parva* is composed of the *Tpr* genes (for *Theileria parva* repeat), with *Tar* being the homologous family in *T. annulata* (Weir *et al.*, 2009). These families encode proteins defined by a C-terminal domain of 245 amino acids that is relatively conserved among copies within and between genomes of different strains and even between *Theileria* species (Palmateer *et al.*, 2023). This conserved protein domain contains five transmembrane motifs, suggesting that the Tpr proteins are membrane-associated, consistent with a role in parasite–host interactions and antigenicity; the N-terminus, when present, is semi-conserved, and the central region is highly variable and can also be absent (Bishop *et al.*, 1997; Weir *et al.*, 2009; Palmateer *et al.*, 2023).

Tpr genes can be classified into two types, according to their genomic location (Palmateer *et al.*, 2023): (i) most belong to the '*Tpr* locus', a species-specific tandem array of at least 29 copies located internally on *T. parva*'s chromosome 3; (ii) 13 other copies are dispersed throughout all four nuclear chromosomes, with two in chromosome 1, three each in chromosomes 2 and 4 and the remainder in chromosome 3, but not in the *Tpr* locus. The copies in the *Tpr* locus share a high degree of sequence similarity, but some are truncated (missing the central regions and/or the N-terminal domain), suggesting that this locus has expanded in copy number relatively recently through duplication and possibly recombination and gene conversion (Bishop *et al.*, 1997; Palmateer *et al.*, 2023). The repetitive nature of the *Tpr* locus prevented the full assembly of this region of chromosome 3 in the original assembly, although the locus was estimated to be ~100 kb (Gardner *et al.*, 2005). One of three gaps present in the *Tpr* locus in the original assembly was closed with the use of long-read PacBio sequencing, and the current length of the locus that has been assembled stands at 65 kb (Fig. 9.3; Palmateer *et al.*, 2023). The tandem arrangement of copies to form the *Tpr* locus is absent in *T. annulata* (Pain *et al.*, 2005; Weir *et al.*, 2009), consistent with its recent emergence in the lineage leading to *T. parva*.

Interestingly, the three *Tpr* copies with the most divergent C-terminus have syntenic

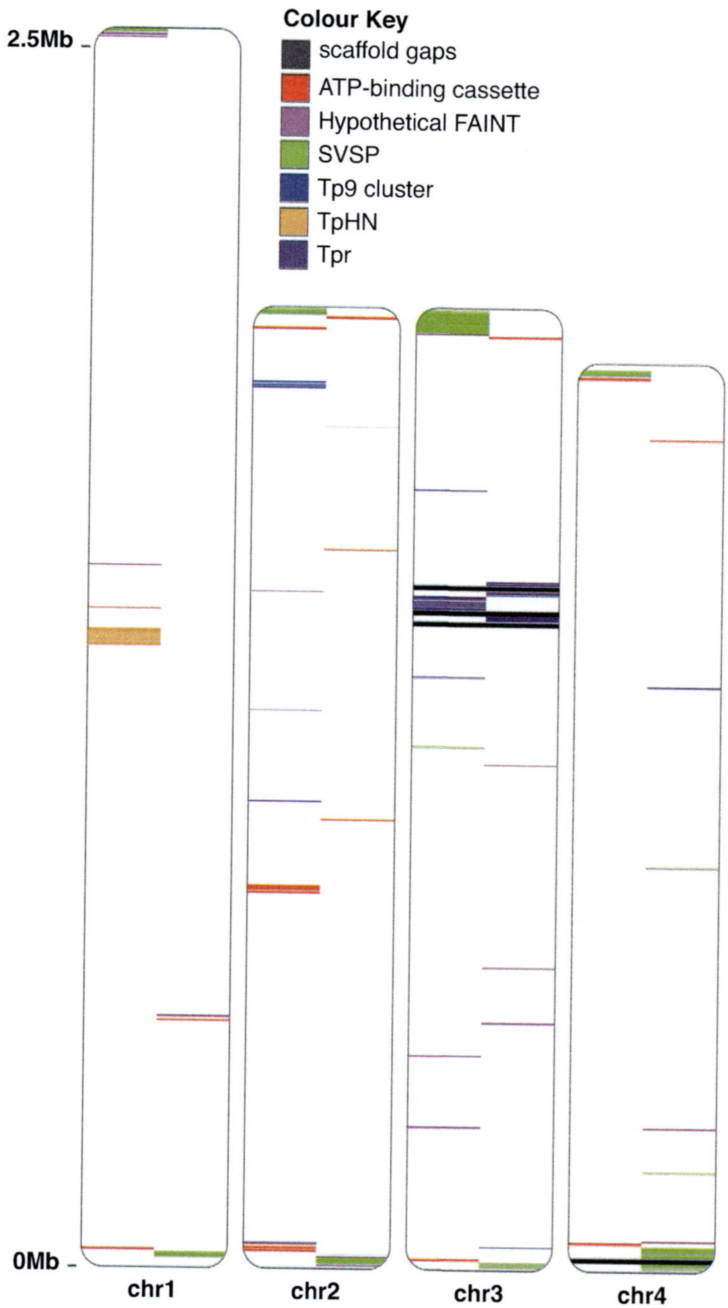

Fig. 9.3. Chromosomal location of members of select *T. parva* multigene families. The distribution of loci encoding members of six *T. parva* gene families is shown by chromosome and strand. Subtelomeric-encoded variable secreted proteins (SVSP) loci (green) are present in all eight subtelomeric regions and are always transcribed towards the end of the chromosome. Genes containing ATP binding cassettes (red) are almost always present in the transition between SVSP loci and the core of each chromosome. Physical gaps in the assembly (black) are located in regions containing genes of the Tpr (chromosome 3) or SVSP (chromosome 4) families. (Figure kindly provided by Jonathan Crabtree.)

homologues in *Theileria* sp. (buffalo) (an undescribed *Theileria* species that infects African Cape buffalo, and likely the species most closely related to *T. parva*), in *T. annulata* and in the more distantly related species *Theileria equi* and *Cytauxzoon felis* (from a genus closely related to *Theileria*), but are absent in *Theileria orientalis* and in *Babesia* species, suggesting gene loss in sole lineages. These three loci behave like orthologues, as suggested by their syntenic chromosome location and with phylogenetic relationships that mirror those between species (Palmateer *et al.*, 2023).

Differential expression analysis in *T. parva* showed that *Tpr* genes from the *Tpr* locus appear to be preferentially expressed in the piroplasm stage (n=16) or the sporozoite stage (n=13), with nine genes highly expressed in both, relative to the schizont stage (Tonui *et al.*, 2018; Atchou *et al.*, 2020). The preferential expression of *Tpr* locus family members in these two stages of the life cycle, together with their high amino acid substitution rate (Weir *et al.*, 2010), led Palmateer and colleagues (2023) to speculate that *Tpr* locus-encoded proteins may be involved in cell invasion, be it the entry of sporozoites into mammalian leukocytes or the establishment of piroplasm infection of the mammalian red blood cells.

Interestingly, two of the *Tpr* genes outside of the *Tpr* locus that have syntenic copies across multiple *Theileria* species, in what Palmateer and colleagues called *Tpr* clades α and γ, are among the most highly expressed genes in the schizont stage (Tonui *et al.*, 2018; Atchou *et al.*, 2020; Palmateer *et al.*, 2023), suggesting a role during intra-lymphocyte multiplication. Two of these phylogenetically conserved *Tpr* genes, those in *Tpr* clades β and δ (Palmateer *et al.*, 2023), are nonetheless absent in *T. orientalis* and *T. equi* (Palmateer *et al.*, 2023). Since the schizont stage is transient in these two species, it is tempting to speculate that their function is essential only for prolonged schizogony.

9.3.2 Subtelomeric-encoded variable secreted proteins (SVSPs)

Polymorphic, paralogous multicopy gene families are frequently located in subtelomeric regions of the genomes of parasitic protozoa, and this is also the case for *T. parva*. Initial sequencing studies of two of the four nuclear chromosomes of *T. parva* revealed that telomere-associated DNA contained long open reading frames (ORFs) with sequence identity >50% across the 5' end, indicating the presence of a multigene family, and that these ORFs were within 3 kb from the telomeric repeats (Bishop *et al.*, 2000). These are among the closest ORFs to telomeres ever found in any organism, again a reflection of the high gene density of the *T. parva* genome. This was the first report of *T. parva*'s SVSPs.

With the original release of the annotated *T. parva* genome, in 2005, a total of 85 SVSP-encoding genes were annotated in the genome of the reference Muguga *T. parva* strain, making this the most abundant multigene family in the species (Gardner *et al.*, 2005). The current release of PiroplasmaDB, the database in VEuPathDB providing genomic resources for piroplasmids (Alvarez-Jarreta *et al.*, 2024), reports 94 genes in the SVSP homologous cluster, as detected by OrthoMCL (Carhuaricra-Huaman and Setubal, 2024). In 2023, Palmateer and colleagues used long-read PacBio sequencing to close the existing gap in chromosome 4, which falls within a cluster of SVSP-encoding genes, and identified four additional SVSP ORFs, bringing to 98 the total number of members of this gene family in the Muguga genome. Even though all eight subtelomeric regions of the nuclear chromosomes of *T. parva* Muguga encode SVSPs, their distribution is uneven. Chromosomes 1 and 2 of the Muguga strain, with nine and 18 SVSP-encoding genes respectively, contain the fewest copies, while chromosomes 3 and 4, with 36 and 35, respectively, encode the largest arrays. Interestingly, five genes in this gene family, two in chromosome 3 (TpMuguga_03g00298 and _03g00498) and three in chromosome 4 (TpMuguga_04g00098, _04g00099 and _04g00406) are located in the core genome, that is, are not subtelomeric. It stands to be determined if these genes have syntenic homologues in *T. annulata* and if their mode of evolution differs from those in tandem arrays in the subtelomeric regions.

Many of the encoded SVSP proteins contained a predicted N-terminal signal peptide, suggesting secretion into the mammalian host cell, and one of these signal peptides was shown to be functional in a heterologous system, complementing secretion in Baker's yeast (Bishop *et al.*, 2000). Some SVSP genes also encode a functional nuclear localization signal, and might target the nucleolus, which has led to the hypothesis that these proteins can be targeted to the host nucleus and modulate gene expression (Schmuckli-Maurer *et al.*, 2009). The PEST motif, a proteolytic signal associated with rapid degradation of nuclear proteins (Rogers *et al.*, 1986), which is enriched in proline (P), glutamic acid (E), serine (S) and threonine (T) residues, can also be found in a subset of SVSP copies. Finally, several copies contain a motif known as FAINT (frequently associated in *Theileria*; Pain *et al.*, 2005), whose function is unknown (hence its alternative PFAM name 'domain of unknown function 529' – DUF529, in the InterPro database). The relative frequency of SVSPs with different combinations of signal peptides and motifs, the genomic distributions of those variants in the reference Muguga genome and whether these features vary among *T. parva* strains remains unknown.

Similar to what is observed with subtelomeric gene families in *P. falciparum*, expression of SVSP-encoding genes is complex. At least some SVSP copies are differentially expressed between different *T. parva* isolates, according to results from PCR assays, and only a minority of parasites appear to express some of the SVSPs (Schmuckli-Maurer *et al.*, 2009). However, it remains to be shown whether multiple SVSPs can be expressed in the same cell.

A study using Southern blots identified extensive between-strain variation in SVSPs due to either presence/absence or sequence divergence, such that some Muguga SVSP ORFs could not be detected in a different *T. parva* strain (Bishop *et al.*, 2000). The reference genome of the relatively closely related species *T. annulata* contains 53 SVSP copies (Pain *et al.*, 2005), and that of the more distantly related (non-host transforming) species *T. orientalis* contains none (Hayashida *et al.*, 2012), reflecting the lineage-specific nature of this protein family.

The presence of these proteins only in host-transforming *Theileria* species, and their potential to alter host gene expression, led to the hypothesis that these proteins can alter host cell phenotypes (Schmuckli-Maurer *et al.*, 2009). Recent experimental studies using a yeast two-hybrid system have demonstrated the ability of specific *T. annulata* SVSP to bind bovine proteins, and microscopy and co-immunoprecipitation were employed to validate the binding in *ex vivo* experiments (Li *et al.*, 2021, 2022; Ma *et al.*, 2024). However, the rapid amino acid sequence evolution of SVSP copies has led to the suggestion that their evolution is consistent with a role in host immune system subversion (Weir *et al.*, 2010), rather than being marked by the substantive sequence conservation associated with functional constraint. The fact that five *T. parva* Muguga SVSPs have been identified as antigens recognized by parasite-specific CD4 T cells (Morrison *et al.*, 2021) is consistent with their immunogenicity.

9.3.3 ATP-binding cassette proteins

ATP-binding cassette transporter genes, a family of proteins that mediate transfer of ions across membranes, are located immediately interior to the multicopy SVSP-encoding genes in seven of the eight subtelomeric regions, the exception being the subtelomeric region in chromosome 1 with the fewest number of SVSP copies (only three copies). However, there are also gene-encoding ATP-binding cassette proteins at other locations in the *T. parva* genome. There is no indication as to why the genes encoding a particular subset within this protein transport superfamily are subtelomerically located or whether the location has any functional significance.

9.3.4 *T. parva* host nuclear (*TpHN*) genes

The genes in the *TpHN* family are present as a cluster of 20 contiguous genes on chromosome 1 (Shiels *et al.*, 2006). An homologous gene family of 17 genes known as *TashAT* (for *T. annulata* macroschizont-specific AT hook-containing protein) is found in *T. annulata*, and the gene families show a high level of conservation between the species (Swan *et al.*, 1999; Shiels *et al.*, 2006). They were initially identified in *T. annulata*, in a screen for genes that are down-regulated during differentiation from the schizont to merozoite stage. They were found to bear an AT hook DNA binding domain (Swan *et al.*, 2001). The genes in both species encode predicted proteins with signal peptides, nuclear localization signals and PEST motifs, similarly to some SVSPs. However, unlike *TashAT* genes, the *TpHN* genes do not encode a consensus AT hook domain (Shiels *et al.*, 2006). The *TashAT* genes in *T. annulata* are expressed in the schizont and their expression is down-regulated during merogony. Expansion of this gene cluster appears to be confined to host-transforming species of *Theileria*. Only one gene in the cluster has an orthologue in *T. orientalis*, and, in contrast to the *TashAT* genes, it shows elevated expression levels during merogony (Hayashida *et al.*, 2012). Functional studies with some of the *TashAT* gene products have confirmed their ability to localize to the host cell nucleus, and transfection of a bovine macrophage cell line with one of the *TashAT* genes was shown to result in altered host gene expression (Swan *et al.*, 1999; Durrani *et al.*, 2023). The function of the products of these gene families is not understood, but available information suggests that they may be involved in host cell transformation and/or in regulating parasite differentiation.

9.3.5 Tp9 cluster

A cluster of nine genes, one of which encodes the Tp9 protein, is present on chromosome 2 of *T. parva*. The genes are predicted to encode polypeptides with a conserved N-terminal signal peptide, two loosely conserved regions towards the C terminus and a highly polymorphic, low-complexity central region rich in proline and glutamine residues, part of which constitutes a predicted PEST domain. An orthologous cluster of four genes is present in *T. annulata*, also on chromosome 2. The *Tp9/Ta9* gene clusters are considered specific to transforming species of *Theileria*; only a single, poorly conserved gene is found in *T. orientalis*. Genes encoding *Ta9* (TA15705) and the *T. parva* orthologue *Tp9* (TpMuguga_02g00895; originally TP02_0895) were first identified while screening for antigens recognized by cytotoxic CD8 T cells from cattle immune to *T. annulata* and *T. parva*, respectively (MacHugh *et al.*, 2011; Hemmink *et al.*, 2016). The antigens encoded by both species induce highly dominant CD8 T cell responses (MacHugh *et al.*, 2009, 2011) and also CD4 T cell responses in the case of *T. parva* (Morrison *et al.*, 2021). They also elicit strong antibody responses (Bilgic *et al.*, 2016; Bastos *et al.*, 2019). *Tp9* and *Ta9* are among the most abundantly expressed genes in the schizont stage of the respective parasites and their expression levels decrease during early merogony. The *Ta9* gene was also identified in a screen of *T. annulata* schizont cDNAs capable of activating the host cell transcription factor AP-1 (Unlu *et al.*, 2018), and the gene product was detected in the cytoplasm of *T. annulata*-infected cells (Brühlmann *et al.*, 2024). Although the function of proteins encoded by *Tp9/Ta9* genes are not understood, preliminary findings suggest that they may be involved as part of the host cell transformation process (see Chapter 10 of this volume).

9.4 Applications of Genotyping and Genome Sequencing

There are several biological properties of *T. parva* and aspects of the epidemiology of disease caused by the parasite that are incompletely understood and for which further application of genome sequencing can advance our understanding. Much has been learned from the sequences that have been studied to date, but they represent a very small sample of a parasite population that is now known to be highly polymorphic. The genome sequences have also been obtained from parasites with a limited geographic range relative to the overall distribution of the species. There have been significant recent advances in sequencing technologies, which, coupled with the availability of high-quality, thoroughly annotated reference *T. parva* genome sequences, now provide a platform for undertaking larger-scale genomic studies of the parasite.

9.4.1 Genotypic heterogeneity in *T. parva* from cattle and buffalo

Cattle infected by *T. parva* transmitted from buffalo develop an acute, usually fatal disease similar to ECF but with lower levels of parasitized cells in lymphoid tissues and few piroplasms (see Chapter 5 of this volume). The latter is responsible for the failure of tick transmission of the buffalo-derived parasites from cattle (discussed further in Section 9.4.2). Clear evidence of immunological differences between buffalo-derived *T. parva* and the parasites maintained in cattle became apparent during studies that led to development of the Infection and Treatment Method (ITM) of vaccination. Although immunization of cattle with the mixture of three parasite isolates (known as the Muguga cocktail) eventually used in the commercialized vaccine provided robust protection against experimental challenge with several parasite isolates and against field challenge, it did not provide protection against challenge with parasites originating from buffalo (Radley *et al.*, 1975). This was demonstrated in early studies in which ITM-immunized cattle introduced into a clean paddock together with an infected buffalo remained susceptible to infection (Radley *et al.*, 1979). Two more recent studies on ranches in the Central and Rift Valley Provinces of Kenya, involving introduction of ITM-vaccinated animals into areas grazed solely or predominantly by buffalo, showed that most vaccinated animals developed severe disease (Bishop *et al.*, 2015; Sitt *et al.*, 2015).

Consistent with the results of these immunological findings, several studies have demonstrated that the parasites in buffalo contain much greater genotypic diversity than those maintained in cattle (Pelle *et al.*, 2011; Hemmink *et al.*, 2018; summarized in Chapter 5 of this volume), supporting the idea that cattle *T. parva* represent a subset that has adapted to maintenance in cattle. Additionally, buffalo are almost invariably infected with multiple parasite genotypes (Oura *et al.*, 2011; Hemmink *et al.*, 2018). The greater genetic diversity in buffalo has been confirmed by whole genome sequencing, initially using DNA isolated from partially purified schizonts from infected T-cell lines (Hayashida *et al.*, 2013) and more recently by oligonucleotide capture from similar samples (Palmateer *et al.*, 2020; Maboko *et al.*, 2021; J.C. Silva *et al.*, unpublished data). Buffalo isolates consistently contained at least twice the number of single nucleotide polymorphisms (SNPs), compared to the reference Muguga genome, than cattle isolates (Palmateer *et al.*, 2020). Capture-based enrichment of *T. parva* DNA was also used by Palmateer *et al.* (2020) to generate the first full genome assembly of a *T. parva* strain from buffalo. At 8.366 Mbp, this assembly was 20 kbp longer than the reference Muguga genome, despite the presence of several gaps in repetitive regions, and contained a number of structural variations, including expansion of repeat regions, deletions and insertions. As mentioned above, 25 additional genes were found in the genome assembly of the buffalo-derived strain, 19 with homology to *T. parva* Muguga genes and a further six genes most similar to genes found in *T. annulata* or *T. orientalis*. The presence of these 25 new genes was substantiated by read coverage from a distinct isolate from buffalo reported by Hayashida and colleagues (2013).

A wider representation of buffalo *T. parva* genome sequences from different geographical sites is required to provide a clearer definition of the distinctive characteristics of cattle and buffalo parasites. Despite the immunological differences between cattle and buffalo parasites discussed above, in Tanzania there are no documented cases of ECF in ITM-vaccinated cattle in the Maasai areas where buffalo graze adjacent to the cattle (Homewood *et al.*, 2006). The only study so far conducted of the genetic diversity of *T. parva* in buffalo in Tanzania was that of Rukambile *et al.* (2016), using satellite DNA typing applied to a limited number of buffalo from several geographically separated national parks. The mean number of alleles per sample (used as a proxy for the number of genotypes in the host animal), at 3.37, was relatively lower than would be expected for *T. parva* parasites circulating in buffalo in Kenya or southern Uganda. However, the animals were present in national parks and not pastoralist areas where buffalo co-graze with vaccinated cattle. The comparative analysis of parasites in buffalo and cattle in areas where cattle are vaccinated and graze in close proximity to buffalo awaits a definitive study. More generally, examination of the genome sequences of *T. parva* parasites in such cattle is warranted to explore whether there has been any introgression of buffalo genotypes into the cattle-maintained parasites.

9.4.2 Parasite differentiation and tick transmissibility

A key feature that distinguishes buffalo-derived *T. parva* from the parasite population maintained in cattle is that infections of cattle with the former are not transmissible by ticks and there is no establishment of a tick-transmissible carrier state (Neitz and Jansen, 1956). This is consistent with detection of few microschizonts (i.e. parasites undergoing merogony) and no or very few piroplasms in cattle infected with parasites from buffalo, findings that indicate a failure of differentiation of the schizont stage of the parasite to generate the tick-infective piroplasms (Lawrence, 1937; Young *et al.*, 1977). As discussed in Chapter 5 of this volume, this finding is not unique to *T. parva*. Sheep are susceptible to infection with *T. annulata*, but the infections do not generate piroplasms and are not transmissible by ticks (Leemans *et al.*, 1999a, b). Hence, the ability of *Theileria* parasites to differentiate from the schizont stage appears to be a critical step in the ability of the parasites to adapt to new host species. Although most attempts to transmit infections with buffalo-derived *T. parva* in cattle with ticks have been unsuccessful, a few experimental studies using large numbers of experimentally infected ticks have achieved transmission and, following further tick passages of these parasites, they have come to resemble cattle-maintained *T. parva* and are readily transmitted by ticks (Brocklesby and Barnett, 1966; Young and Purnell, 1973; Maritim *et al.*, 1989), a phenomenon referred to as 'behavioural transformation'. A possible genetic model to explain these findings, based on the occurrence of multiple recombination events during repeated passage of the genotypically heterogeneous buffalo parasites, is presented in Chapter 5 of this volume. Currently, it is unknown whether there is a similar barrier to establishing infections in buffalo with cattle isolates of *T. parva*. The availability of a larger panel of *T. parva* genome sequences would allow identification of alleles of genes that are largely restricted to cattle or buffalo parasites, which may be involved in regulating tick transmissibility. Raw data exist from a series of such cattle-infective but non-transmissible isolates with partial or near-complete genome sequence data, but have not yet been fully analysed (J.C. Silva and R.P. Bishop, unpublished data). Moreover, sequencing of parasites at different stages of tick passage in experiments to achieve behavioural transformation of buffalo parasites could aid in identification of genes involved in parasite differentiation and tick transmissibility. This would require experiments to repeat the study of buffalo-derived parasites subjected to sequential tick passage in cattle. A cryopreserved stock of the starting parasite population used in one of the previous studies to produce the behaviourally transformed parasites is available.

9.4.3 Cell tropism of the parasite

Detailed studies of the susceptibility of different lineages of cells to infection with *T. parva* using the Muguga isolate have demonstrated that the CD4, CD8 and gamma/delta subsets of T cells, as well as B cells, are infected by the parasite. Sporozoites are able to bind to and invade these cell types and establish cell lines with similar efficiency (Baldwin *et al.*, 1988). These findings have been confirmed with a further two Kenyan isolates, namely Marikebuni and Mariakani. *T. parva* sporozoites can also invade monocytes and dendritic cells but do not undergo further development in these cells. By contrast, investigation of a Zambian isolate (Chitongo) has shown that infection with this parasite is restricted to CD8 T cells and that this parasite is less virulent than the reference Muguga isolate (Tindih *et al.*, 2012).

The parasite and host proteins involved in invasion of lymphocytes by sporozoites are poorly understood. Antibodies specific for an abundant protein (p67, encoded by TpMuguga_03g00287) in the sporozoite surface coat prevent binding of sporozoites to bovine lymphocytes and neutralize their infectivity *in vitro* (Dobbelaere *et al.*, 1984). Strong neutralization has also been obtained with antibodies specific for another two sporozoite proteins (Nyagwange *et al.*, 2018). Somewhat surprisingly, given the expression of host class I MHC (major histocompatibility complex) proteins on most cell types, antibodies specific for these proteins have also been shown to neutralize sporozoite infectivity, and mutated cells lacking class I MHC expression show reduced binding of sporozoites (Shaw *et al.*, 1991, 1995). As discussed in Chapter 3 of this volume, these findings suggest that host cell invasion by *T. parva* involves more than a single molecular interaction.

Despite the marked difference in cell tropism of the Chitongo isolate of *T. parva*, the sequence of the gene encoding the p67 sporozoite protein is identical to that of eastern African parasites. The distinct phenotype of this parasite at a fundamental trait provides an opportunity to examine its genome sequence to investigate differences from the reference Muguga sequence that could influence cell tropism. More generally, there is a need to determine whether the Chitongo phenotype is a feature of other *T. parva* parasites in Zambia and neighbouring countries.

9.4.4 Potential impact of the Muguga cocktail on natural parasite populations

Because natural infections of cattle with *T. parva* typically induce a tick-transmissible carrier state (Bishop *et al.*, 1992; Kariuki *et al.*, 1995; Skilton *et al.*, 2002; Oura *et al.*, 2004), the parasites in the ITM live vaccine may establish a carrier state that would facilitate their transfer into field ticks and cattle. Evidence for the presence of a vaccine component parasite in calves following vaccination by ITM was first reported by Oura *et al.* (2004) during a trial of the Muguga cocktail ITM vaccine at a site near Iganga, in eastern Uganda. The study used nested PCRs to amplify segments of the PIM gene (TpMuguga_04g00051), designed to be specific for the Kiambu or Muguga parasite isolates (based on sequence data available at the time). Vaccinated animals gave positive results with the Muguga primers for a short period following vaccination, whereas the Kiambu primers gave positive results in samples from most animals up to three years after vaccination. These results provided strong evidence that the Kiambu component of the ITM vaccine establishes a carrier state and suggest that the live vaccine, as well as controlling the disease, could spread the parasite into regions where vaccinated herds graze (McKeever, 2007). This hypothesis would be especially relevant to vaccination in areas bordering the known extent of *T. parva* distribution and which are ecologically suitable for the *Rhipicephalus appendiculatus* vector.

The availability of an expanding collection of *T. parva* genome sequences is likely to provide information that will allow the design of specific and more easily applied assays to unequivocally detect the parasite strains in the vaccine, which have been genotyped (Norling *et al.*, 2015).

9.4.5 Spread of *T. parva* in sub-Saharan Africa

The core region where East Coast fever has the greatest impact, causing high levels of mortality, includes Kenya, Uganda, Tanzania and surrounding countries in eastern and central Africa. However, the distribution of *T. parva* is not as wide as that predicted for the tick vector according to climate-based models (Norval *et al.*, 1992). So, there is potential for *T. parva* to spread, especially given the largely unregulated transboundary cattle movements between certain countries within the eastern and central African region.

Two countries which represent contrasting situations have recently been investigated using molecular epidemiology. In South Sudan, *T. parva* is moving northwards (Malak *et al.*, 2012; Marcellino *et al.*, 2017), and in Cameroon, the parasite has recently been discovered for the first time (Silatsa *et al.*, 2020). *T. parva* can therefore be considered an emerging pathogen in these regions. It is likely that cattle movement has played a major role in the spread of the parasite in both instances, but aspects of the epidemiology are distinct between Cameroon and South Sudan. In South Sudan, the tick vector *R. appendiculatus* is present in all four cattle populations surveyed, and 61 (25%) of cattle sampled, using a sensitive nested PCR assay based on the p104 antigen gene (TpMuguga_04g00437), were infected with *T. parva* (Odongo et al., 2010; Marcellino *et al.*, 2017). Genotyping using 14 micro- and minisatellites revealed very high levels of diversity in Sudanese cattle, with an average of 9.57 alleles per locus and a range of between 6 and 15 alleles per locus (Salih *et al.*, 2018). Principal components analysis applied to the Sudanese data indicated a degree of substructure suggesting that the populations were partially distinct, with limited gene flow between them. This indicates that multiple migrations of *T. parva*-infected cattle, together with the tick vector, are likely to have occurred into different regions of South Sudan. In a participatory survey, farmers from one of two districts regarded ECF as their most serious animal health problem (Malak *et al.*, 2012). The fact that the vector is present suggests that the parasite is likely to be maintained and will continue to cause a serious challenge for cattle keepers in South Sudan.

By contrast, in Cameroon, all surveyed animals were asymptomatic and a parallel comprehensive countrywide tick survey did not reveal the presence of the major vector *R. appendiculatus*, although the other expected ixodid tick species associated with livestock were present (Silatsa *et al.*, 2019). Among animals surveyed using a *T. parva*-specific ELISA, 23.76% were serologically positive and, of 1324 DNA samples from blood assessed by PCR using the p104 nested PCR assay, 1.86%, representing 25 animals, were positive. Sequencing of the p104 gene was used to genotype the *T. parva*, although this locus has not typically been used as a polymorphic marker as it usually displays limited polymorphism and is used in a standard diagnostic PCR assay (Skilton *et al.*, 2002; Odongo *et al.*, 2010). The p104 sequences of *T. parva* from Cameroon revealed seven genotypes, some of the rarer ones not having been described previously. What is clear is that *T. parva* is present in asymptomatic cattle in Cameroon, although there is currently no known tick vector in the country. Given this and the asymptomatic nature of the infections in Cameroon, the most obvious explanation is that infection has been introduced by movement of carrier cattle from endemic areas outside Cameroon. However, the presence of positive animals in different regions of the country, and the apparent genotypic diversity of the parasites, would imply frequent movement of infected animals, which seems unlikely given that Cameroon does not border other *T. parva*-endemic countries. An alternative explanation, as suggested by Silatsa *et al.* (2019), is that the parasite is maintained in Cameroon by another tick species.

In both Sudan and Cameroon, additional analyses of parasite genotypes using high-resolution next-generation 'deep' sequencing of variable loci, as preliminarily characterized in Table 2 of Palmateer *et al.* (2020, p. 16), and ideally also whole genome sequencing, will be required to determine the likely origin of the parasites and whether they display any unique features. This is of particular relevance for the parasites detected in Cameroon, which appear to exhibit very different characteristics than *T. parva* in other endemic areas.

9.5 Conclusions

Theileria genomes are generally highly compact, with selection seemingly favouring short introns and intergenic regions. By contrast, *Plasmodium* genomes are considerably larger. There is only a single well-annotated 8.3 Mb *T. parva* genome reference sequence containing 4055 predicted protein encoding regions following recent re-annotation. Several other *T. parva* genomes, from cattle and buffalo origin, have been generated based on capture array technology, using oligonucleotides derived from the reference sequence, an approach that enables enrichment of the parasite DNA relative to that of bovine cells with high specificity and sensitivity (Palmateer *et al.*, 2020; Maboko *et al.*, 2021; R. Bishop and J.C. Silva, unpublished data). These include vaccine stocks, strains with relevant phenotype and unique provenance, and several parasites of buffalo origin. Further exploration of these data may start to shed light into the genetic architecture of phenotypes of interest.

As in other parasitic protozoa, there are numerous multicopy gene families present, but no indication of their function. Knowledge of the role of specific genes in *Theileria* biology, including immortalization of bovine host lymphocytes, would benefit greatly from a system enabling functional genetic manipulations, but methods for genetic manipulation of *Theileria* have not yet been established. *Theileria parva* genomics is under-researched, particularly in a field context. Preliminary investigation suggests high diversity of *T. parva* in the field, including among cattle-derived strains but particularly so among parasites in buffalo. Additional complete genomes are desirable and would allow insight into population genomics, including the extent of the differentiation of cattle and buffalo parasite populations and how population genetic structure is altered locally by live vaccination and monitoring the spread of *T. parva* in central Africa.

References

Akkerman, L.J., Kooij, T.W.A. and Vries, L.E. (2025) The apicoplast transportome of the malaria parasite. *Trends in Parasitology* 41(8), 641–656. DOI: 10.1016/j.pt.2025.06.011.

Alvarez-Jarreta, J., Amos, B., Aurrecoechea, C., Bah, S., Barba, M. *et al.* (2024) VEuPathDB: The eukaryotic pathogen, vector and host bioinformatics resource center in 2023. *Nucleic Acids Research* 52(D1), D808–D816. DOI: 10.1093/nar/gkad1003.

Ashley, E.A. (2021) *The Genome Odyssey: Medical Mysteries and the Incredible Quest to Solve Them*, 1st edn. Celadon Books, New York.

Atchou, K., Ongus, J., Machuka, E., Juma, J., Tiambo, C. *et al.* (2020) Comparative transcriptomics of the bovine apicomplexan parasite *Theileria parva* developmental stages reveals massive gene expression variation and potential vaccine antigens. *Frontiers in Veterinary Science* 7, 287. DOI: 10.3389/fvets.2020.00287.

Baldwin, C.L., Black, S.J., Brown, W.C., Conrad, P.A., Goddeeris, B.M. *et al.* (1988) Bovine T cells, B cells, and null cells are transformed by the protozoan parasite *Theileria parva*. *Infection and Immunity* 56(2), 462–467. DOI: 10.1128/iai.56.2.462-467.1988.

Bastos, R.G., Franceschi, V., Tebaldi, G., Connelley, T., Morrison, W.I. *et al.* (2019) Molecular and antigenic properties of mammalian cell-expressed *Theileria parva* antigen Tp9. *Frontiers in Immunology* 10, 897. DOI: 10.3389/fimmu.2019.00897.

Besteiro, S. (2017) Autophagy in apicomplexan parasites. *Current Opinion in Microbiology* 40, 14–20. DOI: 10.1016/j.mib.2017.10.008.

Bilgic, H.B., Karagenc, T., Bakırcı, S., Shiels, B., Tait, A. *et al.* (2016) Identification and analysis of immunodominant antigens for ELISA-based detection of *Theileria annulata*. *PLoS ONE* 11(6), e0156645. DOI: 10.1371/journal.pone.0156645.

Bishop, R., Sohanpal, B., Kariuki, D.P., Young, A.S., Nene, V. *et al.* (1992) Detection of a carrier state in *Theileria parva*-infected cattle by the polymerase chain reaction. *Parasitology* 104(Pt 2), 215–232. DOI: 10.1017/s0031182000061655.

Bishop, R., Musoke, A., Morzaria, S., Sohanpal, B. and Gobright, E. (1997) Concerted evolution at a multicopy locus in the protozoan parasite *Theileria parva*: Extreme divergence of potential protein-coding sequences. *Molecular and Cellular Biology* 17(3), 1666–1673. DOI: 10.1128/MCB.17.3.1666.

Bishop, R., Morzaria, S. and Gobright, E. (1998) Linkage of two distinct AT-rich minisatellites AT multiple loci in the genome of *Theileria parva*. *Gene* 216(2), 245–254. DOI: 10.1016/s0378-1119(98)00336-9.

Bishop, R., Gobright, E., Nene, V., Morzaria, S., Musoke, A. *et al.* (2000) Polymorphic open reading frames encoding secretory proteins are located less than 3 kilobases from *Theileria parva* telomeres. *Molecular and Biochemical Parasitology* 110(2), 359–371. DOI: 10.1016/S0166-6851(00)00291-7.

Bishop, R., Shah, T., Pelle, R., Hoyle, D., Pearson, T. *et al.* (2005) Analysis of the transcriptome of the protozoan *Theileria parva* using MPSS reveals that the majority of genes are transcriptionally active in the schizont stage. *Nucleic Acids Research* 33(17), 5503–5511. DOI: 10.1093/nar/gki818.

Bishop, R.P., Hemmink, J.D., Morrison, W.I., Weir, W., Toye, P.G. *et al.* (2015) The african buffalo parasite *Theileria* sp. (buffalo) can infect and immortalize cattle leukocytes and encodes divergent orthologues of *Theileria parva* antigen genes. *International Journal for Parasitology: Parasites and Wildlife* 4(3), 333–342. DOI: 10.1016/j.ijppaw.2015.08.006.

Brocklesby, D.W. and Barnett, S.F. (1966) The isolation of "*Theileria lawrencei* (Kenya)" from a wild buffalo (*Syncerus caffer*) and its serial passage through captive buffaloes. *British Veterinary Journal* 122, 387–395. DOI: 10.1016/S0007-1935(17)40405-2.

Brühlmann, F., Perry, C., Griessen, C., Gunasekera, K., Reymond, J.-L. *et al.* (2024) TurboID mapping reveals the exportome of secreted intrinsically disordered proteins in the transforming parasite *Theileria annulata*. *mBio* 15(6), e0341223. DOI: 10.1128/mbio.03412-23.

Carhuaricra-Huaman, D. and Setubal, J.C. (2024) Protein-coding gene families in prokaryote genome comparisons. *Methods in Molecular Biology* 2802, 33–55. DOI: 10.1007/978-1-0716-3838-5_2.

Cerqueira, A.V. and Lemos, B. (2019) Ribosomal DNA and the nucleolus as keystones of nuclear architecture, organization, and function. *Trends in Genetics* 35(10), 710–723. DOI: 10.1016/j.tig.2019.07.011.

Chen, X., Suo, X., Zhu, G. and Shen, B. (2024) The apicoplast biogenesis and metabolism: Current progress and questions. *Trends in Parasitology* 40(12), 1144–1158. DOI: 10.1016/j.pt.2024.10.019.

D'Alfonso, A., Micheli, G. and Camilloni, G. (2024) rDNA transcription, replication and stability in *Saccharomyces cerevisiae*. *Seminars in Cell & Developmental Biology* 159–160, 1–9. DOI: 10.1016/j.semcdb.2024.01.004.

Dobbelaere, D.A., Spooner, P.R., Barry, W.C. and Irvin, A.D. (1984) Monoclonal antibody neutralizes the sporozoite stage of different *Theileria parva* stocks. *Parasite Immunology* 6(4), 361–370. DOI: 10.1111/j.1365-3024.1984.tb00808.x.

Durrani, Z., Kinnaird, J., Cheng, C.W., Brühlmann, F., Capewell, P. *et al.* (2023) A parasite DNA binding protein with potential to influence disease susceptibility acts as an analogue of mammalian HMGA transcription factors. *PLoS ONE* 18(6), e0286526. DOI: 10.1371/journal.pone.0286526.

Fleige, T., Limenitakis, J. and Soldati-Favre, D. (2010) Apicoplast: Keep it or leave it. *Microbes and Infection* 12(4), 253–262. DOI: 10.1016/j.micinf.2009.12.010.

Gardner, M.J., Hall, N., Fung, E., White, O., Berriman, M. *et al.* (2002) Genome sequence of the human malaria parasite *Plasmodium falciparum*. *Nature* 419(6906), 498–511. DOI: 10.1038/nature01097.

Gardner, M.J., Bishop, R., Shah, T., de Villiers, E.P., Carlton, J.M. *et al.* (2005) Genome sequence of *Theileria parva*, a bovine pathogen that transforms lymphocytes. *Science* 309, 134–137. DOI: 10.1126/science.1110439.

Goo, Y.K. (2022) Vivax malaria and the potential role of the subtelomeric multigene *vir* superfamily. *Microorganisms* 10(6), 1083. DOI: 10.3390/microorganisms10061083.

Guo, X. and Silva, J.C. (2008) Properties of non-coding DNA and identification of putative cis-regulatory elements in *Theileria parva*. *BMC Genomics* 9(1), 582. DOI: 10.1186/1471-2164-9-582.

Hakimi, H., Yamagishi, J., Sakaguchi, M., Fathi, A., Lee, J.S. *et al.* (2025) *Ves1α* genes expression is the major determinant of *Babesia bovis*-infected erythrocytes cytoadhesion to endothelial cells. *PLOS Pathogens* 21(4), e1012583. DOI: 10.1371/journal.ppat.1012583.

Harb, O.S., Boehme, U., Crouch, K., Ifeonu, O.O., Roos, D.S. *et al.* (2016) Genomes. In: Walochnik, J. and Duchene, M. (eds) *Molecular Parasitology: Protozoan Parasites and Their Molecules*. Springer, Cham, Switzerland, pp. 3–48.

Hayashida, K., Hara, Y., Abe, T., Yamasaki, C., Toyoda, A. *et al.* (2012) Comparative genome analysis of three eukaryotic parasites with differing abilities to transform leukocytes reveals key mediators of *Theileria*-induced leukocyte transformation. *mBio* 3(5), e00204-12. DOI: 10.1128/mBio.00204-12.

Hayashida, K., Abe, T., Weir, W., Nakao, R., Ito, K. *et al.* (2013) Whole-genome sequencing of *Theileria parva* strains provides insight into parasite migration and diversification in the African continent. *DNA Research* 20(3), 209–220. DOI: 10.1093/dnares/dst003.

Hemmink, J.D., Weir, W., MacHugh, N.D., Graham, S.P., Patel, E. *et al.* (2016) Limited genetic and antigenic diversity within parasite isolates used in a live vaccine against *Theileria parva*. *International Journal for Parasitology* 46(8), 495–506. DOI: 10.1016/j.ijpara.2016.02.007.

Hemmink, J.D., Sitt, T., Pelle, R., de Klerk-Lorist, L.-M., Shiels, B. *et al.* (2018) Ancient diversity and geographical sub-structuring in African buffalo *Theileria parva* populations revealed through metagenetic analysis of antigen-encoding loci. *International Journal for Parasitology* 48(3–4), 287–296. DOI: 10.1016/j.ijpara.2017.10.006.

Homewood, K., Trench, P., Randall, S., Lynen, G. and Bishop, B. (2006) Livestock health and socioeconomic impacts of a veterinary intervention in Maasailand: Infection-and-treatment vaccine against East Coast fever. *Agricultural Systems* 89(2–3), 248–271. DOI: 10.1016/j.agsy.2005.09.004.

Howden, B.P., Giulieri, S.G., Wong Fok Lung, T., Baines, S.L., Sharkey, L.K. *et al.* (2023) *Staphylococcus aureus* host interactions and adaptation. *Nature Reviews Microbiology* 21(6), 380–395. DOI: 10.1038/s41579-023-00852-y.

IGVF Consortium (2024) Deciphering the impact of genomic variation on function. *Nature* 633(8028), 47–57. DOI: 10.1038/s41586-024-07510-0.

Kappmeyer, L.S., Thiagarajan, M., Herndon, D.R., Ramsay, J.D., Caler, E. *et al.* (2012) Comparative genomic analysis and phylogenetic position of *Theileria equi*. *BMC Genomics* 13(1), 603. DOI: 10.1186/1471-2164-13-603.

Kariuki, D.P., Young, A.S., Morzaria, S.P., Lesan, A.C., Mining, S.K. *et al.* (1995) *Theileria parva* carrier state in naturally infected and artificially immunised cattle. *Tropical Animal Health and Production* 27(1), 15–25. DOI: 10.1007/BF02236328.

Kibe, M.K., ole-MoiYoi, O.K., Nene, V., Khan, B., Allsopp, B.A. *et al.* (1994) Evidence for two single copy units in *Theileria parva* ribosomal RNA genes. *Molecular and Biochemical Parasitology* 66(2), 249–259. DOI: 10.1016/0166-6851(94)90152-x.

Lawrence, D.A. (1937) *Report of the Director of Veterinary Research for the Year 1936*. Rhodesian Printing and Publishing Company Ltd, Salisbury, p. 12.

Leemans, I., Brown, D., Fossum, C., Hooshmand-Rad, P., Kirvar, E. *et al.* (1999a) Infectivity and cross-immunity studies of *Theileria lestoquardi* and *Theileria annulata* in sheep and cattle: II. *In vitro* studies. *Veterinary Parasitology* 82(3), 193–204. DOI: 10.1016/S0304-4017(99)00014-X.

Leemans, I., Brown, D., Hooshmand-Rad, P., Kirvar, E. and Uggla, A. (1999b) Infectivity and cross-immunity studies of *Theileria lestoquardi* and *Theileria annulata* in sheep and cattle: *In vitro* studies. *Veterinary Parasitology* 82(3), 179–192. DOI: 10.1016/S0304-4017(99)00013-8.

Li, Z., Liu, J., Ma, Q., Liu, A., Li, Y. *et al.* (2021) Screening and identification of *Theileria annulata* subtelomere-encoded variable secreted protein-950454 (SVSP454) interacting proteins from bovine B cells. *Parasites & Vectors* 14(1), 319. DOI: 10.1186/s13071-021-04820-4.

Li, Z., Liu, J., Zhao, S., Ma, Q., Guo, Z. *et al.* (2022) *Theileria annulata* SVSP455 interacts with host HSP60. *Parasites & Vectors* 15(1), 308. DOI: 10.1186/s13071-022-05427-z.

Lim, L. and McFadden, G.I. (2010) The evolution, metabolism and functions of the apicoplast. *Philosophical Transactions of the Royal Society B* 365(1541), 749–763. DOI: 10.1098/rstb.2009.0273.

Lizundia, R., Werling, D., Langsley, G. and Ralph, S.A. (2009) *Theileria apicoplast* as a target for chemotherapy. *Antimicrobial Agents and Chemotherapy* 53, 1213–1217. DOI: 10.1128/AAC.00126-08.

Ma, Q., Han, Y., Fu, Y., Teng, G., Wang, X. *et al.* (2024) *Theileria annulata* subtelomere-encoded variable secreted protein-TA05560 interacts with bovine RNA binding motif protein 39 (RBM39). *Acta Tropica* 252, 107133. DOI: 10.1016/j.actatropica.2024.107133.

Maboko, B.B., Featherston, J., Sibeko-Matjila, K.P. and Mans, B.J. (2021) Whole genome sequencing of *Theileria parva* using target capture. *Genomics* 113(2), 429–438. DOI: 10.1016/j.ygeno.2020.12.033.

MacHugh, N.D., Connelley, T., Graham, S.P., Pelle, R., Formisano, P. *et al.* (2009) CD8 T cell responses to *Theileria parva* are preferentially directed to a single dominant antigen: Implications for parasite strain-specific immunity. *European Journal of Immunology* 39, 1–11. DOI: 10.1002/eji.200939227.

MacHugh, N.D., Weir, W., Burrells, A., Lizundia, R., Graham, S.P. *et al.* (2011) Extensive polymorphism and evidence of immune selection in a highly dominant antigen recognized by bovine CD8 T cells specific for *Theileria annulata*. *Infection and Immunity* 79(5), 2059–2069. DOI: 10.1128/IAI.01285-10.

Malak, A.K., Mpoke, L., Banak, J., Muriuki, S., Skilton, R.A. *et al.* (2012) Prevalence of livestock diseases and their impact on livelihoods in Central Equatoria State, Southern Sudan. *Preventive Veterinary Medicine* 104(3–4), 216–223. DOI: 10.1016/j.prevetmed.2011.12.001.

Marcellino, W.L., Salih, D.A., Njahira, M.N., Ndiwa, N., Araba, A. *et al.* (2017) The emergence of *Theileria parva* in Jonglei State, South Sudan: Confirmation using molecular and serological diagnostic tools. *Transboundary and Emerging Diseases* 64(4), 1229–1235. DOI: 10.1111/tbed.12495.

Maritim, A.C., Young, A.S., Lesan, A.C., Ndungu, S.G., Mutugi, J.J. *et al.* (1989) Theilerial parasites isolated from carrier cattle after immunization with *Theileria parva* by the Infection and Treatment Method. *Parasitology* 99(Pt 1), 139–147. DOI: 10.1017/s0031182000061126.

McCutchan, T.F., Li, J., McConkey, G.A., Rogers, M.J. and Waters, A.P. (1995) The cytoplasmic ribosomal RNAs of *Plasmodium* spp. *Parasitology Today* 11(4), 134–138. DOI: 10.1016/0169-4758(95)80132-4.

McFadden, G.I. and Roos, D.S. (1999) Apicomplexan plastids as drug targets. *Trends in Microbiology* 7(8), 328–333. DOI: 10.1016/s0966-842x(99)01547-4.

McFadden, G.I. and Yeh, E. (2017) The apicoplast: Now you see it, now you don't. *International Journal for Parasitology* 47(2–3), 137–144. DOI: 10.1016/j.ijpara.2016.08.005.

McKeever, D.J. (2007) Live immunisation against *Theileria parva*: Containing or spreading the disease? *Trends in Parasitology* 23(12), 565–568. DOI: 10.1016/j.pt.2007.09.002.

Morrison, W.I., Aguado, A., Sheldrake, T.A., Palmateer, N.C., Ifeonu, O.O. *et al.* (2021) CD4 T cell responses to *Theileria parva* in immune cattle recognize a diverse set of parasite antigens presented on the surface of infected lymphoblasts. *The Journal of Immunology* 207(8), 1965–1977. DOI: 10.4049/jimmunol.2100331.

Neitz, W.O. and Jansen, B.C. (1956) A discussion on the classification of the *Theileridae*. *Onderstepoort Journal of Veterinary Research* 27, 7–18.

Norling, M., Bishop, R.P., Pelle, R., Qi, W., Henson, S. *et al.* (2015) The genomes of three stocks comprising the most widely utilized live sporozoite *Theileria parva* vaccine exhibit very different degrees and patterns of sequence divergence. *BMC Genomics* 16(1), 729. DOI: 10.1186/s12864-015-1910-9.

Norval, R.A.I., Perry, B.D. and Young, A.S. (1992) *The Epidemiology of Theileriosis in Africa*. Academic Press, London.

Nyagwange, J., Nene, V., Mwalimu, S., Henson, S., Steinaa, L. *et al.* (2018) Antibodies to *in silico* selected GPI-anchored *Theileria parva* proteins neutralize sporozoite infection *in vitro*. *Veterinary Immunology and Immunopathology* 199, 8–14. DOI: 10.1016/j.vetimm.2018.03.004.

Odongo, D.O., Sunter, J.D., Kiara, H.K., Skilton, R.A. and Bishop, R.P. (2010) A nested PCR assay exhibits enhanced sensitivity for detection of *Theileria parva* infections in bovine blood samples from carrier animals. *Parasitology Research* 106(2), 357–365. DOI: 10.1007/s00436-009-1670-z.

Oura, C.A.L., Bishop, R., Wampande, E.M., Lubega, G.W. and Tait, A. (2004) The persistence of component *Theileria parva* stocks in cattle immunized with the 'Muguga cocktail' live vaccine against East Coast fever in Uganda. *Parasitology* 129(Pt 1), 27–42. DOI: 10.1017/s003118200400513x.

Oura, C.A.L., Tait, A., Asiimwe, B., Lubega, G.W. and Weir, W. (2011) *Theileria parva* genetic diversity and *haemoparasite* prevalence in cattle and wildlife in and around Lake Mburo National Park in Uganda. *Parasitology Research* 108(6), 1365–1374. DOI: 10.1007/s00436-010-2030-8.

Pain, A., Renauld, H., Berriman, M., Murphy, L., Yeats, C.A. *et al.* (2005) Genome of the host-cell transforming parasite *Theileria annulata* compared with *T. parva*. *Science* 309(5731), 131–133. DOI: 10.1126/science.1110418.

Palmateer, N.C., Tretina, K., Orvis, J., Ifeonu, O.O., Crabtree, J. *et al.* (2020) Capture-based enrichment of *Theileria parva* DNA enables full genome assembly of first buffalo-derived strain and reveals exceptional intra-specific genetic diversity. *PLOS Neglected Tropical Diseases* 14(10), e0008781. DOI: 10.1371/journal.pntd.0008781.

Palmateer, N.C., Munro, J.B., Nagaraj, S., Crabtree, J., Pelle, R. *et al.* (2023) The hypervariable *Tpr* multigene family of *Theileria* parasites, defined by a conserved, membrane-associated, c-terminal domain, includes several copies with defined orthology between species. *Journal of Molecular Evolution* 91(6), 897–911. DOI: 10.1007/s00239-023-10142-z.

Pelle, R., Graham, S.P., Njahira, M.N., Osaso, J., Saya, R.M. *et al.* (2011) Two *Theileria parva* CD8 T cell antigen genes are more variable in buffalo than cattle parasites, but differ in pattern of sequence diversity. *PLoS ONE* 6(4), e19015. DOI: 10.1371/journal.pone.0019015.

Pieszko, M., Weir, W., Goodhead, I., Kinnaird, J. and Shiels, B. (2015) ApiAP2 factors as candidate regulators of stochastic commitment to merozoite production in theileria annulata. *PLOS Neglected Tropical Diseases* 9(8), e0003933. DOI: 10.1371/journal.pntd.0003933.

Potapova, T.A. and Gerton, J.L. (2019) Ribosomal DNA and the nucleolus in the context of genome organization. *Chromosome Research* 27(1–2), 109–127. DOI: 10.1007/s10577-018-9600-5.

Radley, D.E., Brown, C.G.D., Cunningham, M.P., Kimber, C.D., Musisi, F.L. *et al.* (1975) East Coast fever: 3. Chemoprophylactic immunization of cattle using oxytetracycline and a combination of *theilerial* strains. *Veterinary Parasitology* 1(1), 51–60. DOI: 10.1016/0304-4017(75)90007-2.

Radley, D.E., Young, A.S., Grootenhuis, J.G., Cunningham, M.P., Dolan, T.T. *et al.* (1979) Further studies on the immunization of cattle against *Theileria lawrencei* by infection and chemoprophylaxis. *Veterinary Parasitology* 5(2–3), 117–128. DOI: 10.1016/0304-4017(79)90003-7.

Rodriguez-Algarra, F., Whittaker, E., Del Castillo Del Rio, S. and Rakyan, V.K. (2025) Assessing human Ribosomal DNA variation and its association with phenotypic outcomes. *BioEssays* 47(4), e202400232. DOI: 10.1002/bies.202400232.

Rogers, S., Wells, R. and Rechsteiner, M. (1986) Amino acid sequences common to rapidly degraded proteins: The PEST hypothesis. *Science* 234(4774), 364–368. DOI: 10.1126/science.2876518.

Rukambile, E., Machuka, E., Njahira, M., Kyalo, M., Skilton, R. *et al.* (2016) Population genetic analysis of *Theileria parva* isolated in cattle and buffaloes in Tanzania using minisatellite and microsatellite markers. *Veterinary Parasitology* 224, 20–26. DOI: 10.1016/j.vetpar.2016.04.038.

Sadiq, A., Bostan, N., Yinda, K.C., Naseem, S. and Sattar, S. (2018) Rotavirus: Genetics, pathogenesis and vaccine advances. *Reviews in Medical Virology* 28(6), e2003. DOI: 10.1002/rmv.2003.

Salih, D.A., Mwacharo, J.M., Pelle, R., Njahira, M.N., Odongo, D.O. *et al.* (2018) Genetic diversity and population structure of *Theileria parva* in South Sudan. *Ticks and Tick-Borne Diseases* 9(4), 806–813. DOI: 10.1016/j.ttbdis.2018.03.002.

Schmuckli-Maurer, J., Casanova, C., Schmied, S., Affentranger, S., Parvanova, I. *et al.* (2009) Expression analysis of the *Theileria parva* subtelomere-encoded variable secreted protein gene family. *PLoS ONE* 4(3), e4839. DOI: 10.1371/journal.pone.0004839.

Seehausen, O., Butlin, R.K., Keller, I., Wagner, C.E., Boughman, J.W. *et al.* (2014) Genomics and the origin of species. *Nature Reviews Genetics* 15(3), 176–192. DOI: 10.1038/nrg3644.

Sharma, I., Fang, J., Lewallen, E.A., Deitsch, K.W. and McCutchan, T.F. (2023) Identification of a long non-coding RNA required for temperature induced expression of stage-specific rrna in malaria parasites. *Gene* 877, 147516. DOI: 10.1016/j.gene.2023.147516.

Shaw, M.K., Tilney, L.G. and Musoke, A.J. (1991) The entry of *Theileria parva* sporozoites into bovine lymphocytes: Evidence for MHC class I involvement. *The Journal of Cell Biology* 113(1), 87–101. DOI: 10.1083/jcb.113.1.87.

Shaw, M.K., Tilney, L.G., Musoke, A.J. and Teale, A.J. (1995) MHC class I molecules are an essential cell surface component involved in *Theileria parva* sporozoite binding to bovine lymphocytes. *Journal of Cell Science* 108(Pt 4), 1587–1596. DOI: 10.1242/jcs.108.4.1587.

Shiels, B., Langsley, G., Weir, W., Pain, A., McKellar, S. *et al.* (2006) Alteration of host cell phenotype by *Theileria annulata* and *Theileria parva*: Mining for manipulators in the parasite genomes. *International Journal for Parasitology* 36(1), 9–21. DOI: 10.1016/j.ijpara.2005.09.002.

Silatsa, B.A., Simo, G., Githaka, N., Mwaura, S., Kamga, R.M. *et al.* (2019) A comprehensive survey of the prevalence and spatial distribution of ticks infesting cattle in different agro-ecological zones of cameroon. *Parasites & Vectors* 12(1), 489. DOI: 10.1186/s13071-019-3738-7.

Silatsa, B.A., Simo, G., Githaka, N., Kamga, R., Oumarou, F. *et al.* (2020) First detection of *Theileria parva* in cattle from Cameroon in the absence of the main tick vector *Rhipicephalus appendiculatus*. *Transboundary and Emerging Diseases* 67(Suppl. 1), 68–78. DOI: 10.1111/tbed.13425.

Singh, P., Vydyam, P., Fang, T., Estrada, K., Gonzalez, L.M. *et al.* (2024) Insights into the evolution, virulence and speciation of *Babesia MO1* and *Babesia divergens* through multiomics analyses. *Emerging Microbes & Infections* 13(1), 2386136. DOI: 10.1080/22221751.2024.2386136.

Sitt, T., Poole, E.J., Ndambuki, G., Mwaura, S., Njoroge, T. *et al.* (2015) Exposure of vaccinated and naive cattle to natural challenge from buffalo-derived *Theileria parva*. *International Journal for Parasitology* 4(2), 244–251. DOI: 10.1016/j.ijppaw.2015.04.006.

Skilton, R.A., Bishop, R.P., Katende, J.M., Mwaura, S. and Morzaria, S.P. (2002) The persistence of *Theileria parva* infection in cattle immunized using two stocks which differ in their ability to induce a carrier state: Analysis using a novel blood spot PCR assay. *Parasitology* 124(3), 265–276. DOI: 10.1017/S0031182001001196.

Sohanpal, B., Wasawo, D. and Bishop, R. (2000) Cloning of telomere-associated DNA using single-specific-primer polymerase chain reaction provides evidence for a conserved sequence directly adjacent to *Theileria parva* telomeric repeats. *Gene* 255(2), 401–409. DOI: 10.1016/S0378-1119(00)00284-5.

Sohanpal, B.K., Morzaria, S.P., Gobright, E.I. and Bishop, R.P. (1995) Characterisation of the telomeres at opposite ends of a 3 Mb *Theileria parva* chromosome. *Nucleic Acids Research* 23(11), 1942–1947. DOI: 10.1093/nar/23.11.1942.

Su, X., Lane, K.D., Xia, L., Sá, J.M. and Wellems, T.E. (2019) *Plasmodium* genomics and genetics: New insights into malaria pathogenesis, drug resistance, epidemiology, and evolution. *Clinical Microbiology Reviews* 32(4). DOI: 10.1128/CMR.00019-19.

Swan, D.G., Phillips, K., Tait, A. and Shiels, B.R. (1999) Evidence for localisation of a *Theileria parasite* AT hook DNA-binding protein to the nucleus of immortalised bovine host cells. *Molecular and Biochemical Parasitology* 101(1–2), 117–129. DOI: 10.1016/S0166-6851(99)00064-X.

Swan, D.G., Stern, R., McKellar, S., Phillips, K., Oura, C.A. *et al.* (2001) Characterisation of a cluster of genes encoding *Theileria annulata* AT hook DNA-binding proteins and evidence for localisation to the host cell nucleus. *Journal of Cell Science* 114(Pt 15), 2747–2754. DOI: 10.1242/jcs.114.15.2747.

Tindih, H.S., Geysen, D., Goddeeris, B.M., Awino, E., Dobbelaere, D.A.E. *et al.* (2012) A *Theileria parva* isolate of low virulence infects a subpopulation of lymphocytes. *Infection and Immunity* 80(3), 1267–1273. DOI: 10.1128/IAI.05085-11.

Tonui, T., Corredor-Moreno, P., Kanduma, E., Njuguna, J., Njahira, M.N. *et al.* (2018) Transcriptomics reveal potential vaccine antigens and a drastic increase of upregulated genes during *Theileria parva* development from arthropod to bovine infective stages. *PLoS ONE* 13(10), e0204047. DOI: 10.1371/journal.pone.0204047.

Tretina, K., Pelle, R. and Silva, J.C. (2016) Cis regulatory motifs and antisense transcriptional control in the apicomplexan *Theileria parva*. *BMC Genomics* 17, 128. DOI: 10.1186/s12864-016-2444-5.

Tretina, K., Pelle, R., Orvis, J., Gotia, H.T., Ifeonu, O.O. *et al.* (2020) Re-annotation of the *Theileria parva* genome refines 53% of the proteome and uncovers essential components of N-glycosylation, a conserved pathway in many organisms. *BMC Genomics* 21(1), 279. DOI: 10.1186/s12864-020-6683-0.

Unlu, A.H., Tajeri, S., Bilgic, H.B., Eren, H., Karagenc, T. *et al*. (2018) The secreted *Theileria annulata* Ta9 protein contributes to activation of the AP-1 transcription factor. *PLoS ONE* 13(5), e0196875. DOI: 10.1371/journal.pone.0196875.

van Dooren, G.G. and Striepen, B. (2013) The algal past and parasite present of the apicoplast. *Annual Review of Microbiology* 67, 271–289. DOI: 10.1146/annurev-micro-092412-155741.

Wahlgren, M., Goel, S. and Akhouri, R.R. (2017) Variant surface antigens of *Plasmodium falciparum* and their roles in severe malaria. *Nature Reviews Microbiology* 15(8), 479–491. DOI: 10.1038/nrmicro.2017.47.

Weir, W., Sunter, J., Chaussepied, M., Skilton, R., Tait, A. *et al*. (2009) Highly syntenic and yet divergent: A tale of two theilerias. *Infection, Genetics and Evolution* 9(4), 453–461. DOI: 10.1016/j.meegid.2009.01.002.

Weir, W., Karagenç, T., Baird, M., Tait, A. and Shiels, B.R. (2010) Evolution and diversity of secretome genes in the apicomplexan parasite *Theileria annulata*. *BMC Genomics* 11, 42. DOI: 10.1186/1471-2164-11-42.

Wiesner, J. and Seeber, F. (2005) The plastid-derived organelle of protozoan human parasites as a target of established and emerging drugs. *Expert Opinion on Therapeutic Targets* 9(1), 23–44. DOI: 10.1517/14728222.9.1.23.

Wong, A.K., Sealfon, R.S.G., Theesfeld, C.L. and Troyanskaya, O.G. (2021) Decoding disease: From genomes to networks to phenotypes. *Nature Reviews Genetics* 22(12), 774–790. DOI: 10.1038/s41576-021-00389-x.

Yamagishi, J., Wakaguri, H., Yokoyama, N., Yamashita, R., Suzuki, Y. *et al*. (2014) The *Babesia bovis* gene and promoter model: An update from full-length EST analysis. *BMC Genomics* 15(1), 678. DOI: 10.1186/1471-2164-15-678.

Young, A.S. and Purnell, R.E. (1973) Transmission of *Theileria lawrencei* (Serengeti) by the ixodid tick, *Rhipicephalus appendiculatus*. *Tropical Animal Health and Production* 5(3), 146–152. DOI: 10.1007/BF02251383.

Young, A.S., Radley, D.E., Cunningham, M.P., Musisi, F.L., Payne, R.C. *et al*. (1977) Exposure of immunized cattle to prolonged natural challenge of *Theileria lawrencei* derived from African buffalo (*Syncerus caffer*). *Veterinary Parasitology* 3(4), 283–290. DOI: 10.1016/0304-4017(77)90015-2.

Zhan, Q., Pascual, M. and He, Q. (2025) Evolutionary trade-offs between functional and immune selection shape multigene families in pathogens. *Evolutionary Biology*. DOI: 10.1101/2025.06.24.661038.

10 The Cell Biology of the *Theileria*–Leukocyte Relationship

Brian Shiels[1]* and Kerry Woods[2]

[1]College of Medical, Veterinary and Life Sciences, University of Glasgow, Glasgow, UK; [2]Institute of Animal Pathology, Vetsuisse Faculty, University of Bern, Bern, Switzerland

10.1 Introduction

As detailed in Chapter 4 of this volume, the dominant feature of East Coast fever (ECF) caused by *Theileria parva* is that it resembles a lymphoproliferative disorder. Disease is manifested by a marked expansion of dividing infected leukocytes together with a dysregulated response of host immune cells induced by the infected cell population. How the parasite brings about 'transformation' of bovine leukocytes and induces their proliferation has been the focus of much research. Not only is this research of biological interest, as the ability of a eukaryotic cell to transform another eukaryotic cell is thought to be unique, but understanding how lymphoproliferation occurs and how the host responds to the transformed cell is key to development of novel therapeutics and vaccine strategies against ECF. The aim of this chapter is to document current knowledge gained on the molecular mechanisms deployed by *T. parva* and *T. annulata* to transform their intracellular niche. Host cell pathways and structures co-opted by the parasite and strategies used to identify and characterize parasite-encoded transformation factors will be highlighted. Transformation of the host leukocyte is limited to a small number of *Theileria* species. The two most studied 'transforming' *Theileria* species, *T. parva* and *T. annulata*, are closely related and evolved, relatively recently, from a common ancestor (Allsopp *et al.*, 1994). Subsequently, *T. lestoquardi*, which transforms leukocytes of sheep and goats, has arisen via adaptation of *T. annulata* to a small ruminant cellular environment (Al-Hamidhi *et al.*, 2016). For all three species, shortly after cellular invasion by the tick-inoculated sporozoite, and coincident with differentiation to the schizont stage, transformation of the infected leukocyte generates a marked exponential phase of uncontrolled proliferation of infected cells over the course of at least 10 days (Jarrett *et al.*, 1969; Morrison *et al.*, 1981). Lymph nodes draining the site of tick bites become enlarged, and infected cells disseminate throughout the lymphoid system and infiltrate the gastrointestinal tract, liver and lungs, resembling metastasis of transformed cancer cells (Irvin and Morrison, 1987; see Chapter 4 of this volume). During the phase of infected cell proliferation, parasite-infected cell lines can be established *ex vivo* and have the potential, like transformed cancer cells, to proliferate *in vitro* indefinitely (reviewed by Dobbelaere and Heussler, 1999). Establishment of infected cell lines allowed studies of how the

*Corresponding author: Brian.Shiels@glasgow.ac.uk

 East Coast Fever: The Disease, its Impact and Control (eds W.I. Morrison and P. Toye)
DOI: 10.1079/9781800626324.0010

macroschizont stage coordinates its cellular division with that of its host cell, the parasite physically attaching to the host mitotic spindle to ensure each daughter cell is infected (Hulliger *et al.*, 1964; von Schubert *et al.*, 2010). Thus, the parasite population greatly increases during the phase of infected cell proliferation.

Transformed cancer cells are considered immortal, but *in vivo*, reversal of transformation of at least some *Theileria*-infected leukocytes is required to allow differentiation of the parasite to the tick-transmissible stage and progression to the next life-cycle generation. After the initial rapid proliferation of infected leukocytes, division of some of the infected host cells slows down and the parasite enlarges before undergoing merogony to generate hundreds of merozoites that are released from the destroyed host cell (Hulliger *et al.*, 1966; Jarrett *et al.*, 1969; Shiels *et al.*, 1992). Merozoites rapidly invade erythrocytes to produce piroplasms, the parasite stage ingested by feeding ticks. For *T. parva* and *T. annulata*, respectively, there is either no or limited piroplasm proliferation within erythrocytes (Conrad *et al.*, 1985; Irvin and Morrison, 1987). However, retention of a transformed state by some of the infected leukocytes is required to establish low-level persistent infection (the carrier state). These species are, therefore, dependent on the macroschizont-infected cell and merogony for expansion and persistence of the parasite population within the host. This is in marked contrast to 'non-transforming' *Theileria* species such as *T. orientalis*, which show significant proliferation within, and reinvasion of, erythrocytes. *T. orientalis*-infected leukocytes are very large, containing enlarged macroschizont syncytia, and parasites undergo merogony as soon as 8 days after sporozoite inoculation (Minami *et al.*, 1990; Hagiwara *et al.*, 1997), indicating a more limited phase of infected leukocyte proliferation. It can be concluded that for *T. parva* both parasite expansion and disease pathology are intimately linked to the ability of the parasite to transform its host cell. Infections with *T. annulata* show similar properties, and the disease syndromes induced by both parasite species display similar clinical signs of a lymphoproliferative condition (Irvin and Morrison, 1987; Brown *et al.*, 1990). Animals suffering tropical theileriosis caused by *T. annulata* also display anaemia, whereas only a slight decrease in erythrocyte count is observed in ECF. Presentation of anaemia might relate, in part, to the propensity for *T. annulata* to initiate merogony earlier than *T. parva* (Mehlhorn and Shein, 1984), which can be considered the *Theileria* species that shows greatest host cell-transforming capacity.

The close evolutionary relationship between transforming *Theileria* species indicates they share a range of mechanisms that bring about the transformation event. Thus, parasite molecules deployed to hijack host cell targets are likely to be conserved, and manipulation of host cell gene expression networks and signal transduction pathways can be expected to show similarities across these species. However, it should be noted that, based on the number of pathways and parasite-encoded molecules implicated (see Section 10.4 and 10.6), transformation of the infected cell is likely to be the result of multiple complex interactions, rather than the work of a master oncogenic regulator. The probability of whether the infected cell causes disease almost certainly involves additional modulatory interactions with cells of the host immune response. *T. annulata*-infected cell lines that display attenuated pathogenesis can be selected based on their superior survival and proliferation *in vitro* (Pipano and Shkap, 2000), and it is apparent that infection of *Bos indicus* cattle breeds and buffalo with either *T. parva* or *T. annulata* results in transformed infected cells but generates significantly milder or no overt disease (Baldwin *et al.*, 1986; Jensen *et al.*, 2008; Larcombe *et al.*, 2019; Morrison *et al.*, 2020; Latré de Laté *et al.*, 2021). Although *T. parva* infects and transforms B and T lymphocytes, infected B cells do not produce disease (Morrison *et al.*, 1996), implying that transformation alone does not lead to pathology (see Chapters 4 and 11 of this volume). *T. parva* and *T. annulata* preferentially establish in different cell types – *T. parva* in B and T lymphocytes and *T. annulata* in monocytes, dendritic cells and B lymphocytes. *T. parva* can invade dendritic cells but cannot transform them (Shaw *et al.*, 1993), whereas *T. annulata* can (Stephens and Howard, 2002). Therefore, the mechanisms deployed to generate the fully established phenotype of the transformed cell can be predicted to show a degree of divergence between *Theileria* species that is influenced by the lineage and genetic background of the host cell. It can be concluded that, in addition to proliferation *per se*, the resulting phenotype of the infected cell strongly influences the degree of dysregulation of the bovine immune response that in turn determines the likelihood of disease.

10.2 Methods Available for the Study of *Theileria*-Transformed Cell Lines

The ability of *T. parva* and other transforming *Theileria* species to transform the host leukocyte has the advantage of allowing indefinite culture of infected cell lines *in vitro* (reviewed in Dobbelaere and Heussler, 1999). Cultures are propagated using standard media supplemented with foetal bovine serum, and lines can be stored long-term in liquid nitrogen. Virtually every culture cell is infected with a parasite, and these are very amenable for study by immunolocalization and immunochemistry methodologies. Infected cells can be fractionated into different cellular compartments (Kinnaird *et al.*, 2017) and methods for isolation of schizonts have been developed (Baumgartner *et al.*, 1999). Infected cells can be transiently or stably transfected with gene constructs for expression of tagged parasite or host proteins (Durrani, 2012; Marsolier *et al.*, 2015). A system is available for *T. annulata* whereby bovine lymphosarcoma (BL) lines can be infected with sporozoites *in vitro* and the resulting schizont cell line compared with the uninfected counterpart (Kinnaird *et al.*, 2013; Rchiad *et al.*, 2020). Moreover, the transformation process can be reversed by treatment with the theilericidal drug buparvaquone (reviewed in Dobbelaere and Heussler, 1999). After 48 hours drug treatment, the parasite nuclear number is drastically reduced, infected cell proliferation slows down (Kinnaird *et al.*, 2013) and the cells undergo apoptosis unless given supportive growth factors (reviewed in Dobbelaere and Heussler, 1999). Bovine gene expression differences linked to *T. annulata* infection (for example in the comparison of infected TBL20 cells with their uninfected BL20 counterpart) are altered within 24 hour of adding the drug (Kinnaird *et al.*, 2013). Host genes implicated in the transformed phenotype can be knocked out using CRISPR-Cas9 methodology (Rchiad *et al.*, 2020; Maurizio *et al.*, 2024), and cell lines can be cloned to represent a single host cell type and parasite genotype (Shiels *et al.*, 1992). Transfer of parasites from donor cell line to cells of a recipient animal can readily occur for *T. annulata* (Pipano and Shkap, 2000) and would allow transfer of genetically engineered parasites to cattle, and possibly ticks, if a system for stable transfection of the parasite is developed.

The current lack of stable transfection of the parasite is the major deficiency in the *Theileria* model system. Thus, it is impossible to prove a functional requirement for a gene expressed by the parasite. Other caveats exist. There is a large amount of variability between and within cell lines, which is often unaccounted for (Shiels *et al.*, 1992; Hall *et al.*, 1999), and changes to parasite and host cell gene expression will result from prolonged culture *in vitro*. Study of multiple, early passage cell lines to establish critical, conserved modulatory events is required, and this may not always establish a conclusive answer (see study of Hall *et al.*, 1999). Moreover, it is much more difficult to investigate mechanisms of transformation *in vivo*, and relatively few studies have confirmed that modulation of signal transduction pathways and parasite–host interactions identified for cell lines *in vitro* also occur during natural infection/*ex vivo*. Despite these caveats, the *Theileria*-infected leukocyte provides a unique model system for how a parasite can hijack the molecular machinery of its host leukocyte to generate a cancer-like transformed cell.

10.3 Interior Design – Parasite Interaction with Host Cell Structures and Establishment of the Infected Cell Niche

One of the earliest events that occurs following invasion of a leukocyte is the dissolution of the surrounding host-derived vacuole membrane, allowing the parasite to establish a niche within the host cytoplasm. This occurs within 15 min of invasion and coincides with the release of microsphere and rhoptry contents (Shaw *et al.*, 1991). The absence of a parasitophorous vacuole membrane (PVM) distinguishes *Theileria* from most other *Apicomplexans* and raises intriguing questions about how it evades host-mediated pathogen clearance mechanisms. In a recent study, autophagy was found to be suppressed in *T. annulata*-infected B cells compared to their uninfected counterpart (TBL3 compared to BL3) (Villares *et al.*, 2024). Structures resembling autophagosomes and autolysosomes were strikingly absent from infected cells, as assessed by electron microscopy and fluorescence microscopy, and Western blotting confirmed a reduction in autophagic flux in infected cells. A drug screen carried out by the same authors identified a small molecule compound (MC2646) that reduced parasite load in *T. annulata*-infected B cells or macrophages and *T. parva*-infected T cells (Villares *et al.*, 2024). Autophagy was induced upon treatment with this compound, supporting the notion that *Theileria* suppresses host autophagy to promote its own survival. Intriguingly, the host translation factor eIF5A was found to be recruited close to the schizont surface and to be required for the activation of autophagy upon drug treatment of infected cells, leading to the proposal that schizont sequestration of eIF5A may be a novel mechanism of preventing autophagy-mediated elimination of the parasite. On the other hand, others have detected the autophagy marker LC3 in and around the *T. annulata* schizont in infected macrophages (Latré de Laté *et al.*, 2017), possibly indicating that different mechanisms are employed in different cell types to avoid lysosomal degradation. Further studies are required to unravel the interplay between *Theileria* schizonts and the host autophagy machinery in different cell types.

Very soon after sporozoite invasion and the dissolution of the surrounding host-derived vacuole membrane, host microtubules (MTs) assemble around the parasite next to a layer of 'fuzzy' material that appears at the surface of the sporozoite. It is thought that this layer consists of the secreted contents of sporozoite rhoptries and microspheres, although the protein content has not been determined. The close association between the intracellular parasite and host MTs is maintained throughout the macroschizont stage of development, allowing the *Theileria* schizont to persist in the cytoplasm of the dividing cell by co-opting the host mitotic machinery (Hulliger *et al.*, 1964; von Schubert *et al.*, 2010). Time-lapse imaging of mitotic cells revealed that MTs at the *T. annulata* schizont surface are highly stable compared to those in the host cytoplasm. The interaction of the schizont with both astral and central spindle MTs during mitosis is required for the proper segregation of the parasite into daughter cells following cytokinesis and, therefore, the maintenance of the transformed state. Interestingly, host polo-like kinase (Plk1) associates with the *T. annulata* schizont surface in a cell cycle-dependent manner, and the activity of this kinase is required for the binding of the schizont with host central spindles (von Schubert *et al.*, 2010).

A study to identify *Theileria* molecules involved in the binding of MTs revealed that a *T. annulata* protein (encoded by TA08425), henceforth named p104, previously annotated as '*Theileria parva* microsphere rhoptry antigen', plays a role in regulating MT dynamics at the schizont surface (Woods *et al.*, 2013). *T. parva* p104 (TpMuguga_04g00437), which shares 51% identity and 60% similarity to *T. annulata* p104, was first identified as an immunogenic protein that reacts strongly with monoclonal antibodies raised against sporozoites. Immunoelectron microscopy analysis localized *T. parva* p104 within the rhoptry/microsphere complex of the sporozoite (Iams *et al.*, 1990). Later it was shown that *T. annulata* p104, recognized by the monoclonal antibody 1C12 (Shiels *et al.*, 1986), is expressed on the surface of the schizont and on the surface of internalized sporozoites 30 min following invasion of leukocytes (Woods *et al.*, 2013; Huber *et al.*, 2017). In the schizont stage, *T. annulata* p104 binds to the host MT-associated end-binding protein 1 (EB1) and CLIP-170-associating protein 1 (CLASP1) (Woods *et al.*, 2013; Huber *et al.*, 2017). EB1 is considered a master regulator of MT dynamics as it binds in a transient and highly dynamic manner with numerous interaction partners (Honnappa *et al.*, 2009). A large family of EB1-binding proteins contain a conserved SxIP motif, and both *T. parva* and *T. annulata* p104 contain SxIP motifs. EB1 is enriched at the schizont surface in a cell cycle-dependent manner, and the importance of the *T. annulata* p104 SxIP motif for EB1 binding was confirmed by mutagenesis and co-immunoprecipitation experiments (Woods *et al.*, 2013). It was proposed that the p104-dependent recruitment of EB1 at the schizont surface is required for the binding of MTs to the schizont, although this was difficult to test experimentally due to a lack of transfection tools for *Theileria*, and because EB1-MT interactions are essential for host cell viability. Subsequent studies showed that CLASP1, an MT-stabilizing protein that captures MTs at the kinetochore and the cell cortex (Maiato *et al.*, 2003; Mimori-Kiyosue *et al.*, 2006), coats the surface of the *T. annulata* schizont throughout the entire cell cycle (Huber *et al.*, 2017). It is likely that CLASP1 contributes to the stabilization of MTs at the schizont surface, although again it was difficult to interfere specifically with schizont-associated CLASP1 without disrupting MT dynamics in a more general sense. Another *T. annulata* surface molecule that is part of the p104-CLASP1-EB1 complex at the schizont surface has been named TaMISHIP (*T. annulata* microtubule and SH3 domain-interacting protein, encoded by TA20980) (Huber *et al.*, 2018). TaMISHIP, like p104, is present on the schizont surface throughout the entire intracellular life cycle and contains functional EB1-binding SxIP motifs. In addition to its interaction with the p104-CLASP1-EB1 complex, TaMISHIP binds to the adaptor protein CD2AP, a protein involved in numerous interactions. TaMISHIP has an orthologue in *T. parva* (TpMuguga_01g00380, 42% sequence identity) and *T. lestoquardi* (DQ00498, 68% identity), while no comparative gene exists in the non-transforming *T. orientalis* (Huber *et al.*, 2018). In summary, interaction between the schizont surface and host MTs is critical for the persistence of the parasite within the cytoplasm of the continually dividing cell and is regulated by key host-encoded MT-binding proteins that also bind to schizont surface proteins, including p104 and TaMISHIP.

Theileria-infected leukocytes not only exhibit changes in host MT distribution but also induce rearrangements of cellular organelles. Soon after invasion by a sporozoite, the host Golgi becomes enlarged and highly active, and associates closely with the parasite (Musisi *et al.*, 1981; Stagg *et al.*, 1981). Nuclear pore-embedded membranes termed 'annulate lamellae' (AL) have been observed by electron microscopy in the cytoplasm of *T. annulata*- and *T. parva*-infected lymphoblasts (Musisi *et al.*, 1981; Jura *et al.*, 1983). AL have also been detected in close association with the *T. annulata* schizont surface in infected macrophages, and were shown to consist of host nuclear pore complex proteins (Nups) (Huber *et al.*, 2020). Structures resembling a cytostome exist in the schizont membrane, and fragments of AL can be seen within vacuoles in the schizont cytosol (Jura *et al.*, 1983; Huber *et al.*, 2020). The distribution of AL in infected cells is dynamic, exhibiting a striking alignment along the schizont membrane during host interphase, and dissolving along with the nuclear envelope during mitosis. Along with the structural components of the nuclear envelope, host proteins of the nuclear transport machinery including the small GTPase Ran and the karyopherin importin B were also found to be enriched close to the schizont surface (Huber *et al.*, 2020). AL have been observed in numerous fast-growing cells such as cancer cells and embryonic cells, although their function is still not understood (Kessel, 1992). What role they play in *Theileria*-transformed cells is not known. Host and parasite DNA replication are inversely correlated, with parasite DNA synthesis and nuclear division occurring during host metaphase (Irvin *et al.*, 1982; Wiens *et al.*, 2014). How the timing of host and parasite cell cycle progression is so exquisitely regulated is unknown. An interesting (but untested) hypothesis is that the parasite might monitor changes in host cell cycle stage through the internalization of host AL. While the function of the infection-associated AL remains unknown, it can be concluded that upon invasion the parasite establishes a supportive niche in the infected cell by intimate interaction with cytoskeletal structures of the host leukocyte.

10.4 Turn on the Lights: *Theileria* as an Activator of Cell Cycle Regulators and Janus-Like Transcription Factors

Theileria-induced transformation of the host leukocyte is defined by uncontrolled progression through the cell cycle and is driven by the expression of cell cycle activators and pro-survival signalling molecules. Central to this phenotype is the activation of leukocyte kinases and transcription factors that can be considered signalling hubs due to their influence on multiple cellular pathways. Below we summarize evidence of the role of the primary host cell-derived factors that operate in the transformation event.

10.4.1 Casein kinase II

A significant increase in total phosphorylation has been observed in *T. parva*-infected lymphocytes compared to non-infected IL-2-dependent T lymphoblasts, and a major contributing factor is the increased expression and activity of the pleiotropic serine/threonine-specific casein kinase 2 (CK2) (ole-MoiYoi *et al.*, 1993). Inhibition of CK2 activity blocks DNA synthesis and proliferation of infected cells, underpinning its importance in the clonal expansion of *Theileria*-infected cells (Shayan and Ahmed, 1997).

10.4.2 c-Myc

c-Myc is a transcription factor that targets as many as 15% of all genes (Dang *et al.*, 2006) and is constitutively activated in more than 70% of human cancers (Madden *et al.*, 2021). c-Myc activation and the subsequent expression of the anti-apoptotic protein Mcl-1 is a key feature of *Theileria*-induced transformation (Dessauge *et al.*, 2005c), and ablation of c-Myc expression in *T. parva*-infected B cells with antisense oligonucleotides leads to cell death within 24 hours, accompanied by loss of Mcl-1 expression (Dessauge *et al.*, 2005a). CK2-mediated phosphorylation of the c-Myc C-terminal PEST (**P**roline (P), **E**glutamic acid (E), **S**erine (S), and **T**hreonine (T)) domains reduces proteasomal degradation of c-Myc (Channavajhala and Seldin, 2002), and inhibition of CK2 activity with apigenin in *T. parva*-transformed B cells led to a drop in c-Myc phosphorylation and allowed the subsequent degradation of the protein (Dessauge *et al.*, 2005a). Thus, CK2 kinase activity and c-Myc-driven gene expression are central to the transformed phenotype. Constitutive phosphorylation of signal transducer and activator of transcription 3 (STAT3) by Janus kinase 2 (JAK2) occurs in *T. parva*-infected B cells, and inhibition studies combined with luciferase-based reporter assays confirmed that JAK2-STAT3 signalling promotes high levels of c-Myc expression at the transcriptional level. Inhibition of JAK2 activity resulted in caspase-dependent apoptosis in infected B cells, and this could be rescued by ectopic expression of c-Myc in these cells. Therefore, CK2 activity and JAK2-STAT3 signalling both contribute to c-Myc-dependent survival of *Theileria*-infected cells (Dessauge *et al.*, 2005a). Importantly, c-Myc expression and JAK2 and CK2 activity are strictly dependent upon the presence of a viable parasite and are rapidly reversed upon buparvaquone treatment.

10.4.3 NF-kB

Another signalling hub that is targeted by *Theileria* is the NF-kB signalling cascade. NF-kB is constitutively activated in the nucleus of *T. parva*-infected T cells and *T. annulata*-infected macrophages (Ivanov *et al.*, 1989; Palmer *et al.*, 1997; Heussler *et al.*, 2002; Schmuckli-Maurer *et al.*, 2010). Chemical or genetic inhibition of NF-kB activity induced the onset of apoptosis within 2 hour in *T. parva*-infected T cells (Heussler *et al.*, 1999). The parasite has evolved a unique mechanism of NF-kB activation, whereby signalosomes consisting of the IkB kinase (IKK) complex are enriched at the schizont surface ensuring the continual phosphorylation and degradation of the IkB cytoplasmic inhibitor of NF-kB (Heussler *et al.*, 2002). This allows NF-kB to accumulate in the nucleus of infected cells, where it drives the expression of anti-apoptotic genes including *c-FLIP*, *c-iap* and *xiap* (Heussler *et al.*, 2002; Küenzi *et al.*, 2003). Despite substantial effort, no parasite-encoded binding partner of the IKK signalosomes has been identified and the mechanism of IKK recruitment is still not understood.

10.4.4 AP-1

The transcription factor AP-1 (activator protein 1) has constitutively high DNA-binding activity in all *Theileria*-infected leukocytes tested (Baylis *et al.*, 1995; Botteron and Dobbelaere, 1998; Chaussepied *et al.*, 1998). Increased activity is due to increased expression of the AP-1 subunits c-Jun, Fos and ATF-2 family proteins, and the constitutive phosphorylation of c-Jun and ATF-2 by c-Jun N-terminal kinase (JNK), which is permanently active in infected cells (Galley *et al.*, 1997; Botteron and Dobbelaere, 1998; Chaussepied *et al.*, 1998). Inactivation of JNK with specific inhibitors or expression of a dominant-negative mutant leads to a reduction in AP-1 activity and induces apoptosis within 6 hours, demonstrating that JNK activity has an anti-apoptotic function in infected leukocytes, at least in part mediated via AP-1 (Lizundia *et al.*, 2006). Expression of a dominant-negative c-Jun mutant leads to a drop in the expression of anti-apoptotic proteins Mcl-1 and c-IAP, and sensitizes cells to induction of apoptosis, although it did not induce spontaneous apoptosis nor affect cellular proliferation. Thus, JNK must have other targets, aside from activating AP-1, that are required for suppressing apoptosis in infected leukocytes. *Theileria*-infected leukocytes can form tumours when injected into immunocompromised mice, and the inhibition of c-Jun reduced invasiveness of cells and tumour formation, revealing a role for cJun in metastasis, likely via the AP-1 driven expression of matrix metalloproteinases (MMPs) (Baylis *et al.*, 1995; Hall *et al.*, 1999; Lizundia *et al.*, 2006). Interestingly, inhibition of NF-kB or AP-1 by over-expression of IkB or a JNK dominant-negative mutant, respectively, negatively impacted c-Myc transcriptional activity, indicating that multiple pathways that are hijacked by *Theileria* converge upon c-Myc (Dessauge *et al.*, 2005b).

10.4.5 E2F

E2F family members are transcription factors that play key roles in the mammalian cell cycle, and E2F transcriptional activity is high in *T. parva*-transformed B cells. Treatment with cell-penetrating, parasite-derived peptides that bind to the E2F negative regulator Retinoblastoma-1 (RB) led to an increase in E2F-driven transcription and an accompanying increase in leukocyte proliferation in *T. parva*-infected B cells and *T. annulata*-infected macrophages, underpinning the role that E2F signalling plays in *Theileria*-induced leukocyte proliferation (Tretina *et al.*, 2020). Similarly, phosphoinositide 3-kinase (PI3K) and its downstream target Akt/PBK are found to be constitutively active in *T. parva*- and *T. annulata*-infected cells, and inhibitor studies revealed that PI3K activity is essential for proliferation, but not survival, of *Theileria*-infected cells (Baumgartner *et al.*, 2000; Dobbelaere *et al.*, 2000; Heussler *et al.*, 2001).

10.4.6 P53

P53 is a tumour suppressor protein that plays a crucial role in preventing genomic instability and cancer. In normal cells, p53 accumulates in the nucleus in response to DNA damage or other types of stress and can influence cell cycle progression and initiate apoptosis to prevent the occurrence of genomic mutations. In many cancers p53 is mutated. In *T. parva*-infected cells, the nuclear accumulation of p53 and its activation, as measured by a p21-luciferase reporter, is impaired (Hayashida *et al.*, 2013). Low p53 protein levels in infected cells are correlated with high expression of the negative regulator of p53, mouse double minute 2 (MDM2). Upon inhibition of MDM2, p53 nuclear levels and transcriptional activity were restored. Thus, in *T. parva*-infected T cells, p53 protein levels were kept low by the activity of MDM2. It is important to note that MDM2 levels varied significantly between different *T. parva*-infected cell lines and was sometimes barely detectable, suggesting that MDM2-mediated degradation of p53 is probably not the only mechanism employed by *Theileria* to ensure low p53 activity (Hayashida *et al.*, 2013). In a separate study, it was reported that p53 is excluded from the nucleus of *T. annulata*-infected macrophages by the sequestration of the p53 protein at the schizont surface (Haller *et al.*, 2010). In some other *T. annulata*-infected cell lines, p53 is undetectable at the schizont surface (unpublished observations from our laboratories), suggesting that different mechanisms have evolved to ensure low p53 activity in different infected cell lineages.

10.4.7 Warburg glycolysis

Tumour cells exhibit changes in their cellular metabolism compared to normal cells, which is characterized by increased glycolytic rate and decreased oxidative respiration, even in the presence of sufficient oxygen. This is known as the 'Warburg effect' and is driven by expression and stabilization of the transcription factor hypoxia inducible factor HIF1α (Koh and Powis, 2012). *Theileria*-infected cells consume higher levels of glucose than non-infected cells, and, like many cancer cells, are highly susceptible to glucose deprivation, in a phenomenon known as 'glucose addiction' (Medjkane and Weitzman, 2013). HIF1α expression is induced and stabilized in *T. annulata*-infected cells, and its sustained expression is required for maintenance of the transformed phenotype (Medjkane *et al.*, 2014; Metheni *et al.*, 2014; Marsolier *et al.*, 2019).

10.4.8 Cytokines

As reviewed previously (Dobbelaere and Heussler, 1999), both *T. parva*- and *T. annulata*-infected leukocytes modulate expression of genes encoding an array of cytokines. Stimulation of infected cells by cytokines in an autocrine manner has been proposed as a mechanism of enhancing the proliferation of *T. parva*-infected cells. This activity has been demonstrated for TNF-α and GM-CSF for some infected cell lines (Baumgartner *et al.*, 2000; Guergnon *et al.*, 2003). *T. parva*-infected cell lines constitutively express the IL2 receptor, and their proliferation is enhanced by addition of IL2, but a role for this cytokine in autocrine stimulation has not been confirmed (Shayan *et al.*, 1999). Significant variability in the profile of cytokine gene expression has been reported between *T. parva*-infected cell lines and between *T. parva*- and *T. annulata*-infected lines, raising doubts about the general relevance of autocrine stimulation. However, it remains possible that expression of cytokine receptors on infected cells functions to support proliferation of infected cells in a paracrine manner, *in vivo*. Evidence of a role for induction of transforming growth factor beta-2 (TGFb2) in conferring a metastasis phenotype has been obtained for *T. annulata*-infected cells (Chaussepied *et al.*, 2010) and may also operate for *T. parva* (Latré de Laté *et al.*, 2021).

From the results of the studies outlined above, it is clear that constitutive activation of pathways with potential to reorder host cell gene expression networks operates to promote the survival, proliferation and metastasis of leukocytes infected by *T. parva* and *T. annulata*. An overview of some of the pathways modulated by infection with *T. parva* is shown in Fig. 10.1.

10.5 A Mighty Makeover – Parasite-Dependent Rewiring of Host Cell Gene Expression Pathways

The constitutive activation of host cell transcription factors by *T. parva* and *T. annulata* has the potential to generate wide-scale changes in gene expression. For example, it has been estimated that NF-kB recognizes more than 3000 binding sites in DNA of monocytes (Lim *et al.*, 2007). Wide-scale alteration of the host cell transcriptome has been confirmed by microarray studies and more recently by RNA-seq. A comparison of the gene expression profile between *T. annulata*-infected and uninfected BL20 cells identified over 3000 differentially expressed (DE) host cell genes encoding cytokines, cellular receptors (including elevated IL2RA and B), oncogenes and transcriptional regulators (Kinnaird *et al.*, 2013). More than a third of the DE genes showed reversal in gene expression upon buparvaquone treatment, but reversal to the non-infected expression value was not obtained for others, and for some genes, death of the parasite coincided with a change opposite to that predicted. How this irreversible rewiring of host cell gene expression is achieved is not fully understood. It is likely to involve altered expression of host chromatin modifiers and was predicted to alter networks involved in regulation of haematopoietic cell fate (Kinnaird *et al.*, 2013), supporting previous work indicating that *T. annulata* infection induces a de-differentiated myeloid-type phenotype (Jensen *et al.*, 2009). A less pronounced de-differentiation phenotype has been proposed for *T. parva*-transformed lymphoid cells (Dobbelaere and Heussler, 1999), with changes to the differentiation state and cell surface markers recorded (Naessens *et al.*, 1985). The gene expression networks involved would be expected to show differences compared to those of *T. annulata* myeloid-derived lines.

Several of the host transcription factors activated in the *Theileria*-transformed

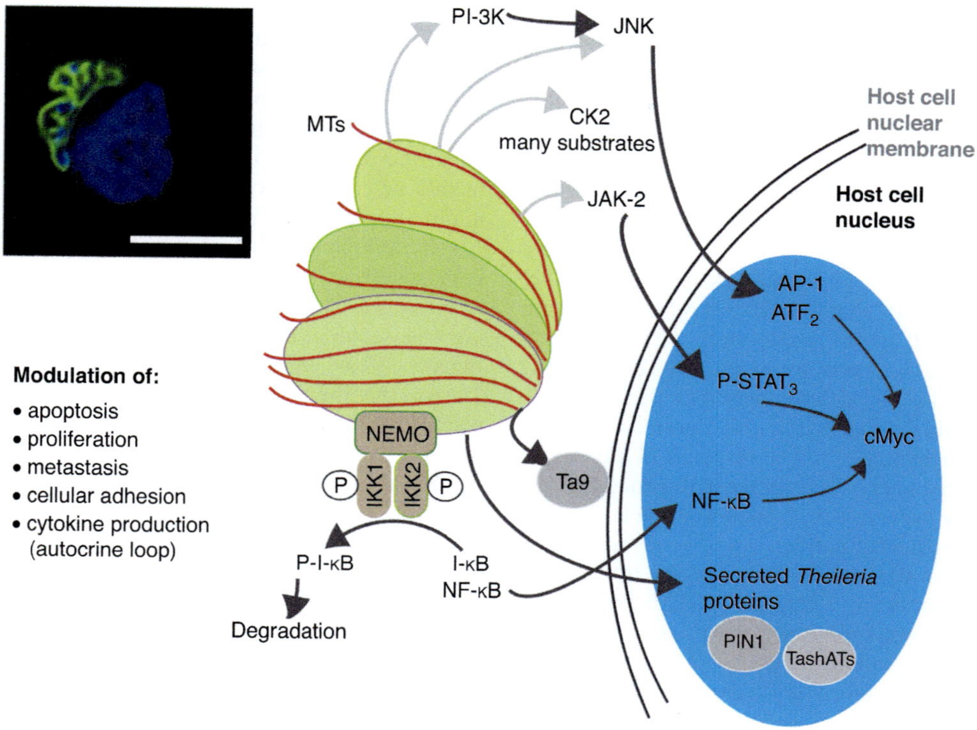

Fig. 10.1. Schematic overview of selected pathways modulated by *Theileria* infection. MTs: microtubules (shown in red). *Theileria* schizont shown in green. Several kinases (PI-3K, JNK, CK2, JAK-2) and transcription factors (e.g. AP-1, ATF2, cMyc and NF-kB) have been shown to be constitutively activated in infected cells. Light grey lines indicate that it is unknown how the parasite modifies these pathways. The IkB kinase (IKK) complex is sequestered at the schizont surface, leading to the constitutive activation of NF-kB. A few *Theileria* exported proteins have been detected in the bovine nucleus or cytoplasm and are likely to contribute to phenotype alteration. Examples shown are the *T. annulata* peptidyl prolyl isomerase (PIN1), proteins of the TashAT family (TashATs), and Ta9. The fluorescence image is *T. parva* (Marikebuni)-infected γIV T cells (951-F31; Katzer *et al.*, 2006) labelled with anti-*T. parva* monoclonal antibody ILS-40 at a dilution of 1 μg/ml (green, a kind gift from Tim Connelley). Scale bar = 10 μm.

leukocytes are known as 'Janus-type' because they have been shown to either protect against or induce cellular destruction. NF-kB is a classic Janus transcription factor, with activation either protecting cells from, or inducing, apoptosis, depending on cellular context (Lipton, 1997). NF-kB is a key modulator of genes involved in innate immunity and inflammation, and a causative factor in inflammatory disease (Atreya *et al.*, 2008). Similar properties are characteristic of AP-1 (Durchdewald *et al.*, 2009). Thus, constitutive transcription factor activation could have detrimental consequences for parasite viability or the infected host cell (Heussler *et al.*, 2002).

That *T. annulata* can moderate the outcome of these activation events was demonstrated by comparing the gene expression profile of uninfected and infected cells following stimulation by lipopolysaccharide, a known activator of NF-kB (Durrani *et al.*, 2012). NF-kB target genes elevated in uninfected BL20 cells were expressed at a lower level in infected cells, including the pro-inflammatory response genes *CXCL10*, *CCL4* and *IL15*. In contrast, genes predicted to be beneficial to the infected cell were elevated. *SPARC* (secreted protein acidic and rich in cysteine), for example, may promote degradation of the tumour suppressor p53 (Fenouille *et al.*, 2011), while *ICAM1* (intercellular adhesion molecule 1), which like *SPARC* is expressed at a significantly higher level in infected TBL20 relative to LPS (lipopolysaccharide)-stimulated (NF-kB-activated) BL20, has been linked to metastasis (Lin *et al.*, 2006).

A major reorganization of gene expression networks that operate in inflammation and cancer can be proposed for *T. parva*-infected leukocytes. A recent study that profiled peripheral blood leukocytes from naturally infected Boran cattle over a 15-day time course (Chepkwony *et al.*, 2022) identified over 10,000 differentially expressed genes. It should be noted that these profiles represent changes linked to the response of uninfected white blood cells together with genes differentially expressed in *T. parva*-infected leukocytes. Nevertheless, pathways and genes were highlighted that can be linked to the transformed cell, including E2F, MYC, p53, IL2RA and B, and pro-inflammatory cytokines.

Comparing the RNA-seq data from Boran cattle that survived *T. parva* infection to those of animals that died provided a set of differentially expressed genes potentially linked to tolerance of infection (Chepkwony *et al.*, 2022). The data were enriched for genes predicted to function in cellular proliferation and metastasis, which are expressed at lower levels in surviving animals, while genes induced by interferon (IFN) were expressed at a higher level relative to animals that died. Related work was performed comparing *T. annulata* RNA-seq data derived from infected cell lines established from susceptible Holstein cattle with that from tolerant Sahiwal cattle (Larcombe *et al.*, 2022). The results revealed moderated expression of genes stimulated by type 1 IFN (e.g. *MX1*, *MX2*, *OAS1Y/Z*, *OAS2*, *ISG15*, *IFI6*, *IFI44* and *RSAD2*), all of which were expressed at lower levels in Holstein relative to Sahiwal, whereas genes that are oncogenic (e.g. *UBD (FAT10)*, *SLIT2*, *PRUNE2* and *CLU*) were expressed at higher levels in Holstein. A separate study also highlighted elevation of *ICAM1* expression in Holstein infected cells (Jensen *et al.*, 2008). It can be concluded that the extensive rewiring of the host transcriptome in *Theileria*-infected cells is variable, and that the resulting expression profile will have a bearing on whether infection will be tolerated or cause acute disease. How the variability arises is not known. It could involve infection of different host cell lineages, and possibly the differentiation or activation status of the cell when infected, which would in turn influence differential activity of host transcription factors and modulation of infected cell chromatin architecture.

It has been accepted for some time that the pathogenesis of ECF and tropical theileriosis is associated with dysregulation of the bovine immune response (reviewed in Dobbelaere and Heussler, 1999; see Chapter 11 of this volume). The role that the transformed infected leukocyte plays in the aberrant stimulation of the immune response is not fully understood. It is likely to involve altered expression of genes encoding cell surface receptors/adhesion molecules, and genes encoding secreted cytokines and chemokines. For *T. parva*-infected lines, variable expression of lymphocyte cell surface antigens has been described and this has been linked to variable pathogenicity (Irvin and Morrison, 1987). Expression of genes encoding cytokines is also variable in *T. parva*-infected cell lines. However, expression of the gene encoding IL10 was found to be consistent for all lines tested and is also expressed by *T. annulata* cell lines (Brown *et al.*, 1995; McKeever *et al.*, 1997). IL-10 is known to be a key anti-inflammatory mediator that inhibits activation and effector function of T cells, monocytes and macrophages (Moore *et al.*, 2001) and has been proposed to contribute to pathology of theileriosis (Dobbelaere and Heussler, 1999). Some *T. parva*-infected cells also express IFNγ (DeMartini and Baldwin, 1991), a critical regulator of the innate and adaptive immune responses.

Modulated expression of genes encoding surface receptors, surface markers and cytokines has been reported for *T. annulata*-infected cells. The surface markers CD14, CD11b, M-M7 and TH57A are all down-regulated, corresponding with de-differentiation of the infected myeloid cell (Sager *et al.*, 1997). Moreover, in contrast to responses of uninfected macrophages, *T. annulata*-infected cells do not produce IFNα following stimulation with poly (I-C), although they do produce IFNβ (Sager *et al.*, 1998). More recent work indicated that modulated expression of genes encoding polypeptides located to the infected cell surface is extensive (Kinnaird *et al.*, 2013). Alterations include a marked reduction in expression of genes encoding Toll receptors involved in perception of inflammatory stimulation (Durrani *et al.*, 2012; Kinnaird *et al.*, 2013). Differential expression of infection-modulated receptor genes has also been linked to disease susceptibility. In the study of Larcombe *et al.* (2022), differential expression of genes encoding CCR1 (a receptor for the chemokine CCL5), CRLF2 (cytokine receptor-like factor 2), IL10RA (but not the IL10 cytokine), TLR2, CD2, CD48 and IL7R was identified between Holstein and Sahiwal infected cell lines. Likewise, modulation of genes encoding secreted proteins that could disrupt regulation of the immune response was reported. These included SLIT2 (known to function in leukocyte chemotaxis/infiltration), C1QTNF6 (complement C1q tumour necrosis related protein: anti-inflammatory), TNFSF10 (a cytokine that induces apoptosis) and CCL5 (a chemo-attractant for monocytes and memory T helper cells). In addition, elevated expression of the pro-inflammatory *IFNB1* gene was detected in infected cells from disease-susceptible Holstein cattle, implying a greater stimulation of an inflammatory response. Other studies have implicated a role for IL-1, IL-6 and TNF-α in generation of a pro-inflammatory cytokine storm (Glass *et al.*, 2003; McGuire *et al.*, 2004). Although not confirmed by qRT-PCR (quantitative reverse transcription polymerase chain reaction) due to variability within the breeds, expression of IL-6 was identified by RNA-seq as higher in infected Holstein cells (Larcombe *et al.*, 2022). It can be proposed that, in susceptible cattle breeds, rewiring of the host cell gene expression network by transforming *Theileria* results in altered production of receptors and secreted proteins that could promote pathological stimulation of the immune response. Modulation and aberrant stimulation of immune cells via the cargo of extracellular vesicles produced by *T. annulata*-transformed cells may also operate (Gillan *et al.*, 2019; Chai *et al.*, 2025). In contrast, co-evolution over millennia of both *T. parva* and *T. annulata* with buffalo is likely to have resulted in an infected cell phenotype that favours both parasite and host survival by limiting inflammatory stimulation and causing no overt pathology.

10.6 The Holy Grail – Screening for and Characterization of Parasite-Encoded Transformation Candidates

The Holy Grail for the understanding of *Theileria*-mediated host cell transformation is to identify factors encoded by the parasite genome that regulate this event. To date, due to the lack of a transfection system to functionally screen for candidates, the approach taken has primarily used bioinformatic prediction as the selection criterion. It is widely accepted that, since the parasite is not enclosed in a parasitophorous vacuole, then proteins that possess a signal peptide (SP) will be either deployed at the schizont surface membrane or, if the SP has a predicted cleavage site, secreted into the host cell cytoplasm. Surface membrane proteins possessing a GPI anchor or with large regions that are predicted to be exposed to the host side of the parasite plasma membrane may be more attractive candidates than integral membrane proteins. Secreted (and surface) parasite proteins that also possess domains that provide a function known to be associated with cell growth would clearly meet criteria as transformation candidates. The caveat to this approach, however, is that the algorithms are predictive, and proteins fundamental to controlling cellular proliferation might also function within the parasite as it proliferates within the infected cell. For example, the parasite-encoded cell cycle protein ThCRK2 (CDK) generated some interest as a potential transformation candidate (Kramer and Johnston, 1997), but immunofluorescence firmly identified this protein as only located within the parasite (Kinnaird *et al.*, 1996). It is imperative, in the authors' view, that the SP prediction is: (i) of high significance and generated by multiple algorithms, (ii) validated by localization studies, preferably by more than one experimental method, and (iii) supported by additional characteristics that point to a possible role in the transformation process. Two obvious characteristics that can be employed for candidate selection are: (i) given that proliferation of schizont-infected cells is limited for 'non-transforming' species such as *T. orientalis* and schizont-infected cell lines cannot be established *in vitro*, it can be predicted that the genomes of transforming species like *T. parva* would encode additional unique genes, protein motifs or expanded gene families that confer the fully transformed phenotype (Hayashida *et al.*, 2012); (ii) because during merogony host cell proliferation slows and eventually stops, parasite genes that promote host cell transformation can be predicted to display peak RNA expression values in the macroschizont stage, followed by a significant reduction as the schizont transitions to the merozoite. Recently, a TurboID-based proximity labelling approach was used to experimentally identify *T. annulata* proteins exported to the host cell cytoplasm and/or nucleus (Brühlmann *et al.*, 2024). In total, 179 *T. annulata* proteins were detected with at least one peptide in host cell compartments. Following stringent selection criteria including the above-mentioned bioinformatic criteria, nine candidate proteins were assigned with high confidence to the host nucleus, and four to the cytoplasm. Several bioinformatic screens have generated a reasonable number of candidates with lists published (Shiels *et al.*, 2006; Hayashida *et al.*, 2012; Marsolier *et al.*, 2015), and some recent reviews have summarized data on parasite factors that play a role in host cell transformation (Tretina *et al.*, 2015; Tajeri and Langsley, 2021; Woods *et al.*, 2021). Below we consider the merit of these candidates.

10.6.1 HSP90

HSP90 proteins were identified as transformation candidates based on possession of a signal peptide and a known role in oncogenesis, including promotion of proliferation and inhibition of apoptosis (Shiels *et al.*, 2006). HSP90 is a known component of the IKK signalosome and is required for activation of NF-kB. A parasite HSP90 secreted into the host compartment might therefore be a key component of the transformation mechanism. Subsequent detailed characterization of the *Theileria* HSP90 gene family in *T. annulata*, which comprises four members (with orthologues identified for *T. parva*), failed to validate a role as transformation candidates (Kinnaird *et al.*, 2017). TA12105 was located to the schizont cytoplasm, TA10720 to the apicoplast, TA06470 to the schizont endoplasmic reticulum and TA06845 was concluded to be a parasite mitochondrial chaperone. All four *HSP90* genes showed constitutive expression at the mRNA level during differentiation to the merozoite. HSP90 serves as an example that sequence analysis and possession of a signal peptide are not sufficient to conclude a parasite molecule is a *bona fide* transformation candidate.

10.6.2 *Tp*GcpE

Proliferation of eukaryotic cells is regulated by the transcription factor E2F and the Retinoblastoma-1 (RB) tumour suppressor protein that negatively regulates E2F signalling. It is of interest, therefore, that a bioinformatic screen identified a putative *T. parva*-secreted protein encoding a LxCxE motif predicted to bind RB (Tretina *et al.*, 2020). Subsequent experiments demonstrated that the peptide motif and recombinant protein bind the RB pocket domain with nanomolar affinity. In addition, incubation of *T. annulata*-infected cells with LxCxE peptide could elevate E2F activity and cellular proliferation. Unfortunately, immunolocalization experiments failed to demonstrate conclusively that *Tp*GcpE is secreted into the host cell compartment, and the signal peptide predicts translocation of the protein to the parasite apicoplast. Thus, while perturbation of E2F signalling is likely to operate in transformation of host cells by *T. parva* and *T. annulata*, it remains to be proven that this is performed by *Tp*GcpE or any of the other 14 parasite proteins predicted to bind RB.

10.6.3 Casein kinase II

Casein Kinase II (CKII) is an important modulator of cellular metabolism and implicated in cellular transformation. Constitutive activation of CKII in *T. parva*-infected leukocytes has been demonstrated (ole-MoiYoi *et al.*, 1993) and considered central to the transformed phenotype (Dessauge *et al.*, 2005a). Based on identification of a putative signal peptide, it was proposed that a parasite-encoded CKIIα subunit is secreted into the host cytosol (ole-MoiYoi *et al.*, 1992) to regulate host cell proliferation (ole-MoiYoi, 1995). Detailed analysis of the *T. annulata* CKIIα gene and immunolocalization failed to confirm this hypothesis. The predicted signal peptide is not translated, and the protein was located within the schizont (Biermann *et al.*, 2003). The mechanism whereby constitutive activation of CKII occurs in the *Theileria*-transformed leukocyte remains unknown.

10.6.4 Prolyl isomerases

An initial bioinformatic screen for transformation candidates identified several prolyl isomerases as potential candidates (Shiels *et al.*, 2006). However, no prolyl isomerases were found to be specific to the transforming lineage (Hayashida *et al.*, 2012). A refined bioinformatic screen for transformation candidates predicted a signal peptide (SP) specific for the *T. annulata* and *T. parva* homologues of the mammalian peptidyl-prolyl isomerase PIN1, designated as *TaPIN1/TpPIN1* (Marsolier *et al.*, 2015). The SP was not predicted for the *T. orientalis* orthologue. Supporting evidence for secretion of TaPIN1 was generated by identification of the protein in the nuclear fraction of infected cells by immunoblotting and immunofluorescence, although the highest concentration of antibody reactivity in the infected cell was within the schizont. Further experiments provided evidence that TaPIN1 acts as a homologue of its mammalian counterpart and promotes transformation by activating AP-1 via destabilization of the FBW7 ubiquitin ligase that targets c-Jun (a component of the AP-1 heterodimer) for degradation. In a follow-up study, evidence was generated for a role of TaPIN1 in stabilization of pyruvate kinase isoform M2 (PKM2). PKM2 leads to HIF1α-dependent regulation of metabolic enzymes that promote a Warburg-like aerobic glycolysis described for *Theileria*-transformed leukocytes and cancer cells (Medjkane and Weitzman, 2013; Metheni *et al.*, 2015). Clearly, identification of a secreted form of this parasite prolyl isomerase is an important finding. It should be noted, however, that it is not known whether the parasite protein plays a dual function and is required for viability of the parasite *per se*. This could explain why the gene has been retained in the non-transforming *T. orientalis* (lacking an SP) and why the TaPIN1 protein appears to be most abundant within the schizont. Alternatively, a non-secreted paralogous protein could provide this function in transforming *Theileria* species.

Marsolier *et al.* (2015) also identified a gene encoding cyclophilin1, *TaCyp-1* (TA19600, TP01_0244), as a transformation candidate. In a separate study, TaCyp-1 was shown by immunofluorescence to be located at the schizont surface (Zhao *et al.*, 2018). Yeast-2 hybrid screening demonstrated interaction with host MED21 (Mediator of RNA polymerase II transcription subunit 21), a regulator of RNA polymerase II-dependent gene expression, and experiments were performed to investigate a role in activation of NF-kB. Knock-down of *MED21* expression showed no effect on the level of either NF-kB components or the phosphorylation status of the IkB inhibitor. *TaCyp-1* is conserved across the Piroplasmida (EuPath DB). A role in leukocyte transformation remains to be demonstrated.

10.6.5 Prohibitin

Prohibitin can act as a tumour suppressor but has also been associated with tumour development (Li *et al.*, 2011). Prohibitin genes that encode a signal peptide are present within the *T. parva* and *T. annulata* genomes but are not designated as specific to the transforming lineage. A recent study has proposed that a parasite-encoded prohibitin, *Ta*PHB-1 (TA04375), is secreted into the transformed leukocyte cytosol (Aravetia *et al.*, 2023). Confocal microscopy using antibody affinity-purified against recombinant *Ta*PHB-1 indicated that this parasite prohibitin is located to both schizont surface and host cell cytosol, while bovine prohibitin is confined to the nucleus in infected cells. *Ta*PHB-1 detected in infected cell extract appears to be significantly larger than its recombinant form or host prohibitin. Yeast-2 hybrid and co-immunoprecipitation experiments identified bovine RUVBL1 (Bo-RUVBL1) as an interacting partner. It is proposed that this interaction takes place on the schizont surface and that the associated protein interactome has potential to manipulate several functions, including protein folding, catalytic activity, transporter activity and actin cytoskeleton organization. Further localization and functional validation of this interactome at the parasite surface is necessary.

10.6.6 Peptidases

A number of peptidases have been proposed as putative transformation candidates (Shiels *et al.*, 2006). None are specific to the transforming lineage, and subsequent *in silico* analyses failed to identify a secreted peptidase as a transformation candidate. A membrane-bound peptidase, TA18300/Tp03_0804, was reported as expressed specifically by the schizont stage and predicted to cleave signal peptides of secreted parasite proteins, thus contributing indirectly to the transformed phenotype (Weir *et al.*, 2009). More recent work investigated a *T. annulata* cysteine proteinase, TaCP, using yeast-2 hybrid methodology (Zhao *et al.*, 2017). Interacting partners with a proposed role in the transformation process were identified. No data confirming either a surface location or secretion of TaCP into the host cytosol were presented. The direct involvement of *Theileria* peptidases in the transformation process remains to be proven.

10.6.7 SVSPs

The subtelomere-encoded variable secreted protein (SVSP) gene family is a large multigene family that has been markedly expanded in the genomes of transforming *Theileria* species (Hayashida *et al.*, 2012). SVSPs are a major component of the predicted schizont secretome and a number are postulated to translocate to the host cell nucleus, with one (TP03_0882) locating to the nucleus of mammalian cells when over-expressed. However, immunofluorescence against TP03_0882 showed that only a small (< 5%) proportion of parasites expressed detectable protein and that staining was internal to the parasite. Native protein was not detected in infected cell extracts. The pattern of SVSP mRNA expression was reported to be variable across *T. parva*-infected cloned cell lines, with the gene expression pattern linked to parasite genotype (Schmuckli *et al.*, 2009). A paper investigating SVSP allelic diversity in *T. annulata* reported that SVSP genes show atypical codon usage compared to other major secretome gene families and are evolving neutrally, with high levels of nucleotide substitutions and multiple insertions and deletions. It was proposed that, like other subtelomeric gene families, SVSPs act as contingency genes to evade/subvert a protective T cell immune response, although this is not supported by experimental evidence (Weir *et al.*, 2010). In marked contrast, recent work indicated that SVSP455 (*TA05545*) is located on the parasite surface, secreted into the host cytosol, reacts with host HSP60 and functions to protect the infected cell against apoptosis (Li *et al.*, 2022), whereas a second SVSP (TA05575) was concluded to be mainly in the host nucleus and interact with a host RBMX2-like protein (Li *et al.*, 2021). Additional work is required to demonstrate whether these interactions are specific to these two SVSPs and operate via binding domains that are encoded in all alleles of TA05545 and TA05575 and orthologues identified in *T. parva*.

10.6.8 Ta9/Tp9

Genes encoding Ta9 (TA15705) and the *T. parva* orthologue Tp9 (TP02_0895) were first identified while screening for antigens recognized by cytotoxic CD8 T cells from cattle immune to *T. annulata* and *T. parva*, respectively (MacHugh *et al.*, 2011; Hemmink *et al.*, 2016). Both genes encode highly dominant CD8 antigens and both antigens also appear to be immunodominant for an antibody response (Bilgic *et al.*, 2016; Bastos *et al.*, 2019). The Ta9 gene was also identified in a screen of *T. annulata* schizont cDNAs capable of activating the host cell transcription factor AP-1 (Unlu *et al.*, 2018) and was identified in the host cytoplasm as part of the *T. annulata* 'exportome' by TurboID proximity-based labelling (Brühlmann *et al.*, 2024). *Ta9* mRNA is highly expressed at the schizont stage, with expression levels decreasing significantly early in merogony (Fig. 10.2A), and *Ta9/Tp9* family genes are classed as specific to the transforming

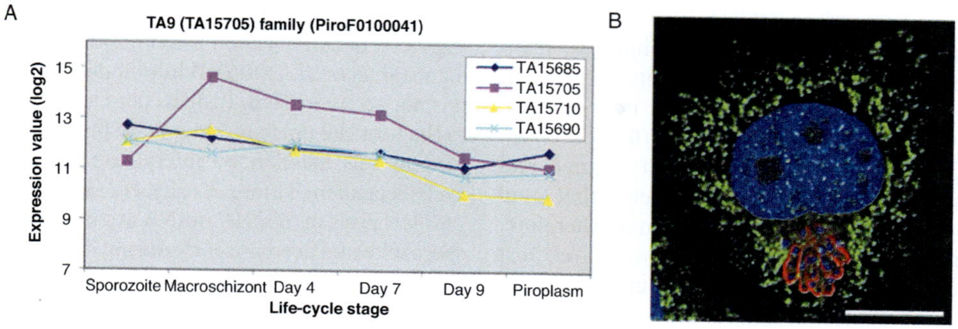

Fig. 10.2. A: mRNA expression profile of Ta9 gene family. B: Immunofluorescence of *T. annulata* schizont-infected cell with antisera against Ta9 (green) and p104 (red). Ta9 shows a vesicular pattern in host cytosol while p104 detects schizont membrane. Scale bar = 10 µm.

Theileria lineage (Hayashida *et al.*, 2012). Affinity purified antibodies from immune sera (Unlu *et al.*, 2018) and antisera raised against Ta9 fusion proteins detect a vesicular pattern in the host cytosol (Fig. 10.2B), supporting the conclusion that the protein interacts with the host endosomal pathway and is exported out of the infected cell as a component of extracellular vesicles (EV) (Chai *et al.*, 2025). The finding that divergent regions of the protein are under selection to evade killer T cell recognition validates that presentation of Ta9/Tp9 peptides at the cell surface is detrimental to survival of the infected leukocyte (MacHugh *et al.*, 2011). It can be concluded, therefore, that the conservation of Ta9/Tp9 and expansion of the gene family across transforming species, including *T. lestoquardi* (Goh *et al.*, 2016), is likely because Ta9/Tp9 (and paralogous genes) perform an important function for the transformed phenotype. This function could be limited to induction of *AP-1* gene expression by the semi-conserved C-terminal region (Unlu *et al.*, 2018). However, it is possible that Ta9/Tp9, and other members of the gene family, perform additional functions to modify the infected leukocyte niche.

10.6.9 TashAT/TpHN

T. annulata genes encoding parasite-secreted proteins bearing AT-hook DNA-binding domains (*TashAT*) were first identified in a screen for genes down-regulated during schizont to merozoite stage differentiation. TashAT2 was located to the host nucleus of infected leukocytes by immunofluorescence, cell fractionation and immunoblotting (Swan *et al.*, 1999). Three proteins of the Tash family, including TashAT2, were identified with confidence in the TurboID-based exportome screen (Brühlmann *et al.*, 2024). *TashAT* genes are arranged in a cluster of 17 contiguous genes (in the reference *T. annulata* genome) and encode proteins that bind to AT-rich DNA motifs (Swan *et al.*, 2001; Pain *et al.*, 2005). An orthologous cluster of 20 genes (*TpHN* cluster) was identified for *T. parva* (Shiels *et al.*, 2006). The *TashAT/TpHN* cluster is markedly expanded in transforming species. Only one gene in the cluster has an orthologue in *T. orientalis* and, in contrast to all other *TashAT* genes, shows elevated expression levels during merogony (Hayashida *et al.*, 2012). Although genes in the *TpHN* cluster of *T. parva* do not encode consensus AT-hook domains, orthologues of *TashAT* genes encoding predicted proteins with signal peptides, nuclear localization signals and PEST sequences have been identified, and a serum raised against TashAT2 detects the host nucleus of *T. parva*-infected cells (Swan *et al.*, 1999; Shiels *et al.*, 2006; Hayashida *et al.*, 2012). Thus, the *TashAT/TpHN* clusters have evolved with the transforming lineage and are likely to perform an important function in modulating the host leukocyte, with diversification of function required for the different cellular niches preferentially transformed by different *Theileria* species.

The function of TashAT cluster genes is not fully known. TashAT2 and TashAT3 show similarity in the AT-hook domain arrangement with mammalian HMGA proteins. HMGA1 and 2 alter chromatin accessibility to transcription factors and modulate expression of genes involved in stem cell development, innate immunity and cancer (Reeves *et al.*, 2001; Schuldenfrei *et al.*, 2011; Vignali and Marracci, 2020). TashAT proteins that bind to host AT-rich DNA motifs may, therefore, generate wide-scale modulation of the host cell epigenome/transcriptome and moderate the outcome of host cell transcription factor activation. Studies to investigate modulation of bovine gene expression have utilized cells from a transformed macrophage cell line (BoMac) stably expressing a *TashAT2* transgene. Alteration of BoMac gene expression was identified by differential display analysis but only a few genes were characterized (Oura *et al.*, 2006). These initial findings have been extended by a recent study performing RNA-seq on three TashAT2 expressing BoMac lines relative to three control lines (reverse orientation/non-expressing). Over 800 bovine genes were found to show significant alteration, with a subset of overlapping genes also modulated by parasite infection of BL20 cells (Durrani *et al.*, 2023). Comparison with pathways altered by mammalian HMGA factors supports the premise that TashAT2 acts as an analogue of these important chromatin modifiers. Moreover, modulation of host gene expression by TashAT2 has been tentatively linked to disease severity. Substantial differences in the number and pattern of the host nucleotide motif that TashAT2 binds were identified in the reference *Bos taurus* vs *Bos indicus* genomes (Larcombe *et al.*, 2022). There is also variability in the number, arrangement and amino acid sequence of the AT-hook DNA-binding domains encoded by different *TashAT2* alleles, with geographical sub-structuring of alleles reported (Weir *et al.*, 2010). It was proposed that TashAT family genes could have co-evolved with their target host genomes (Weir *et al.*, 2010). Furthermore, recent work suggests that the diversity in its DNA-binding domains, together with a variable pattern of the nucleotide motif in the host genome to which TashAT2 binds, could differentially mould the epigenome of the infected cell and influence the degree of disease severity (Larcombe *et al.*, 2022; Durrani *et al.*, 2023).

The *TashAT* cluster gene *TashHN* shows a high level of conservation with its *T. parva* orthologue (Shiels *et al.*, 2006). While binding to DNA has not been reported, TashHN does translocate to the host cell nucleus and may be phosphorylated in this location by interaction with cell cycle-dependent kinase 2 (CDK2) (Swan *et al.*, 2003). Levels of *TashHN* mRNA are high in the sporozoite and decrease early during differentiation from schizont to merozoite. *TashHN* mRNA levels are elevated in attenuated *T. annulata* cell lines that show reduced ability to undergo merogony, indicating association between *TashHN* and selection for growth of schizont-infected cells *in vitro*. Taken together, these data suggest that TashHN could function early in the transformation event, possibly by promoting survival or proliferation of the infected cell.

10.7 A Tapestry of Transformation – Conclusions and Future Perspectives

Transformation of the host leukocyte by *T. parva* and related *Theileria* species is considered a unique event in eukaryotic biology. Based on the studies outlined in this chapter, it appears unlikely that transformation is induced by a single master regulator: the evidence suggests that a tapestry of co-dependent events must operate to generate the resulting infected cell phenotype. Whether multiple overlapping pathways and the discovery of several expanded gene families in the genomes of transforming *Theileria* species indicate a degree of mechanistic redundancy remains to be determined. Transformation events include interaction with the host cell cytoskeleton and cytokinesis, establishment of platforms that initiate signal transduction cascades, activation of host transcription factors and modulation of the activation phenotype to promote proliferation and survival of both the parasite and the infected leukocyte. Candidate parasite molecules that operate in these events have been identified. However, the role each candidate plays and whether their activities must be coordinated to generate the fully transformed phenotype needs to be established. One glaring gap is the identification of the putative parasite-encoded ligand for the IKK signalosome complex. Numerous studies have failed to identify any candidates. The study of Hayashida *et al.* (2010) identified the schizont surface molecule TpSCOP (*Theileria parva* schizont-derived cytoskeleton-binding protein) as a modulator of NF-kB activity, but a direct association with parasite-associated signalosome complexes was not reported. Why this has been so difficult could relate to a requirement for a transient interactome involving parasite surface, IKK signalosome components and host cell cytoskeletal structures. Other putative regulators that are missing are the proposed ligand on the schizont that recruits p53 and the parasite–host interaction that promotes degradation of this molecule, although an involvement of p104-sequestered host JNK2 has been proposed for modulation of p53 (Latré de Laté *et al.*, 2019). Likewise, how the pRB/E2F axis is manipulated requires further research, and it is not understood how host CKII is modulated or precisely how c-Myc is activated by the parasite. Nor is it known how the parasite sequesters essential nutrients and lipids from the host niche, but this may show similarities to strategies used by related apicomplexans (reviewed in Woods *et al.*, 2021). Mining for more manipulators may be required, and there is much still to be discovered, including the role of the infected cell epigenome and how modulated expression of cytokines and receptors induce dysregulation of the immune response to cause pathology. Future studies should aim to validate that mechanisms and pathways discovered *in vitro* also operate *in vivo*. Difficulties in profiling expression changes *in vivo* should be overcome by the adoption of single-cell sequencing methodology (Agboraw *et al.*, 2025). Moreover, future studies aiming to unravel the transformation tapestry will be made substantially easier if a reverse genetics system can be developed. Solving the technical barriers that have prevented its establishment is essential if functional validation of parasite-encoded transformation candidates is to be achieved. In addition, stable transfection has the potential to generate genetically manipulated parasites attenuated for virulence that can be used to vaccinate animals, via macroschizont transfer (*T. annulata*) or sporozoite infection (*T. parva*), in place of current methods that require long-term cell line passage or sporozoite infection and treatment.

References

Agboraw, E., Haese-Hill, W., Hentzschel, F., Briggs, E., Aghabi, D. *et al.* (2025) ParaCell: A novel software tool for the interactive analysis and visualization of standard and dual host-parasite single-cell RNA-seq data. *Nucleic Acids Research* 53(4), gkaf091. DOI: 10.1093/nar/gkaf091.

Al-Hamidhi, S., Weir, W., Kinnaird, J., Tageledin, M., Beja-Pereira, A. *et al.* (2016) *Theileria lestoquardi* displays reduced genetic diversity relative to sympatric *Theileria annulata* in Oman. *Infection, Genetics and Evolution* 43, 297–306. DOI: 10.1016/j.meegid.2016.05.007.

Allsopp, M.T., Cavalier-Smith, T., De Waal, D.T. and Allsopp, B.A. (1994) Phylogeny and evolution of the *piroplasms*. *Parasitology* 108(Pt 2), 147–152. DOI: 10.1017/s0031182000068232.

Aravetia, P.B., Kar, P.P., Kuriakosea, A., Sanju, A., Kumar, K. *et al.* (2023) Identification of a novel interaction between *Theileria* prohibitin (*Ta*PHB-1) and bovine RuvB-like AAA ATPase 1. *Microbiology Spectrum* 11(1), e02502–2522. DOI: 10.1128/spectrum.02502-22.

Atreya, I., Atreya, R. and Neurath, M.F. (2008) NF-kappaB in inflammatory bowel disease. *Journal of Internal Medicine* 263(6), 591–596. DOI: 10.1111/j.1365-2796.2008.01953.x.

Baldwin, C.L., Malu, M.N., Kinuthia, S.W., Conrad, P.A. and Grootenhuis, J.G. (1986) Comparative analysis of infection and transformation of lymphocytes from African buffalo and Boran cattle with *Theileria parva* subsp. *parva* and *T. parva* subsp. *lawrencei*. *Infection and Immunity* 53(1), 186–191. DOI: 10.1128/iai.53.1.186-191.1986.

Bastos, R.G., Franceschi, V., Tebaldi, G., Connelley, T., Morrison, W.I. *et al.* (2019) Molecular and antigenic properties of mammalian cell-expressed *Theileria parva* antigen Tp9. *Frontiers in Immunology* 10, 897. DOI: 10.3389/fimmu.2019.00897.

Baumgartner, M., Tardieux, I., Ohayon, H., Gounon, P. and Langsley, G. (1999) The use of nocodazole in cell cycle analysis and parasite purification from *Theileria parva*-infected B cells. *Microbes and Infection* 1(14), 1181–1188. DOI: 10.1016/s1286-4579(99)00244-0.

Baumgartner, M., Chaussepied, M., Moreau, M.F., Werling, D., Davis, W.C. *et al.* (2000) Constitutive PI3-k activity is essential for proliferation, but not survival, of *Theileria parva*-transformed B cells. *Cellular Microbiology* 2(4), 329–339. DOI: 10.1046/j.1462-5822.2000.00062.x.

Baylis, H.A., Megson, A. and Hall, R. (1995) Infection with *Theileria annulata* induces expression of matrix metalloproteinase 9 and transcription factor AP-1 in bovine leucocytes. *Molecular and Biochemical Parasitology* 69(2), 211–222. DOI: 10.1016/0166-6851(94)00216-a.

Biermann, R., Schnittger, L., Beyer, D. and Ahmed, J.S. (2003) Initiation of translation and cellular localization of *Theileria annulata* casein kinase IIalpha: Implication for its role in host cell transformation. *Journal of Cellular Physiology* 196(3), 444–453. DOI: 10.1002/jcp.10291.

Bilgic, H.B., Karagenc, T., Bakırcı, S., Shiels, B., Tait, A. *et al.* (2016) Identification and analysis of immunodominant antigens for ELISA-based detection of *Theileria annulata*. *PLoS ONE* 11(6), e0156645. DOI: 10.1371/journal.pone.0156645.

Botteron, C. and Dobbelaere, D. (1998) AP-1 and ATF-2 are constitutively activated via the JNK pathway in *Theileria parva*-transformed T-cells. *Biochemical and Biophysical Research Communications* 246(2), 418–421. DOI: 10.1006/bbrc.1998.8635.

Brown, C.G.D., Hunter, A.G. and Luckins, A.G. (1990) Diseases caused by protozoa. In: Sewell, M.M.H. and Brocklesby, D.W. (eds) *Handbook on Animal Diseases in the Tropics*, 4th edn. Baillière Tindall, London, pp. 161–226.

Brown, D.J., Campbell, J.D., Russell, G.C., Hopkins, J. and Glass, E.J. (1995) T cell activation by *Theileria annulata*-infected macrophages correlates with cytokine production. *Clinical and Experimental Immunology* 102(3), 507–514. DOI: 10.1111/j.1365-2249.1995.tb03845.x.

Brühlmann, F., Perry, C., Griessen, C., Gunasekera, K., Reymond, J.L. *et al.* (2024) TurboID mapping reveals the exportome of secreted intrinsically disordered proteins in the transforming parasite *Theileria annulata*. *mBio* 15(6): e0341223. DOI: 10.1128/mbio.03412-23.

Chai, Y., Che, J., Wang, J., Guan, G. and Yin, H. (2025) Systematic proteomic and small RNA profiling of extracellular vesicles from cattle infected with a naturally occurring buparvaquone-resistant strain of *Theileria annulata* and from uninfected controls. *Parasites & Vectors* 18(1), 221. DOI: 10.1186/s13071-025-06834-8.

Channavajhala, P. and Seldin, D.C. (2002) Functional interaction of protein kinase CK2 and C-Myc in lymphomagenesis. *Oncogene* 21(34), 5280–5288. DOI: 10.1038/sj.onc.1205640.

Chaussepied, M., Lallemand, D., Moreau, M.F., Adamson, R., Hall, R. *et al.* (1998) Upregulation of Jun and Fos family members and permanent JNK activity lead to constitutive AP-1 activation in *Theileria*-transformed leukocytes. *Molecular and Biochemical Parasitology* 94(2), 215–226. DOI: 10.1016/s0166-6851(98)00070-x.

Chaussepied, M., Janski, N., Baumgartner, M., Lizundia, R., Jensen, K. *et al.* (2010) TGF-b2 induction regulates invasiveness of *Theileria*-transformed leukocytes and disease susceptibility. *PLoS Pathogens* 6(11), e1001197. DOI: 10.1371/journal.ppat.1001197.

Chepkwony, M., Wragg, D., Latré de Laté, P., Paxton, E., Cook, E. *et al.* (2022) Longitudinal transcriptome analysis of cattle infected with *Theileria parva*. *International Journal for Parasitology* 52(13–14), 799–813. DOI: 10.1016/j.ijpara.2022.07.006.

Conrad, P.A., Kelly, B.G. and Brown, C.G. (1985) Intraerythrocytic schizogony of *Theileria annulata*. *Parasitology* 91(Pt 1), 67–82. DOI: 10.1017/s0031182000056523.

Dang, C.V., O'Donnell, K.A., Zeller, K.I., Nguyen, T., Osthus, R.C. *et al.* (2006) The c-Myc target gene network. *Seminars in Cancer Biology* 16(4), 253–264. DOI: 10.1016/j.semcancer.2006.07.014.

DeMartini, J.C. and Baldwin, C.L. (1991) Effects of gamma-interferon, tumour necrosis factor alpha, and interleukin-2 on infection and proliferation of *Theileria parva*-infected bovine lymphoblasts and production of interferon by parasitized cells. *Infection and Immunity* 59(12), 4540–4546. DOI: 10.1128/iai.59.12.4540-4546.1991.

Dessauge, F., Lizundia, R., Baumgartner, M., Chaussepied, M. and Langsley, G. (2005c) Taking the Myc is bad for *Theileria*. *Trends in Parasitology* 21(8), 377–385. DOI: 10.1016/j.pt.2005.06.003.

Dessauge, F., Hilaly, S., Baumgartner, M., Blumen, B., Werling, D. *et al.* (2005a) C-Myc activation by *Theileria parasites* promotes survival of infected B-lymphocytes. *Oncogene* 24(6), 1075–1083. DOI: 10.1038/sj.onc.1208314.

Dessauge, F., Lizundia, R. and Langsley, G. (2005b) Constitutively activated CK2 potentially plays a pivotal role in *Theileria*-induced lymphocyte transformation. *Parasitology* 130(S1), S37–S44. DOI: 10.1017/S0031182005008140.

Dobbelaere, D. and Heussler, V. (1999) Transformation of leukocytes by *Theileria parva* and *T. annulata*. *Annual Review of Microbiology* 53, 1–42. DOI: 10.1146/annurev.micro.53.1.1.

Dobbelaere, D.A.E., Fernandez, P.C. and Heussler, V.T. (2000) *Theileria parva*: Taking control of host cell proliferation and survival mechanisms. *Cellular Microbiology* 2(2), 91–99. DOI: 10.1046/j.1462-5822.2000.00045.x.

Durchdewald, M., Angel, P. and Hess, J. (2009) The transcription factor Fos: A Janus-type regulator in health and disease. *Histology and Histopathology* 24(11), 1451–1461. DOI: 10.14670/HH-24.1451.

Durrani, Z. (2012) Investigation of *Theileria annulata* as modulator of activation associated host cell gene expression. PhD thesis, University of Glasgow, UK. Available at: http://theses.gla.ac.uk/3430 (accessed 4 December 2025).

Durrani, Z., Weir, W., Pillai, S., Kinnaird, J. and Shiels, B. (2012) Modulation of activation-associated host cell gene expression by the apicomplexan parasite *Theileria annulata*. *Cellular Microbiology* 14(9), 1434–1454. DOI: 10.1111/j.1462-5822.2012.01809.x.

Durrani, Z., Kinnaird, J., Cheng, C.W., Brühlmann, F., Capewell, P. *et al.* (2023) A parasite DNA binding protein with potential to influence disease susceptibility acts as an analogue of mammalian HMGA transcription factors. *PLoS ONE* 18(6), e0286526. DOI: 10.1371/journal.pone.0286526.

Fenouille, N., Puissant, A., Tichet, M., Zimniak, G., Abbe, P. *et al.* (2011) SPARC functions as an anti-stress factor by inactivating p53 through Akt-mediated MDM2 phosphorylation to promote melanoma cell survival. *Oncogene* 30(49), 4887–4900. DOI: 10.1038/onc.2011.198.

Galley, Y., Hagens, G., Glaser, I., Davis, W., Eichhorn, M. *et al.* (1997) Jun NH_2-terminal kinase is constitutively activated in T cells transformed by the intracellular parasite *Theileria parva*. *Proceedings of the National Academy of Sciences* 94(10), 5119–5124. DOI: 10.1073/pnas.94.10.5119.

Gillan, V., Simpson, D.M., Kinnaird, J., Maitland, K., Shiels, B. *et al.* (2019) Characterisation of infection associated microRNA and protein cargo in extracellular vesicles of *Theileria annulata* infected leukocytes. *Cellular Microbiology* 21(1), e12969. DOI: 10.1111/cmi.12969.

Glass, E.J., Craigmile, S.C., Springbett, A., Preston, P.M., Kirvar, E. *et al.* (2003) The protozoan parasite, *Theileria annulata*, induces a distinct acute phase protein response in cattle that is associated with pathology. *International Journal for Parasitology* 33(12), 1409–1418. DOI: 10.1016/s0020-7519(03)00166-8.

Goh, S., Ngugi, D., Lizundia, R., Hostettler, I., Woods, K. *et al.* (2016) Identification of *Theileria lestoquardi* antigens recognized by CD8+ T cells. *PLoS ONE* 11(9), e0162571. DOI: 10.1371/journal.pone.0162571.

Guergnon, J., Chaussepied, M., Sopp, P., Lizundia, R., Moreau, M.F. *et al.* (2003) A tumour necrosis factor alpha autocrine loop contributes to proliferation and nuclear factor-kappaB activation of *Theileria parva*-transformed B cells. *Cell Microbiology* 5(10), 709–716. DOI: 10.1046/j.1462-5822.2003.00314.x.

Hagiwara, K., Takahashi, K., Taniyama, H., Kawamoto, S., Kurosawa, T. *et al.* (1997) Detection of *Theileria sergenti* schizonts in bovine lymph node. *International Journal for Parasitology* 27(11), 1375–1378. DOI: 10.1016/S0020-7519(97)00092-1.

Hall, R., Ilhan, T., Kirvar, E., Wilkie, G., Preston, P.M. *et al.* (1999) Mechanism(s) of attenuation of *Theileria annulata* vaccine cell lines. *Tropical Medicine & International Health* 4(9), A78–A84. DOI: 10.1046/j.1365-3156.1999.00454.x.

Haller, D., Mackiewicz, M., Gerber, S., Beyer, D., Kullmann, B. *et al.* (2010) Cytoplasmic sequestration of p53 promotes survival in leukocytes transformed by *Theileria*. *Oncogene* 29(21), 3079–3086. DOI: 10.1038/onc.2010.61.

Hayashida, K., Hattori, M., Nakao, R., Tanaka, Y., Kim, J.Y. *et al.* (2010) A schizont-derived protein, TpSCOP, is involved in the activation of NF-kappaB in *Theileria parva*-infected lymphocytes. *Molecular and Biochemical Parasitology* 174(1), 8–17. DOI: 10.1016/j.molbiopara.2010.06.005.

Hayashida, K., Hara, Y., Abe, T., Yamasaki, C., Toyoda, A. *et al.* (2012) Comparative genome analysis of three eukaryotic parasites with differing abilities to transform leukocytes reveals key mediators of *Theileria*-induced leukocyte transformation. *mBio* 3(5), e00204–212. DOI: 10.1128/mBio.00204-12.

Hayashida, K., Kajino, K., Hattori, M., Wallace, M., Morrison, I. *et al.* (2013) MDM2 regulates a novel form of incomplete neoplastic transformation of *Theileria parva* infected lymphocytes. *Experimental and Molecular Pathology* 94, 228–238. DOI: 10.1016/j.yexmp.2012.08.008.

Hemmink, J.D., Weir, W., MacHugh, N.D., Graham, S.P., Patel, E. *et al.* (2016) Limited genetic and antigenic diversity within parasite isolates used in a live vaccine against *Theileria parva*. *International Journal for Parasitology* 46(8), 495–506. DOI: 10.1016/j.ijpara.2016.02.007.

Heussler, V.T., Machado, J., Fernandez, P.C., Botteron, C., Chen, C.G. *et al.* (1999) The intracellular parasite *Theileria parva* protects infected T cells from apoptosis. *Proceedings of the National Academy of Sciences* 96(13), 7312–7317. DOI: 10.1073/pnas.96.13.7312.

Heussler, V.T., Kuenzi, P., Fraga, F., Schwab, R., Hemmings, B. *et al*. (2001) The Akt/PKB pathway is constitutively activated in *Theileria*-transformed leucocytes, but does not directly control constitutive NF-kappaB activation. *Cellular Microbiology* 3(8), 537–550. DOI: 10.1046/j.1462-5822.2001.00134.x.

Heussler, V.T., Rottenberg, S., Schwab, R., Küenzi, P., Fernandez, P.C. *et al*. (2002) Hijacking of host cell IKK signalosomes by the transforming parasite *Theileria*. *Science* 298(5595), 1033–1036. DOI: 10.1126/science.1075462.

Honnappa, S., Gouveia, S.M., Weisbrich, A., Damberger, F.F., Bhavesh, N.S. *et al*. (2009) An EB1-binding motif acts as a microtubule tip localization signal. *Cell* 138(2), 366–376. DOI: 10.1016/j.cell.2009.04.065.

Huber, S., Theiler, R., de Quervain, D., Wiens, O., Karangenc, T. *et al*. (2017) The microtubule-stabilizing protein CLASP1 associates with the *Theileria annulata* schizont surface via its kinetochore-binding domain. *mSphere* 2(4), e00215–17. DOI: 10.1128/mSphere.00215-17.

Huber, S., Karagenc, T., Ritler, D., Rottenberg, S. and Woods, K. (2018) Identification and characterisation of a *Theileria annulata* proline-rich microtubule and SH3 domain-interacting protein (TaMISHIP) that forms a complex with CLASP1, EB1, and CD2AP at the schizont surface. *Cellular Microbiology* 20(7), e12838. DOI: 10.1111/cmi.12838.

Huber, S., Bär, A., Epp, S., Schmuckli-Maurer, J., Eberhard, N. *et al*. (2020) Recruitment of host nuclear pore components to the vicinity of *Theileria* schizonts. *mSphere* 5(1), e00709–719. DOI: 10.1128/mSphere.00709-19.

Hulliger, L., Wilde, K.H., Brown, C.G. and Turner, L. (1964) Mode of multiplication of *Theileria* in cultures of bovine lymphocytic cells. *Nature* 203, 728–730. DOI: 10.1038/203728a0.

Hulliger, L., Brown, C.G. and Wilde, J.K. (1966) Transition of developmental stages of *Theileria parva in vitro* at high temperature. *Nature* 211(5046), 328–329. DOI: 10.1038/211328a0.

Iams, K.P., Young, J.R., Nene, V., Desai, J., Webster, P. *et al*. (1990) Characterisation of the gene encoding a 104-kilodalton microneme-rhoptry protein of *Theileria parva*. *Molecular and Biochemical Parasitology* 39(1), 47–60. DOI: 10.1016/0166-6851(90)90007-9.

Irvin, A.D. and Morrison, W.I. (1987) Immunopathology, immunology, and immuno- prophylaxis of *Theileria* infections. In: Soulsby, E.J.L. (ed.) *Immune Responses in Parasitic Infections: Immunology, Immunopathology and Immunoprophylaxis, Vol III: Protozoa*. CRC Press, Baton Rouge, Florida, pp. 223–274.

Irvin, A.D., Ocama, J.G.R. and Spooner, P.R. (1982) Cycle of bovine lymphoblastoid cells parasitised by *Theileria parva*. *Research in Veterinary Science* 33(3), 298–304. DOI: 10.1016/S0034-5288(18)32305-1.

Ivanov, V., Stein, B., Baumann, I., Dobbelaere, D.A.E., Herrlich, P. *et al*. (1989) Infection with the intracellular protozoan parasite *Theileria parva* induces constitutively high levels of NF-KB in bovine T lymphocytes. *Molecular and Cellular Biology* 9(11), 4677–4686. DOI: 10.1128/mcb.9.11.4677-4686.1989.

Jarrett, W.F.H., Crighton, G.W. and Pirie, H.M. (1969) *Theileria parya*: Kinetics of replication. *Experimental Parasitology* 24(1), 9–25. DOI: 10.1016/0014-4894(69)90215-X.

Jensen, K., Paxton, E., Waddington, D., Talbot, R., Darghouth, M.A. *et al*. (2008) Differences in the transcriptional responses induced by *Theileria annulata* infection in bovine monocytes derived from resistant and susceptible cattle breeds. *International Journal for Parasitology* 38(3–4), 313–325. DOI: 10.1016/j.ijpara.2007.08.007.

Jensen, K., Makins, G.D., Kaliszewska, A., Hulme, M.J., Paxton, E. *et al*. (2009) The protozoan parasite *Theileria annulata* alters the differentiation state of the infected macrophage and suppresses musculoaponeurotic fibrosarcoma oncogene (MAF) transcription factors. *International Journal for Parasitology* 39(10), 1099–1108. DOI: 10.1016/j.ijpara.2009.02.020.

Jura, W.G.Z.O., Brown, C.G.D. and Rowland, A.C. (1983) Ultrastructural characteristics of *in vitro* parasite-lymphocyte behaviour in invasions with *Theileria annulata* and *Theileria parva*. *Veterinary Parasitology* 12(2), 115–134. DOI: 10.1016/0304-4017(83)90001-8.

Katzer, F., Ngugi, D., Oura, C., Bishop, R.P., Taracha, E.L. *et al*. (2006) Extensive genotypic diversity in a recombining population of the apicomplexan parasite *Theileria parva*. *Infection and Immunity* 74, 5456–5464. DOI: 10.1128/IAI.00472-06.

Kessel, R.G. (1992) Annulate lamellae: A last frontier in cellular organelles. *International Review of Cytology* 133, 43–120. DOI: 10.1016/s0074-7696(08)61858-6.

Kinnaird, J.H., Logan, M., Kirvar, E., Tait, A. and Carrington, M. (1996) The isolation and characterization of genomic and cDNA clones coding for a cdc2-related kinase (ThCRK2) from the bovine protozoan parasite *Theileria*. *Molecular Microbiology* 22(2), 293–302. DOI: 10.1046/j.1365-2958.1996.00124.x.

Kinnaird, J.H., Weir, W., Durrani, Z., Pillai, S.S., Baird, M. *et al*. (2013) A bovine lymphosarcoma cell line infected with *Theileria annulata* exhibits an irreversible reconfiguration of host cell gene expression. *PLoS ONE* 8(6), e66833. DOI: 10.1371/journal.pone.0066833.

Kinnaird, J.H., Singh, M., Gillan, V., Weir, W., Calder, E.D. *et al*. (2017) Characterization of HSP90 isoforms in transformed bovine leukocytes infected with *Theileria annulata*. *Cellular Microbiology* 19(3), e12669. DOI: 10.1111/cmi.12669.

Koh, M.Y. and Powis, G. (2012) Passing the baton: The HIF switch. *Trends in Biochemical Sciences* 37(9), 364–372. DOI: 10.1016/j.tibs.2012.06.004.

Kramer, K.M. and Johnston, L.H. (1997) An unwelcome partner: Parasitic choreography of the host cell cycle? *Trends in Microbiology* 5(5), 169–170. DOI: 10.1016/S0966-842X(97)01016-0.

Küenzi, P., Schneider, P. and Dobbelaere, D.A.E. (2003) *Theileria parva*-transformed T cells show enhanced resistance to Fas/Fas ligand-induced apoptosis. *The Journal of Immunology* 171(3), 1224–1231. DOI: 10.4049/jimmunol.171.3.1224.

Larcombe, S.D., Kolte, S.W., Ponnudurai, G., Kurkure, N., Magar, S. *et al*. (2019) The impact of tick-borne pathogen infection in Indian bovines is determined by host type but not the genotype of *Theileria annulata*. *Infection, Genetics and Evolution* 75, 103972. DOI: 10.1016/j.meegid.2019.103972.

Larcombe, S.D., Capewell, P., Jensen, K., Weir, W., Kinnaird, J. *et al*. (2022) Susceptibility to disease (tropical theileriosis) is associated with differential expression of host genes that possess motifs recognised by a pathogen DNA binding protein. *PLoS ONE* 17(1), e0262051. DOI: 10.1371/journal.pone.0262051.

Latré de Laté, P., Pineda, M., Harnett, M., Harnett, W., Besteiro, S. *et al*. (2017) Apicomplexan autophagy and modulation of autophagy in parasite-infected host cells. *Biomedical Journal* 40(1), 23–30. DOI: 10.1016/j.bj.2017.01.001.

Latré de Laté, P., Haidar, M., Ansari, H., Tajeri, S., Szarka, E. *et al*. (2019) *Theileria* highjacks JNK2 into a complex with the macroschizont GPI (GlycosylPhosphatidylInositol)-anchored surface protein p104. *Cellular Microbiology* 21(3), e12973. DOI: 10.1111/cmi.12973.

Latré de Laté, P., Cook, E.A.J., Wragg, D., Poole, E.J., Ndambuki, G. *et al*. (2021) Inherited tolerance in cattle to the apicomplexan protozoan *Theileria parva* is associated with decreased proliferation of parasite-infected lymphocytes. *Frontiers in Cellular and Infection Microbiology* 11(11), 751671. DOI: 10.3389/fcimb.2021.751671.

Lipton, S.A. (1997) Janus faces of NF-κB: Neurodestruction versus neuroprotection. *Nature Medicine* 3(1), 20–22. DOI: 10.1038/nm0197-20.

Li, Q.-F., Liang, Y., Shi, S.-L., Liu, Q.-R., Xu, D.-H. *et al*. (2011) Localization of prohibitin in the nuclear matrix and alteration of its expression during differentiation of human neuroblastoma SK-N-SH cells induced by retinoic acid. *Cellular and Molecular Neurobiology* 31(2), 203–211. DOI: 10.1007/s10571-010-9608-7.

Li, Z., Liu, J., Zhao, S., Ma, Q., Liu, A. *et al*. (2021) *Theileria annulata* subtelomere-encoded variable secreted protein-TA05575 binds to bovine RBMX2. *Frontiers in Cellular and Infection Microbiology* 11, 11. DOI: 10.3389/fcimb.2021.644983.

Li, Z., Liu, J., Zhao, S., Ma, Q., Guo, Z. *et al*. (2022) *Theileria annulata* SVSP455 interacts with host HSP60. *Parasites & Vectors* 15(1), 308. DOI: 10.1186/s13071-022-05427-z.

Lim, C.-A., Yao, F., Wong, J.J.-Y., George, J., Xu, H. *et al*. (2007) Genome-wide mapping of RELA(p65) binding identifies E2F1 as a transcriptional activator recruited by NF-kappaB upon TLR4 activation. *Molecular Cell* 27(4), 622–635. DOI: 10.1016/j.molcel.2007.06.038.

Lin, Y.C., Shun, C.T., Wu, M.S. and Chen, C.C. (2006) A novel anticancer effect of thalidomide: Inhibition of intercellular adhesion molecule-1-mediated cell invasion and metastasis through suppression of nuclear factor-kappaB. *Clinical Cancer Research* 12(23), 7165–7173. DOI: 10.1158/1078-0432.CCR-06-1393.

Lizundia, R., Chaussepied, M., Huerre, M., Werling, D., Santo, J.P. *et al*. (2006) C-Jun NH2-terminal kinase/c-Jun signaling promotes survival and metastasis of B lymphocytes transformed by *Theileria*. *Cancer Research* 66(12), 6105–6110. DOI: 10.1158/0008-5472.CAN-05-3861.

MacHugh, N.D., Weir, W., Burrells, A., Lizundia, R., Graham, S.P. *et al*. (2011) Extensive polymorphism and evidence of immune selection in a highly dominant antigen recognized by bovine CD8 T cells specific for *Theileria annulata*. *Infection and Immunity* 79(5), 2059–2069. DOI: 10.1128/IAI.01285-10.

Madden, S.K., de Araujo, A.D., Gerhardt, M., Fairlie, D.P. and Mason, J.M. (2021) Taking the Myc out of cancer: Toward therapeutic strategies to directly inhibit c-Myc. *Molecular Cancer* 20(1), 3. DOI: 10.1186/s12943-020-01291-6.

Maiato, H., Fairley, E., Rieder, C., Swedlow, J., Sunkel, C. *et al.* (2003) Human CLASP1 is an outer kinetochore component that regulates spindle microtubule dynamics. *Cell* 113(7), 891–904. DOI: 10.1016/s0092-8674(03)00465-3.

Marsolier, J., Perichon, M., DeBarry, J.D., Villoutreix, B.O., Chluba, J. *et al.* (2015) *Theileria* parasites secrete a prolyl isomerase to maintain host leukocyte transformation. *Nature* 520(7547), 378–382. DOI: 10.1038/nature14044.

Marsolier, J., Perichon, M., Weitzman, J. and Medjkane, S. (2019) Secreted parasite Pin1 isomerase stabilizes host PKM2 to reprogram host cell metabolism. *Communications Biology* 2(1), 152. DOI: 10.1038/s42003-019-0386-6.

Maurizio, M., Masid, M., Woods, K., Caldelari, R., Doench, J.G. *et al.* (2024) Host cell CRISPR genomics and modelling reveal shared metabolic vulnerabilities in the intracellular development of *Plasmodium falciparum* and related hemoparasites. *Nature Communications* 15(1), 6145. DOI: 10.1038/s41467-024-50405-x.

McGuire, K., Manuja, A., Russell, G.C., Springbett, A., Craigmile, S.C. *et al.* (2004) Quantitative analysis of pro-inflammatory cytokine mRNA expression in *Theileria annulata*-infected cell lines derived from resistant and susceptible cattle. *Veterinary Immunology and Immunopathology* 99(1–2), 87–98. DOI: 10.1016/j.vetimm.2004.01.003.

McKeever, D.J., Nyanjui, J.K. and Ballingall, K.T. (1997) *In vitro* infection with *Theileria parva* is associated with IL10 expression in all bovine lymphocyte lineages. *Parasite Immunology* 19(7), 319–324. DOI: 10.1046/j.1365-3024.1997.d01-214.x.

Medjkane, S. and Weitzman, J.B. (2013) A reversible Warburg effect is induced by *Theileria* parasites to transform host leukocytes. *Cell Cycle* 12(14), 2167–2168. DOI: 10.4161/cc.25540.

Medjkane, S., Perichon, M., Marsolier, J., Dairou, J. and Weitzman, J.B. (2014) *Theileria* induces oxidative stress and HIF1α activation that are essential for host leukocyte transformation. *Oncogene* 33(14), 1809–1817. DOI: 10.1038/onc.2013.134.

Mehlhorn, H. and Shein, E. (1984) The piroplasms: Life cycle and sexual stages. *Advances in Parasitology* 23, 37–103. DOI: 10.1016/s0065-308x(08)60285-7.

Metheni, M., Echebli, N., Chaussepied, M., Ransy, C., Chéreau, C. *et al.* (2014) The level of H_2O_2 type oxidative stress regulates virulence of *Theileria*-transformed leukocytes. *Cellular Microbiology* 16(2), 269–279. DOI: 10.1111/cmi.12218.

Metheni, M., Lombes, A., Bouillaud, F., Batteux, F. and Langsley, G. (2015) HIF-1 alpha induction, proliferation, and glycolysis of *Theileria*-infected leukocytes. *Cellular Microbiology* 17, 467–472. DOI: 10.1111/cmi.12421.

Mimori-Kiyosue, Y., Grigoriev, I., Sasaki, H., Matsui, C., Akhmanova, A. *et al.* (2006) Mammalian CLASPs are required for mitotic spindle organization and kinetochore alignment. *Genes to Cells* 11(8), 845–857. DOI: 10.1111/j.1365-2443.2006.00990.x.

Minami, T., Kawazu, S., Shimura, K., Fujisaki, K., Kamio, T. *et al.* (1990) Detection of the schizont stage in experimentally infected cattle with Japanese *Theileria sergenti*. *The Japanese Journal of Veterinary Science* 52(3), 601–604. DOI: 10.1292/jvms1939.52.601.

Moore, K.W., de Waal Malefyt, R., Coffman, R.L. and O'Garra, A. (2001) Interleukin-10 and the interleukin-10 receptor. *Annual Review of Immunology* 19, 683–765. DOI: 10.1146/annurev.immunol.19.1.683.

Morrison, W.I., Buscher, G., Murray, M., Emery, D.L., Masake, R.A. *et al.* (1981) *Theileria parva*: Kinetics of infection in the lymphoid system of cattle. *Experimental Parasitology* 52(2), 248–260. DOI: 10.1016/0014-4894(81)90080-1.

Morrison, W.I., MacHugh, N.D. and Lalor, P.A. (1996) Pathogenicity of *Theileria parva* is influenced by the host cell type infected by the parasite. *Infection and Immunity* 64(2), 557–562. DOI: 10.1128/iai.64.2.557-562.1996.

Morrison, W.I., Hemmink, J.D. and Toye, P.G. (2020) *Theileria parva*: A parasite of African buffalo, which has adapted to infect and undergo transmission in cattle. *International Journal for Parasitology* 50(5), 403–412. DOI: 10.1016/j.ijpara.2019.12.006.

Musisi, F.L., Bird, R.G., Brown, C.G.D. and Smith, M. (1981) The fine structural relationship between *Theileria* schizonts and infected bovine lymphoblasts from cultures. *Zeitschrift Für Parasitenkunde Parasitology Research* 65(1), 31–41. DOI: 10.1007/BF00926551.

Naessens, J., Newson, J., Bensaid, A., Teale, A.J., Magondu, J.G. *et al.* (1985) De novo expression of T cell markers on *Theileria parva*-transformed lymphoblasts in cattle. *The Journal of Immunology* 135(6), 4183–4188. DOI: 10.4049/jimmunol.135.6.4183.

ole-MoiYoi, O.K. (1995) Casein kinase II in theileriosis. *Science* 267(5199), 834–836. DOI: 10.1126/science.7846527.

ole-MoiYoi, O.K., Sugimoto, C., Conrad, P.A. and Macklin, M.D. (1992) Cloning and characterization of the casein kinase II alpha subunit gene from the lymphocyte-transforming intracellular protozoan parasite theileria parva. *Biochemistry* 31(27), 6193–6202. DOI: 10.1021/bi00142a004.

ole-MoiYoi, O.K., Brown, W.C., Iams, K.P., Nayar, A., Tsukamoto, T. *et al.* (1993) Evidence for the induction of casein kinase II in bovine lymphocytes transformed by the intracellular protozoan parasite *Theileria parva*. *The EMBO Journal* 12(4), 1621–1631. DOI: 10.1002/j.1460-2075.1993.tb05807.x.

Oura, C.A.L., McKellar, S., Swan, D.G., Okan, E. and Shiels, B.R. (2006) Infection of bovine cells by the protozoan parasite *Theileria annulata* modulates expression of the ISGylation system. *Cellular Microbiology* 8(2), 276–288. DOI: 10.1111/j.1462-5822.2005.00620.x.

Pain, A., Renauld, H., Berriman, M., Murphy, L., Yeats, C.A. *et al.* (2005) Genome of the host-cell transforming parasite *Theileria annulata* compared with *T. parva*. *Science* 309(5731), 131–133. DOI: 10.1126/science.1110418.

Palmer, G.H., Machado, J., Fernandez, P., Heussler, V., Perinat, T. *et al.* (1997) Parasite-mediated nuclear factor kappaB regulation in lymphoproliferation caused by *Theileria parva* infection. *Proceedings of the National Academy of Sciences* 94(23), 12527–12532. DOI: 10.1073/pnas.94.23.12527.

Pipano, E. and Shkap, V. (2000) Vaccination against tropical theileriosis. *Annals of the New York Academy of Sciences* 916(1), 484–500. DOI: 10.1111/j.1749-6632.2000.tb05328.x.

Rchiad, Z., Haidar, M., Ansari, H.R., Tajeri, S., Mfarrej, S. *et al.* (2020) Novel tumour suppressor roles for GZMA and RASGRP1 in *Theileria annulata*-transformed macrophages and human B lymphoma cells. *Cellular Microbiology* 22(12), e13255. DOI: 10.1111/cmi.13255.

Reeves, R., Edberg, D.D. and Li, Y. (2001) Architectural transcription factor HMGI(Y) promotes tumor progression and mesenchymal transition of human epithelial cells. *Molecular and Cellular Biology* 21(2), 575–594. DOI: 10.1128/MCB.21.2.575-594.2001.

Sager, H., Davis, W.C., Dobbelaere, D.A. and Jungi, T.W. (1997) Macrophage-parasite relationship in theileriosis. Reversible phenotypic and functional de-differentiation of macrophages infected with *Theileria annulata*. *Journal of Leukocyte Biology* 61(4), 459–468. DOI: 10.1002/jlb.61.4.459.

Sager, H., Brunschwiler, C. and Jungi, T.W. (1998) Interferon production by *Theileria annulata*-transformed cell lines is restricted to the beta family. *Parasite Immunology* 20(4), 175–182. DOI: 10.1046/j.1365-3024.1998.00141.x.

Schmuckli-Maurer, J., Casanova, C., Schmied, S., Affentranger, S., Parvanova, I. *et al.* (2009) Expression analysis of the *Theileria parva* subtelomere-encoded variable secreted protein gene family. *PLoS ONE* 4(3), e4839. DOI: 10.1371/journal.pone.0004839.

Schmuckli-Maurer, J., Kinnaird, J., Pillai, S., Hermann, P., McKellar, S. *et al.* (2010) Modulation of NF-kappaB activation in *Theileria annulata*-infected cloned cell lines is associated with detection of parasite-dependent IKK signalosomes and disruption of the actin cytoskeleton. *Cellular Microbiology* 12(2), 158–173. DOI: 10.1111/j.1462-5822.2009.01386.x.

Schuldenfrei, A., Belton, A., Kowalski, J., Talbot, C.C., Jr, Cello, F. *et al.* (2011) HMGA1 drives stem cell, inflammatory pathway, and cell cycle progression genes during lymphoid *tumorigenesis*. *BMC Genomics* 12, 549. DOI: 10.1186/1471-2164-12-549.

Shaw, M.K., Tilney, L.G. and Musoke, A.J. (1991) The entry of *Theileria parva* sporozoites into bovine lymphocytes: Evidence for MHC class I involvement. *The Journal of Cell Biology* 113(1), 87–101. DOI: 10.1083/jcb.113.1.87.

Shaw, M.K., Tilney, L.G. and McKeever, D.J. (1993) Tick salivary gland extract and interleukin-2 stimulation enhance susceptibility of lymphocytes to infection by *Theileria parva* sporozoites. *Infection and Immunity* 61(4), 1486–1495. DOI: 10.1128/iai.61.4.1486-1495.1993.

Shayan, P. and Ahmed, J.S. (1997) *Theileria*-mediated constitutive expression of the casein kinase II-α subunit in bovine lymphoblastoid cells. *Parasitology Research* 83(6), 526–532. DOI: 10.1007/s004360050293.

Shayan, P., Schop, B., Conze, G., Schein, E. and Ahmed, J.S. (1999) Is interleukin 2 necessary for the autocrine proliferation of *Theileria*-infected bovine cells? *Parasitology Research* 85(5), 409–412. DOI: 10.1007/s004360050567.

Shiels, B., Kinnaird, J., McKellar, S., Dickson, J., Miled, L.B. *et al.* (1992) Disruption of synchrony between parasite growth and host cell division is a determinant of differentiation to the merozoite in *Theileria annulata*. *Journal of Cell Science* 101(Pt 1), 99–107. DOI: 10.1242/jcs.101.1.99.

Shiels, B., Langsley, G., Weir, W., Pain, A., McKellar, S. *et al.* (2006) Alteration of host cell phenotype by *Theileria annulata* and *Theileria parva*: Mining for manipulators in the parasite genomes. *International Journal for Parasitology* 36(1), 9–21. DOI: 10.1016/j.ijpara.2005.09.002.

Shiels, B.R., McDougall, C., Tait, A. and Brown, C.G. (1986) Identification of infection-associated antigens in *Theileria annulata* transformed cells. *Parasite Immunology* 8(1), 69–77. DOI: 10.1111/j.1365-3024.1986.tb00834.x.

Stagg, D.A., Dolan, T.T., Leitch, B.L. and Young, A.S. (1981) The initial stages of infection of cattle cells with *Theileria parva* sporozoites *in vitro*. *Parasitology* 83(1), 191–197. DOI: 10.1017/s0031182000050150.

Stephens, S.A. and Howard, C.J. (2002) Infection and transformation of dendritic cells from bovine afferent lymph by *Theileria annulata*. *Parasitology* 124(Pt 5), 485–493. DOI: 10.1017/s003118200200152x.

Swan, D.G., Phillips, K., Tait, A. and Shiels, B.R. (1999) Evidence for localisation of a *Theileria parasite* AT hook DNA-binding protein to the nucleus of immortalised bovine host cells. *Molecular and Biochemical Parasitology* 101(1–2), 117–129. DOI: 10.1016/S0166-6851(99)00064-X.

Swan, D.G., Stern, R., McKellar, S., Phillips, K., Oura, C.A. *et al.* (2001) Characterisation of a cluster of genes encoding *Theileria annulata* AT hook DNA-binding proteins and evidence for localisation to the host cell nucleus. *Journal of Cell Science* 114(Pt 15), 2747–2754. DOI: 10.1242/jcs.114.15.2747.

Swan, D.G., Stadler, L., Okan, E., Hoffs, M., Katzer, F. *et al.* (2003) TashHN, a *Theileria annulata* encoded protein transported to the host nucleus displays an association with attenuation of parasite differentiation. *Cellular Microbiology* 5(12), 947–956. DOI: 10.1046/j.1462-5822.2003.00340.x.

Tajeri, S. and Langsley, G. (2021) *Theileria* secretes proteins to subvert its host leukocyte. *Biology of the Cell* 113(4), 220–233. DOI: 10.1111/boc.202000096.

Tretina, K., Gotia, H.T., Mann, D.J. and Silva, J.C. (2015) Theileria-transformed bovine leukocytes have cancer hallmarks. *Trends in Parasitology* 31(7), 306–314. DOI: 10.1016/j.pt.2015.04.001.

Tretina, K., Haidar, M., Madsen-Bouterse, S.A., Sakura, T., Mfarrej, S. *et al.* (2020) *Theileria* parasites subvert E2F signaling to stimulate leukocyte proliferation. *Scientific Reports* 10(1), 3982. DOI: 10.1038/s41598-020-60939-x.

Unlu, A.H., Tajeri, S., Bilgic, H.B., Eren, H., Karagenc, T. *et al.* (2018) The secreted *Theileria annulata* Ta9 protein contributes to activation of the AP-1 transcription factor. *PLoS ONE* 13(5), e0196875. DOI: 10.1371/journal.pone.0196875.

Vignali, R. and Marracci, S. (2020) HMGA genes and proteins in development and evolution. *International Journal of Molecular Sciences* 21(2), 654. DOI: 10.3390/ijms21020654.

Villares, M., Lourenço, N., Ktorza, I., Berthelet, J., Panagiotou, A. *et al.* (2024) Theileria parasites sequester host eIF5A to escape elimination by host-mediated autophagy. *Nature Communications* 15(1), 2235. DOI: 10.1038/s41467-024-45022-7.

von Schubert, C., Xue, G., Schmuckli-Maurer, J., Woods, K.L., Nigg, E.A. *et al.* (2010) The transforming parasite *Theileria* co-opts host cell mitotic and central spindles to persist in continuously dividing cells. *PLoS Biology* 8(9), e1000499. DOI: 10.1371/journal.pbio.1000499.

Weir, W., Sunter, J., Chaussepied, M., Skilton, R., Tait, A. *et al.* (2009) Highly syntenic and yet divergent: A tale of two *Theilerias*. *Infection, Genetics and Evolution* 9(4), 453–461. DOI: 10.1016/j.meegid.2009.01.002.

Weir, W., Karagenç, T., Baird, M., Tait, A. and Shiels, B.R. (2010) Evolution and diversity of secretome genes in the apicomplexan parasite *Theileria annulata*. *BMC Genomics* 11(1), 42. DOI: 10.1186/1471-2164-11-42.

Wiens, O., Xia, D., von Schubert, C., Wastling, J.M., Dobbelaere, D.A.E. *et al.* (2014) Cell cycle-dependent phosphorylation of *Theileria annulata* schizont surface proteins. *PLoS ONE* 9(7), e103821. DOI: 10.1371/journal.pone.0103821.

Woods, K., Perry, C., Brühlmann, F. and Olias, P. (2021) *Theileria's* strategies and effector mechanisms for host cell transformation: From invasion to immortalization. *Frontiers in Cell and Developmental Biology* 9, 662805. DOI: 10.3389/fcell.2021.662805.

Woods, K.L., Theiler, R., Mühlemann, M., Segiser, A., Huber, S. *et al.* (2013) Recruitment of EB1, a master regulator of microtubule dynamics, to the surface of the *Theileria annulata* schizont. *PLoS Pathogens* 9(5), e1003346. DOI: 10.1371/journal.ppat.1003346.

Zhao, S., Guan, G., Liu, J., Liu, A., Li, Y. *et al.* (2017) Screening and identification of host proteins interacting with *Theileria annulata* cysteine proteinase (TaCP) by yeast-two-hybrid system. *Parasites & Vectors* 10(1), 536. DOI: 10.1186/s13071-017-2421-0.

Zhao, S., Liu, J., Guan, G., Liu, A., Li, Y. *et al.* (2018) *Theileria annulata* cyclophilin1 (TaCyp1) interacts with host cell MED21. *Frontiers in Microbiology* 9, 2973. DOI: 10.3389/fmicb.2018.02973.

11 Immunity to *Theileria parva*

W. Ivan Morrison* and Timothy Connelley
Roslin Institute, University of Edinburgh, Edinburgh, UK

11.1 Introduction

The antigenic complexity of apicomplexan parasites and their intricate life cycles present major challenges to the host immune system. These parasites have evolved strategies to modify their host cells, allowing them to survive in the face of cellular defence mechanisms and to progress through their different developmental stages. This frequently involves modulation of host immune responses, in order to suppress or delay immune elimination. In the case of vector-borne parasites such as *Theileria parva*, the parasites must survive until the stages that infect the arthropod vector have developed, and persistence of low levels of infection usually occurs beyond the acute phase of infection to provide a source of parasites for transmission by the vector. Hence, host–parasite relationships have evolved that result in immune responses that accommodate survival of the parasite as well as protecting the host. This is exemplified by *T. parva* in the African buffalo, which causes a low-level persistent infection without causing disease. By contrast, cattle, which have been introduced into Africa relatively recently (see Chapter 5 of this volume), suffer severe disease when infected by the same parasite.

Because of the acute and frequently fatal nature of East Coast fever (ECF) in cattle, it has long been recognized that vaccination would offer the most effective method of controlling the disease. The early recognition that animals that recover from the disease develop robust immunity to parasite challenge encouraged the belief that vaccination should be a realistic option. A live vaccine, involving infection of cattle with sporozoites and simultaneous treatment with oxytetracycline (termed the Infection and Treatment Method (ITM) for immunization), was developed in the 1970s (Radley *et al.*, 1975a, b; Uilenberg *et al.*, 1976) and eventually licenced for field use in several East African countries between 2007 and 2009 (Peters *et al.*, 2020), but difficulties in production and distribution of this vaccine have limited its widespread use (discussed in Chapters 12 and 13 of this volume). Hence there is a need for a more easily applied and sustainable method of vaccination. Over the past 40 years, this has driven research aimed at understanding the nature and specificity of immune responses that mediate immunity to the parasite, with a view to developing alternative methods of vaccination. This work has provided insight into the mechanisms of immunity to the parasite and identified some of the antigens involved. It has also indicated that modulation of the immune response by the parasite contributes to the pathogenesis of the disease.

This chapter will discuss our current knowledge of the basis of immunity to *T. parva* and the antigens known to be recognized by protective immune responses. Attempts to immunize cattle

*Corresponding author: Ivan.Morrison@ed.ac.uk

 East Coast Fever: The Disease, its Impact and Control (eds W.I. Morrison and P. Toye)
DOI: 10.1079/9781800626324.0011

with defined parasite antigens will be described, and the main obstacles that need to be addressed to translate the findings to a practical vaccine against ECF will be considered.

11.2 Early Studies Indicated that Live Parasites are Required to Induce Immunity

11.2.1 Immunization with cells from infected animals

Over the years, attempts to immunize cattle against *T. parva* using various preparations of inactivated parasites or crude parasite antigens, including sporozoites in adjuvant, irradiated sporozoites, non-infective schizont-infected cells, or semi-purified schizont or piroplasm antigens in adjuvant, have all proved unsuccessful (Wilde *et al.*, 1968; Cunningham *et al.*, 1973a; Purnell *et al.*, 1974; Wagner *et al.*, 1974; Emery *et al.*, 1981b). By contrast, immunity could be induced using live parasitized cells. The initial demonstration in 1909 (Meyer, 1909) that infection with *T. parva* could be transferred by transplanting pieces of lymphoid tissue from infected cattle and that some surviving animals were immune to parasite challenge led to attempts to determine whether such material could be used to produce mild infections with recovery and subsequent immunity. Multiple studies carried out over the next six decades (starting with Theiler in 1912) attempted to immunize cattle by administering various preparations of live infected cells harvested from lymphoid tissues of animals suffering from ECF (reviewed in Wilde, 1967; Pirie *et al.*, 1970). However, the results were highly variable: immunity to parasite challenge was usually achieved in a variable proportion of the animals, but in many studies the inoculum produced lethal ECF in some of the animals and failed to induce immunity in others. These studies included a large-scale immunization trial reported by Spreull in 1914, which was undertaken in an attempt to combat a field outbreak of ECF in South Africa. In this heroic exercise, 283,000 susceptible cattle were inoculated with spleen and lymph node cells from cases of ECF. However, the inoculum caused lethal ECF in approximately 25% of the recipient animals, although 70% of the survivors were considered to have been protected. While these studies demonstrated that use of this method of vaccination was clearly impractical, they reinforced the evidence that immunity could be generated with live schizont-infected cells.

In the 1960s, the development of methods to cryopreserve the parasite in the form of homogenized infected ticks (Cunningham *et al.*, 1973b) provided large batches of parasites of defined infectivity and pathogenicity, which allowed further investigation of immunization with live parasites. However, infection of cattle with low doses of parasites from cryopreserved stocks was found to result in severe infections in a proportion of animals (Cunningham *et al.*, 1974). Further studies eventually led to the development of the ITM of immunization (discussed in Chapter 12 of this volume).

11.2.2 Use of cultured parasitized cells for immunization

The advent in the 1960s of cell culture systems to propagate *Theileria*-infected cells as continuously growing cell lines *in vitro* (Tsur and Adler, 1962; Malmquist *et al.*, 1970; Brown *et al.*, 1973) opened up an obvious opportunity to investigate the use of these cells for vaccination. This was initially investigated with *Theileria annulata*, the causative agent of tropical theileriosis. Administration of 10^5 or fewer *T. annulata*-infected cells resulted in immunity to parasite challenge, although prolonged *in vitro* passage of the cell lines was required to avoid production of clinical disease by the inoculated cells (Pipano and Tsur, 1966; Pipano, 1981, 1989). Studies in Israel in the early 1970s resulted in a national vaccine programme for *T. annulata* using a dose of $1–5 \times 10^6$ cultured cells. Similar vaccines were subsequently developed in several other countries using cell lines derived from local parasite isolates (Gill *et al.*, 1976).

A similar approach was investigated for *T. parva*, but yielded different results (Brown, 1981). Administration of 10^8 infected cells was required to achieve immunity in the majority of animals, and, as observed with *T. annulata*, use of cells from early passages of cell lines resulted in clinical disease in some of the animals. Culture of the donor-infected cell lines for at least 50 passages attenuated their virulence and allowed them to be used safely for immunization. For example, one group of 37 cattle that received 10^8 cells from between passages 49 and 205 of the same cell line all developed mild infections and all were immune to parasite challenge (Brown, 1981). However, the large number of cells required for immunization, equivalent to about 100 ml of culture cell suspension per dose, is economically prohibitive for the commercial use of this method of vaccination

11.2.3 Parasites need to establish in the cells of recipient animals

Subsequent studies of animals immunized with parasitized cells from *in vitro* cultures demonstrated that, for both *T. annulata* and *T. parva*, transfer of the parasites from the donor culture cells into cells of the recipient animals is required for successful induction of immunity. This was initially shown by immunization of animals with cells of different sex and use of cell karyotyping to confirm infection of the recipient animal cells. Typing of infected cells for the major histocompatibility complex (MHC) genotype has been used in subsequent studies to confirm parasite transfer. An anti-graft cellular response to the inoculated cells was detected prior to the emergence of infection in the recipient animals' cells (Fig. 11.1).

The ability to immunize cattle with smaller numbers of *T. annulata*-infected cells, compared to *T. parva*, appears to reflect a greater capacity of *T. annulata* to transfer into the cells of recipient animals (Emery *et al.*, 1982; Innes *et al.*, 1989). The schizont stage of the parasites lacks the organelles and surface proteins utilized by sporozoites for cell invasion. However, recent *in vitro* studies with *T. annulata* have indicated that transfer of the parasite can occur by spontaneous cell fusion between the infected cells and recipient leukocytes (W.I. Morrison, unpublished data). However, the reason for the difference between the two *Theileria* species in frequency of parasite transfer is not understood.

11.3 General Features of Immunity

11.3.1 Immunity is directed primarily against infected lymphocytes

The ability to induce immunity by administering schizont-infected cells clearly indicates that

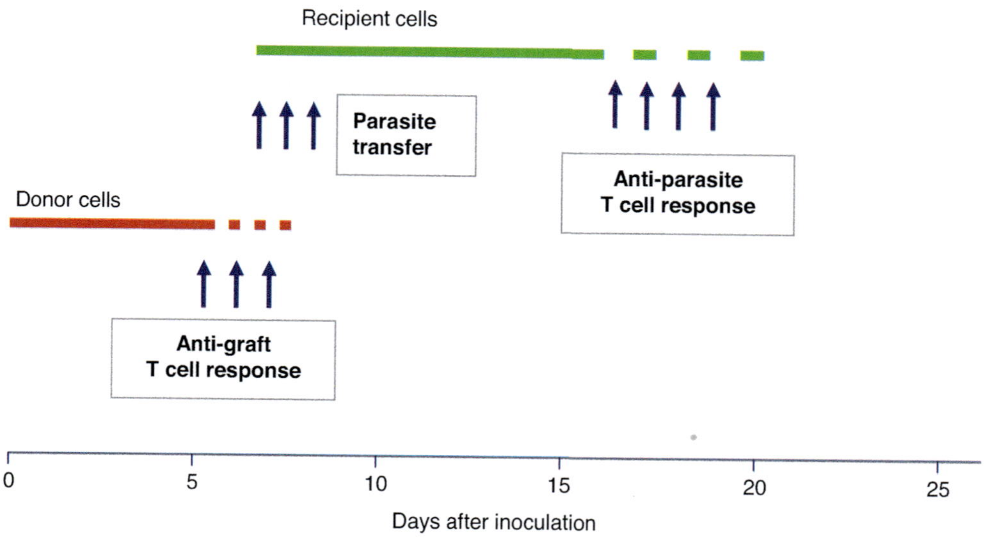

Fig. 11.1. Schematic representation of the events leading to transfer of *T. parva* into the cells of recipient animals following administration of allogeneic infected cells.

the induction of immunity does not depend on exposure to pre-schizont stages of the parasite (Pirie *et al.*, 1970; Emery *et al.*, 1982; Büscher *et al.*, 1984). Moreover, following challenge of animals immunized by infection and treatment or animals that have recovered from infection, parasitized lymphoblasts are transiently detected in the regional lymph node at the same time or only slightly later than they arise in unimmunized controls, indicating that the immunity engendered by infection and treatment does not prevent establishment of infection but operates by controlling infection at the level of the parasitized lymphoblast. The strict intracellular nature of this stage of the parasite and lack of any evidence of parasite-encoded antigens detectable by immune sera on the surface of infected cells (Creemers, 1982) indicated that immunity is likely to involve T cell-mediated mechanisms. This contention was supported by the demonstration of protection following adoptive transfer of thoracic duct lymphocytes from immune to naïve twin calves (Emery, 1981). Earlier studies had failed to show protection by passive transfer of immune serum to susceptible animals (Muhammed *et al.*, 1975), and calves that had received colostrum from cows immunized by infection and treatment and repeatedly challenged with the parasite remained fully susceptible to parasite challenge (Cunningham *et al.*, 1989).

The first direct evidence of T cell-mediated immune responses against parasitized cells was presented by Pearson *et al.* (1979, 1982), who showed that irradiated infected cells stimulated proliferative responses *in vitro* in autologous peripheral blood mononuclear cells (PBM) from immune animals, accompanied by cell-mediated cytotoxic activity against the infected cells. Subsequent studies demonstrated cytotoxic T cell responses *in vivo* in animals immunized by infection and treatment and in immune animals undergoing parasite challenge (Eugui and Emery, 1981; Emery *et al.*, 1981a). In these animals, the emergence of the cytotoxic T cell response coincided with control of the infection, implying that this response plays an important role in mediating immunity (reviewed in Morrison *et al.*, 2015).

11.3.2 Parasite strain restriction of immunity

For many decades it was believed that immunity acquired following recovery from ECF provided broad protection against challenge from all strains of *T. parva*. However, during the course of studies to investigate immunization by infection and treatment, it became apparent that this was not the case (discussed more fully in Chapter 12 of this volume). Immunization with a given parasite isolate resulted in solid immunity to challenge with the same parasite isolate but often incomplete protection against other isolates (Radley *et al.*, 1975a; Cunningham, 1977). Typically, among a group of immunized animals challenged with a heterologous parasite strain, some animals were fully protected whereas others remained susceptible. The immunological basis of this complex pattern of strain heterogeneity has been the subject of much research and is discussed further below.

11.4 Potential for Generating Immunity against the Sporozoite

11.4.1 Stimulation of sporozoite-specific neutralizing antibodies

Cattle that recover from a primary infection with *T. parva* generate a weak antibody response of the IgM isotype to sporozoites that does not provide protection against parasite challenge (Musoke *et al.*, 1982). This weak response is not surprising, given the small number of sporozoites required to produce a lethal infection (discussed in Chapter 4 of this volume). However, repeated challenge of immunized animals with sporozoites induces a strong IgG antibody response, and incubation of serum from such animals with sporozoites *in vitro* has been shown to neutralize the infectivity of the sporozoites, based on testing their infectivity when administered to naïve animals (Musoke *et al.*, 1982). The neutralizing activity of the serum resided in the IgG2 subclass of antibody. Further studies produced monoclonal antibodies against sporozoites, some of which showed similar neutralizing activity, and neutralization was effective against different isolates of the parasite (Dobbelaere *et al.*, 1984; Musoke *et al.*, 1984).

In the initial experiments reported by Musoke *et al.* (1982), sporozoites were incubated with antibody *in vitro* for 90 min prior to testing infectivity *in vivo*. However, *in vitro* studies have shown that attachment to and invasion of host cells by sporozoites occurs within a few minutes (Fawcett *et al.*, 1984; Shaw, 1997). During natural infection, sporozoites are released by the feeding tick into the site of an inflammatory cellular response, which includes lymphocytes, and therefore invasion of target cells *in vivo* is also likely to occur very rapidly. Given the results of previous studies indicating that antibodies from serum or colostrum of immune animals fail to confer protection (Muhammed *et al.*, 1975; Cunningham *et al.*, 1989), it remains unclear whether or not the detection of antibodies that neutralize infectivity *in vitro* reflects a protective role of such antibodies in natural infections. Nevertheless, the results of these studies have encouraged efforts to determine whether immunity can be induced artificially using sporozoite antigens.

11.4.2 Antigenic specificity of anti-sporozoite antibodies

Monoclonal antibodies produced by immunizing mice with sporozoites were found to recognize a dominant protein with a relative molecular mass of 67 kDa, referred to as p67 (Musoke *et al.*, 1984; Dobbelaere *et al.*, 1984, 1985b). Immuno-electron microscopy demonstrated that the protein was present within a loosely arranged proteinaceous coat on the surface of the sporozoites (Dobbelaere *et al.*, 1985a). Similar to immune serum, some of the antibodies were found to neutralize the infectivity of sporozoites for lymphocytes in *in vitro* cultures. Subsequent studies showed that p67 is a 709 amino acid polypeptide encoded by a single copy gene (Tp03_0287) (Iams *et al.*, 1990; Nene *et al.*, 1992), the sequence of which appears to be conserved among all cattle-derived isolates of *T. parva* examined to date (Nene *et al.*, 1996), although some sequence diversity is observed in parasites derived from buffalo (Sibeko *et al.*, 2010; Sitt *et al.*, 2019). Around the same time that p67 was identified, studies of *T. annulata* identified a similar sporozoite surface antigen referred to as SPAG-1, which is somewhat larger (907 amino acids) but shows 47% sequence identity with p67 (Williamson *et al.*, 1989). SPAG-1 also elicits neutralizing antibodies and, indeed, two of the epitopes recognized by neutralizing antibodies were found to be conserved between *T. parva* and *T. annulata* (Boulter *et al.*, 1994; Knight *et al.*, 1996).

Ultrastructural studies of *T. parva* sporozoites invading host lymphocytes have shown that invasion is initiated by binding of the sporozoite surface coat to target cells, following which there is progressively a more intimate interaction between the sporozoite surface and the host cell membrane, leading to a zippering process that results in rapid internalization into the host cell (Fawcett *et al.*, 1984). Internalization occurs within a few minutes of initial cell contact. Neutralizing antibodies prevent the initial cell binding by sporozoites. Studies involving immuno-labelling of p67 have shown that all or part of p67 is cleaved and shed from the sporozoite surface during cell invasion (Webster *et al.*, 1985).

Cattle that recover from infection with *T. parva* generate strong antibody responses against a protein known as the polymorphic immunodominant molecule (PIM; Toye *et al.*, 1991; Toye *et al.*, 1995a, b), which is expressed on the surface of the schizont and is used in sero-diagnostic assays for epidemiological studies. However, PIM is also expressed by the sporozoite stage of the parasite, in which it can be detected intracellularly within microspheres (Toye *et al.*, 1996, 2014). Some PIM-specific murine monoclonal antibodies have been shown to partially neutralize the infectivity of sporozoites *in vitro*. As with p67, neutralization prevents binding of sporozoites to the host cells. Although not readily detectable on the surface of free sporozoites, PIM appears to be transported to the parasite surface following contact with bovine lymphocytes (Toye *et al.*, 2014). Unlike the murine monoclonal antibodies, sera from immune cattle lack neutralizing activity despite having high levels of PIM-specific antibodies. It has also been shown that recombinant versions of PIM can inhibit the attachment and internalization of sporozoites *in vitro*, presumably by binding to a putative PIM-specific ligand on lymphocytes (Toye *et al.*, 2014).

A more recent study sought to identify further sporozoite antigens based on a bioinformatics search of the *T. parva* genome for genes encoding proteins likely to be expressed on the sporozoite surface. Genes predicted to encode a C-terminal GPI (glycosyl-phosphatidyl-inositol) membrane anchor and an N-terminal signal peptide were identified (Nyagwange *et al.*, 2018), and recombinant protein produced for segments of six of these genes was used to produce antisera in mice. The resultant antibodies against two of the proteins (encoded by Tp01_0876 and Tp01_0939) strongly neutralized the infectivity of sporozoites *in vitro*, and antibodies against a further two antigens exhibited weak neutralizing activity. The antigen encoded by Tp01_0939 had previously been described as a protein on the surface of schizonts referred to as p34 (Xue *et al.*, 2010). These findings suggest that multiple host–parasite ligand interactions are involved in infection of bovine lymphocytes by *T. parva* sporozoites.

11.5 The Nature of the T Cell Response against Infected Cells

11.5.1 Experimental systems used to study cellular immune responses

The ability to induce immunity by infection and treatment, coupled with the capacity to generate parasite-infected cell lines *in vitro*, has provided a robust experimental system to study the mechanisms of immunity to *T. parva*. Animals immunized by infection and treatment have been shown to withstand challenge with 1000 ticks infected with the same parasite isolate used for immunization (i.e. equivalent to > 1000 LD_{50} doses; Morzaria *et al.*, 1987). Immunity has also been shown to persist for at least 3 years in the absence of parasite challenge (Burridge *et al.*, 1972). Establishment of *T. parva*-infected cell lines from animals prior to infection or immunization provided autologous infected cells against which T cell responses could be monitored *ex vivo*. *T. parva*-infected cell lines express high levels of surface class I and class II MHC and are efficient antigen-presenting cells, enabling them to be used to activate parasite-specific T cells from immune animals *in vitro* (Goddeeris and Morrison, 1988). Repeated *in vitro* stimulation of immune T cells with irradiated autologous parasitized cells has been used successfully to generate parasite-specific T cell lines and clones from immune cattle, allowing detailed characterization of the effector cell population and dissection of the specificity of the T cell responses (Goddeeris and Morrison, 1988).

11.5.2 A role for CD8 T cell responses in protection

The generation of reagents specific for bovine leukocyte surface markers in the 1980s allowed more in-depth analyses of the T cell response to *T. parva*. Immune animals were shown to generate strong CD4 and CD8 T cell responses against infected lymphocytes, and the cytotoxic activity of PBM from immune animals was found to be mediated by class I MHC-restricted CD8 T cells (Goddeeris *et al.*, 1986a, 1990; Morrison *et al.*, 1987). These were among the first studies to demonstrate MHC-restricted T cell killing of parasite-infected cells. Use of a limiting dilution cytotoxicity assay to provide a semi-quantitative measure of cytotoxic T cells demonstrated the potent nature of the response: in immune animals undergoing parasite challenge, up to 1:2500 of cells in PBM at the peak of the response (i.e. > 1:500 of the CD8 T cells) were parasite-specific cytotoxic T cells, and cytotoxic T cells represented approximately 2.5% of the CD8 T cells in efferent lymph from the lymph node draining the site of infection (Taracha *et al.*, 1992).

Testing of CD8 T cell lines and clones from immune animals on target cells infected with different parasite isolates demonstrated that the response was frequently parasite strain-restricted (Goddeeris *et al.*, 1986b) and that CD8 T cells restricted by different class I MHC proteins differed in their strain specificity (Goddeeris *et al.*, 1990). Given the known lack of cross-protection between some parasite isolates, a series of experiments was undertaken to examine the relationship of strain specificity of the cytotoxic T cell response with protection (Taracha *et al.*, 1995a, b). These experiments utilized animals immunized with the Muguga isolate or a cloned derivative of the Marikebuni isolate of *T. parva* and subsequently challenged with the reciprocal parasite isolate. The results showed that the parasite strain specificity of the cytotoxic T cell responses following immunization correlated closely with the susceptibility of the animals to parasite challenge, i.e. those animals that exhibited a cross-reactive cytotoxic T cell response were solidly immune to challenge with the heterologous parasite, whereas those with a strain-specific response developed clinical disease of varying severity.

The central role of CD8 T cells in immunity was underscored by adoptive transfer experiments using sets of identical twin calves produced by embryo splitting, which demonstrated that transfer of highly enriched CD8 T cells collected from immune animals undergoing parasite challenge and administered to the naïve co-twins 6–9 days after parasite challenge conferred protection (McKeever *et al.*, 1994). Further depletion of CD8 T cells from the transferred cells removed the protective activity, indicating that protection did not reside in the contaminating lymphocyte population. Separate experiments also showed that transfer of similarly enriched populations of CD4 T cells did not confer protection. Collectively, these findings provided compelling evidence that CD8 T cells play an important role in immunity to *T. parva*.

The cytotoxic activity of CD8 T cells is mediated by proteins released by exocytosis following recognition of the target cells; a protein known as perforin creates small pores in the cell membrane of the target cell, through which granzymes are introduced into the cells to initiate programmed cell death. Although death of the target cells was originally described as apoptosis, more recent studies have indicated that killing by CD8 T cells frequently involves a process known as necroptosis (reviewed by de Miguel *et al.*, 2022). Killing of *T. parva*-infected cells by CD8 T cells has been shown to be dependent on perforin and granzyme B and involves activation of the pro-apoptotic molecule Bid, but is independent of caspases (Yang *et al.*, 2019). These features, coupled with the observed rapid disintegration of the *T. parva*-infected cells with release of cytoplasmic contents (Fig. 11.2), are consistent with killing by necroptosis, rather than classical apoptosis, which involves caspases and results in shrinkage and pyknosis of the target cells.

CD8 T cell responses are also key mediators of immunity against a number of other apicomplexan parasites, including *Toxoplasma gondii* and the liver stages of *Plasmodium* species. In addition to expressing cytotoxic activity, the CD8 T cells produce cytokines that have an effector role against these parasites (Tsitsiklis *et al.*, 2019; Lefebvre and Harty, 2020). In particular, interferon-γ (IFNγ) has been shown to be an essential mediator of immunity in murine models

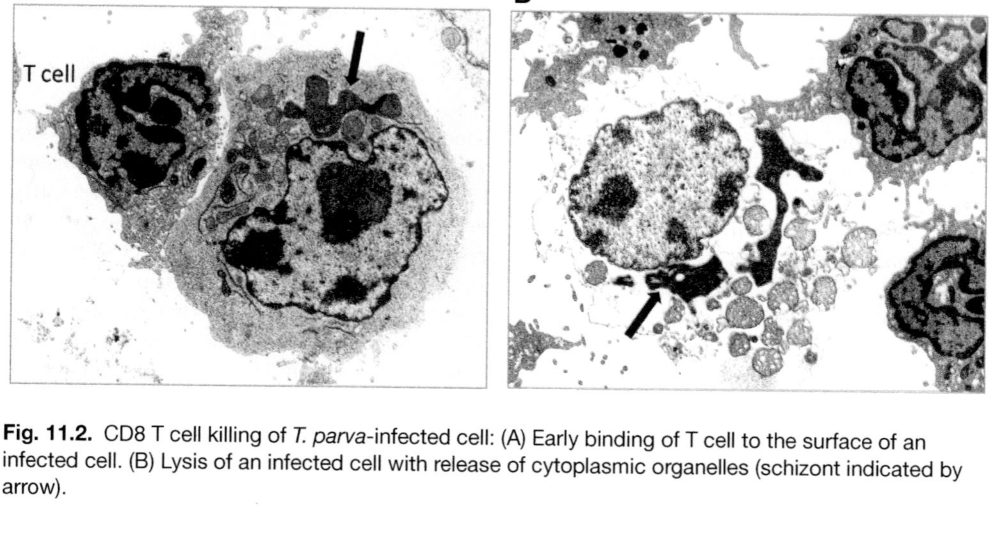

Fig. 11.2. CD8 T cell killing of *T. parva*-infected cell: (A) Early binding of T cell to the surface of an infected cell. (B) Lysis of an infected cell with release of cytoplasmic organelles (schizont indicated by arrow).

of malaria and *Toxoplasma gondii* (Schofield *et al.*, 1987; Suzuki *et al.*, 1988). However, although *T. parva*-specific CD8 T cells release IFNγ and tumour necrosis factor α (TNFα) upon antigenic stimulation, these cytokines do not appear to have direct effector activity against the parasite (DeMartini and Baldwin, 1991). Indeed, both cytokines are produced by some *T. parva*-infected cell lines (McKeever *et al.*, 1997). Thus, it remains unclear what other properties of CD8 T cells, apart from their cytotoxic activity, play a role in mediating control of *T. parva*.

11.5.3 CD4 T cell responses

Studies of responses of immune animals to *T. parva* have also revealed strong parasite-specific CD4 T cell responses against parasitized cells (Baldwin *et al.*, 1987, 1992; Brown *et al.*, 1989, 1990). Indeed, CD4 T cells usually represent a majority of cells (80–85%) within parasite-specific T cell lines established from PBM of immune cattle. Most of them release IFNγ following antigenic stimulation. Although some CD4 T cell clones displaying low levels of cytotoxic activity against infected cells have been reported (Baldwin *et al.*, 1992), most CD4 T cell lines lack cytolytic activity.

In the adoptive transfer studies discussed above (McKeever *et al.*, 1994), the transferred CD8 T cells that provided protection were from an active response in the donor animals and therefore it is possible that other cell types were involved in their activation. Studies of other intracellular pathogens have indicated that CD4 T cell responses often have an important role in generating an effective CD8 T cell response. In laboratory animal disease models, the extent to which CD4 T cells influence the induction of an effective CD8 T cell response varies dependent on the pathogen involved. In some cases, such as *Listeria monocytogenes*, CD8 T cell responses are induced in CD4 T cell-deficient mice, although there is a reduced CD8 T cell response following bacterial challenge of such animals (Sun and Bevan, 2003; Lara-Tejero and Pamer, 2004). In mice infected with *Plasmodium yoelii*, CD8 T cell responses are substantially reduced in the absence of CD4 T cells, due to reduced expansion and survival of the specific memory CD8 T cells, and the mice are not protected against parasite challenge (Overstreet *et al.*, 2011). Results from clinical human trials involving therapy of Epstein-Barr virus(EBV)-associated disease in immune-deficient patients by administering EBV-specific CD8 T cell lines (Haque *et al.*, 2007) provided evidence that the presence of virus-specific CD4 T cells in the CD8 T cell lines improved the survival of the transferred CD8 T cells in the recipients and enhanced their protective activity. Taracha *et al.* (1997) investigated the role of CD4 T cells in induction of *T. parva*-specific CD8 T cell responses *in vitro* from immune animals, using different combinations of purified naïve and immune CD4 and CD8 T cells from pairs of identical twin calves. They demonstrated that CD4 T cells were required for activation of specific CD8 T cells and that recognition of antigen on the same antigen-presenting cells by the CD4 and CD8 T cells was required. Given the acute nature of *T. parva* infections, these findings indicated that CD4 T cell responses will be required *in vivo* for efficient recall of CD8 T cell responses following challenge of immunized animals.

11.5.4 Responses of other lymphocyte subsets

T. parva-infected cells have been shown to stimulate responses in γ/δ T cells and NK (natural killer) cells, although most of the available information has been derived from *in vitro* studies and their role in immunity remains unclear.

11.5.4.1 γ/δ T cells

There has only been one detailed study of the responses of γ/δ T cells to *T. parva*. Purified γ/δ T cells from both naïve and immune cattle were shown to proliferate *in vitro* in response to irradiated autologous *T. parva*-infected cells in the presence of added IL-2 (Daubenberger *et al.*, 1999). The response appeared to be parasite specific, in that there was no proliferation induced by uninfected lymphoblasts and the responding cells showed killing of infected cells but not uninfected cells. Demonstration of inhibition of cytotoxicity by a monoclonal antibody specific for the γ/δ T cell receptor (TCR) indicated specific ligand recognition, but there was no evidence of parasite strain restriction. Limiting dilution analyses of responses of γ/δ T cells harvested following primary infection with *T. parva* revealed an increase in frequency of responding cells shortly after infection and a further increase following curative treatment, providing evidence of an *in vivo* response.

The specificities and functions of γ/δ T cells are in general poorly defined, but in humans and mice they have been shown to interact with non-classical class I MHC and class I MHC-like molecules with or without bound epitopes (usually glycolipids), and the kinetics of their responses are considered characteristic of innate immune responses (Vantourout and Hayday, 2013). Specific responses by bovine γ/δ T cells to *Mycobacterium bovis* proteins and peptides have been reported (McGill *et al.*, 2014). Bovine γ/δ T cells also express a unique family of scavenger receptor-like surface proteins known as WC1 (Chen *et al.*, 2009), which are involved in activating γ/δ T cell responses to *Leptospira* and have been proposed to function as ligands for stimulating innate immune responses (Wang *et al.*, 2011). Similarly, detailed high-throughput sequencing analysis of the γδ TCR repertoire suggests that in the response to *Leptospira* the γδV TCR functions as an 'innate-like' receptor (Gillespie *et al.*, 2022). The precise role of these cells in immunity to *T. parva* remains to be determined.

11.5.4.2 NK cells and NK-like T cells

Although early studies described non-MHC restricted killing of parasitized cells by PBM from cattle in the advanced stages of ECF, described as NK-like activity (Emery *et al.*, 1981a), the nature of the cells mediating this killing could not be determined. The development of antibodies specific for the NK cell surface marker NKp46 (Storset *et al.*, 2004) for the first time facilitated studies of NK cell responses. $NKp46^+$ lymphocytes purified from PBM of naïve or immune cattle were shown to proliferate *in vitro* in response to autologous parasitized cells (Connelley *et al.*, 2014). Prior to this study, NKp46 had been considered a definitive marker for NK cells. However, the responding $NKp46^+$ cells in *T. parva*-stimulated cultures contained a subpopulation that expressed the T cell-specific marker CD3. Purified populations of $NKp46^+$ $CD3^-$ and $NKp46^+$ $CD3^+$ cells both exhibited non-MHC-restricted cytotoxic activity against parasitized cells. Careful analyses of the phenotype of resting PBM identified a small discrete population (0.1–1.7%) of $NKp46^+$ $CD3^+$ cells, which, when purified, responded *in vitro* to parasitized cells, confirming that the responding cells are a phenotypically distinct subset rather than the product of activation-induced upregulation of NKp46 on conventional T cells. They show several functional and cell surface phenotypic features that distinguish them from conventional T cells and NK cells. Similar to NK cells, they express CD16 and a range of NK receptors, and unlike conventional T cells, they are negative for CD5 and CD6. Antibody ligation of surface receptors demonstrated that both the TCR and NKp46 are functionally intact, although unlike NK cells, NKp46 ligation did not stimulate IFNγ production.

The characteristics of these $NKp46^+$ T cells indicate that they may be able to participate in both innate and adaptive immune responses to *T. parva*. Although cultures of *T. parva*-specific T cells obtained from immune cattle are usually dominated by conventional CD4 and CD8 T cells, they sometimes contain small numbers of $NKp46^+$ $CD3^+$ cells. The role played by both $NKp46^+$ subsets of lymphocytes in immunity to *T. parva* remains to be determined. They could potentially contribute as effectors in controlling the infection or, as described in other model systems, help to promote induction of the specific T cell response. Further understanding of the ligands engaged in their activation by parasitized cells might help to clarify their function.

11.6 Antigens Recognized by *T. parva*-Specific T Cell Responses

11.6.1 Systems used for antigen identification

Compared to antibody responses, the identification of antigens recognized by T cell responses is a much more challenging task, particularly when dealing with large complex pathogens such as protozoa. Screening requires actively responding T cells and for candidate antigens to be presented on the relevant MHC backgrounds. The ability to generate parasite-specific T cell lines and clones from cattle immunized with *T. parva* proved invaluable for antigen screening and for investigating the precise antigenic specificities of the T cell responses. Publication of the genome sequence of *T. parva* in 2005 (Gardner *et al.*, 2005) also provided a catalogue of the functional genes, revealing that the parasite encodes just over 4000 proteins. The first successful identification of antigens involved use of parasite-specific CD8 T cell lines from immune cattle to perform a high-throughput screen of Cos-7 cells co-transfected with parasite cDNAs together with cDNAs encoding the class I MHC alleles expressed by the respective CD8 T cell lines (Graham *et al.*, 2006). Measurement of IFNγ release by responding T cells was used as the read-out to detect a positive response. These experiments utilized a cDNA library prepared from schizonts purified from parasitized cells, initially screened as a series of pools each containing 20 cDNAs. An additional set of cDNAs selected from the recently sequenced *T. parva* genome, which were predicted to encode proteins with a signal peptide, were also included in the screen. Eight CD8 T cell antigens (designated Tp1–Tp8) were identified in this study (Graham *et al.*, 2006) and a further two antigens (Tp9 and Tp10) were identified subsequently using the same parasite cDNA library (Hemmink *et al.*, 2016). More recently, a library of overlapping synthetic peptides representing 499 proteins encoded by genes selected from the parasite genome was used in further screens using both CD4 and CD8 T cell lines (Morrison *et al.*, 2021; W.I. Morrison, unpublished data). Initial screens were conducted using pools of 50 peptides added directly to immune T cells, again using production of IFNγ as the read-out for a positive response.

11.6.2 CD8 T cell antigens

Screens using the library of synthetic peptides referred to above identified a further five CD8 antigens (W.I. Morrison, unpublished data). CD8 T cell lines of different class I MHC types from immune Boran and Holstein cattle were used for the various antigen screens. Holstein animals are increasingly being used for milk production in Africa and are highly susceptible to ECF. The Holstein CD8 T cell lines included lines representing nine of the most frequently expressed class I MHC types in Holstein cattle. A striking feature of the results was that animals of different MHC genotypes tended to detect different antigens, and, within the animals studied, only a few of the antigens were recognized by T cells from animals of more than one MHC genotype. Some of the antigens were detected by lines from both Boran and Holstein cattle and others by only one of the breeds. Characterization of the class I MHC alleles expressed by Holstein cattle allowed detailed analyses of the specificities of the nine antigens recognized by animals of this breed. The results summarized in Table 11.1, which shows the MHC restriction specificities of the antigens and the epitopes within the antigens recognized by the CD8 T cells, clearly illustrate the divergent antigenic specificities of the CD8 T cell responses in animals of different MHC types. No antigens have so far been detected by T cells from Holstein animals expressing four of the MHC class I types used for screening (A13, A19, A20 and A31). Mapping of the CD8 T cell epitopes, in most cases, identified one or occasionally two epitopes recognized by T cells restricted by a given MHC allele (Graham *et al.*, 2008). Each epitope was presented by only one of the class I gene products expressed by the respective MHC haplotype. The results of these studies collectively indicate that a large number of *T. parva* proteins are capable of eliciting CD8 T cell responses but that many of the target antigens have not yet been identified.

11.6.3 CD4 T cell antigens

More recent studies have also identified a series of *T. parva* proteins recognized by CD4 T cells from immune cattle (Morrison *et al.*, 2021). CD4 T cell lines from animals expressing 12 different class II MHC types were used to screen the synthetic peptide library referred to above, which represented approximately 12.5% of the *T. parva* genome. The results were very different from those obtained with CD8 T cells. Multiple antigens were detected by all CD4 T cell lines used in the screens, with up to 12 antigens detected per

Table 11.1. *Theileria parva* antigens recognized by bovine CD8 T cells in Holstein cattle.

MHC I haplotype		Antigens (encoding gene)	Epitope regions
Serological specificities	Genotype		
A10	00201 01201	Tp10 (4_00772) Tp2 (1_00056)	$_{419}$NNPELIPVL$_{427}$ $_{49}$KSSHGMGKVGK$_{59}$ $_{50}$SSHGMGKVGK$_{59}$ $_{98}$QSLVCVLMK$_{106}$
A11	01701 01801	Tp9 (2_00895) Tp12 (1_01091)	Repeat region $_{-121\text{-}204}$ $_{245}$TPQTKMVEI$_{253}$
A12	00801 01901	Tp35 (1_ 00612) Tp12 (1_01091)	$_{177}$TEKSDPIEAT$_{186}$ $_{345}$QLLNQFYQL$_{353}$
A13[a]	03101		
A14	02301 02401 02501 00401	Tp9 (2_00895) Tp5 (2_00767) Tp32 (2_00123)	$_{67}$AKFPGMKKS$_{75}$ $_{87}$SKADVIAKY$_{95}$ $_{301}$GQKERDLIM$_{309}$
A15	00901 02401 02501	Tp5 (2_00767)	$_{87}$SKADVIAKY$_{95}$
A18	01301	Tp1 (3_00849) Tp33 (3_00263)	$_{214}$VGYPKVKEEML$_{224}$ $_{460}$VQFLKITKI$_{469}$
A19[a]	01401 01601		
A20[a]	02601 02701		
A31[a]	02101 02201		
N5	03601 03701	Tp34 (4_00164) Tp9 (2_00895)	($_{187}$KEEPIYEEMRSI$_{198}$) ($_{41}$PHQRSSMFRDDLGSSFTSGYT$_{61}$)

[a]No antigens detected in antigen screens.

animal. A total of 26 antigens were identified, 6 of which had also been detected in CD8 T cell screens. Examples of the antigens recognized by individual animals are shown in Table 11.2. However, as with the CD8 antigens, the antigenic specificity of the CD4 T cell response differed in animals of different MHC types, although some of the antigens were recognized on multiple MHC backgrounds.

11.6.4 Properties of the T cell antigens

The antigens recognized by CD4 and CD8 T cells are encoded by a variety of mostly unrelated genes distributed across the parasite genome. The CD4 antigens include members of two multi-gene families, namely five members of the haloacid dehydrogenase family and five members of the subtelomere-encoded variable secreted protein (SVSP) family, which comprises proteins of unknown function with conserved N-terminal and C-terminal regions and a central QP-rich region (Schmuckli-Maurer *et al.*, 2009). Genes encoding some of the antigens are predicted to be orthologues of other parasite and/or mammalian genes, whereas others have no identifiable orthologues. Comparison of the genome sequences of different *T. parva* isolates has revealed that some of the antigens display extensive sequence polymorphism whereas others have highly conserved sequences (Nene and Morrison, 2016; Morrison *et al.*, 2021). At the outset of these antigen screening

Table 11.2. *Theileria parva* antigens recognized by CD4 T cells from eight immune animals.

Class II DR types of immune animals	Antigens recognized by CD4 T cells[a]
10:01/10:01	Tp1, Tp7, Tp9, Tp13, Tp16, Tp18, Tp19, Tp20
11:01/11:01	Tp7, Tp9, Tp16, Tp18, Tp20, Tp24, Tp28, Tp36,
16:01/16:01	Tp9, Tp14, Tp15, Tp17, Tp20, Tp21, Tp22, Tp23, Tp29, Tp30, Tp31
20:02/20:02	Tp14, Tp15, Tp16, Tp19, Tp20, Tp24, Tp25, Tp33,
11:01/16:01	Tp2, Tp9, Tp14, Tp16, Tp17, Tp21, Tp22, Tp23
01:01/15:01	Tp1, Tp9, Tp20, Tp24, Tp31, Tp33,
12:01/15:01	Tp9, Tp20, Tp28, Tp31
14:01/27:03	Tp2, Tp9, Tp13, Tp26, Tp29

[a]Based on screening synthetic peptides representing 499 gene products in the *T. parva* genome. Frequently recognized antigens highlighted in yellow and green (Morrison *et al.* 2021).

experiments, it was considered likely that proteins secreted by the parasite into the host cell cytosol would be preferentially recognized by T cell responses. Consequently, possession of a predicted signal peptide, indicating likely secretion, was one of the parameters used to select parasite gene products for some of the antigen screens. However, a significant number of the T cell antigens (both CD4 and CD8) lacked a detectable signal peptide and, given the bias in selection of the proteins used in some of the antigen screens, it was not possible to conclude whether possession of a signal peptide favoured antigenicity. Nor was it possible to identify other parameters that reliably predict antigenicity.

11.6.5 Polymorphism of CD8 T cell antigens

Detailed studies of the CD8 T cell responses to two of the antigens (Tp1 and Tp2) demonstrated that CD8 T cells specific for these antigens from cattle immunized with the Muguga isolate of *T. parva* showed differential recognition of cells infected with heterologous parasite isolates (MacHugh *et al.*, 2009; Connelley *et al.*, 2011), indicating polymorphism in the epitopes within the antigens. A study of the nucleotide sequences of Tp1 and Tp2 in ~80 *T. parva* isolates from cattle and buffalo identified 35 alleles of Tp1 and 43 alleles of Tp2 (Pelle *et al.*, 2011). However, only a subset of these alleles was found in the isolates derived from cattle, consistent with the idea that the parasites in cattle represent a subset of *T. parva* that have adapted to maintenance in cattle (discussed in further detail in Chapter 5 of this volume). Further studies of the first 10 identified CD8 antigens (including Tp1 and Tp2), involving sequencing of the genes in a series of field isolates of *T. parva* from cattle and buffalo, demonstrated marked variation in their degree of polymorphism, with levels of amino acid identity ranging from 52% to 98% (Nene and Morrison, 2016). Some antigens had conserved amino acid sequences, whereas others, notably Tp1, Tp2 and Tp9, were particularly variable, displaying multiple antigenic variants, and including variation in the CD8 T cell epitopes recognized by immune cattle (MacHugh *et al.*, 2009; Connelley *et al.*, 2011). However, as mentioned above, these antigens show much greater diversity in buffalo population of *T. parva* compared to cattle parasites (Pelle *et al.*, 2011; Hemmink *et al.*, 2018; Sitt *et al.*, 2018).

The high level of polymorphism of some of the antigens raised the question of whether these antigens are undergoing rapid contemporary mutational changes. Although this has not been addressed directly, available evidence suggests that the genes are not subject to rapid change. Thus, parasites examined from different tick passages of the same parasite isolate retain identical antigen gene nucleotide sequences. Moreover, in a study of Tp1 and Tp2 gene sequences in parasites from buffalo in Kenya and South Africa, many identical alleles of the antigens were identified in both populations and included alleles identical to those found in cattle-maintained populations of *T. parva* (Hemmink *et al.*, 2018). These findings suggest that sequence diversification in these genes occurred prior to adaptation of *T. parva* to maintenance in cattle.

11.6.6 Immunodominance and strain specificity of the CD8 T cell response

Given the antigenic complexity of parasites such as *T. parva* and the knowledge that many proteins are conserved among different parasite isolates, the induction of parasite strain-restricted CD8 T cell responses seems counter-intuitive. However, studies carried out prior to identification of target antigens had suggested that the CD8 T cell response in individual animals is directed against a limited number of antigenic specificities (Taracha *et al.*, 1995b).

Analyses of responses to antigens recognized on defined MHC backgrounds confirmed that the CD8 T cell responses of individual animals are focused on a limited number of antigens (Connelley *et al.*, 2008). Using pairs of Holstein animals homozygous for the A18 and A10 MHC haplotypes, which respond to Tp1 and Tp2, respectively, screening of large panels of CD8 T cell clones revealed that in each case approximately 70% of the CD8 T cells were specific for the respective antigen. No recognition of the reciprocal antigen or three additional antigens (Tp4, Tp5 and Tp8) was detected in these animals, although subsequent work revealed that a minor component (< 2%) of the T cell lines from both A10 + animals recognized Tp10. Subsequent experiments involving the use of fluorescently labelled class I MHC tetramer complexes incorporating the target epitopes to identify epitope-specific T cells confirmed the dominant nature of the responses to Tp1 and Tp2. An obvious concern regarding these findings was that certain antigen specificities may become preferentially enriched in CD8 T cell lines following repeated *in vitro* stimulation. Molecular tools to analyse the expressed TCR Vβ gene repertoire of the responding T cells, reflecting the clonal composition of the T cell response, were developed to address this issue (Connelley *et al.*, 2011). Comparison of the expressed TCR Vβ gene repertoire of the *in vitro*-generated CD8 T cell lines with that of CD8 T cells harvested *ex vivo* from the active CD8 T cell response to parasite challenge in the corresponding animal revealed that they were remarkably similar, confirming that the T cell lines were representative of the CD8 T cell response.

The phenomenon of immunodominance is a recognized feature of CD8 T cell responses to a number of pathogens, both in mice and in humans (reviewed in Yewdell, 2006). It does not reflect an inability to respond to other epitopes but rather is indicative of a strong hierarchy in dominance among the epitopes against which a response can be generated. This is most strikingly illustrated by human responses to HIV, in which CD8 T cell responses to one or a few dominant epitopes result in selection of mutations in the target epitopes, and the response then switches to other epitopes not previously recognized (Goulder *et al.*, 1997; Im *et al.*, 2011; Killian and Levy, 2011). Hence, although an individual possesses a T cell repertoire capable of generating CD8 T cell responses to many different peptides, responses are focused on a few of the most dominant available epitopes in the hierarchy. An early indication of dominance hierarchy in *T. parva* was the observation that, in identical twin calves immunized with different parasite strains, one calf generated a CD8 T cell response that recognized only the immunizing strain, whereas the other calf mounted a cross-reactive CD8 T cell response (Taracha *et al.*, 1995b). This was interpreted as the presence of a highly dominant, strain-restricted epitope in one of the parasite isolates that precluded induction of the response to the conserved epitope. The factors that determine immunodominance are complex. Epitope abundance, affinity of peptide-MHC binding, the frequencies of epitope reactive T cells in the naïve repertoire and the affinity of the specific TCRs for the peptide-MHC complex have all been implicated in determining dominance, but its basis is still not fully understood (Yewdell, 2006).

As discussed in further detail below, this focusing of the CD8 T cell response on highly dominant polymorphic T cell epitopes is a key determinant of parasite strain specificity of CD8 T cell responses in cattle immunized with *T. parva*.

Immunodominance of CD8 T cell responses probably also accounts for the difficulty experienced in immunizing cattle with allogeneic *T. parva*-infected cells. Studies in laboratory animals have demonstrated that CD8 T cell responses can be induced with exogenous antigen taken up and presented by a subset of dendritic cells, a phenomenon referred to as 'cross-priming' (Joffre *et al.*, 2012). However, the T cell repertoire contains a high frequency of T cells capable of recognizing allogeneic MHC molecules, which enables generation of powerful CD8 T cell responses to allogeneic cells. In the case of immunization with allogeneic *T. parva*-infected cells, dominance of the T cell responses to alloantigens may well prohibit stimulation of CD8 T cell responses to parasite antigens by cross-priming before the parasitized cells are eliminated.

11.6.7 Identification of MHC-bound parasite peptides

Immunodominance of the CD8 T cell response to *T. parva* almost certainly accounts for the smaller number of antigens detected in antigen screens using CD8 T cells compared to screens with CD4 T cells. This also implies that the CD8 T cell lines used for antigen screening do not recognize some antigens potentially capable of inducing CD8 T cell responses. In the past few years, advances in biochemical technologies have allowed isolation and identification of MHC-bound peptides from infected cells. The characterization of the MHC-presented peptides (termed 'immunopeptidomics') has the potential to permit a more comprehensive description of the *T. parva*-derived peptides that are available for presentation to CD8 and CD4 T cells. Application of this technology to a series of *T. parva*-infected cells has led to the identification of 74 MHC I- and 15 MHC II-DR-presented *T. parva* peptides (Connelley *et al.*, 2022). This offers a potentially alternative route to antigen identification that may assist in attempts to circumvent the effects of immunodominance and facilitate the development of a recombinant vaccine that has broader specificity. Although the preliminary data generated to date from these peptide elution studies has identified a large number of candidate antigens, it has not yet been demonstrated that administration of these antigens by a vaccine delivery vehicle will elicit parasite-specific CD4/CD8 T cell responses.

11.6.8 Sexual recombination: An added level of antigenic complexity

In common with other apicomplexan protozoa, *T. parva* can undergo sexual recombination. All stages of the parasite in the mammalian host have a haploid genome. As discussed in Chapter 3 of this volume, ingested piroplasms in the tick develop into gametes, which fuse to form zygotes. The zygotes enter the gut epithelium of the tick, where they undergo meiosis to generate haploid kinetes. Kinetes released into the haemolymph migrate to the salivary glands where sporogony occurs, generating sporozoites (Shaw, 2002). The occurrence of frequent recombination events in *T. parva* during this process has been confirmed experimentally by genotyping of parasites produced in ticks fed on calves co-infected with two genotypically distinct cloned *T. parva* populations (Katzer *et al.*, 2011; Henson *et al.*, 2012). Studies involving genotyping of field populations of *T. parva* in Uganda and Kenya, using a panel of satellite DNA markers, have also indicated that there is frequent genetic exchange in the field (Oura *et al.*, 2005; Odongo *et al.*, 2006). The results of these studies also revealed that most infected cattle harbour parasites of several genotypes. This epidemiological state is highly favourable for ingestion of mixed parasite genotypes by feeding ticks and hence provides the opportunity for sexual recombination during transmission. In such circumstances, it seems unlikely that stable clonal strains of parasites could be maintained; rather, constant genome reassortment is likely to be the norm.

The obvious practical significance of recombination in *T. parva* is its influence on the antigenic makeup of the parasites. Since the CD8 target antigens are encoded by genes distributed across all four chromosomes, there is a huge potential to generate parasites expressing different combinations of alleles of polymorphic antigens.

11.6.9 Relevance of parasite population structure to strain-restricted immunity

Available data on responses to the antigens identified to date indicate that the polymorphic nature of the dominant target antigens recognized by the protective CD8 T cell response is a key determinant of the strain-restricted immunity to *T. parva*. However, immunodominance of the response, whereby a large proportion of the response is focused on one or a few polymorphic antigenic epitopes, is also likely to be an important contributory factor, ensuring that CD8 T cells specific for variable epitopes dominate the response. This is particularly so given the apparent high rate of genetic recombination in the *T. parva* population. Whereas on the one hand such recombination can lead to enormous genetic diversity in the parasite population, on the other, it increases the likelihood (compared to a clonal non-recombining population) that any two parasite clones will share at least some alleles of the polymorphic antigen-encoding genes. Hence, if the CD8 T cell response were to target a wider range of antigens, there would be an increased chance of cross-reactivity of the response and less obvious strain-restricted immunity. Based on these arguments, merely broadening the antigenic specificity of the CD8 T cell response to include responses to more antigens, even if these are polymorphic, may overcome the strain specificity of immunity (Morrison, 2007).

Broadening of the antigenic specificity of T cell responses by simultaneous infection with different parasite strains may account for the protection achieved with the ITM vaccine using the Muguga cocktail. Although protection was originally thought to be a consequence of antigenic diversity among the three parasite isolates that make up the cocktail, more recent sequencing of the genomes and selected CD8 T cell antigens of the parasites has indicated that they contain limited antigenic diversity (Norling *et al.*, 2015; Hemmink *et al.*, 2016). Immune protection may, therefore, be the result of each of the component parasites independently inducing a CD8 T cell response, collectively producing a response of broader antigenic specificity than achieved with the individual parasites. This phenomenon is discussed more fully in Chapter 12 of this volume.

11.7 Cellular Responses to Primary Infection

In contrast to the robust immunity induced following immunization by infection and treatment, primary infection of susceptible cattle with *T. parva* usually fails to induce a protective immune response but results in unconstrained multiplication of parasitized cells leading to severe disease, usually with a fatal outcome. The cellular immune response in animals undergoing primary infection has not been investigated in the same level of detail as that in immune animals. A study reported by Houston *et al.* (2008), involving analyses of cells aspirated from the lymph node draining the site of infection, demonstrated that there is an early vigorous T cell response coinciding with initial detection of parasites in the node. By the time parasitosis reaches 1%, the lymph node contains 15–25% lymphoblasts. These activated cells comprise both CD4 and CD8 T cells, but there is a particularly dramatic increase in the content of CD8 T cells, which represent 60–70% of the total cells at this time. These T cells include a large population (~70% of CD8 cells) that lack expression of CD2, a phenotype that is uncommon in resting or antigen-specific bovine T cell populations. The cells did not express $\gamma\delta$ T cell markers, implying they belonged to the $\alpha\beta$ T cell lineage. Purified populations of the $CD2^{-}$ $CD8^{+}$ cells failed to proliferate *in vitro* in response to stimulation with autologous *T. parva*-infected cells, with or without added cytokines. Moreover, the unfractionated lymph node cells did not exhibit cytotoxic activity against infected cells, nor did they develop cytotoxic activity following *in vitro* stimulation with infected cells (Houston *et al.*, 2008). They contained abundant transcripts for IFNγ and IL-10, the latter of which is a regulatory cytokine. IL-10 is often expressed as a feedback response to high levels of IFNγ and has been shown to down-regulate type 1 T cell responses. Given that the development of this T cell response to infection coincides with a period of rapid multiplication of the infected cells and is followed by unconstrained growth of the infected cells, the response clearly lacks any effector activity against the parasitized cells.

Progression to severe disease is not an inevitable consequence of infection with *T. parva*.

Cattle inoculated with purified autologous T cells incubated *in vitro* with sporozoites for 48 h develop severe disease (Morrison *et al.*, 1996), whereas inoculation with autologous infected T cells passaged *in vitro* for 8 weeks or more results in mild self-limiting infection and immunity to subsequent parasite challenge. Moreover, infection of cattle with autologous purified B cells incubated *in vitro* with sporozoites also results in similar self-limiting infection and immunity to parasite challenge (Morrison *et al.*, 1996). In both of these situations, the infected cells multiply *in vivo* to give detectable infection in the local lymph node prior to control of the infection by the immune response, but the immune response clearly differs from that induced by freshly infected T cells. These findings have, therefore, been taken as evidence that infected T cells modulate the primary T cell response to *T. parva*, in order to suppress control of infection. This is discussed in further detail in Chapter 4 of this volume.

11.8 Attempts to Vaccinate with Defined Antigens

11.8.1 Immunization of cattle with the p67 sporozoite antigen

Over the past 30 years, the use of recombinant forms of p67 for immunization of cattle against parasite challenge has been evaluated extensively in experimental immunization and challenge experiments (Musoke *et al.*, 1992; Nene *et al.*, 1996; Bishop *et al.*, 2003; Lacasta *et al.*, 2021). These studies have shown that protection can be achieved in a proportion of the immunized animals. The majority of the studies used recombinant versions of p67 generated in *E. coli*, which were recognized by all except one of the p67-specific neutralizing monoclonal antibodies. By using the neutralizing antibodies to screen overlapping synthetic peptides, it was shown that they recognized five distinct epitopes, three epitopes towards the N-terminus (amino acid residues 105–229) and two towards the C-terminus of the protein (residues 615–639) (Nene *et al.*, 1999). Since preparation of purified full-length p67 protein in *E. coli* proved problematic because of degradation of the antigen during the production process, later immunization experiments used fragments of the protein containing neutralizing epitopes, which could be produced in a more stable form in *E. coli*. Polypeptides representing N-terminal and C-terminal segments (205 and 80 residues, respectively) of the protein both induced neutralizing antibody responses, and the C-terminal fragment (residues 572–651) was shown to generate similar levels of protection to that achieved with the full-length protein (Bishop *et al.*, 2003). Most of the subsequent studies used this 80-amino acid polypeptide.

The immunization and challenge protocols with p67 generally took the form of three to five monthly immunizations using antigen incorporated in proprietary adjuvant formulations, followed by subcutaneous needle challenge with an LD_{70} dose of cryopreserved sporozoites 2–3 weeks after the final boost. A minimum of three doses of antigen was found to be required to achieve maximal antibody responses. Almost invariably, these experiments resulted in about 70% of immunized animals surviving parasite challenge without suffering severe disease, which, given the challenge dose, is roughly equivalent to 50% protection (Ballingall *et al.*, 2004). Approximately 30% showed no signs of clinical disease and the remainder underwent infections of varying severity. Although the underlying concept behind the vaccine is neutralization of infection, no clear correlation has been found between the level of protection and antibody levels; ELISA (enzyme-linked immunosorbent assay) antibody titres of the order of 10^4–10^5 are equally common in animals that develop severe disease and those that remain clinically normal. Similarly, analyses of the isotype and avidity of the antibodies in these responses have revealed no significant differences between the two reaction phenotypes; in all cases, isotype profiles have been characteristic of a mature, T cell-dependent response (Musoke *et al.*, 1995). In spite of this, specific CD4 T cell responses are detected *in vitro* only intermittently and with low intensity in immunized animals (Musoke *et al.*, 1995; Ballingall *et al.*, 2004). Finally, when the epitope specificity of the antibody response in protected animals was compared with that of animals undergoing severe disease, by testing reactivity with overlapping synthetic peptides, no clear differences were observed (Musoke *et al.*, 1995; Nene *et al.*, 1999).

The finding of epitopes that are conserved between p67 and the *T. annulata* orthologue (SPAG-1) prompted experiments to test the capacity of the antigens to elicit protection against the reciprocal parasite species (Hall *et al.*, 2000). Immunization of calves with recombinant SPAG-1 was found to result in a degree of protection against challenge with *T. parva*, although the level of protection appeared to be inferior to that obtained with p67.

Production of p67 in other expression systems has also been investigated. Use of the C-terminal polypeptide of the antigen expressed in insect cells and in the envelope of inactivated baculovirus have been evaluated (Nene *et al.*, 1995; Kaba *et al.*, 2004, 2005). Live antigen delivery systems offer potential advantages over conventional adjuvant formulations in that they abrogate the need for large quantities of purified antigen and may only require one or two doses of vaccine. Laboratory immunization and challenge experiments have been conducted in cattle using various p67 expression constructs delivered in recombinant vaccinia virus and *Salmonella typhimurium* (Gentschev *et al.*, 1998; Heussler *et al.*, 1998; Honda *et al.*, 1998). These trials yielded results similar to or less effective than those obtained previously with *E. coli*-expressed antigen.

More recently, two types of nanoparticles, namely hepatitis B core virus-like particles and silica vesicles incorporated in adjuvant, have been investigated as antigen delivery systems for vaccinating cattle using the C-terminal component of p67 (Lacasta *et al.*, 2021). Animals immunized with the former produced high levels of antibody but poor CD4 T cell responses, whereas the antigen in silica particles stimulated modest antibody responses but strong CD4 T cell responses. Animals immunized with a combination of the two formulations generated strong antibody and T cell responses, but, as in previous studies, variable protection against parasite challenge was observed.

Experimental challenge of cattle with suspensions of sporozoites differs in several aspects from natural challenge from infected ticks. During natural challenge, the parasite is delivered in a trickle fashion over a period of days, during which a substantial inflammatory reaction is present at the attachment site (Walker and Fletcher, 1986). A study to examine the performance of the p67 vaccine in the face of tick-delivered challenge in the field was undertaken by Musoke *et al.* (2005) at three sites in endemically infected areas of Kenya. The immunization protocol essentially mirrored that of the laboratory trials, with animals receiving three inoculations of recombinant p67 in adjuvant at monthly intervals, followed by field exposure to challenge 2 weeks after the final boost along with age-matched unimmunized controls. Field exposure was allowed to continue until all control animals had developed patent infection, which resulted in variation between sites in the duration of challenge. The intensity of challenge also varied between the sites, as indicated by the incidence of severe disease in the control animals. The outcomes of the trials were somewhat ambivalent, with severe disease being observed in both control and immunized groups in each case. Although no significant differences were observed between the groups in the incidence of severe disease at two of the sites, when data from the three trial sites were combined, a significant reduction of 50% was apparent in the overall incidence of severe disease in immunized animals. Nonetheless, when the effective challenge at each site was taken into account, this equated to a level of protection that is somewhat lower than that observed in the laboratory trials. Significantly, specific antibody titres were observed to decline by an order of magnitude in immunized animals during the challenge period, indicating that the responses to p67 were not boosted by natural challenge.

11.8.2 Implications for an anti-sporozoite vaccine

In common with *T. parva*, the sporozoite stage of *Plasmodium falciparum* expresses an abundant surface protein (the circumsporozoite protein – CSP), which has been used to induce neutralizing antibodies and is being investigated as a potential vaccine antigen (Wahl and Wardemann, 2022). However, unlike p67, which is restricted in expression to the sporozoite stage of *T. parva*, the CSP is also expressed in the early liver stages of the malaria parasite and stimulates a CD8 T cell response that is implicated in immune protection (Kumar *et al.*, 1988). Hence, p67 relies largely on induction of anti-sporozoite antibody responses to provide immune protection.

The interpretation of results of the immunization trials using p67 discussed above is in part complicated by the use of an LD_{70} dose of sporozoites for challenge of the immunized animals. The response of both the unimmunized control animals and the immunized animals to this challenge dose can be highly variable, making it difficult to draw conclusions regarding what immune parameters determine variation in protection achieved in the immunized animals. Given the small numbers of parasites in the LD_{70} challenge dose, this variation may well be due to stochastic variation in the number of parasites that make contact with target cells and establish infection, or may reflect subtle genetic differences in susceptibility to this low level of parasite challenge. An obvious question that remains unanswered is whether protection can be achieved against challenge with higher doses of sporozoites. If not, this would imply that achieving complete protection against field challenge by immunizing with p67 will be extremely difficult to achieve.

The results obtained in studies of p67 raise questions as to whether p67 on its own is a valid candidate antigen for vaccination. As discussed above, there is no evidence that maternal antibody in colostrum provides protection in calves. Moreover, studies of the genotypes of *T. parva* in cattle residing in endemically infected areas using satellite DNA markers have shown that carrier animals acquire increasing numbers of genotypes with advancing age, indicating sequential acquisition of infections with different genotypes (Oura *et al.*, 2011). Collectively, the findings suggest that antibody responses to p67 do not prevent infection upon parasite challenge, although they may reduce the level of infection. Hence, it could be argued that despite the relative immunodominance of p67 as a sporozoite antigen, the parasite may have evolved a relationship with the host that allows some infection of host cells in the presence of antibody to p67.

As discussed above, evidence that other sporozoite antigens can induce neutralizing antibodies (Nyagwange *et al.*, 2018), and that neutralization can be achieved with antibodies specific for host class 1 MHC proteins, indicates that multiple proteins are likely to be involved in host cell invasion by the parasite. Given the apparent immunodominance of p67, it is possible that p67 in the sporozoite surface coat masks other potential antibody targets on the sporozoite until p67 is cleaved from the cell surface. Alternatively, engagement of p67 with its host cell ligand may stimulate mobilization of other immunogenic parasite proteins to the sporozoite surface. Investigation of the immunogenicity of these proteins, either singly or in combination with p67, is worth pursuing to determine whether more efficient neutralization can be achieved compared to that obtained with p67. Antigens that are also expressed in the schizont stage, such as the p34 antigen (encoded by Tp01_0939; Xue *et al.*, 2010), may be of particular relevance, as they offer the possibility that antibody responses will be boosted by natural parasite challenge and they might also be used to elicit T cell responses against the schizont stage.

However, irrespective of the immunogens used, the small number of sporozoites required to produce a fatal infection with *T. parva*, together with the limited amount of time the parasite is exposed extracellularly after inoculation, present a significant challenge for a vaccine relying on antibodies against the sporozoite stage of the parasite. Since protection appears to require complete or near-complete neutralization of sporozoite infectivity by antibodies, at least some of the animals protected against parasite challenge will remain susceptible to infection following subsequent decline in the levels of antibodies. Hence, any successful vaccine using sporozoite antigens, in addition to providing protection in most animals, is likely to require long-term maintenance of high levels of antibody.

11.8.3 Immunization with schizont antigens

The capacity to induce immunity against *T. parva* using CD8 T cell target antigens has been investigated in two studies. Both involved prime-boost protocols employing DNA plasmids and/or viral vectors, which had been developed for vaccine testing in humans. In the first of these studies, animals were immunized with five *T. parva* antigens (Tp1, Tp2, Tp4, Tp5 and Tp8) by priming with plasmid DNA or recombinant canarypox viruses followed by a boost with recombinant vaccinia viruses (the replication-defective Ankara strain) (Graham *et al.*, 2006). The five antigens were incorporated in separate DNA or viral constructs, and the animals were challenged 3 weeks later with a lethal dose of sporozoites. Following further improvement of viral vectors, a second study, involving prime-boost with replication-defective vaccinia and human adenovirus-5 vectors, was undertaken using the Tp1 antigen (Svitek *et al.*, 2018). In both studies, cattle of MHC types known to respond to the antigens were selected for the experiments. Most of the immunized animals in both studies exhibited readily detectable antigen-specific CD8 T cell responses following immunization, based on detection of IFNγ release *in vitro* following antigen stimulation. The study by Svitek *et al.* (2018) also demonstrated induction of parasite-specific CD4 T cell responses to Tp1. However, only a few of the immunized animals in both studies were substantially protected against parasite challenge, although some other animals showed reduced severity of disease. A follow-up experiment to the studies reported by Graham *et al.* (2006), in which similarly immunized cattle were treated with DNA-encoded FLT3L and GM-CSF in an attempt to increase targeting of the expressed antigen to dendritic cells, failed to enhance protection (Mwangi *et al.*, 2011). Analyses of the immune responses of cattle following immunization with vaccinia and adenovirus vectors (Svitek *et al.*, 2018) indicated that the CD8 T cell responses were of similar magnitude to those detected following immunization by infection and treatment. However, both in this study and in the findings reported by Graham *et al.* (2006), CD8 T cells from most of the immunized animals did not display cytotoxic activity following *in vitro* stimulation with parasitized cells, indicating that they differ functionally from CD8 cells induced by live parasites. Although Svitek *et al.* (2018) found that the CD8 T cells did display cytotoxicity when stimulated with Tp1 peptides, the concentration of peptides used is likely to have resulted in much higher (non-physiological) levels of presentation of the Tp1 epitope than occurs in infected cells.

The reasons for the failure to obtain robust protection against parasite challenge, despite induction of specific CD8 T cell responses, remain unclear. Given that the CD8 T cell response to some of the currently identified antigens represents a major component of the CD8 T cell response in immune cattle, and that the strain specificity of the measurable CD8 T cell response in immune animals correlates closely with the strain specificity of immunity, it is clear that these antigens are involved in generating protective immune responses. Evidence that T cells induced by experimental prime-boost protocols differ from those induced by immunization with live parasites indicates that the T cell response in the former is in some way functionally defective. Such a defect may lie in the CD8 T cells themselves or in responses of other lymphocyte populations such as CD4 T cells that regulate the activation and differentiation of CD8 T cell responses. Further detailed studies to clarify the functional differences in the responses of immune and (non-immune) experimentally immunized animals are required to identify features of the response that are associated with protection, which can be used as markers to investigate alternative methods of vaccine delivery.

11.8.4 Challenges to development of a vaccine with defined schizont antigens

As implied from the above discussion, the major initial challenge is to identify an antigen delivery system that can be used to induce a protective T cell response. The ability to exploit such a system for a practical vaccine would then depend on whether it will be possible to induce responses that recognize different parasite strains in animals of diverse MHC genotypes, using only a few antigens. The nature of the immunodominant immune responses observed in animals immunized with live parasites might at first sight suggest that this will be difficult to achieve. However, the antigenic specificity of immunodominant CD8 T cell responses to live parasites does not reflect an inability to respond to other antigens, but rather a hierarchy in dominance of available antigens that restricts the response to only a few of the potentially immunogenic antigens. The antigens that have been identified to date include a number of antigens that have highly conserved amino acid sequences (Nene and Morrison, 2016). As discussed above, the application of immunopeptidomics to identify class I MHC-bound parasite peptides provides a means of obtaining a more complete picture of the CD8 antigen repertoire. Finally, among the conserved antigens, there will be a need to identify those that are capable of inducing CD8 T cell responses in animals of different class 1 MHC types. Again, the immunodominance of the CD8 T cell response against intact parasites gives the impression that antigens are only capable of being recognized on certain MHC backgrounds. However, studies of CD8 T cell responses in mice and humans have shown that single proteins frequently contain epitopes presented by different MHC types. Hence, identification of a restricted set of antigens that can elicit CD8 T cell responses restricted by a broad range of MHC types and accommodate diversity between *T. parva* strains may be more feasible than would be inferred by direct extrapolation from currently available data.

11.9 Concluding Remarks

Studies of the nature and specificity of the immune responses to *T. parva* in immune cattle have provided an understanding of the mechanisms of immunity and identified some of the target antigens. Immunity is mediated primarily by T cell responses against the intracellular schizont stage of the parasite. Parasite-specific CD8 T cell responses play a pivotal role in immunity, and parasite strain specificity of immunity is associated with strain specificity of the CD8 T cell response. Strain-restricted immunity appears to be the result of focusing of CD8 T cell responses in individual animals on a few of the most dominant antigens (immunodominance), coupled with polymorphism of the target antigens. In contrast to the robust immunity achieved in animals vaccinated by infection and treatment, primary infection with *T. parva* in susceptible breeds of cattle usually results in progressive disease despite generating an early and vigorous T cell response. Available evidence indicates that this response is functionally defective, suggesting that the parasite modulates the primary T cell response to subvert control of the infection.

Although repeated exposure of cattle to *T. parva* in the field results in induction of antibodies that neutralize the infectivity of sporozoites *in vitro*, available evidence indicates that such antibodies do not prevent establishment of reinfection by the parasite. Nevertheless, a series of experimental immunization studies have attempted to generate immunity with a recombinant sporozoite surface coat antigen (p67), which was shown to induce neutralizing antibodies. However, despite achieving high titres of neutralizing antibodies using different formulations of the antigen, the level of protection obtained against challenge with a relatively low dose (LD_{70}) of sporozoites never exceeded 50%. As discussed earlier, these findings raise doubts about the feasibility of immunization with p67. The recent identification of other sporozoite antigens capable of inducing neutralizing antibodies indicates that invasion of bovine lymphocytes involves multiple host–parasite ligand interactions. Further studies are required to determine whether one or more of these antigens induce more robust neutralizing antibody responses that could be exploited for vaccination. However, it should be borne in mind that, in the absence of protection against the schizont stage, any such vaccine would require sustained high levels of neutralizing antibodies, which will be difficult to achieve in practice.

Attempts to immunize cattle with schizont antigens recognized by immune T cells have successfully induced parasite-specific CD8 and CD4 T cell responses, but only a small proportion of the immunized animals were protected against parasite challenge. In contrast to the responses in animals vaccinated by infection and treatment, the CD8 T cells exhibited little cytotoxic activity against infected cells, indicating that the vaccine-induced response is functionally defective. Testing of alternative methods of antigen delivery will be required to identify protocols that generate responses providing more robust immunity. However, in the absence of information on the functional features of the T cell response associated with immune protection, such testing will be empirical and therefore potentially open-ended. There is, therefore, an urgent need to undertake studies to identify functional differences between the protective and non-protective T cell responses (both CD4 and CD8 T cells) induced by live parasites and parasite antigen immunization, respectively. Such information should provide useful markers for monitoring vaccine testing. The difficulty in achieving protective T cell responses by immunizing with parasite proteins may well be related to the apparent capacity of the parasite to modulate T cell responses, as indicated by the aberrant non-functional T cell responses observed in primary infections with *T. parva*. This is a neglected area of research that requires further investigation. In this regard, comparison of the responses induced by infected B cells (which produce self-limiting infections) with those induced by infected T cells would be particularly informative and could also provide useful input into the design of a more effective vaccine protocol.

References

Baldwin, C.L., Goddeeris, B.M. and Morrison, W.I. (1987) Bovine helper T-cell clones specific for lymphocytes infected with *Theileria parva* (Muguga). *Parasite Immunology* 9(4), 499–513. DOI: 10.1111/j.1365-3024.1987.tb00526.x.

Baldwin, C.L., Iams, K.P., Brown, W.C. and Grab, D.J. (1992) *Theileria parva*: CD4+ helper and cytotoxic T-cell clones react with a schizont-derived antigen associated with the surface of *Theileria parva*-infected lymphocytes. *Experimental Parasitology* 75(1), 19–30. DOI: 10.1016/0014-4894(92)90118-T.

Ballingall, K.T., Luyai, A., Rowlands, G.J., Sales, J., Musoke, A.J. *et al.* (2004) Bovine leukocyte antigen major histocompatibility complex class II DRB3*2703 and DRB3*1501 alleles are associated with variation in levels of protection against *Theileria parva* challenge following immunization with the sporozoite p67 antigen. *Infection and Immunity* 72(5), 2738–2741. DOI: 10.1128/IAI.72.5.2738-2741.2004.

Bishop, R., Nene, V., Staeyert, J., Rowlands, J., Nyanjui, J. *et al.* (2003) Immunity to East Coast fever in cattle induced by a polypeptide fragment of the major surface coat protein of *Theileria parva* sporozoites. *Vaccine* 21(11–12), 1205–1212. DOI: 10.1016/s0264-410x(02)00621-7.

Boulter, N., Knight, P.A., Hunt, P.D., Hennessey, E.S., Katzer, F. *et al.* (1994) *Theileria annulata* sporozoite surface antigen (SPAG-1) contains neutralizing determinants in the C terminus. *Parasite Immunology* 16(2), 97–104. DOI: 10.1111/j.1365-3024.1994.tb00328.x.

Brown, C.G.D., Stagg, D.A., Purnell, R.E., Kanhai, G.K. and Payne, R.C. (1973) Infection and transformation of bovine lymphoid cells *in vitro* by infective particles of *Theileria parva*. *Nature* 245(5420), 101–103. DOI: 10.1038/245101a0.

Brown, C.G.D. (1981) Application of *in vitro* techniques to vaccination against theileriosis. In: Irvin, A.D., Cunningham, M.P. and Young, A.S. (eds) *Advances in the Control of Theileriosis. Current Topics in Veterinary Medicine and Animal Science*, Vol. 14. Martinus Nijhoff, The Hague, The Hague, The Netherlands, pp. 104–119.

Brown, W.C., Sugimoto, C., Conrad, P.A. and Grab, D.J. (1989) Differential response of bovine T-cell lines to membrane and soluble antigens of *Theileria parva* schizont-infected cells. *Parasite Immunology* 11(6), 567–583. DOI: 10.1111/j.1365-3024.1989.tb00921.x.

Brown, W.C., Lonsdale-Eccles, J.D., DeMartini, J.C. and Grab, D.J. (1990) Recognition of soluble *Theileria parva* antigen by bovine helper T cell clones: Characterization and partial purification of the antigen. *The Journal of Immunology* 144(1), 271–277. DOI: 10.4049/jimmunol.144.1.271.

Burridge, M.J., Morzaria, S.P., Cunningham, M.P. and Brown, C.G. (1972) Duration of immunity to East Coast fever (*Theileria parva* infection of cattle). *Parasitology* 64(3), 511–515. DOI: 10.1017/s0031182000045571.

Büscher, G., Morrison, W.I. and Nelson, R.T. (1984) Titration in cattle of infectivity and immunogenicity of autologous cell lines infected with *Theileria parva*. *Veterinary Parasitology* 15(1), 29–38. DOI: 10.1016/0304-4017(84)90107-9.

Chen, C., Herzig, C.T.A., Telfer, J.C. and Baldwin, C.L. (2009) Antigenic basis of diversity in the γδ T cell co-receptor WC1 family. *Molecular Immunology* 46(13), 2565–2575. DOI: 10.1016/j.molimm.2009.05.010.

Connelley, T., MacHugh, N.D., Burrells, A. and Morrison, W.I. (2008) Dissection of the clonal composition of bovine alpha/beta T cell responses using T cell receptor Vbeta subfamily-specific PCR and heteroduplex analysis. *Journal of Immunological Methods* 335(1–2), 28–40. DOI: 10.1016/j.jim.2008.02.015.

Connelley, T., Nicastri, A., Sheldrake, T., Vrettou, C., Fisch, A. *et al.* (2022) Immunopeptidomic analysis of BoLA-I and BoLA-DR presented peptides from *Theileria parva* infected cells. *Vaccines* 10, 11. DOI: 10.3390/vaccines10111907.

Connelley, T.K., MacHugh, N.D., Pelle, R., Weir, W. and Morrison, W.I. (2011) Escape from $CD8^+$ T cell response by natural variants of an immunodominant epitope from *Theileria parva* is predominantly due to loss of TCR recognition. *The Journal of Immunology* 187(11), 5910–5920. DOI: 10.4049/jimmunol.1102009.

Connelley, T.K., Longhi, C., Burrells, A., Degnan, K., Hope, J. *et al.* (2014) NKp46+CD3+ cells: A novel nonconventional T cell subset in cattle exhibiting both NK cell and T cell features. *The Journal of Immunology* 192(8), 3868–3880. DOI: 10.4049/jimmunol.1302464.

Creemers, P. (1982) Lack of reactivity of sera from *Theileria parva*-infected and recovered cattle against cell membrane antigens of *Theileria parva* transformed cell lines. *Veterinary Immunology and Immunopathology* 3(4), 427–438. DOI: 10.1016/0165-2427(82)90025-3.

Cunningham, M.P., Brown, C.G., Burridge, M.J., Musoke, A.J., Purnell, R.E. *et al.* (1973a) East coast fever of cattle: ^{60}Co irradiation of infective particles of *Theileria parva*. *The Journal of Protozoology* 20(2), 298–300. DOI: 10.1111/j.1550-7408.1973.tb00881.x.

Cunningham, M.P., Brown, C.G.D., Burridge, M.J. and Purnell, R.E. (1973b) Cryopreservation of infective particles of *Theileria parva*. *International Journal for Parasitology* 3(5), 583–587. DOI: 10.1016/0020-7519(73)90082-9.

Cunningham, M.P., Brown, C.G.D., Burridge, M.J., Musoke, A.J., Purnell, R.E. *et al.* (1974) East Coast fever: Titration in cattle of suspensions of *Theileria parva* derived from ticks. *British Veterinary Journal* 130(4), 336–345. DOI: 10.1016/S0007-1935(17)35836-0.

Cunningham, M.P. (1977) Immunization of cattle against *Theileria parva*. In: Miller, L.H., Pino, J.A. and McKelvey, J.J. (eds) *Immunity to Blood Parasites of Animals and Man*, Vol. 93. Advances in Experimental Medicine and Biology, Springer, Boston, Massachusetts, pp. 189–207.

Cunningham, M.P., Brown, C.G.D., Burridge, M.J., Morzaria, S.P. and Urquhart, G.M. (1989) *Theileria parva*: The immune status of calves born of dams immunised against East Coast fever. *Research in Veterinary Science* 46(1), 90–94. DOI: 10.1016/S0034-5288(18)31124-X.

Daubenberger, C.A., Taracha, E.L.N., Gaidulis, L., Davis, W.C. and McKeever, D.J. (1999) Bovine γδ T-cell responses to the intracellular protozoan parasite *Theileria parva*. *Infection and Immunity* 67(5), 2241–2249. DOI: 10.1128/IAI.67.5.2241-2249.1999.

DeMartini, J.C. and Baldwin, C.L. (1991) Effects of gamma interferon, tumor necrosis factor alpha, and interleukin-2 on infection and proliferation of *Theileria parva*-infected bovine lymphoblasts and production of interferon by parasitized cells. *Infection and Immunity* 59(12), 4540–4546. DOI: 10.1128/iai.59.12.4540-4546.1991.

de Miguel, D., Ramirez-Labrada, A., Uranga, I., Hidalgo, S., Santiago, L. *et al.* (2022) Inflammatory cell death induced by cytotoxic lymphocytes: A dangerous but necessary liaison. *The FEBS Journal* 289(15), 4398–4415. DOI: 10.1111/febs.16093.

Dobbelaere, D.A., Spooner, P.R., Barry, W.C. and Irvin, A.D. (1984) Monoclonal antibody neutralizes the sporozoite stage of different *Theileria parva* stocks. *Parasite Immunology* 6(4), 361–370. DOI: 10.1111/j.1365-3024.1984.tb00808.x.

Dobbelaere, D.A.E., Webster, P., Leitch, B.L., Voigt, W.P. and Irvin, A.D. (1985a) *Theileria parva*: Expression of a sporozoite surface coat antigen. *Experimental Parasitology* 60(1), 90–100. DOI: 10.1016/S0014-4894(85)80026-6.

Dobbelaere, D.A.E., Shapiro, S.Z. and Webster, P. (1985b) Identification of a surface antigen on *Theileria parva* sporozoites by monoclonal antibody. *Proceedings of the National Academy of Sciences* 82(6), 1771–1775. DOI: 10.1073/pnas.82.6.1771.

Emery, D.L. (1981) Adoptive transfer of immunity to infection with *Theileria parva* (East Coast fever) between cattle twins. *Research in Veterinary Science* 30(3), 364–367.

Emery, D.L., Eugui, E.M., Nelson, R.T. and Tenywa, T. (1981a) Cell-mediated immune responses to *Theileria parva* (East Coast fever) during immunization and lethal infections in cattle. *Immunology* 43(2), 323–336.

Emery, D.L., Morrison, W.I., Nelson, R.T. and Murray, M. (1981b) The induction of cell-mediated immunity in cattle inoculated with cell lines parasitized with *Theileria parva*. In: Irvin, A.D., Cunningham, M.P. and Young, A.S. (eds) *Advances in the Control of Theileriosis: Proceedings of an International Conference Held at the International Laboratory for Research on Animal Diseases in Nairobi*. Martinus Nijhoff, The Hague, The Netherlands, pp. 295–310.

Emery, D.L., Morrison, W.I., Büscher, G. and Nelson, R.T. (1982) Generation of cell-mediated cytotoxicity to *Theileria parva* (East Coast fever) after inoculation of cattle with parasitized lymphoblasts. *Journal of Immunology* 128(1), 195–200. DOI: 10.4049/jimmunol.128.1.195.

Eugui, E.M. and Emery, D.L. (1981) Genetically restricted cell-mediated cytotoxicity in cattle immune to *Theileria parva*. *Nature* 290(5803), 251–254. DOI: 10.1038/290251a0.

Fawcett, D.W., Musoke, A. and Voigt, W. (1984) Interaction of sporozoites of *Theileria parva* with bovine lymphocytes *in vitro*. 1. Early events after invasion. *Tissue and Cell* 16(6), 873–884. DOI: 10.1016/0040-8166(84)90068-5.

Gardner, M.J., Bishop, R., Shah, T., Villiers, E.P., Carlton, J.M. *et al*. (2005) Genome sequence of *Theileria parva*, a bovine pathogen that transforms lymphocytes. *Science* 309(5731), 134–137. DOI: 10.1126/science.1110439.

Gentschev, I., Glaser, I., Goebel, W., McKeever, D.J., Musoke, A. *et al*. (1998) Delivery of the p67 sporozoite antigen of *Theileria parva* by using recombinant *Salmonella dublin*: Secretion of the product enhances specific antibody responses in cattle. *Infection and Immunity* 66(5), 2060–2064. DOI: 10.1128/IAI.66.5.2060-2064.1998.

Gill, B.S., Bhattacharyulu, Y., Kaur, D. and Singh, A. (1976) Vaccination against bovine tropical theileriasis (*Theileria annulata*). *Nature* 264(5584), 355–356. DOI: 10.1038/264355a0.

Goddeeris, B.M. and Morrison, W.I. (1988) Techniques for the generation, cloning, and characterization of bovine cytotoxic T cells specific for the protozoan *Theileria parva*. *Journal of Tissue Culture Methods* 11(2), 101–110. DOI: 10.1007/BF01404140.

Gillespie, A.E., Loonie, K., Lefevre, L., Hope, J.C., Baldwin, C.L. *et al*. (2022) γ/δ T cells function as innate-like receptors in the bovine γ/δ T cell response against *leptospira*. *The Journal of Immunology* 209(10), 1870–1879. DOI: 10.4049/jimmunol.2200319.

Goddeeris, B.M., Morrison, I.W. and Teale, A.J. (1986a) Generation of bovine cytotoxic cell lines, specific for cells infected with the protozoan parasite *Theileria parva* and restricted by products of the major histocompatibility complex. *European Journal of Immunology* 16(10), 1243–1249. DOI: 10.1002/eji.1830161010.

Goddeeris, B.M., Morrison, W.I., Teale, A.J., Bensaid, A. and Baldwin, C.L. (1986b) Bovine cytotoxic T-cell clones specific for cells infected with the protozoan parasite *Theileria parva*: Parasite strain specificity and class I major histocompatibility complex restriction. *Proceedings of the National Academy of Sciences* 83(14), 5238–5242. DOI: 10.1073/pnas.83.14.5238.

Goddeeris, B.M., Morrison, W.I., Toye, P.G. and Bishop, R. (1990) Strain specificity of bovine *Theileria parva*-specific cytotoxic T cells is determined by the phenotype of the restricting class I MHC. *Immunology* 69(1), 38–44.

Goulder, P.J., Sewell, A.K., Lalloo, D.G., Price, D.A., Whelan, J.A. *et al*. (1997) Patterns of immunodominance in HIV-1-specific cytotoxic T lymphocyte responses in two human histocompatibility leukocyte antigens (HLA)-identical siblings with HLA-A*0201 are influenced by epitope mutation. *The Journal of Experimental Medicine* 185(8), 1423–1433. DOI: 10.1084/jem.185.8.1423.

Graham, S.P., Pellé, R., Honda, Y., Mwangi, D.M., Tonukari, N.J. *et al*. (2006) *Theileria parva* candidate vaccine antigens recognized by immune bovine cytotoxic T lymphocytes. *Proceedings of the National Academy of Sciences* 103(9), 3286–3291. DOI: 10.1073/pnas.0511273103.

Graham, S.P., Yamage, M., Mwangi, D.M., Honda, Y., Mwakubambanya, R.S. *et al*. (2008) Characterization of the fine specificity of bovine CD8 T-cell responses to defined antigens from the protozoan parasite *Theileria parva*. *Infection and Immunity* 76(2), 685–694. DOI: 10.1128/IAI.01244-07.

Hall, R., Boulter, N.R., Brown, C.G., Wilkie, G., Kirvar, E. *et al*. (2000) Reciprocal cross-protection induced by sporozoite antigens SPAG-1 from *Theileria annulata* and p67 from *Theileria parva*. *Parasite Immunology* 22(5), 223–230. DOI: 10.1046/j.1365-3024.2000.00302.x.

Haque, T., Wilkie, G.M., Jones, M.M., Higgins, C.D., Urquhart, G. *et al*. (2007) Allogeneic cytotoxic T-cell therapy for EBV-positive post-transplantation lymphoproliferative disease: Results of a phase 2 multicenter clinical trial. *Blood* 110(4), 1123–1131. DOI: 10.1182/blood-2006-12-063008.

Hemmink, J.D., Weir, W., MacHugh, N.D., Graham, S.P., Patel, E. *et al.* (2016) Limited genetic and antigenic diversity within parasite isolates used in a live vaccine against *Theileria parva*. *International Journal for Parasitology* 46(8), 495–506. DOI: 10.1016/j.ijpara.2016.02.007.

Hemmink, J.D., Sitt, T., Pelle, R., Klerk-Lorist, L.-M., Shiels, B. *et al.* (2018) Ancient diversity and geographical sub-structuring in African buffalo *Theileria parva* populations revealed through metagenetic analysis of antigen-encoding loci. *International Journal for Parasitology* 48(3–4), 287–296. DOI: 10.1016/j.ijpara.2017.10.006.

Henson, S., Bishop, R.P., Morzaria, S., Spooner, P.R., Pelle, R. *et al.* (2012) High-resolution genotyping and mapping of recombination and gene conversion in the protozoan *Theileria parva* using whole genome sequencing. *BMC Genomics* 13, 503. DOI: 10.1186/1471-2164-13-503.

Heussler, V.T., Taracha, E.L., Musoke, A., Duchateau, L. and McKeever, D.J. (1998) Immunisation with live attenuated *Salmonella dublin* expressing a sporozoite protein confers partial protection against *Theileria parva*. *Vaccine* 16(8), 834–841. DOI: 10.1016/s0264-410x(97)00263-6.

Honda, Y., Waithaka, M., Taracha, E.L.N., Duchateau, L., Musoke, A.J. *et al.* (1998) Delivery of the *Theileria parva* p67 antigen to cattle using recombinant vaccinia virus: IL-2 enhances protection. *Vaccine* 16(13), 1276–1282. DOI: 10.1016/s0264-410x(98)00041-3.

Houston, E.F., Taracha, E.L., Brackenbury, L., MacHugh, N.D., McKeever, D.J. *et al.* (2008) Infection of cattle with *Theileria parva* induces an early CD8 T cell response lacking appropriate effector function. *International Journal for Parasitology* 38(14), 1693–1704. DOI: 10.1016/j.ijpara.2008.05.014.

Iams, K.P., Hall, R., Webster, P. and Musoke, A.J. (1990) Identification of λ gt11 clones encoding the major antigenic determinants expressed by *Theileria parva* sporozoites. *Infection and Immunity* 58(6), 1828–1834. DOI: 10.1128/iai.58.6.1828-1834.1990.

Im, E.-J., Hong, J.P., Roshorm, Y., Bridgeman, A., Létourneau, S. *et al.* (2011) Protective efficacy of serially up-ranked subdominant CD8+ T cell epitopes against virus challenges. *PLoS Pathogens* 7(5), e1002041. DOI: 10.1371/journal.ppat.1002041.

Innes, E.A., Millar, P., Brown, C.G. and Spooner, R.L. (1989) The development and specificity of cytotoxic cells in cattle immunized with autologous or allogeneic *Theileria annulata*-infected lymphoblastoid cell lines. *Parasite Immunology* 11(1), 57–68. DOI: 10.1111/j.1365-3024.1989.tb00648.x.

Joffre, O.P., Segura, E., Savina, A. and Amigorena, S. (2012) Cross-presentation by dendritic cells. *Nature Reviews Immunology* 12(8), 557–569. DOI: 10.1038/nri3254.

Kaba, S.A., Schaap, D., Roode, E.C., Nene, V., Musoke, A.J. *et al.* (2004) Improved immunogenicity of novel baculovirus-derived *Theileria parva* p67 subunit antigens. *Veterinary Parasitology* 121(1–2), 53–64. DOI: 10.1016/j.vetpar.2004.02.013.

Kaba, S.A., Musoke, A.J., Schaap, D., Schetters, T., Rowlands, J. *et al.* (2005) Novel baculovirus-derived p67 subunit vaccines efficacious against East Coast fever in cattle. *Vaccine* 23(21), 2791–2800. DOI: 10.1016/j.vaccine.2004.10.043.

Katzer, F., Lizundia, R., Ngugi, D., Blake, D. and McKeever, D. (2011) Construction of a genetic map for *Theileria parva*: Identification of hotspots of recombination. *International Journal for Parasitology* 41(6), 669–675.

Killian, M.S. and Levy, J.A. (2011) HIV/AIDS: 30 years of progress and future challenges. *European Journal of Immunology* 41(12), 3401–3411. DOI: 10.1002/eji.201142082.

Knight, P., Musoke, A.J., Gachanja, J.N., Nene, V., Katzer, F. *et al.* (1996) Conservation of neutralizing determinants between the sporozoite surface antigens of *Theileria annulata* and *Theileria parva*. *Experimental Parasitology* 82(3), 229–241. DOI: 10.1006/expr.1996.0030.

Kumar, S., Miller, L.H., Quakyi, I.A., Keister, D.B., Houghten, R.A. *et al.* (1988) Cytotoxic T cells specific for the circumsporozoite protein of *Plasmodium falciparum*. *Nature* 334(6179), 258–260. DOI: 10.1038/334258a0.

Lacasta, A., Mody, K.T., Goeyse, I., Yu, C., Zhang, J. *et al.* (2021) Synergistic effect of two nanotechnologies enhances the protective capacity of the *Theileria parva* sporozoite p67c antigen in cattle. *The Journal of Immunology* 206(4), 686–699. DOI: 10.4049/jimmunol.2000442.

Lara-Tejero, M. and Pamer, E.G. (2004) T cell responses to *Listeria monocytogenes*. *Current Opinion in Microbiology* 7(1), 45–50. DOI: 10.1016/j.mib.2003.12.002.

Lefebvre, M.N. and Harty, J.T. (2020) You shall not pass: Memory CD8 T cells in liver-stage malaria. *Trends in Parasitology* 36(2), 147–157. DOI: 10.1016/j.pt.2019.11.004.

MacHugh, N.D., Connelley, T., Graham, S.P., Pelle, R., Formisano, P. *et al.* (2009) CD8+ T-cell responses to *Theileria parva* are preferentially directed to a single dominant antigen: Implications for parasite strain-specific immunity. *European Journal of Immunology* 39(9), 2459–2469. DOI: 10.1002/eji.200939227.

Malmquist, W.A., Nyindo, M.B.A. and Brown, C.G.D. (1970) East coast fever: Cultivation *in vitro* of bovine spleen cell lines infected and transformed by *Theileria parva*. *Tropical Animal Health and Production* 2(3), 139–145. DOI: 10.1007/BF02359680.

McGill, J.L., Sacco, R.E., Baldwin, C.L., Telfer, J.C., Palmer, M.V. *et al.* (2014) Specific recognition of mycobacterial protein and peptide antigens by γδ T cell subsets following infection with virulent *Mycobacterium bovis*. *Journal of Immunology* 192(6), 2756–2769. DOI: 10.4049/jimmunol.1302567.

McKeever, D.J., Taracha, E.L., Innes, E.L., MacHugh, N.D., Awino, E. *et al.* (1994) Adoptive transfer of immunity to *Theileria parva* in the CD8+ fraction of responding efferent lymph. *Proceedings of the National Academy of Sciences* 91(5), 1959–1963. DOI: 10.1073/pnas.91.5.1959.

McKeever, D.J., Nyanjui, J.K. and Ballingall, K.T. (1997) *In vitro* infection with *Theileria parva* is associated with IL10 expression in all bovine lymphocyte lineages. *Parasite Immunology* 19(7), 319–324. DOI: 10.1046/j.1365-3024.1997.d01-214.x.

Meyer, K.F. (1909) Preliminary note on the transmission of East Coast fever to cattle by intra-peritoneal inoculation of the spleen or portions of the spleen of a sick animal. *Journal of Comparative Pathology and Therapeutics* 22, 213–217. DOI: 10.1016/S0368-1742(09)80048-9.

Morrison, W.I. (2007) The biological and practical significance of antigenic variability in protective T cell responses against *Theileria parva*. *Veterinary Parasitology* 148(1), 21–30. DOI: 10.1016/j.vetpar.2007.05.007.

Morrison, W.I., Goddeeris, B.M., Teale, A.J., Groocock, C.M., Kemp, S.J. *et al.* (1987) Cytotoxic T-cells elicited in cattle challenged with *Theileria parva* (Muguga): Evidence for restriction by class I MHC determinants and parasite strain specificity. *Parasite Immunology* 9(5), 563–578. DOI: 10.1111/j.1365-3024.1987.tb00530.x.

Morrison, W.I., MacHugh, N.D. and Lalor, P.A. (1996) Pathogenicity of *Theileria parva* is influenced by the host cell type infected by the parasite. *Infection and Immunity* 64(2), 557–562. DOI: 10.1128/iai.64.2.557-562.1996.

Morrison, W.I., Connelley, T., Hemmink, J.D. and MacHugh, N.D. (2015) Understanding the basis of parasite strain-restricted immunity to *Theileria parva*. *Annual Review of Animal Biosciences* 3(1), 397–418. DOI: 10.1146/annurev-animal-022513-114152.

Morrison, W.I., Aguado, A., Sheldrake, T.A., Palmateer, N.C., Ifeonu, O.O. *et al.* (2021) CD4 T cell responses to *Theileria parva* in immune cattle recognize a diverse set of parasite antigens presented on the surface of infected lymphoblasts. *The Journal of Immunology* 207(8), 1965–1977. DOI: 10.4049/jimmunol.2100331.

Morzaria, S.P., Irvin, A.D., Voigt, W.P. and Taracha, E.L.N. (1987) Effect of timing and intensity of challenge following immunization against East Coast fever. *Veterinary Parasitology* 26(1–2), 29–41. DOI: 10.1016/0304-4017(87)90074-4.

Muhammed, S.I., Lauerman, L.H. and Johnson, L.W. (1975) Effect of humoral antibodies on the course of *Theileria parva* infection (East Coast fever) of cattle. *American Journal of Veterinary Research* 36, 399–402.

Musoke, A., Morzaria, S., Nkonge, C., Jones, E. and Nene, V. (1992) A recombinant sporozoite surface antigen of *Theileria parva* induces protection in cattle. *Proceedings of the National Academy of Sciences* 89(2), 514–518. DOI: 10.1073/pnas.89.2.514.

Musoke, A., Rowlands, J., Nene, V., Nyanjui, J., Katende, J. *et al.* (2005) Subunit vaccine based on the p67 major surface protein of *Theileria parva* sporozoites reduces severity of infection derived from field tick challenge. *Vaccine* 23(23), 3084–3095. DOI: 10.1016/j.vaccine.2004.09.039.

Musoke, A.J., Nantulya, V.M., Büscher, G., Masake, R.A. and Otim, B. (1982) Bovine immune response to *Theileria parva*: Neutralizing antibodies to sporozoites. *Immunology* 45(4), 663–668.

Musoke, A.J., Nene, V. and McKeever, D.J. (1995) Epitope specificity of bovine immune responses to the major surface antigen of *Theileria parva* sporozoites. In: Chanock, R.M., Brown, F., Ginsberg, H.S. and Norrby, E. (eds) *Molecular Approaches to the Control of Infectious Diseases*. Cold Spring Harbor Laboratory Press, Cold Spring Harbor, New York, pp. 57–61.

Musoke, A.J., Nantulya, V.M., Rurangirwa, F.R. and Büscher, G. (1984) Evidence for a common protective antigenic determinant on sporozoites of several *Theileria parva* strains. *Immunology* 52(2), 231–238.

Mwangi, D.M., Honda, Y., Graham, S.P., Pelle, R., Taracha, E.L.N. *et al.* (2011) Treatment of cattle with DNA-encoded flt3l and GM-CSF prior to immunization with *Theileria parva* candidate vaccine antigens induces CD4 and CD8 T cell IFN-γ responses but not CTL responses. *Veterinary Immunology and Immunopathology* 140(3–4), 244–251. DOI: 10.1016/j.vetimm.2010.12.013.

Nene, V. and Morrison, W.I. (2016) Approaches to vaccination against *Theileria parva* and *Theileria annulata*. *Parasite Immunology* 38(12), 724–734. DOI: 10.1111/pim.12388.

Nene, V., Iams, K.P., Gobright, E. and Musoke, A.J. (1992) Characterisation of the gene encoding a candidate vaccine antigen of *Theileria parva* sporozoites. *Molecular and Biochemical Parasitology* 51(1), 17–27. DOI: 10.1016/0166-6851(92)90196-q.

Nene, V., Inumaru, S., McKeever, D., Morzaria, S., Shaw, M. *et al.* (1995) Characterization of an insect cell-derived *Theileria parva* sporozoite vaccine antigen and immunogenicity in cattle. *Infection and Immunity* 63(2), 503–508. DOI: 10.1128/iai.63.2.503-508.1995.

Nene, V., Musoke, A., Gobright, E. and Morzaria, S. (1996) Conservation of the sporozoite p67 vaccine antigen in cattle-derived *Theileria parva* stocks with different cross-immunity profiles. *Infection and Immunity* 64(6), 2056–2061. DOI: 10.1128/iai.64.6.2056-2061.1996.

Nene, V., Gobright, E., Bishop, R., Morzaria, S. and Musoke, A. (1999) Linear peptide specificity of bovine antibody responses to p67 of *Theileria parva* and sequence diversity of sporozoite-neutralizing epitopes: Implications for a vaccine. *Infection and Immunity* 67(3), 1261–1266. DOI: 10.1128/IAI.67.3.1261-1266.1999.

Norling, M., Bishop, R.P., Pelle, R., Qi, W., Henson, S. *et al.* (2015) The genomes of three stocks comprising the most widely utilized live sporozoite *Theileria parva* vaccine exhibit very different degrees and patterns of sequence divergence. *BMC Genomics* 16(1), 729. DOI: 10.1186/s12864-015-1910-9.

Nyagwange, J., Nene, V., Mwalimu, S., Henson, S., Steinaa, L. *et al.* (2018) Antibodies to *in silico* selected GPI-anchored *Theileria parva* proteins neutralize sporozoite infection *in vitro*. *Veterinary Immunology and Immunopathology* 199, 8–14. DOI: 10.1016/j.vetimm.2018.03.004.

Odongo, D.O., Oura, C.A.L., Spooner, P.R., Kiara, H., Mburu, D. *et al.* (2006) Linkage disequilibrium between alleles at highly polymorphic mini- and micro-satellite loci of *Theileria parva* isolated from cattle in three regions of Kenya. *International Journal for Parasitology* 36(8), 937–946. DOI: 10.1016/j.ijpara.2006.01.008.

Oura, C.A.L., Asiimwe, B.B., Weir, W., Lubega, G.W. and Tait, A. (2005) Population genetic analysis and sub-structuring of *Theileria parva* in Uganda. *Molecular and Biochemical Parasitology* 140(2), 229–239. DOI: 10.1016/j.molbiopara.2004.12.015.

Oura, C.A.L., Tait, A., Asiimwe, B., Lubega, G.W. and Weir, W. (2011) *Theileria parva* genetic diversity and haemoparasite prevalence in cattle and wildlife in and around Lake Mburo National Park in Uganda. *Parasitology Research* 108(6), 1365–1374. DOI: 10.1007/s00436-010-2030-8.

Overstreet, M.G., Chen, Y.-C., Cockburn, I.A., Tse, S.-W. and Zavala, F. (2011) CD4+ T cells modulate expansion and survival but not functional properties of effector and memory CD8+ T cells induced by malaria sporozoites. *PloS One* 6(1), e15948. DOI: 10.1371/journal.pone.0015948.

Pearson, T.W., Lundin, L.B., Dolan, T.T. and Stagg, D.A. (1979) Cell-mediated immunity to *Theileria*-transformed cell lines. *Nature* 281(5733), 678–680. DOI: 10.1038/281678a0.

Pearson, T.W., Hewett, R.S., Roelants, G.E., Stagg, D.A. and Dolan, T.T. (1982) Studies on the induction and specificity of cytotoxicity to *Theileria*-transformed cell lines. *Journal of Immunology* 128(6), 2509–2513. DOI: 10.4049/jimmunol.128.6.2509.

Pelle, R., Graham, S.P., Njahira, M.N., Osaso, J., Saya, R.A. *et al.* (2011) Two *Theileria parva* CD8 T cell antigens both exhibit higher polymorphism in buffalo parasites than those maintained in cattle, but differ in pattern of sequence diversity. *PloS One* 6(4), e19015. DOI: 10.1371/journal.pone.0019015.

Peters, A.R., Toye, P., Spooner, P., Di Giulio, G. and Lynen, G. (2020) Registration of the East Coast fever infection and treatment vaccine (Muguga cocktail) in East Africa. *Gates Open Research* 4, 100.

Pipano, E. and Tsur, I. (1966) Experimental immunisation against *Theileria annulata* with a tissue culture vaccine. I. Laboratory trials. *Refuah Veterinarith* 23, 186–194.

Pipano, E. (1981) Schizonts and tick stages in immunisation against *Theileria annulata* infection. In: Irvin, A.D., Cunningham, M.P. and Young, A.S. (eds) *Advances in the Control of Theileriosis*, Vol. 14. Current Topics in Veterinary Medicine and Animal Science. Martinus Nijhoff, The Hague, The Netherlands, pp. 242–252.

Pipano, E. (1989) Vaccination against *Theileria annulata* theileriosis. In: Wright, I.G. (ed.) *Veterinary Protozoan and Hemoparasite Vaccines*. CRC Press, Boca Raton, pp. 203–234.

Pirie, H.M., Jarrett, W.F.H. and Crighton, G.W. (1970) Studies on vaccination against East Coast fever using macroschizonts. *Experimental Parasitology* 27(3), 343–349. DOI: 10.1016/0014-4894(70)90037-8.

Purnell, R.E., Brown, C.G.D., Burridge, M.J., Cunningham, M.P., Emu, H. *et al.* (1974) East coast fever: ^{60}Co-irradiation of *Theileria parva* in its tick vector, *Rhipicephalus appendiculatus*. *International Journal for Parasitology* 4(5), 507–511. DOI: 10.1016/0020-7519(74)90068-X.

Radley, D.E., Brown, C.G.D., Burridge, M.J., Cunningham, M.P., Kirimi, I.M. *et al.* (1975a) East Coast fever: 1. Chemoprophylactic immunization of cattle against *Theileria parva* (Muguga) and five Theilerial strains. *Veterinary Parasitology* 1(1), 35–41. DOI: 10.1016/0304-4017(75)90005-9.

Radley, D.E., Brown, C.G.D., Cunningham, M.P., Kimber, C.D., Musisi, F.L. *et al.* (1975b) East Coast fever: 3. Chemoprophylactic immunization of cattle using oxytetracycline and a combination of *Theilerial* strains. *Veterinary Parasitology* 1(1), 51–60. DOI: 10.1016/0304-4017(75)90007-2.

Schmuckli-Maurer, J., Casanova, C., Schmied, S., Affentranger, S., Parvanova, I. *et al.* (2009) Expression analysis of the *Theileria parva* subtelomere-encoded variable secreted protein gene family. *PLoS ONE* 4(3), e4839. DOI: 10.1371/journal.pone.0004839.

Schofield, L., Villaquiran, J., Ferreira, A., Schellekens, H., Nussenzweig, R. *et al.* (1987) γ interferon, CD8+ T cells and antibodies required for immunity to malaria sporozoites. *Nature* 330(6149), 664–666. DOI: 10.1038/330664a0.

Shaw, M.K. (1997) The same but different: The biology of *Theileria* sporozoite entry into bovine cells. *International Journal for Parasitology* 27(5), 457–474. DOI: 10.1016/S0020-7519(97)00015-5.

Shaw, M.K. (2002) *Theileria* development and host cell invasion. In: Theileria, Dirk Dobbelaere and Declan McKeever,(eds) *World Class Parasites*, Vol. 3. Kluwer Academic, Boston, Massachusetts, pp. 1–22.

Sibeko, K.P., Geysen, D., Oosthuizen, M.C., Matthee, C.A., Troskie, M. *et al.* (2010) Four p67 alleles identified in South African *Theileria parva* field samples. *Veterinary Parasitology* 167(2–4), 244–254. DOI: 10.1016/j.vetpar.2009.09.026.

Sitt, T., Pelle, R., Chepkwony, M., Morrison, W.I. and Toye, P. (2018) *Theileria parva* antigens recognized by CD8+ T cells show varying degrees of diversity in buffalo-derived infected cell lines. *Parasitology* 145(11), 1430–1439. DOI: 10.1017/S0031182018000264.

Sitt, T., Henson, S., Morrison, W.I. and Toye, P. (2019) Similar levels of diversity in the gene encoding the p67 sporozoite surface protein of *Theileria parva* are observed in blood samples from buffalo and cattle naturally infected from buffalo. *Veterinary Parasitology* 269, 21–27. DOI: 10.1016/j.vetpar.2019.04.006.

Spreull, J. (1914) East Coast fever inoculation in the Transkeian territories, South Africa. *Journal of Comparative Pathology and Therapeutics* 27, 299–304. DOI: 10.1016/S0368-1742(14)80052-0.

Storset, A.K., Kulberg, S., Berg, I., Boysen, P., Hope, J.C. *et al.* (2004) NKp46 defines a subset of bovine leukocytes with natural killer cell characteristics. *European Journal of Immunology* 34(3), 669–676. DOI: 10.1002/eji.200324504.

Sun, J.C. and Bevan, M.J. (2003) Defective CD8 T cell memory following acute infection without CD4 T cell help. *Science* 300(5617), 339–342. DOI: 10.1126/science.1083317.

Suzuki, Y., Orellana, M.A., Schreiber, R.D. and Remington, J.S. (1988) Interferon-γ: The major mediator of resistance against *Toxoplasma gondii*. *Science* 240(4851), 516–518. DOI: 10.1126/science.3128869.

Svitek, N., Saya, R., Awino, E., Munyao, S., Muriuki, R. *et al.* (2018) An Ad/MVA vectored *Theileria parva* antigen induces schizont-specific $CD8^+$ central memory T cells and confers partial protection against a lethal challenge. *Npj Vaccines* 3(1), 35. DOI: 10.1038/s41541-018-0073-5.

Taracha, E.L., Awino, E. and McKeever, D.J. (1997) Distinct CD4+ T cell helper requirements in *Theileria parva*-immune and -naive bovine CTL precursors. *The Journal of Immunology* 159(9), 4539–4545. DOI: 10.4049/jimmunol.159.9.4539.

Taracha, E.L.N., Goddeeris, B.M., Scott, J.R. and Morrison, W.I. (1992) Standardization of a technique for analysing the frequency of parasite-specific cytotoxic T lymphocyte precursors in cattle immunized with *Theileria parva*. *Parasite Immunology* 14(2), 143–154. DOI: 10.1111/j.1365-3024.1992.tb00457.x.

Taracha, E.L.N., Goddeeris, B.M., Morzaria, S.P. and Morrison, W.I. (1995a) Parasite strain specificity of precursor cytotoxic T cells in individual animals correlates with cross-protection in cattle challenged with *Theileria parva*. *Infection and Immunity* 63(4), 1258–1262. DOI: 10.1128/iai.63.4.1258-1262.1995.

Taracha, E.L.N., Goddeeris, B.M., Teale, A.J., Kemp, S.J. and Morrison, W.I. (1995b) Parasite strain specificity of bovine cytotoxic T cell responses to *Theileria parva* is determined primarily by immunodominance. *The Journal of Immunology* 155(10), 4854–4860. DOI: 10.4049/jimmunol.155.10.4854.

Theiler, A. (1912) The immunisation of cattle against east coast fever. In: *Second Report of the Director of Veterinary Research, Union of South Africa, Department of Agriculture*. Cape Times Limited, Government Printer.

Toye, P.G., Goddeeris, B.M., Iams, K., Musoke, A.J. and Morrison, W.I. (1991) Characterization of a polymorphic immunodominant molecule in sporozoites and schizonts of *Theileria parva*. *Parasite Immunology* 13(1), 49–62. DOI: 10.1111/j.1365-3024.1991.tb00262.x.

Toye, P., Gobright, E., Nyanjui, J., Nene, V. and Bishop, R. (1995a) Structure and sequence variation of the genes encoding the polymorphic, immunodominant molecule (PIM), an antigen of *Theileria parva* recognized by inhibitory monoclonal antibodies. *Molecular and Biochemical Parasitology* 73(1–2), 165–177. DOI: 10.1016/0166-6851(95)00110-m.

Toye, P.G., Metzelaar, M.J., Wijngaard, P.L., Nene, V., Iams, K. *et al.* (1995b) Characterization of the gene encoding the polymorphic immunodominant molecule, a neutralizing antigen of *Theileria parva*. *Journal of Immunology* 155(3), 1370–1381.

Toye, P.G., Nyanjui, J.K., Goddeeris, B.M. and Musoke, A.J. (1996) Identification of neutralization and diagnostic epitopes on PIM, the polymorphic immunodominant molecule of *Theileria parva*. *Infection and Immunity* 64(5), 1832–1838. DOI: 10.1128/iai.64.5.1832-1838.1996.

Toye, P., Musoke, A.J. and Naessens, J. (2014) Role of the polymorphic immunodominant molecule in entry of *Theileria parva* sporozoites into bovine lymphocytes. *Infection and Immunity* 82(5), 1786–1792. DOI: 10.1128/IAI.01029-13.

Tsitsiklis, A., Bangs, D.J. and Robey, E.A. (2019) CD8$^+$ T cell responses to *Toxoplasma gondii*: Lessons from a successful parasite. *Trends in Parasitology* 35(11), 887–898. DOI: 10.1016/j.pt.2019.08.005.

Tsur, I. and Adler, S. (1962) Cultivation of *Theileria annulata* schizonts in monolayer cell cultures. *Refuah Veterinarith* 19, 224–225.

Uilenberg, G., Schreuder, B.E.C., Silayo, R.S. and Mpangala, C. (1976) Studies on *Theileriidae (Sporozoa)* in Tanzania. IV. A field trial on immunisation against East Coast fever (*Theileria parva* infection in cattle). *Tropenmedicin Parasitologie* 27, 329–336.

Vantourout, P. and Hayday, A. (2013) Six-of-the-best: Unique contributions of γδ T cells to immunology. *Nature Reviews Immunology* 13(2), 88–100. DOI: 10.1038/nri3384.

Wagner, G.G., Duffus, W.P.H. and Burridge, M.J. (1974) The specific immunoglobulin response in cattle immunized with isolated *Theileria parva* antigens. *Parasitology* 69(1), 43–53. DOI: 10.1017/S0031182000046163.

Wahl, I. and Wardemann, H. (2022) How to induce protective humoral immunity against *Plasmodium falciparum* circumsporozoite protein. *Journal of Experimental Medicine* 219(2), e20201313. DOI: 10.1084/jem.20201313.

Walker, A.R. and Fletcher, J.D. (1986) Histological study of the attachment sites of adult *Rhipicephalus appendiculatus* on rabbits and cattle. *International Journal for Parasitology* 16(4), 399–413. DOI: 10.1016/0020-7519(86)90121-9.

Wang, F., Herzig, C.T.A., Chen, C., Hsu, H., Baldwin, C.L. *et al.* (2011) Scavenger receptor WC1 contributes to the γδ Tcell response to *Leptospira*. *Molecular Immunology* 48(6–7), 801–809. DOI: 10.1016/j.molimm.2010.12.001.

Webster, P., Dobbelaere, D.A. and Fawcett, D.W. (1985) The entry of sporozoites of *Theileria parva* into bovine lymphocytes *in vitro*: Immunoelectron microscopic observations. *European Journal of Cell Biology* 36(2), 157–162.

Wilde, J.K.H. (1967) East Coast fever. *Advances in Veterinary Science* 11, 207–259.

Wilde, J.K.H., Brown, C.G.D., Hulliger, L., Gall, D. and MacLeod, W.G. (1968) East Coast fever: Experiments with the tissues of infected ticks. *British Veterinary Journal* 124(5), 196–208. DOI: 10.1016/S0007-1935(17)39402-2.

Williamson, S., Tait, A., Brown, D., Walker, A., Beck, P. *et al.* (1989) *Theileria annulata* sporozoite surface antigen expressed in *Escherichia coli* elicits neutralizing antibody. *Proceedings of the National Academy of Sciences* 86(12), 4639–4643. DOI: 10.1073/pnas.86.12.4639.

Xue, G., Schubert, C., Hermann, P., Peyer, M., Maushagen, R. *et al.* (2010) Characterisation of gp34, a GPI-anchored protein expressed by schizonts of *Theileria parva* and *T. annulata*. *Molecular and Biochemical Parasitology* 172(2), 113–120. DOI: 10.1016/j.molbiopara.2010.03.018.

Yang, J., Pemberton, A., Morrison, W.I. and Connelley, T. (2019) Granzyme B is an essential mediator in CD8+ T cell killing of *Theileria parva*-infected cells. *Infection and Immunity* 87(1), e00386–18. DOI: 10.1128/IAI.00386-18.

Yewdell, J.W. (2006) Confronting complexity: Real-world immunodominance in antiviral CD8+ T cell responses. *Immunity* 25(4), 533–543. DOI: 10.1016/j.immuni.2006.09.005.

12 Immunization against East Coast Fever Using Live Parasites: Development of an Infection and Treatment Vaccine

Philip Toye[1]* and W. Ivan Morrison[2]
[1]*International Livestock Research Institute, Nairobi, Kenya;* [2]*Roslin Institute, University of Edinburgh, Edinburgh, UK*

12.1 Introduction

Vaccination remains one of the most successful methods of controlling infectious diseases of humans and animals. Most notably, vaccination played a paramount role in the eradication of two diseases, smallpox and rinderpest. The development of a practical method of immunization against East Coast fever (ECF) has been a primary goal of research into the disease, stimulated by the early observation that cattle that survived an episode of the disease were highly unlikely to experience further clinical episodes. As discussed in detail in Chapter 11 of this volume, all attempts to immunize cattle with inactivated parasites have failed and more recent attempts to vaccinate with isolated parasite antigens have been only partially successful. On the other hand, cattle have been successfully immunized with live parasites. These efforts began over 100 years ago, when Theiler (1912) and Spreull (1914) used infected cells harvested from the lymph nodes and spleens of ECF cases. Although a large proportion of the recipient animals were immunized, the inoculum either produced ECF or failed to induce immunity in the remaining animals, which precluded the use of this method in the field. This limitation was overcome in the 1970s in the form of the Infection and Treatment Method (ITM) of vaccination, which remains the only commercial vaccine against ECF.

In essence, the ITM procedure involves infecting cattle with live sporozoites, usually by inoculation with a cryopreserved, semi-purified homogenate of infected ticks, and preventing severe disease by the simultaneous administration of an anti-theilerial compound, typically long-acting oxytetracycline. The procedure has been viewed as crude, even primitive, and its status as a 'vaccine' has been questioned. It undoubtedly serves as a vaccine, as its effectiveness relies on its ability to induce a powerful protective immune response. Remarkably, ITM is routinely administered as a single inoculation in the life of an animal, as immunity in animals that have recovered from infection has been shown to last for at least 3 years, even in the absence of field challenge (Burridge *et al.*, 1972). At the same time, there is little doubt that, in its current form, the vaccine has several drawbacks. It is expensive, it has a complicated and lengthy production process, it requires a cold chain from production to inoculation and it can be lethal if not administered correctly.

*Corresponding author: pgtoye@gmail.com

 East Coast Fever: The Disease, its Impact and Control (eds W.I. Morrison and P. Toye)
DOI: 10.1079/9781800626324.0012

Nevertheless, the fact that over 2 million cattle have been vaccinated successfully by ITM indicates that it is a commercially viable control option (see Chapter 13 of this volume).

The aim of this chapter is to review the development of the ITM vaccine, the more recent studies to understand how it provides broad protection, detailed analyses of the parasites comprising the vaccine and the development of processes used to manufacture 'commercial-scale' batches of the vaccine stabilate. The chapter will focus on the most widely used version of the ITM vaccine, the Muguga cocktail (MC), with allusions to other formats where appropriate.

12.2 Development of the Muguga Cocktail

In 1953, Neitz reported the results of a study aimed primarily at investigating the therapeutic efficacy of chlortetracycline (Aureomycin™) for ECF. As well as documenting the effect of the compound on the development of the schizont stage of the parasite, Neitz observed that the animals that had recovered from an otherwise lethal infection subsequently displayed a solid immunity (Neitz, 1953, 1957). He made no mention of its potential use for immunization and in fact concluded, 'It is self-evident from these chemotherapeutic tests that this form of treatment cannot be applied in practice' (Neitz, 1957, p. 301).

To make practical use of these findings, three primary challenges had to be overcome. The first was to develop a method to deliver a constant dose of infective sporozoites as opposed to infected ticks, which Neitz and others had used. The solution was the development of procedures for cryopreserving sporozoites in the form of homogenized infected ticks (Cunningham *et al.*, 1973). Second, Neitz had used a treatment regime comprising intravenous injections of Aureomycin™ at frequent intervals after infection. As detailed below, a series of studies was undertaken by Radley and co-workers to develop a more practical therapeutic regime, one outcome of which was the use of a single inoculation of a long-acting formulation of oxytetracycline. The third major challenge was that inoculation with one strain of the parasite did not always confer protection against heterologous strains. This prompted the experiments described below, which ultimately resulted in the MC.

In the 1970s, the United Nations Development Programme (UNDP) funded a major ECF research programme under the leadership of Dr Matt Cunningham at the East African Veterinary Research Organization (EAVRO) in Muguga, Kenya. The programme included a series of immunization and challenge experiments with stabilates of various *T. parva* isolates. The experiments had been prompted by results reported by Snodgrass *et al.* (1972) and Cunningham *et al.* (1974), who had shown that animals immunized with the Muguga stock of *T. parva* had died of ECF when exposed to field challenge. This conflicted with protection observed following experimental homologous challenge of *T. parva* Muguga-immunized animals and contradicted a view current at the time that all *T. parva* strains were cross-immunizing (Wilde, 1967). The Muguga isolate had been chosen as the reference parasite isolate, as it had been extensively characterized at EAVRO (Brocklesby *et al.*, 1961). The aim of the experiments carried out by Radley and colleagues was to examine the cross-reactivity among *T. parva* isolates and to identify a 'master' isolate or combination of isolates that would protect animals against field challenge with *T. parva*.

The first experiments (Radley *et al.*, 1975a) did not reflect the results obtained in the field (Snodgrass *et al.*, 1972; Cunningham *et al.*, 1974), in that 25 animals immunized with the Muguga stabilate survived challenge with the homologous stabilate or with one of five heterologous stabilates. In contrast, 22 out of 25 unimmunized animals succumbed to the challenges. However, in the second set of experiments (Radley *et al.*, 1975b), immunization with the Muguga stabilate provided incomplete protection against challenge with a buffalo-derived stabilate (three survivors out of six animals). Three other immunizing stabilates (the cattle-derived *T. parva* Kiambu 5 stabilate, the *T. parva* Serengeti-transformed stabilate, which had been isolated from buffalo and passaged through cattle, and the buffalo-derived stabilate KB5) provided better protection (survival rates: 3/4, 3/4 and 6/6, respectively). When reviewing the

Table 12.1. Clinical outcomes in cattle immunized with various stabilates and challenged with the cattle-derived Kiambu 1 stabilate or the buffalo-derived KB 1 stabilate. The immunizing stabilates comprised various combinations of stabilates from the Muguga (Mug), Serengeti-transformed (ST) and Kiambu 5 (K5) isolates. The table is adapted from Radley *et al.*, 1975c.

Immunizing stabilate	Challenge stabilate	No. cattle	No. severe reactors	No. deaths
Mug + ST +K5	Kiambu 1	5	0	0
Mug + Ki 5	"	5	3	1
Mug + ST	"	4	3	0
Mug	"	5	3	1
ST	"	5	4	4
None	"	5	5	5
Mug + ST + K5	Solio KB 1	5	0	0
None	"	5	5	0

Table 12.2. Clinical outcomes in cattle immunized with a trivalent combination of Muguga, Serengeti-transformed and Kiambu 5 stabilates (MC) and challenged with various cattle-derived stabilates. The table is adapted from Radley *et al.*, 1975c.

Immunizing stabilate	Challenge stabilate	No. cattle	No. severe reactors	No. deaths
MC	Entebbe 1	6	0	0
None	"	5	5	3
MC	Entebbe 2	6	0	0
None	"	5	5	5
MC	Entebbe 3	5	0	0
None	"	5	5	5

results of these experiments, the authors proposed that a combination of strains may prove more effective than a single immunizing strain and, if so, 'a practicable field vaccine against the East Coast fever syndrome may be in sight' (Radley *et al.*, 1975b, p. 49).

Experiments reported in the third publication in the series (Radley *et al.*, 1975c) tested this idea by immunizing cattle with the Muguga isolate complemented with the Kiambu 5 and Serengeti-transformed isolates. The cattle received parasites from stabilates of all three isolates as separate inoculations. They were compared to two other groups of cattle that had been immunized with *T. parva* Muguga and had then survived challenge with one or other of the complementing strains, and two other groups recovered from infection with either *T. parva* Muguga alone or *T. parva* Serengeti-transformed alone. The animals were challenged with a cattle-derived stabilate (Kiambu 1). The results, summarized in Table 12.1, showed that the only group for which no deaths or severe reactions were recorded was that in which the animals had received all three stabilates. Three other groups had zero or one death, but also three severe reactors. A second group of cattle immunized with the trivalent vaccine was protected against death and severe reaction when challenged with the buffalo-derived KB 1 isolate, although no deaths were recorded in the unvaccinated control group either.

In a second experiment reported in the same publication, groups of cattle immunized with the trivalent combination of Muguga, Serengeti-transformed and Kiambu 5 (MC) and challenged with one of three cattle-derived isolates were all protected against death and severe reactions, whereas all unvaccinated animals underwent severe reactions and all but two cattle died when challenged with one of the three cattle-derived isolates (Table 12.2).

There were two transforming features of this last experiment. The first was that the trivalent stabilate was administered as a single inoculum, rather than the three separate inoculations as previously used. Second, an experimental, long-acting formulation of oxytetracycline ('Terramycin ECF experimental formulation, Pfizer Inc., New York') was used and administered as a single inoculation at the time of infection, as opposed to the series of four inoculations of shorter-acting oxytetracycline used previously. These changes substantially enhanced the prospects of field application of the vaccine. The overall conclusion of the authors was that 'a combination of theilerial strains and a limited oxytetracycline regimen' was proposed as a 'method of immunizing cattle before exposure in the field' (Radley *et al.*, 1975c, p. 51). It was in a later publication that the combination of parasite isolates was named the Muguga 'cocktail' (Radley *et al.*, 1979).

Radley *et al.* (1979) tested the MC for its ability to protect against three other buffalo-derived isolates. In general, although there were far fewer mortalities in the immunized animals (3/20) compared to unimmunized control animals (18/20), ten immunized animals reacted severely to challenge. Subsequent experiments presented in the same publication examined the protection afforded by the MC or two buffalo-derived stabilates when cattle were grazed in a paddock infested with ticks derived from infected buffalo. All groups showed high levels of mortality, except the group of surviving cattle from the first experiment, which had been immunized with the MC and had subsequently survived challenge with the paddock-derived stabilate. All five animals in the group survived exposure in the paddock.

The overall outcome of the experiments conducted by Radley and colleagues at Muguga in the 1970s was that a combination of three *T. parva* stabilates offered adequate protection against challenge with all cattle-derived strains that were tested, but incomplete protection against buffalo-derived parasites. The stabilates could be combined and delivered as a single inoculation. Further, immunization with buffalo-derived parasites provided protection against homologous challenge but incomplete protection against heterologous challenge. The results were interpreted as being due to greater antigenic diversity in buffalo-derived parasites, which was supported by results of later, more detailed studies (see Section 12.3.2 and Chapter 11 of this volume). Finally, there was no evidence for the existence of a 'master strain' of the parasite that provided broad protection.

The first field study involving the MC was undertaken in northern Tanzania by Uilenberg *et al.* (1977) in close collaboration with the UNDP programme at Muguga. The study showed that 40 of 50 animals immunized with the MC survived exposure to a natural infestation of *T. parva*-infected ticks. The remaining 10 immunized animals died from causes unrelated to ECF, and all 19 unimmunized control animals succumbed to ECF. The authors 'recommended that this method of immunization be routinely applied to protect valuable animals at risk' (Uilenberg *et al.*, 1977, p. 499).

It could be argued that the evidence from the studies that were the basis for developing the MC as a commercial product is somewhat limited. The numbers of animals in each group were quite small, ranging from four to six. The number of parasite isolates used for either immunization or challenge was also limited (eight each of cattle-derived and buffalo-derived stocks), which most likely comprise a small representation of the population of parasites encountered in the field. Thus, it is possible, even likely, that other combinations of isolates apart from those selected for the trivalent vaccine may have proven equally effective. Further, the protection against mortality provided by the MC was sometimes only marginally better than that afforded by other immunizing stabilates. As shown in Table 12.1, although there were no deaths in the MC-immunized cattle, there were also no deaths in the group immunized with Muguga combined with Serengeti-transformed, and only one death in two of the other groups, including that immunized with Muguga alone. It should also be noted that incomplete protection involved only a proportion of animals dying or undergoing a severe reaction. Subsequent studies by other workers demonstrated that the level of cross-protection among parasite strains is strongly influenced by the MHC genotype of the animal (see Chapter 11 of this volume). Thus, variation in the proportion of animals within immunized groups that were protected against heterologous challenge in the experiments reported by Radley and colleagues is likely to have been influenced by the MHC genotypes of the experimental cattle. Nevertheless, these experiments, together with the vital field trial conducted by Uilenberg *et al.* (1977), provided enough evidence to move forward with the MC, although it was more than 20 years before this happened on a scale approaching routine commercial use (see Section 12.9 and Chapter 13 of this volume).

The MC has proven to be very effective at providing protection in the field (reviewed in Allan and Peters, 2021). A report in 2009 revealed that several hundred thousand cattle have been vaccinated and the protection afforded by the vaccine was over 98% (Di Giulio *et al.*, 2009). There have been other, smaller, more controlled studies. For example, Martins *et al.* (2010) studied the effect of immunization with the MC in northern Tanzania in two groups of 50 zebu cattle. There was a single clinical case of ECF in the immunized group compared to 24 cases in the unimmunized group. As the animals were treated when ECF cases appeared, no statistical association between mortality and immunization could be established. Interestingly, the animals were routinely treated with acaricide, suggesting that the acaricide regime was not completely effective. A study conducted during the period 1997–2000, involving smallholder cross-bred dairy herds, also revealed substantial benefits associated with immunization with the MC (Lynen *et al.*, 2012). A total of five ECF cases and three ECF deaths were recorded among the 1434 immunized animal years compared to 108 cases and 75 deaths among the 744 non-immunized animal years. This translated into efficacies of ITM preventing ECF cases and death due to ECF at 97.6 and 97.9%, respectively.

12.3 Genetic and Antigenic Diversity in the Muguga Cocktail Component Stocks Compared to Field Isolates

A key question that arose from the studies of the EAVRO group is why a combination of stabilates derived from different isolates provided broader protection than that conferred by a single stabilate. An obvious answer is that a vaccine containing several parasite strains offers exposure to greater antigenic diversity, leading to broader protection against heterologous challenge. To provide evidence for this, there have been several studies that have attempted to determine the extent of antigenic diversity in the MC components compared to that observed in field isolates.

12.3.1 Diversity in Muguga cocktail component stabilates

Although CD8 T cell responses had been shown to play an important role in immunity to *T. parva* at the time these studies were initiated, the identity of the antigens recognized by the CD8 T cells was not yet known. Accordingly, these initial studies used an array of techniques to examine other differences among the three component stocks of the MC. These included anti-schizont monoclonal antibodies, restriction fragment length polymorphism of repetitive DNA regions and PCR amplification of genes encoding antigens recognized by sera from infected animals (Bishop *et al.*, 2001). Later analyses employed microsatellite and minisatellite markers that detect substantial diversity in both cattle- and buffalo-derived parasites (Oura *et al.*, 2004; Patel *et al.*, 2011). The surprising outcome from all these studies was that the Muguga and Serengeti-transformed stabilates appeared to be very similar although clearly distinct from the Kiambu 5 parasites. This led Oura *et al.* (2004) to propose that the close similarity of the Muguga and Serengeti-transformed stabilates may have arisen by complete loss of the Serengeti stock from the vaccine and its replacement by a different passage of the Muguga stock at some stage in the cattle–tick production cycles.

The results suggested that the inclusion of both Muguga and Serengeti-transformed stocks in the cocktail is redundant. However, in a practical sense, removal of a component for commercial production of the vaccine stock is not straightforward, as the product would require a new registration process and there would be no major cost reduction in production as similar numbers of cattle are required to produce an equivalent number of infective acini for a two- or three-component stabilate.

The limitation of the above studies was that they could not directly address the extent of diversity among antigens recognized by CD8 T cells, which are the main effectors of immunity against ECF. The identification of several CD8 T cell antigens (Graham *et al.*, 2006) prompted studies to investigate antigenic polymorphism and to identify the precise specificity of CD8 T cell responses. As discussed in detail in Chapter 11 of this volume, the antigenic specificity of CD8 T cell responses of immune cattle is complex. A profound MHC-dependent hierarchy of dominance of the antigens results in responses to only a few antigenic epitopes in individual animals, with different antigens being recognized by animals of different MHC types. Fifteen antigens have been identified to date (see Chapter 11 of this volume), but some animals do not generate responses to any of these antigens. Some but not all of the antigens display extensive polymorphism and induce strain-restricted CD8 T cell responses. It is almost certainly the case that, due to the restricted specificity of CD8 T cells used for antigen screening, the antigens identified to date represent only a small proportion of the total set of antigens that can be recognized by CD8 T cells from *T. parva*-infected cattle.

The identification of these antigens also allowed a first insight into the diversity of antigens within the MC. Pelle *et al.* (2011) sequenced two antigens, Tp1 and Tp2, in cell lines generated by *in vitro* infection of lymphocytes with sporozoites from each of the three components of the MC, as well as in infected cell lines derived from field isolates of *T. parva*. The analysis of the field isolates revealed that both antigens displayed extensive polymorphism, as discussed below (Section 12.3.2). In contrast, cell lines from all three component stocks expressed the same Tp1 allele, and the Muguga and Serengeti-transformed parasites expressed the same Tp2 allele, with a second allele present in Kiambu 5 (summarized in Table 12.1). Thus, this initial and very limited investigation offered little evidence of extensive antigenic diversity within the MC.

The analysis of known CD8 T cell antigens in the MC was extended by using the Muguga reference genome sequence, which had been generated previously from a cloned Muguga stock, to compare genome sequences obtained from piroplasm DNA isolated from cattle infected with the Kiambu 5 or Serengeti-transformed stocks or with a second cloned Muguga stock (Norling *et al.*, 2015). A comparison of single nucleotide polymorphisms (SNPs) confirmed the close similarity but not the identity of the Muguga and Serengeti-transformed parasites, in that the number of SNPs in the Serengeti-transformed parasites (586) was of a similar order of magnitude to that detected in the second Muguga clone (957). By contrast, the Kiambu 5 stabilate contained 39,296 SNPs. The sequences of 14 *T. parva* antigens were also compared, including seven known CD8 T cell antigens. The Serengeti-transformed antigen sequences were identical to those in the Muguga reference stabilate, whereas non-synonymous mutations were seen in the Tp2, Tp4 and Tp8 genes of Kiambu 5, but only two, one and one, respectively. Thus, this study also failed to find evidence of extensive antigenic diversity in the Muguga cocktail and provided further clear evidence of the close similarity of the Muguga and Serengeti-transformed parasites.

Hemmink *et al.* (2016) undertook high-throughput, multi-locus sequencing of amplicons of nine CD8 T cell antigen genes in the components of the Muguga cocktail to examine sequence polymorphism. The results confirmed and extended the previous observations that there is very little antigenic diversity among the component stocks. At each antigen gene locus in each component stabilate, 90% of the obtained sequences were identical, apart from the Tp3 antigen gene locus in the Kiambu 5 stabilate (Fig. 12.1). Non-synonymous mutations were seen in only four of the antigens (Tp2, Tp3, Tp7 and Tp10), which are predicted to yield only a single protein variant for Tp2, Tp7 and Tp10 and two variants for Tp3. Analysis of a tenth antigen gene (Tp9) by traditional sequencing of cloned cell lines from each stock revealed identical antigen sequences in the Muguga and Serengeti stocks, and a single, different allele in the Kiambu 5 stock.

12.3.2 Diversity in field isolates

As mentioned above, the study of Pelle *et al.* (2011) analysed 79 samples, including parasites from buffalo and from cattle that co-grazed with buffalo, and bovine cell lines infected *in vitro* or derived from cattle undergoing clinical ECF. In total, the study detected 35 and 43 different alleles of the Tp1 and Tp2 genes, which are

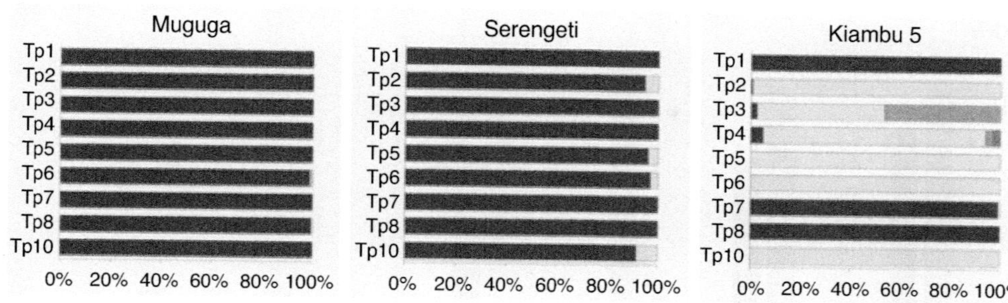

Fig. 12.1. The relative frequencies of alleles of genes encoding CD8 antigens in the three components of the MC vaccine stabilate. For each locus, alleles are denoted by different fill patterns, with the black shading representing the most abundant allele in the Muguga stabilate. (Adapted and reproduced with permission from Hemmink *et al*., 2016.)

Table 12.3. Sequence diversity in the genes encoding Tp1 and Tp2 in the Muguga cocktail compared to that in a series of cattle-derived and buffalo-derived *T. parva* stocks or infected cell lines. Nucleotide sequences were obtained from PCR amplicons of a 432 bp segment (26.5%) of the Tp1 gene and the full length Tp2 gene. Data extracted with permission from Pelle *et al*., 2011, Table S1.

	Buffalo-derived *T. parva* [a]N: 38 (Tp1), 41 (Tp2)		Cattle-derived *T. parva* N: 38 (Tp1), 36 (Tp2)		Muguga cocktail	
Antigen genes	Allelic variants	Protein variants	Allelic variants	Protein variants	Allelic variants	Protein variants
Tp1	26	26	12	9	1	1
Tp2	38	36	4	4	2	2

[a]N indicates the number of readable sequences obtained for each gene in each sample population.

predicted to encode 30 and 42 protein variants, respectively. Substantially more antigenic diversity was detected in the buffalo-derived parasite populations compared to the cattle-derived ones (Table 12.3). As mentioned above, the study included the MC components. Interestingly, the most common allele of the Tp1 antigen detected in the field samples was expressed by 30% of these cell lines and was also expressed by all three MC components. The Muguga and Serengeti-transformed stabilates also expressed the most common Tp2 allele, present in 62% of the cell lines. Of major relevance to this discussion was the analysis of the known CD8 T cell epitopes of Tp1 and Tp2. Four variants of the single known Tp1 epitope were identified in the field samples. Tp2 has six known CD8 T cell epitopes, and a total of 125 variants were detected among these epitopes.

The considerable antigenic diversity in buffalo-derived parasites was explored in two further studies. Hemmink *et al*. (2018) employed high-throughput sequencing of PCR amplicons from genes encoding 6 CD8 T cell antigens (Tp1, Tp2, Tp4, Tp5, Tp6 and Tp10) from blood samples of 14 buffalo. As shown in Fig. 12.2, extensive allelic polymorphism was detected in the nucleotide sequences of all genes. In contrast to the high level of diversity in the Tp1 and Tp2 predicted protein sequences, there were considerably fewer non-synonymous mutations in the coding regions of the other four genes, as reflected in the limited number of protein variants.

In the second study, Sitt *et al*. (2018) performed conventional (Sanger) sequencing of PCR amplicons from genes encoding 10 CD8 T cell antigens (Tp1–Tp10) obtained from 23 buffalo-derived cell lines. The results confirmed that the nucleotide polymorphism reported elsewhere was a feature of all of the genes analysed (Fig. 12.3). The polymorphism of the predicted protein sequence of the Tp9 gene was as extensive as that observed with the Tp1 and Tp2 genes, whereas that of the other antigens was substantially less.

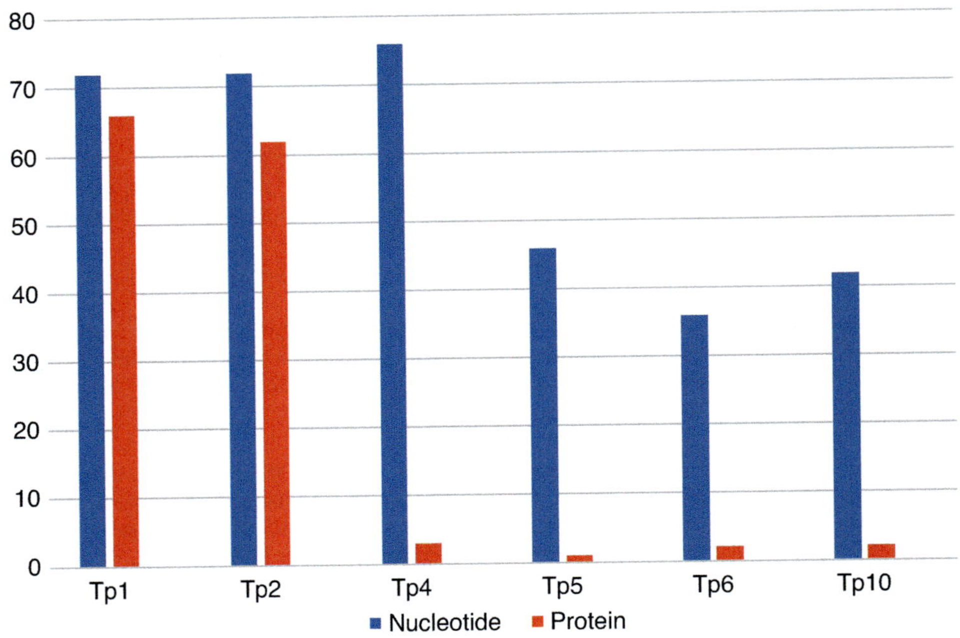

Fig. 12.2. Numbers of nucleotide and protein sequences of CD8 T cell antigens from 14 buffalo obtained by high-throughput sequencing of PCR amplicons derived from blood samples. The *y*-axis figures represent the number of individual sequences obtained. (Data derived from Hemmink *et al.*, 2018, and used with permission.)

With respect to diversity in epitopes known to be recognized by known CD8 T cells, both studies revealed a remarkable level of polymorphism in the six Tp2 epitopes and more restricted diversity in the Tp1 epitope. Sitt *et al.* (2018) also observed polymorphism in the Tp9 epitope. Only a single version of the epitopes on Tp4, Tp5, Tp7 and Tp8 was detected. (The epitopes within the other antigens are yet to be identified.)

In summary, although it is almost certain that only a small fraction of the antigens that can be recognized by CD8 T cells have been identified to date, the conclusion from these studies is that the MC contains only a small proportion of the antigenic diversity that exists in the *T. parva* parasite population. Therefore, the broad protection seen following administration of the vaccine cannot currently be attributed to its ability to elicit CD8 T cell responses to a substantial proportion of the variants of antigens encountered in the field.

12.4 *In Vitro* Analysis of the Specificity of the CD8 T Cell Response Induced by the Muguga Cocktail

The complementary approach to address this question is to analyse the specificity of the immune response induced by the MC. As discussed in Chapter 11 of this volume, immunity to ECF is mediated by CD8 T cells, both in animals that recover from natural infection and those that are immunized by ITM. Crucially, the specificity of the CD8 T cell response, as detected using *in vitro* cytotoxicity assays, has been shown to mimic that observed in *in vivo* cross-protection studies (Taracha *et al.*, 1995). Thus, if the broader protection conferred by the MC in the field is due to greater antigenic diversity within the vaccine stabilate, one would expect a greater level of cross-reactivity exhibited by CD8 T cells from animals vaccinated with the MC compared to those exposed to a single component stabilate.

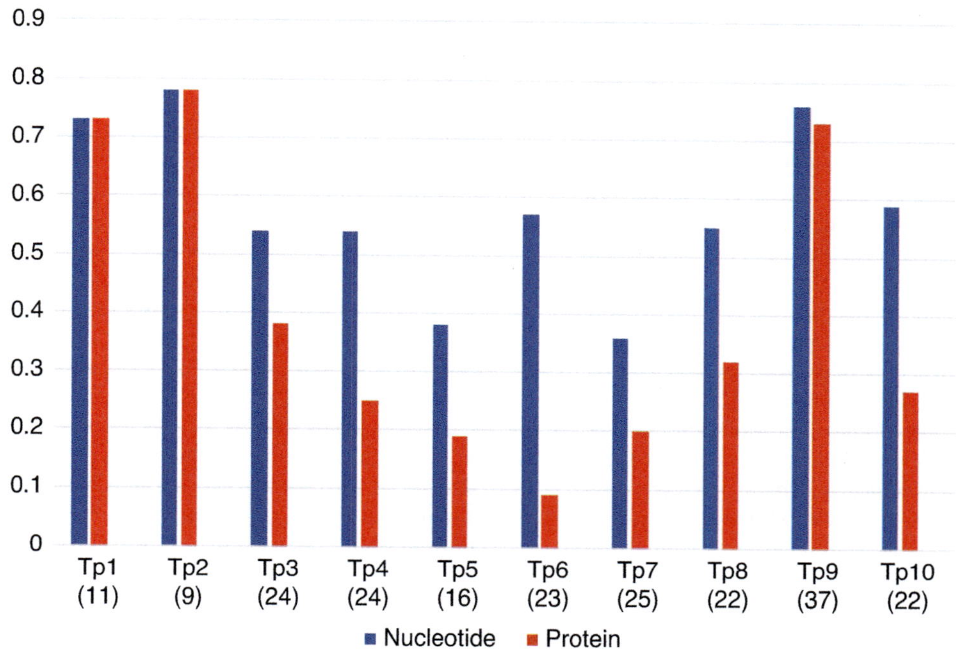

Fig. 12.3. Nucleotide and protein diversity in CD8 T cell antigen genes in buffalo cell lines. The *y*-axis figures represent the number of variant sequences expressed as a fraction of the total number of sequences obtained, which is indicated in brackets below the antigen label on the *x*-axis. (Data derived with permission from Sitt *et al*., 2018.)

Steinaa *et al*. (2018) attempted to demonstrate this by comparing the specificities of CD8 T cells from animals immunized with the MC (the ILRI 08 stabilate, which has been used widely in the field) to those from animals that had received the Muguga stabilate only. To avoid any influence of the MHC, four pairs of haplo-identical animals were used, with one of each pair immunized with either the MC or the Muguga stabilate. The expectation was that the CD8 T cell responses of Muguga-immunized animals that remained susceptible to challenge with the trivalent MC would exhibit narrower specificity compared to those of the MC-immunized twin. However, none of the animals were susceptible when challenged with the MC stabilate, and there was no obvious difference in the antigenic specificity of the CD8 T cell responses of each set of twins. The results likely reflected the MHC genotypes of the animals used in the experiment, resulting in responses to antigens conserved between the MC component parasites. Thus, little evidence could be obtained to confirm if the breadth of protection afforded by the MC was due to broader antigenic specificity within the CD8 T cell response. Further studies are therefore required using twins expressing other MHC haplotypes.

12.5 A Model to Explain the Broad Protection Provided by the Muguga Cocktail

Prior to the demonstration of parasite strain restriction in immunity in the 1970s, it was generally considered that recovery from ECF naturally acquired in the field provided broad protection against the parasite. The reason for this belief is unclear, but it may reflect the presence of greater antigenic diversity among parasites infecting cattle in the field compared to the isolates in the MC, which may enable the initial field challenge to stimulate T cell responses of broader antigenic specificity in animals that survive infection. In this regard, the absence of any detectable antigenic diversity in the Muguga stock may reflect its unusual isolation history, namely that it was isolated in the early 1950s (Brocklesby *et al.*, 1961) and subsequently maintained by regular tick–cattle transmission until the early 1970s when methods of cryopreservation were established. This may have enabled selection of a dominant parasite genotype from the original parasite isolate.

Given that the MC appears to contain only a small component of the antigenic diversity found in field populations of *T. parva*, it is not immediately apparent how it is able to protect against field challenge. A model to explain this has been proposed by Morrison *et al.* (2015). As discussed in Chapter 11 of this volume, immunodominance is a major characteristic of the immune response to *T. parva*, where most of the CD8 T cells in an immunized animal are directed towards one or a few epitopes at most. In other similar systems, the available evidence indicates that immunodominance is determined at the level of the interaction of T cells with infected cells or antigen-presenting cells during induction of a CD8 T cell response (Yewdell, 2006). Hence, the different parasites used in the MC would each be expected to induce independent CD8 T cell responses, and because the antigen dominance hierarchy can vary between parasite isolates, the outcome would be broadening of the antigenic specificity of the response. Since the alleles of different dominant polymorphic antigens are likely to have different distributions among field parasite strains, such immune responses could provide broad strain coverage, at least against the more limited diversity found in cattle-maintained *T. parva*. An additional possibility is that immunization with a mixture of parasites might bias the CD8 T cell responses toward antigens that are conserved between the immunizing parasites. Further work to elucidate the antigenic specificities within the CD8 T cell responses induced by the MC is required to clarify these issues and to provide a sound scientific basis for any further refinement of the composition of the vaccine.

Unlike experimental cross-challenge experiments with *T. parva*, which typically have involved challenge of separate groups of immunized cattle with parasites derived from different isolates, field challenge of vaccinated cattle consists of a sequential series of challenges with infected ticks, which are likely to carry different parasite genotypes. Moreover, the genotypes capable of 'breaking through' the immunity induced by the MC may not be initially encountered as a lethal dose. Immunity induced by infection and treatment does not prevent infection upon challenge, and challenged immune cattle generate a strong CD8 T cell response to the challenge parasites (Morrison *et al.*, 1987; Oura *et al.*, 2007). Hence, initial field challenge of vaccinated animals, in addition to stimulating recall of the vaccine-induced CD8 T cell responses, is likely to elicit CD8 T cell responses to other antigenic specificities. Thus, sequential, non-lethal challenges with infected ticks will broaden the antigenic specificity and protective activity of the memory CD8 T cell pool. In this situation, it may be sufficient for the vaccine to provide protection against a proportion of the parasites encountered upon field challenge.

12.6 The Carrier State and ITM

A carrier state in theileriosis has been defined as a 'persistent, tick-transmissible infection' (Oura *et al.*, 2004, p. 27). The carrier state in general has been discussed elsewhere in this volume (see Chapter 3). With respect to use of the MC, carrier animals are of potential concern due to the possibility that parasite types in the vaccine stabilates can be transmitted to sympatric, unvaccinated cattle and thus become established in a region where these types did not previously exist. It has been suggested that this situation might cause disease outbreaks in cattle that have developed immunity to local strains only, a perceived threat that has been used as an argument against the use of the ITM vaccine (discussed in McKeever, 2007). It should be noted that this situation has never been definitively documented and is not different to that which would occur after the movement of naturally infected cattle into areas with no or different circulating parasites. There was a reported observation that vaccinated cattle brought onto the island of Grand Comore, located off the east coast of Africa, in the early 2000s were responsible for an outbreak of ECF (de Deken *et al.*, 2007). Although DNA from parasites from two infected cattle showed similarities to DNA from parasites in the MC, an unequivocal connection could not be established. Nevertheless, a review of the evidence for transmission of ITM-induced carrier state is warranted.

Most carrier infections are not detectable by microscopic examination of blood. The most direct way of detecting a carrier state is by xenodiagnosis, where ticks that have been allowed to feed on previously infected or vaccinated animals are placed on naïve cattle and evidence for subsequent infection is sought. As this approach is expensive and cumbersome, more recent methods have been based on the detection of parasite DNA in blood by PCR. It should also be noted that PCR assays may not always be sufficiently sensitive to detect all carriers, as indicated by results reported by Olds *et al.* (2018).

The first reported evidence that cattle immunized by the MC were carriers of parasites derived from the vaccine was by Oura *et al.* (2004) in Uganda. Blood samples obtained from 15 cattle at various times after vaccination were analysed by PCR using primers for the gene encoding the polymorphic immunodominant molecule (PIM). Parasites with PIM sequences resembling those in the Kiambu 5 and Muguga stocks were detected in cattle up to 303 and 48 days after vaccination, respectively. A follow-up study (Oura *et al.*, 2007) showed that, based on PCR amplification of the PIM gene and minisatellite 7, most (70%) of the same cattle harboured parasites that were similar to the Kiambu 5 stock 4 years after vaccination, although evidence for the presence of parasites from either the Muguga or Serengeti-transformed stabilates was not detected.

The study also addressed the important question of whether the vaccine parasites were transmitted from the persistently infected vaccinated animals to co-grazing unvaccinated animals, using PCR amplification of the PIM and satellite genes, in samples from cattle on a farm in central Uganda. No vaccine parasite types were detected in ten unvaccinated cattle that had co-grazed with cattle vaccinated 11 months previously. Analysis of a second group of 13 unvaccinated cattle after more than 4 years of exposure to vaccinated cattle detected DNA similar to the Kiambu 5 genotype in four of the unvaccinated animals. The authors considered that difference between the two groups was due to there being an increased number of vaccinated animals on the farm and the longer time between vaccination and analysis of the unvaccinated animals. This result provided evidence that components of the Muguga cocktail could be transmitted from vaccinated animals to co-grazing unvaccinated animals, although there was no report of ECF in these animals.

In summary, while there is some evidence that parasites may be transmitted from vaccinated cattle that have become carriers, there is no definitive evidence to suggest that such transmission has caused outbreaks of ECF. Further studies and monitoring are required to resolve this issue.

12.7 The Muguga Cocktail Does Not Fully Protect against Buffalo-Derived Challenge

As mentioned above, Radley and his co-workers observed incomplete protection when MC-immunized cattle were challenged with various stabilates prepared from ticks harvested from captured wild buffalo (Radley *et al.*, 1979). Additionally, when 11 MC-immunized animals were introduced into a paddock that had previously been free of *T. parva* and was then seeded with ticks infected from buffalo, six of the cattle died. Cattle immunized with buffalo-derived *T. parva* stabilates were also only partially protected, with five out of ten animals succumbing, indicating antigenic heterogeneity in the buffalo *T. parva* population. An earlier experiment in the same paddock obtained complete protection in cattle immunized with a mixture of buffalo-derived stabilates collected over several months from infected buffalo in the paddock, which presumably contained a wider representation of the parasite genotypes present in the paddock (Young *et al.*, 1977). These results demonstrated that the MC does not provide complete protection against buffalo-derived parasites. A more recent study by Bishop *et al.* (2015) also indicated lack of complete protection against buffalo-derived parasites in animals immunized with the MC.

A more detailed and graphic demonstration of the lack of protection provided by the MC against natural buffalo-derived field challenge was recorded at a site in the Ol Pejeta Conservancy (OPC) in the Laikipia District in Kenya (Sitt *et al.*,

2015). A site was selected in which buffalo but not cattle were previously allowed to graze. The study was prompted by reports that ECF-related deaths were occurring in MC-vaccinated cattle on other parts of the conservancy. When 12 MC-immunized and 12 control cattle were exposed at the site, nine cattle from each group succumbed to *T. parva* infection (discussed in more detail in Chapter 7 of this volume).

Conversely, there has been one report from the field which noted that the MC was equally effective in preventing ECF in cattle co-grazing with buffalo as in those that were grazing away from buffalo (Homewood *et al.*, 2006). It is not clear why there was no difference. The amount of interaction between the buffalo and cattle was not reported, and it may have been due to the cattle being initially exposed to cattle derived-parasites, which broadened the specificity of their immunity and provided some protection against a subsequent buffalo-derived challenge.

As highlighted in Section 12.3.2, the lack of protection provided by the MC against challenge with buffalo-derived *T. parva* is most likely due to the much greater antigenic heterogeneity of the parasite population circulating in buffalo.

The inability of the MC to protect cattle from buffalo-derived challenge seriously limits the use of the vaccine in mixed livestock–wildlife farming systems. Although it is tempting to propose the inclusion of buffalo-derived parasites in the vaccine stabilate as a way to broaden the immune response, there are several challenges to this approach. First, the failure of buffalo-derived parasites to develop to the tick-transmissible piroplasm stage in cattle would make it impossible to produce a vaccine stabilate with such parasites, and the use of African buffalo for vaccine production is clearly not feasible. Second, even if vaccine production were possible, buffalo-derived strains are not always cross-protective and so broad protection against buffalo challenge may well require the inclusion of several buffalo-derived stocks.

12.8 The Use of Tetracycline in ITM

Tetracycline has been used as the treatment of choice in ITM since the earliest experiments (Neitz, 1953; Stobbs, 1966; Radley *et al.*, 1975a, b, c). Initially, the use of long-acting oxytetracycline in the field at a standard dose of 20 mg/kg resulted in some animals showing severe clinical signs as a result of vaccination, which necessitated the close monitoring of animals after immunization. Melewas *et al.* (1999) reported a mean of 3.9% clinical reactors in animals immunized as part of a vaccination campaign in Tanzania between 1990 and 1997. One region reported an exceptionally high rate of clinical reactors (36%), which was attributed to inexperienced vaccinators (Melewas *et al.*, 1999). The use of oxytetracycline at 30 mg/kg, together with more standardized batches of vaccine stabilate, reduced the rate to less than 0.05% (Di Giulio *et al.*, 2009). This allows the vaccination of larger numbers of cattle at a single event, as resources are not required to undertake close monitoring of animals to detect reactors. The oxytetracycline dose of 30 mg/kg remains the recommended protocol for immunization with the MC.

The requirement to administer tetracycline very close to the time of infection suggested that the compound acts on the early stages of infection of the host lymphocytes. McHardy (1978) did not discern any effect of oxytetracycline on already established *T. parva*-infected lymphocytes *in vitro* at concentrations as high as 100 μg/ml. In a later study, Spooner (1990a) showed that oxytetracycline inhibited the development of the parasite to mature schizonts and host cell transformation *in vitro*, if given immediately following infection of lymphocytes with sporozoites. There appeared to be no effect on the infectivity of the sporozoites, and in line with McHardy's earlier observation, no effect was noted on established infected cells. The compound was considered to have an inhibitory effect on cytochrome oxidase C activity in infected lymphocytes (Spooner, 1990b), although there is no immediate explanation as to why this effect does not occur in mature infected cells. Inhibition of parasite mitochondrial protein synthesis was also observed. It should be noted that treatment with oxytetracycline does not completely prevent the development of the parasite to the erythrocytic stages *in vivo*, consistent with the occurrence of carrier infections.

By preventing the uncontrolled proliferation of lymphocytes, treatment with oxytetracycline allows the animal to survive and develop a protective immune response. However, for immunization, a balance must be reached between the potency of the sporozoite inoculum and the dose of antibiotic to ensure survival of the animal and the presence of enough infected cells to induce a protective immune response. This necessitates the titration of each batch of the vaccine stabilate in immunization and challenge experiments (see Section 12.9.2).

12.9 Development of Methodology for Commercial Production of the Muguga Cocktail Vaccine Stabilate

Although the efficacy of the MC was demonstrated in the 1970s, large-scale commercial production of the vaccine did not begin until the late 1990s. The reasons for this are discussed in Chapter 13 of this volume. One of the key factors was the complexity of the production process and uncertainty about whether it could be established as a commercial undertaking, a factor that deterred animal health companies from taking up manufacture of the vaccine. At the time of writing, there have been six commercial-scale productions of the MC vaccine stabilate, two (FAO 1/2 and ILRI 08) at the International Livestock Research Institute (ILRI), Kenya, and four (MCL 01–04) at the Centre for Ticks and Tick-Borne Diseases (CTTBD), Malawi (see Chapter 13 of this volume for details). The sections below summarize the development of the manufacturing process that was used in these productions.

12.9.1 Vaccine stabilate production at scale

The initial challenge in deploying the MC for widespread uptake was to adapt the methodology used to produce small batches of the vaccine for research purposes to develop a robust and reproducible production protocol that could yield high numbers of sporozoites free of other pathogens and suitable for use in a commercial vaccine.

In its simplest form, the production of a sporozoite stabilate begins with the infection of naïve cattle (previously unexposed to *T. parva* and other relevant pathogens) by application of infected ticks or needle inoculation with a sporozoite suspension. After allowing sufficient time for the parasitaemia to develop in the cattle, clean uninfected nymphal ticks are applied to the animals and are subsequently harvested after feeding for 4–6 days. Following moulting, the infected ticks are fed on rabbits for four to five days to stimulate maturation of the parasites to the infective sporozoite stage. After harvesting, the ticks are washed extensively with ethanol and homogenized. The resultant suspension is enriched for sporozoites by centrifugation and filtration to remove particulate tick material. The semi-purified suspension is aliquoted into suitable receptacles and stored frozen in liquid nitrogen. Various *in vivo* tests are subsequently employed to determine the infectivity and potency of the final stabilate.

The first initiative involving production of the ITM vaccine at a commercial scale was a request to ILRI from the Food and Agricultural Organization of the United Nations (FAO) to produce a commercial-scale batch of the MC to be funded by the FAO (see Chapter 13 of this volume). This provided an opportunity to develop an optimized protocol fit for commercial production of the MC vaccine stabilate. ILRI consulted widely with other organizations and experts on the protocol, and was guided by the standards, including quality control, set out by the then Office International des Epizooties, now the World Organisation for Animal Health (Morzaria *et al.*, 1999). The resultant protocol incorporated several modifications to protocols existing at the time.

One of the key modifications to the previously used procedures was to pool the ticks before homogenization, rather than subsequently thawing the three individually prepared stabilates, mixing and re-freezing them. This avoided a freeze-thaw-freeze cycle, which would cause some loss of sporozoite viability. The ticks were collected over several days to ensure that any parasites that appear early or late in the parasitaemic phase were included. Samples of dissected salivary glands from each tick batch were screened by microscopic enumeration of infected salivary gland acini. Batches with high infection rates were preferentially included to maximize the sporozoite concentration and minimize the relative concentration of tick material in the field inoculum. The batches derived from the three component isolates were mixed to ensure there were approximately equal numbers of infected acini from each in the final stabilate. In-process characterization of the materials, including analysis of the homogenates with DNA probes and the use of monoclonal antibodies to screen cells infected with the vaccine parasites was introduced at several stages in the process (described in detail in Section 12.9.3). Finally, the stabilate was placed in plastic straws, which are more suited to transport and field use than the previously used glass capillaries or vials.

12.9.2 Dose determination

Experience had shown that the vaccine stabilate produced as described above is highly virulent and must be diluted to avoid death of recipient animals, even when administered with oxytetracycline. The diluted stabilate must be sufficiently potent to induce a protective immunity in the presence of oxytetracycline but not overcome the curative action of the antibiotic. From a commercial perspective, the more the vaccine stabilate can be diluted and retain its protective capacity, the more doses are available per vaccine batch. This can increase the financial return to the manufacturer and/or vaccinator depending on the sales structure, that is, whether the vaccine is sold at a fixed price per straw or per dose. However, an increased number of doses per straw can present a problem, that is, wastage of vaccine in situations where only small numbers of vaccine doses are required (discussed in Chapter 13 of this volume, Section 13.8.1).

In the absence of an *in vitro* method to determine the infectivity of the vaccine stabilates, the potency of each batch needs to be assessed *in vivo* through a series of immunization and challenge experiments (Morzaria *et al.*, 1999; Patel *et al.*, 2016). Cattle immunized with serial dilutions of vaccine stabilate and the recommended dose of oxytetracycline are subsequently challenged with a lethal dose of a previously characterized batch of vaccine stabilate. The dose of parasites used for vaccination is determined based on the clinical responses of the cattle following immunization and after the challenge.

12.9.3 Quality control

12.9.3.1 *Reproducibility*

The seed stabilates used to infect cattle for production of batches of vaccine were originally derived from stabilates used by Radley *et al.* (1975c) in the 1970s, held at the EAVRO laboratories in Kenya. They had been maintained by cattle–tick passage, initially at Muguga and then at the Central Veterinary Laboratory, Malawi (Patel *et al.*, 2016). The known history of the stabilates is shown in Table 12.4.

Since the parasites in these stabilates are uncloned, one concern is that the parasite genotype composition of the vaccine may not be retained in each production batch of vaccine. Morzaria *et al.* (1999) described a series of in-process characterization tests employing monoclonal antibodies and DNA probes (based on sequences for the *Tpr*, telomeric, *LA6* and minisatellite genes) that were introduced at several stages in the production of FAO 1/2. In brief, the assays involved comparing the DNA and monoclonal antibody profiles of cells infected with the seed stocks with those of the individual seed stabilates during production, with the reference stabilates made from ticks before pooling and with the final trivalent stabilate. The assays confirmed that the integrity of the stabilate had been maintained, namely that parasites from all three components were present.

Satellite DNA typing has also been used to compare the different vaccine batches made at ILRI in 1996 and 2007 (FAO and ILRI 08, respectively) and with the original seed stabilates and with the reference stabilates made with ILRI 08. The results did not reveal any major loss of genotypes following the single cattle–tick passage (Patel *et al.*, 2011). Whether there was any functional change in terms of loss or alteration of important antigen genes could not be assessed, although the dose determination studies described above provide confirmation that the vaccine stabilates retain their ability to protect against the component parasites. Advances in molecular techniques for analysis of parasite populations, including high-throughput sequencing, now provide a means of interrogating the content of vaccine batches in greater detail.

Table 12.4. Origins of the seed stabilates[a] used in the MC. Adapted from Patel *et al.*, 2016.

Muguga	Serengeti-transformed	Kiambu 5
15 April 1970 EAVRO[b], Muguga, Kenya Muguga 10	Unknown date EAVRO, Muguga, Kenya ST 72	1971 EAVRO, Muguga, Kenya K5 E542[c]
17 April 1976 EAVRO, Muguga, Kenya Muguga 147	1 November 1972 EAVRO, Muguga, Kenya ST 47	Unknown EAVRO, Muguga, Kenya K5 32
9 November 1984 CVL[d], Lilongwe, Malawi Muguga 57	28 October 1977 EAVRO, Muguga, Kenya ST 161[e]	9 May 1975 EAVRO, Muguga, Kenya K5 102
1 October 1991 CVL, Lilongwe, Malawi Muguga 73	23 October 1981 VPC[f], Lilongwe, Malawi ST 17	28 October 1977 EAVRO, Muguga, Kenya K5 160
	14 September 1989 VPC, Lilongwe, Malawi ST 69	20 September 1989 CVL, Lilongwe, Malawi K5 68

[a]For each stabilate, the date and place of production and the stabilate name are provided.
[b]EAVRO – East African Veterinary Research Organization.
[c]An infected steer (FS114) was found in the Kiambu district and moved to EAVRO. Clean nymphal ticks were applied onto this animal to result in infected adult ticks.
[d]CVL – Central Veterinary Laboratory, Lilongwe, Malawi.
[e]Ticks infected with ST 161 were transferred from EAVRO to CVL.
[f]VPC – Vaccine Production Centre, Lilongwe, Malawi.

12.9.3.2 Contamination with extraneous pathogens

Clearly, it is essential that the cattle, ticks and seed stabilates used in the production of vaccine stabilate are free of other bovine pathogens. As it is not feasible to screen for every possible pathogen, a rational approach has been adopted. Cattle were sourced from ECF-free regions and were screened serologically for *T. parva*, *T. mutans*, *Anaplasma* spp. and *Babesia* spp., while the vaccine stabilate itself was screened for Enzootic Bovine Leucosis and Bovine Viral Diarrhoea viruses by serological testing of cattle inoculated with the stabilate.

The production of ILRI 08 also involved cattle that were negative to the same tick-borne diseases on blood smear examination, while blood smears were also examined for the presence of *Ehrlichia* spp. A serological assay was carried out to screen for Bovine Leukosis Virus. The seed stabilates and sera from cattle infected with the seed stabilates were examined by PCR for arboviruses known to be present in *Rhipicephalus appendiculatus* in the region from where the cattle were sourced, and for fungal and bacterial contamination (see Patel *et al.*, 2016, for a full list). Finally, all cattle used in the infectivity testing and dose determination stages of the production were monitored for untoward clinical signs indicative of pathogen contamination. Although the authors are not aware of any reports of infections from extraneous pathogens in the vaccine stabilate, more stringent testing of vaccine stabilates may be warranted for future batches.

12.10 Natural Exposure and Treatment (NEAT)

An approach that has been considered as an alternative to ITM is to treat animals naturally exposed to *T. parva* and before the development of severe disease, a protocol known as NEAT (natural exposure and treatment). There are several advantages to this approach. It avoids the expense involved in manufacturing and delivering a defined *T. parva* vaccine stabilate. It results in immunity to the local parasite strains and negates concerns about potential introduction of the vaccine parasites into local tick populations. It also has the potential to be effective against buffalo-derived challenge, which the MC is not.

On the other hand, there are several challenges that make NEAT impractical except under specific circumstances. Apart from its use in endemic areas where there is constant and guaranteed exposure to the parasite, the system requires continual, close monitoring of animals to ensure treatment is administered at an appropriate time and the use of expensive anti-theilerial treatment in animals that develop clinical signs. The alternative approach of long-term administration of tetracycline without monitoring for disease is expensive and presents a risk of facilitating the emergence of antibiotic resistance in bacteria carried by the treated cattle populations.

In an early use of the approach, Stobbs (1966) reported the immunization of Kenyan Boran cattle introduced into Uganda to improve the local cattle genotypes. The animals were treated daily with chlortetracycline (Aurofac™) delivered orally and allowed to graze on infected paddocks. An initial group of ten animals received the antibiotic for a period of 1 month. Although most of the animals in the group were reported to have displayed mild clinical signs during this period, seven animals (70%) died of ECF after the drug was withdrawn. Consequently, the protocol was changed to deliver treatment of the animals for 3 months. This reduced the mortality rate to 15%, which was still not acceptable for routine use.

NEAT is currently being employed successfully on the OPC in central Kenya (G. Prettejohn and A. Butt, Laikipia, personal communication). This ranch is in a highly endemic region where there is a constant and severe *T. parva* challenge. Buffalo co-graze with cattle, which invariably results in fatal infections in the latter if exposed, that is, in the absence of tick control (Latré de Laté *et al.*, 2021). Acaricide treatment, delivered by spray race, is required every 5–7 days. Even with this intensive spraying regime, clinical episodes of ECF occur in young calves, with case rates approaching 100% on some occasions. As mentioned above (Section 12.7), use of vaccination by ITM was ineffective in this setting.

The NEAT method was employed on OPC in an attempt to reduce mortality and the high costs associated with buparvaquone treatment. The protocol entails removing calves from the routine acaricide application at 3–4 months of age for a period of 2 weeks. The animals are treated with an initial dose of short-acting oxytetracycline (10 mg/kg) on day 15 followed by a second dose of long-acting oxytetracycline (20–30 mg/kg) the next day. The calves are then returned to the normal spray regime with their dams. The need for treatment with buparvaquone and the losses of young animals have reduced substantially, which has led to the implementation of the protocol as standard practice on OPC. It should be emphasized that the NEAT approach is feasible on OPC due to the constant, high infection pressure, as discussed in Chapter 7 of this volume.

12.11 Conclusions

It is estimated that the MC has been delivered safely and effectively to over 2 million cattle in eastern Africa (see Chapter 13 of this volume). However, there are several aspects concerning the vaccine that would benefit from further study. Many of these relate to practical considerations regarding the production and distribution of the vaccine, and these are addressed in Chapter 13 of this volume. There are other, more fundamental questions concerning the characteristics of the parasites in the stocks and the immunity that is induced in cattle. For example, it is still uncertain how a vaccine stabilate in which very little antigenic diversity has been detected can protect against a parasite population that is known to demonstrate strain-restricted immunity due to antigenic variability. The model that has been proposed to explain this needs to be tested. The lack of protection afforded by the MC against buffalo-derived challenge has been amply demonstrated and is presumably due to the much greater antigenic diversity in buffalo parasites. Hence, it appears that the lesser degree of antigenic diversity of *T. parva* in cattle allows the vaccine to be effective against cattle-maintained parasites but not those transmitted from buffalo. Finally, there may be scope for deploying the NEAT approach more widely, although it may not be applicable in epidemiological settings where infection pressure is low and prolonged administration of the drug is therefore required.

What is clear is that the powerful immunity induced in cattle after infection with *T. parva* needs to be harnessed as a valuable tool to combat ECF. At a time when there are no immediate prospects for alternative vaccination methods, infection with live parasites followed by treatment remains the most viable approach.

References

Allan, F.K. and Peters, A.R. (2021) Safety and efficacy of the East Coast fever Muguga cocktail vaccine: A systematic review. *Vaccines* 9(11), 1318. DOI: 10.3390/vaccines9111318.

Bishop, R., Geysen, D., Spooner, P., Skilton, R., Nene, V. *et al.* (2001) Molecular and immunological characterisation of *Theileria parva* stocks which are components of the "Muguga cocktail" used for vaccination against East Coast fever in cattle. *Veterinary Parasitology* 94(4), 227–237. DOI: 10.1016/s0304-4017(00)00404-0.

Bishop, R.P., Hemmink, J.D., Morrison, W.I., Weir, W., Toye, P.G. *et al.* (2015) The African buffalo parasite *Theileria* sp. (buffalo) can infect and immortalize cattle leukocytes and encodes divergent orthologues of *Theileria parva* antigen genes. *International Journal for Parasitology: Parasites and Wildlife* 4(3), 333–342. DOI: 10.1016/j.ijppaw.2015.08.006.

Brocklesby, D.W., Barnett, S.F. and Scott, G.R. (1961) Morbidity and mortality rates in East Coast fever (*Theileria parva* infection) and their application to drug screening procedures. *British Veterinary Journal* 117(12), 529–531. DOI: 10.1016/S0007-1935(17)43303-3.

Burridge, M.J., Morzaria, S.P., Cunningham, M.P. and Brown, C.G.D. (1972) Duration of immunity to East Coast fever (*Theileria parva* infection of cattle). *Parasitology* 64, 511–551. DOI: 10.1017/s0031182000045571.

Cunningham, M.P., Brown, C.G.D., Burridge, M.J. and Purnell, R.E. (1973) Cryopreservation of infective particles of *Theileria parva*. *International Journal for Parasitology* 3(5), 583–587. DOI: 10.1016/0020-7519(73)90082-9.

Cunningham, M.P., Brown, C.G.D., Burridge, M.J., Irvin, A.D., Kirimi, I.M. *et al.* (1974) Theileriosis: The exposure of immunized cattle in a *Theileria lawrencei* enzootic area. *Tropical Animal Health and Production* 6(1), 39–43. DOI: 10.1007/BF02380747.

Deken, R., Martin, V., Saido, A., Madder, M., Brandt, J. *et al.* (2007) An outbreak of East Coast fever on the Comoros: A consequence of the import of immunised cattle from Tanzania? *Veterinary Parasitology* 143(3–4), 245–253. DOI: 10.1016/j.vetpar.2006.08.018.

Di Giulio, G., Lynen, G., Morzaria, S., Oura, C. and Bishop, R. (2009) Live immunization against East Coast fever – current status. *Trends in Parasitology* 25(2), 85–92. DOI: 10.1016/j.pt.2008.11.007.

Graham, S.P., Pellé, R., Honda, Y., Mwangi, D.M., Tonukari, N.J. *et al.* (2006) *Theileria parva* candidate vaccine antigens recognized by immune bovine cytotoxic T lymphocytes. *Proceedings of the National Academy of Sciences USA* 103(9), 3286–3291. DOI: 10.1073/pnas.0511273103.

Hemmink, J.D., Weir, W., MacHugh, N.D., Graham, S.P., Patel, E. *et al.* (2016) Limited genetic and antigenic diversity within parasite isolates used in a live vaccine against *Theileria parva*. *International Journal for Parasitology* 46(8), 495–506. DOI: 10.1016/j.ijpara.2016.02.007.

Hemmink, J.D., Sitt, T., Pelle, R., Klerk-Lorist, L.-M., Shiels, B. *et al.* (2018) Ancient diversity and geographical sub-structuring in African buffalo *Theileria parva* populations revealed through metagenetic analysis of antigen-encoding loci. *International Journal for Parasitology* 48(3–4), 287–296. DOI: 10.1016/j.ijpara.2017.10.006.

Homewood, K., Trench, P., Randall, S., Lynen, G. and Bishop, B. (2006) Livestock health and socio-economic impacts of a veterinary intervention in Maasailand: Infection-and-treatment vaccine against East Coast fever. *Agricultural Systems* 89(2–3), 248–271. DOI: 10.1016/j.agsy.2005.09.004.

Latré de Laté, P., Cook, E.A.J., Wragg, D., Poole, E.J., Ndambuki, G. *et al.* (2021) Inherited tolerance in cattle to the apicomplexan protozoan *Theileria parva* is associated with decreased proliferation of parasite-infected lymphocytes. *Frontiers in Cellular and Infection Microbiology* 11, 751671. DOI: 10.3389/fcimb.2021.751671.

Lynen, G., Yrjö-Koskinen, A.E., Bakuname, C., Di Giulio, G., Mlinga, N. *et al.* (2012) East Coast fever immunisation field trial in crossbred dairy cattle in Hanang and Handeni districts in Northern Tanzania. *Tropical Animal Health and Production* 44(3), 567–572. DOI: 10.1007/s11250-011-9936-8.

Martins, S.B., Di Giulio, G., Lynen, G., Peters, A. and Rushton, J. (2010) Assessing the impact of East Coast fever immunisation by the Infection and Treatment Method in Tanzanian pastoralist systems. *Preventive Veterinary Medicine* 97(3–4), 175–182. DOI: 10.1016/j.prevetmed.2010.09.018.

McHardy, N. (1978) *In vitro* studies on the action of menoctone and other compounds on *Theileria parva* and *T. annulata*. *Annals of Tropical Medicine and Parasitology* 72(6), 501–511. DOI: 10.1080/00034983.1978.11719354.

McKeever, D.J. (2007) Live immunisation against *Theileria parva*: Containing or spreading the disease? *Trends in Parasitology* 23(12), 565–568. DOI: 10.1016/j.pt.2007.09.002.

Melewas, J., Majaliwa, M. and Lynen, L. (1999) ECF immunisation in Tanzania. In: Morzaria, S. and Williamson, S. (eds) *Live Vaccines for Theileria parva: Deployment in Eastern, Central and Southern Africa. Proceedings of an FAO/ILRI/OAU-IBAR Workshop Held at ILRI (International Livestock Research Institute)*, Nairobi, Kenya, pp. 16–25.

Morrison, W.I., Goddeeris, B.M., Teale, A.J., Groocock, C.M., Kemp, S.J. *et al.* (1987) Cytotoxic T-cells elicited in cattle challenged with *Theileria parva* (Muguga): Evidence for restriction by class I MHC determinants and parasite strain specificity. *Parasite Immunology* 9(5), 563–578. DOI: 10.1111/j.1365-3024.1987.tb00530.x.

Morrison, W.I., Connelley, T., Hemmink, J.D. and MacHugh, N.D. (2015) Understanding the basis of parasite strain-restricted immunity to *Theileria parva*. *Annual Review of Animal Biosciences* 3, 397–418. DOI: 10.1146/annurev-animal-022513-114152.

Morzaria, S., Spooner, P., Bishop, R. and Mwaura, S. (1999) The preparation of a composite stabilate for immunization against East Coast fever. In: Morzaria, S. and Williamson, S. (eds) *Live Vaccines for Theileria parva: Deployment in Eastern, Central and Southern Africa. Proceedings of an FAO, OAU–IBAR and ILRI Workshop Held at ILRI (International Livestock Research Institute)*, Nairobi, Kenya, pp. 56–61.

Neitz, W.O. (1953) Aureomycin in *Theileria parva* infection. *Nature* 171(4340), 34–35. DOI: 10.1038/171034a0.

Neitz, W.O. (1957) Theileriosis, gonderioses and cytauxzoonoses: A review. *Onderstepoort Journal of Veterinary Research* 27, 275–318.

Norling, M., Bishop, R.P., Pelle, R., Qi, W., Henson, S. *et al.* (2015) The genomes of three stocks comprising the most widely utilized live sporozoite *Theileria parva* vaccine exhibit very different degrees and patterns of sequence divergence. *BMC Genomics* 16, 729. DOI: 10.1186/s12864-015-1910-9.

Olds, C.L., Mason, K.L. and Scoles, G.A. (2018) *Rhipicephalus appendiculatus* ticks transmit *Theileria parva* from persistently infected cattle in the absence of detectable parasitemia: Implications for East Coast fever epidemiology. *Parasites & Vectors* 11(1), 126. DOI: 10.1186/s13071-018-2727-6.

Oura, C.A.L., Bishop, R., Wampande, E.M., Lubega, G.W. and Tait, A. (2004) The persistence of component *Theileria parva* stocks in cattle immunized with the "Muguga cocktail" live vaccine against East Coast fever in Uganda. *Parasitology* 129(Pt 1), 27–42. DOI: 10.1017/s003118200400513x.

Oura, C.A.L., Bishop, R., Asiimwe, B.B., Spooner, P., Lubega, G.W. *et al.* (2007) *Theileria parva* live vaccination: Parasite transmission, persistence and heterologous challenge in the field. *Parasitology* 134(Pt 9), 1205–1213. DOI: 10.1017/S0031182007002557.

Patel, E., Mwaura, S., Kiara, H., Morzaria, S., Peters, A. *et al.* (2016) Production and dose determination of the Infection and Treatment Method (ITM) Muguga cocktail vaccine used to control East Coast fever in cattle. *Ticks and Tick-Borne Diseases* 7(2), 306–314. DOI: 10.1016/j.ttbdis.2015.11.006.

Patel, E.H., Lubembe, D.M., Gachanja, J., Mwaura, S.M., Spooner, P. *et al.* (2011) Molecular characterization of live *Theileria parva* sporozoite vaccine stabilates reveals extensive genotypic diversity. *Veterinary Parasitology* 179(1–3), 62–68. DOI: 10.1016/j.vetpar.2011.01.057.

Pelle, R., Graham, S.P., Njahira, M.N., Osaso, J., Saya, R.M. *et al.* (2011) Two *Theileria parva* CD8 T cell antigen genes are more variable in buffalo than cattle parasites, but differ in pattern of sequence diversity. *PLoS ONE* 6(4), e19015. DOI: 10.1371/journal.pone.0019015.

Radley, D.E., Brown, C.G.D., Burridge, M.J., Cunningham, M.P., Kirimi, I.M. *et al.* (1975a) East Coast fever: 1. Chemoprophylactic immunization of cattle against *Theileria parva* (Muguga) and five theilerial strains. *Veterinary Parasitology* 1(1), 35–41. DOI: 10.1016/0304-4017(75)90005-9.

Radley, D.E., Young, A.S., Brown, C.G.D., Burridge, M.J., Cunningham, M.P. *et al.* (1975b) East Coast fever: 2. Cross-immunity trials with a Kenya strain of *Theileria lawrencei*. *Veterinary Parasitology* 1(1), 43–50. DOI: 10.1016/0304-4017(75)90006-0.

Radley, D.E., Brown, C.G.D., Cunningham, M.P., Kimber, C.D., Musisi, F.L. *et al.* (1975c) East Coast fever: 3. Chemoprophylactic immunization of cattle using oxytetracycline and a combination of *Theilerial strains*. *Veterinary Parasitology* 1(1), 51–60. DOI: 10.1016/0304-4017(75)90007-2.

Radley, D.E., Young, A.S., Grootenhuis, J.G., Cunningham, M.P., Dolan, T.T. *et al.* (1979) Further studies on the immunization of cattle against *Theileria lawrencei* by infection and chemoprophylaxis. *Veterinary Parasitology* 5(2–3), 117–128. DOI: 10.1016/0304-4017(79)90003-7.

Sitt, T., Poole, E.J., Ndambuki, G., Mwaura, S., Njoroge, T. *et al.* (2015) Exposure of vaccinated and naive cattle to natural challenge from buffalo-derived *Theileria parva*. *International Journal for Parasitology: Parasites and Wildlife* 4(2), 244–251. DOI: 10.1016/j.ijppaw.2015.04.006.

Sitt, T., Pelle, R., Chepkwony, M., Morrison, W.I. and Toye, P. (2018) *Theileria parva* antigens recognized by CD8+ T cells show varying degrees of diversity in buffalo-derived infected cell lines. *Parasitology* 145(11), 1430–1439. DOI: 10.1017/S0031182018000264.

Snodgrass, D.R., Trees, A.J., Bowyer, W.A., Bergman, J.R., Daft, J. *et al.* (1972) East Coast fever: Field challenge of cattle immunised against *Theileria parva* (Muguga). *Tropical Animal Health and Production* 4(3), 142–151. DOI: 10.1007/BF02359762.

Spooner, P.R. (1990a) The effects of oxytetracycline on *Theileria parva in vitro*. *Parasitology* 100(1), 11–17. DOI: 10.1017/S0031182000060066.

Spooner, P.R. (1990b) Oxytetracycline inhibition of mitochondrial protein synthesis in bovine lymphocytes infected with *Theileria parva* or stimulated by mitogen. *Parasitology* 101(3), 387–393. DOI: 10.1017/S0031182000060583.

Spreull, J. (1914) East Coast fever inoculation in the Transkeian Territories, South Africa. *Journal of Comparative Pathology and Therapeutics* 27, 299–304. DOI: 10.1016/S0368-1742(14)80052-0.

Steinaa, L., Svitek, N., Awino, E., Njoroge, T., Saya, R. *et al.* (2018) Immunization with one *Theileria parva* strain results in similar level of CTL strain-specificity and protection compared to immunization with the three-component Muguga cocktail in MHC-matched animals. *BMC Veterinary Research* 14(1), 145. DOI: 10.1186/s12917-018-1460-x.

Stobbs, T.H. (1966) The introduction of Boran cattle into an E.C.F. endemic area. *East African Agricultural and Forestry Journal* 31(3), 298–304. DOI: 10.1080/00128325.1966.11662057.

Taracha, E.L.N., Goddeeris, B.M., Morzaria, S.P. and Morrison, W.I. (1995) Parasite strain specificity of precursor cytotoxic T cells in individual animals correlates with cross-protection in cattle challenged with *Theileria parva*. *Infection and Immunity* 63(4), 1258–1262. DOI: 10.1128/iai.63.4.1258-1262.1995.

Theiler, A. (1912) The immunisation of cattle against East Coast fever. In: *Second Report of the Director of Veterinary Research, Union of South Africa, Department of Agriculture*. Department of Agriculture. Cape Times Limited, Government Printer, Cape Town, pp. 266–314.

Uilenberg, G., Silayo, R.S., Mpangala, C., Tondeur, V.W., Tatchell, R.J. *et al.* (1977) Studies on Theileriidae (Sporozoa) in Tanzania. X. A large-scale field trial on immunization against cattle theileriosis. *Tropenmedizin Und Parasitologie* 28, 499–506.

Wilde, J.K.H. (1967) East Coast fever. *Advances in Veterinary Sciences* 11, 223–274.

Yewdell, J.W. (2006) Confronting complexity: Real-world immunodominance in antiviral CD8+ T cell responses. *Immunity* 25(4), 533–543. DOI: 10.1016/j.immuni.2006.09.005.

Young, A.S., Radley, D.E., Cunningham, M.P., Musisi, F.L., Payne, R.C. *et al.* (1977) Exposure of immunized cattle to prolonged natural challenge of *Theileria lawrencei* derived from African buffalo (*Syncerus caffer*). *Veterinary Parasitology* 3(4), 283–290. DOI: 10.1016/0304-4017(77)90015-2.

13 The Commercialization of a Vaccine for *Theileria parva* Based on Infection and Treatment

Andrew Peters[1] and Philip Toye[2*]
[1]*Arpexas (Scotland) Ltd, Edinburgh, UK;* [2] *International Livestock Research Institute, Nairobi, Kenya*

We live and learn but not the wiser grow
(John Pomfret, 1667–1702)

13.1 Introduction

The Infection and Treatment Method (ITM) of vaccination against East Coast fever (ECF) using the Muguga cocktail (MC) was developed over 50 years ago (see Chapter 11 of this volume). However it was not until 1996 that the first large, 'commercial-scale' batch of the vaccine became available. It was produced at the International Livestock Research Institute (ILRI) at the request of the Food and Agriculture Organization of the United Nations (FAO) and comprised a total of about 660,000 doses (Morzaria *et al.*, 1999). In the intervening years, small batches of the MC were produced and used in immunization trials in various countries. In addition, other vaccine stabilates had been produced in small batches, including the Marikebuni isolate in Kenya (Payne, 1999) and local isolates, most notably the Katete and Chitongo isolates from Zambia (Mangani, 1999). The Boleni isolate from Zimbabwe has been used under an infection and treatment regime and has also been administered at a titrated dose without oxytetracycline (Ushewokunze-Obatolu, 1999; Latif and Hove, 2011). However, for various reasons, the widespread, commercial implementation of ITM did not occur. These reasons have been well documented by Perry (2016) and are summarized here.

First, the complexity of the procedures for producing the vaccine stabilate raised doubts as to whether consistent, commercial-scale batches could be produced. Second, there were epidemiological concerns that vaccine stabilates, including the MC, would not induce protection against field strains found in all geographical locations. Third, as immunization with live parasites can result in persistently infected (carrier) animals, the possibility exists for the vaccine strains to be introduced into areas previously free of them (De Castro, 1997, 1998; Berkvens *et al.*, 1998; McKeever, 2007). Fourth, there are significant logistical challenges in the distribution of a vaccine that requires storage in liquid nitrogen until administration to target animals. Fifth, the product had not been taken up by a private commercial organization, which would be required to maintain sustainable distribution channels. There was also the, as yet unfulfilled, prospect of

*Corresponding author: pgtoye@gmail.com

 East Coast Fever: The Disease, its Impact and Control (eds W.I. Morrison and P. Toye)
DOI: 10.1079/9781800626324.0013

a more conventional, subunit vaccine which, in theory at least, would be easier to manufacture and deliver. Attempts to develop such a vaccine are discussed in detail in Chapter 10 of this volume and have been the focus of the majority of the research effort on ECF vaccines in the past few decades.

Several of the fears listed above have proved unfounded, and this chapter explores in greater detail the efforts to develop a sustainable manufacturing and distribution system to promote the commercial deployment of the MC vaccine stabilate, including an analysis of the successes and failures. Although other vaccine stabilates have been used in commercial settings, the focus of the chapter is on the MC, as this combination of parasite isolates is found in the most widely used and commercially developed vaccine stabilate. Specifically, the chapter concentrates on a major effort beginning around 2007 to commercialize the product, which involved several international entities.

13.2 The Institutes and Organizations Involved in the Commercial Deployment of the MC

This section briefly summarizes the activities and histories of the key entities that led ultimately to the commercialization of the ITM based on the MC. Some of this is dealt with in detail in an article by Perry (2016), to which the reader is referred. What follows here is a summary of and additional information about these activities.

13.2.1 EAVRO

The East African Veterinary Research Organization (EAVRO), in Kenya, was a major centre for research into ECF and operated under the auspices of the East African Community (Kenya, Uganda and Tanzania) until 1977. The United Nations Development Programme funded a large project on ticks and tick-borne diseases, including ECF, at EAVRO. The project was administered by the FAO. An early achievement of the ECF research was the demonstration that cryopreserved sporozoite suspensions derived from infected ticks could be reliably used to infect cattle by needle inoculation (Cunningham *et al.*, 1973). In the following years, the group at EAVRO conducted the seminal experiments demonstrating the effectiveness of the ITM approach using the MC (see Chapter 12 of this volume).

13.2.2 ILRAD/ILRI

In the early 1970s, discussions took place to establish an international livestock research centre for Africa. One of the key objectives proposed for the new institute was to undertake basic research into immunity to *T. parva*, with a view to developing a conventional vaccine against ECF. The centre was ultimately established in Nairobi, Kenya, in 1974, as ILRAD (the International Laboratory for Research on Animal Diseases) as part of the CGIAR (Consultative Group on International Agricultural Research). In 1995, ILRAD merged with another CGIAR institute, the International Livestock Centre for Africa (ILCA), to become a single entity designated ILRI, the International Livestock Research Institute. It must be stated that the primary aim of ECF research at ILRAD/ILRI was on research underpinning vaccine development and not on the field application of the ITM vaccine. However, the ECF research programme did lead to the establishment of considerable scientific expertise and facilities at the Institue which were subsequently applied to the production of the MC vaccine stabilate.

13.2.3 CTTBD

The Centre for Ticks and Tick-Borne Diseases (CTTBD) was incorporated as a Trust in 2001 from its predecessor, the Vaccine Production Centre, which had been established in 1978 by the Government of Malawi following a resolution of the African Union (AU), then known as the Organisation of the African Unity. The FAO was the Executing Agency at the time, with assistance from the governments of the Netherlands, Denmark and Belgium. The ownership history of CTTBD since then is unclear, at least to outsiders. It operated under the auspices of the Southern African Development Corporation until 2012, when the AU Executive Council proposed integration into the AU. In 2019, the AU's Commission for the Department of Rural Economy and Agriculture tasked the Africa Capacity Building Foundation (ACBF), an agency of the AU based in Harare, to conduct a feasibility study on integration of CTTBD into AU structures. The ACBF concluded that, as CTTBD was a commercial entity with utility for only a limited number of countries in central and eastern Africa, it could not operate as an AU Council-affiliated organization. Although a request was made to the AU in 2020 to prepare a full proposal on the future of CTTBD, a decision on this has not yet been taken, and so CTTBD continues to generate its own funds from the sale of vaccines and other products and services under the administration of AU's Southern African Regional Office.

In the context of this chapter, although CTTBD had been established to produce vaccines for tick-borne diseases and had produced small batches of country-specific ECF vaccine stabilates (e.g. Katete and Chitongo for Zambia), it had not manufactured large-scale, commercial batches of the MC.

13.2.4 GALVmed

In the early 2000s, the UK's Department for International Development (DFID), now the Foreign and Commonwealth Development Office (FCDO), instigated a new approach to improve the control of livestock diseases to help in the alleviation of poverty in low- and middle-income countries, particularly sub-Saharan Africa. A major aim was to establish public–private partnerships (PPP) to drive field application of promising vaccine technologies. An organization, known initially as the Global Alliance on Livestock Vaccines, was established in 2004 and charged with its implementation. In 2005, the organization became known as the Global Alliance on Livestock Veterinary Medicines (GALVmed), following the inclusion of promising therapeutics and diagnostic assays in its portfolio. The initial funding was provided by DFID (see Perry, 2016), and this was followed by substantial funding and involvement by the Bill and Melinda Gates Foundation. The concept was that GALVmed would work towards moving suitable research products in animal health from the laboratory to the field, and several high-impact livestock diseases were initially targeted. ECF, and specifically the ITM vaccine, were identified as fitting readily into the GALVmed portfolio, and GALVmed subsequently became a major coordinating player in the effort to fully commercialize the MC vaccination technology, including production, registration and distribution.

13.3 Initial Steps towards Full Commercialization

In the mid-1990s, the FAO asked ILRI to produce a commercial-scale batch of the MC. ILRI was recognized as being the most suitable entity at the time with the necessary skills and facilities to undertake this. In consultation with other workers, ILRI developed a modified protocol for production of the MC and used it to produce an initial batch of the vaccine (FAO 1), which was packaged into a total of about 10,000 plastic straws of 0.5 ml capacity. The recommended dosage was subsequently determined to be 1 ml of a 1:80 dilution of the stabilate (Table 13.1). As agreed with the FAO, the first batch (FAO 1) was sent to the Vaccine Production Centre in Malawi for distribution to vaccinators.

With the material remaining after the production of FAO 1, ILRI made a second batch of approximately equal size (called FAO 2), which was made available after the FAO 1 stocks in Malawi were exhausted. The distributors collected the FAO 2 vaccine directly from ILRI's Nairobi campus. The last collection for commercial use of FAO 2 was made in 2009.

In 2007, it became apparent that stocks of the MC vaccine were diminishing and a shortage of the vaccine was inevitable in the near future. There was clearly a continued demand for the vaccine, despite concerns about the complexities of its storage and administration and the relatively high retail price of about US$8–12 per animal. The vaccination package included the MC vaccine, oxytetracycline, ear tags and anthelmintic. As no public or private vaccine manufacturer had appeared, ILRI decided to

Table 13.1. Commercial-scale batches of MC vaccine stabilate produced at ILRI and CTTBD.

Year of production	Designation	No. straws	Recommended dilution[a]	Doses per straw	Total number of doses[b]
ILRI					
1996	FAO 1 & 2	20,000[c]	1:80	32	640,000[c]
2007	ILRI 08 1-4	29,648	1:100	40	1,185,920
CTTBD					
2013	MCL – 01	6,875	1:100	40	275,000
2014	MCL – 02	21,204	1:100	40	848,160
2016	MCL – 03	19,164	1:100	40	766,560
2022	MCL – 04	5,803	1:25[d]	10	58,030

[a]The dilution of the straw contents in the diluent immediately before inoculation.
[b]Theoretical calculation of the maximum number of doses based on dilution, number of straws and minimum usable stabilate volume (0.4 ml) available in each straw.
[c]Approximate figures only.
[d]The bulk MCL04 stabilate was pre-diluted 1:4 to produce 10-dose straws.

undertake a second, commercial-scale production of the MC. This decision was later endorsed by other public entities responsible for animal health in eastern Africa (see below).

The production process was essentially the same as that used in the production of FAO 1 and 2, although more cattle were used to produce the stabilate (see Patel *et al.*, 2016 for details). The same seed stabilates were used as in the FAO production, and the stabilate was made as four separate batches. A total of 29,648 straws were produced, and the recommended dosage was determined to be 1 ml of a 1:100 dilution (Table 13.1). The batch was designated ILRI 08 and, as for FAO 2, it was distributed directly from ILRI from 2009 until 2013.

As part of the production of ILRI 08, new stocks of the seed stabilates were produced to supplement the dwindling stocks of the extant seed stabilates. This was undertaken by producing individual component stabilates from the ticks remaining after production of the composite vaccine stabilate. A total of 1934, 1869 and 2151 straws (0.5 ml capacity) were filled for the Muguga, Serengeti-transformed and Kiambu 5 isolates, respectively. As each production animal was inoculated with the contents of no more than three straws for the ILRI 08 production, these seed stabilates should provide sufficient material for decades, if properly stored.

Although ILRI had shown that production of a commercial-scale batch of the MC stabilate was feasible, it had always been clear that ILRI, as a CGIAR institute, could not act as a long-term commercial manufacturer, and therefore an alternative manufacturer was required. In addition, it was not within ILRI's mandate or sphere of expertise to establish a network of distributors and vaccinators in affected areas or to promote awareness of the vaccine among livestock owners.

Consequently, a stakeholder workshop was held at the headquarters of the African Union-Interafrican Bureau for Animal Resources (AU-IBAR) in Nairobi, Kenya, in February 2007 to determine a future strategy for the commercialization of ITM. The meeting included the Directors of Veterinary Services from relevant countries and representatives from AU-IBAR, AU-Panafrican Veterinary Vaccine Centre (AU-PANVAC), GALVmed and ILRI. Several recommendations emerged from the meeting, one of which was that a Task Force be established to develop a long-term strategy for vaccine production and distribution. It also supported the decision by ILRI to undertake a second commercial-scale production of the MC to avoid an impending shortfall in vaccine supply.

A further recommendation from the meeting was that GALVmed should assist in the overall deployment of the vaccine and assess the currently available infrastructure for vaccine production. In response to this, a tendering exercise was launched by GALVmed in October 2008 by advertising a request for proposals (RFP) for vaccine distributors and vaccine manufacturers in the *EastAfrican* newspaper. The Task Force met in January 2009 at ILRI, Nairobi, to consider the applications. It comprised representatives from the ministries responsible for animal health in Kenya, Uganda, Tanzania and Malawi, the AU-Panafrican Veterinary Vaccine Centre, GALVmed and ILRI. The Task Force recommended that the CTTBD become the next production centre for the vaccine, with assistance from both GALVmed and ILRI. Recommendations were also made for the appointment of distributors, as discussed in Section 13.6.

In June 2009, following the recommendation that CTTBD be the next production centre for the MC, a joint ILRI-GALVmed team visited CTTBD to carry out a due diligence inspection and needs analysis of the manufacturing facility together with an estimate of the likely costs. This followed an earlier visit (October 2007) by one of the authors (AP), a consultant in veterinary vaccines, who was commissioned by GALVmed to visit CTTBD with a view to recommending whether or not it would be an appropriate site for further investment to manufacture the MC. That report concluded that CTTBD had the potential capability to produce the MC, but that investment was needed in laboratory refurbishment and re-equipping, upgrading of farm facilities and employment of additional trained staff. In addition, further review and formalization of in-process quality assurance (QA) procedures, including batch documentation, was strongly recommended to ensure product quality. After the 2009 inspection, the decision was made and endorsed by the GALVmed board that GALVmed would invest resources to bring the CTTBD facility up to the required standard for commercial production of MC.

In early 2011, ILRI transferred portions of each of the reference stabilates made during the production of ILRI 08 to CTTBD for use in the production of the MC. Given the importance of using a highly susceptible strain of *Rhipicephalus appendiculatus* ticks in order to minimize the amount of tick material in the final stabilate, ILRI also transferred nymphs and male and female adult ticks to CTTBD. Production of the first batch of the MC vaccine stabilate began in May 2013 and it was released for sale in 2015. Four batches of the MC have now been produced, comprising a total of almost 3.8 million doses (Table 13.1).

13.4 Intellectual Property

As part of the process to establish full commercialization, it was considered essential to review the intellectual property (IP) rights surrounding the ITM technology and the Muguga cocktail components to determine if there were any IP restrictions in the production or use of the MC as a vaccine. A review carried out in 2008 on behalf of GALVmed concluded that there was no formal IP such as patents that would restrict any party from operating in this area. However, considerable IP resided in the vaccine seed stabilates, the tick colonies and the knowledge and associated facilities required for manufacture, all of which were present at ILRI at the time. The seed stabilates and ticks were freely available on request from ILRI.

13.5 Registration

A more challenging obstacle to full commercialization was the registration of the vaccine. As with the previous, small-scale batches of the MC, FAO 1 and 2 were not formally registered but their use was allowed by special sanction of the Directors of Veterinary Services (DVSs) in the respective countries. In order to facilitate the full commercialization of the MC vaccine, GALVmed undertook to register the product through the national regulatory processes in the key target countries of Kenya, Tanzania, Uganda and Malawi. One of the authors (AP) was commissioned by GALVmed to prepare a registration dossier and effect the registration in these countries. It was recognized that there was no precedent for the registration of a live vaccine like the MC in African countries. It was also decided that the registration dossier would be constructed so that it could potentially be used by any national authority, or at least its modular parts used as necessary, to meet individual national requirements. This was to allow for the production of the vaccine in more than one facility. The dossier was also intended to be used as a technology transfer document to enable the production of the MC vaccine at other sites.

International registration of medicines (including veterinary medicines) universally relies on the principles of product Quality,

Safety and Efficacy. The format for the MC registration dossier was based on the format for a European registration dossier, as it was considered that this would be sufficiently comprehensive to cover all likely requirements. However, the dossier was prepared in the knowledge that the ITM vaccine is an unusual if not unique product in veterinary medicine, from the perspectives of both its potential pathogenicity and the complexities of production, storage and administration. Therefore the dossier was written with a certain pragmatic fitness-for-purpose always in mind.

It was decided to build the dossier primarily around the procedures used to produce the FAO batches at ILRI in 1996, as they had proved to be very effective and safe during many years of field use. It should be noted that the production of these batches was in many ways a scientific undertaking to confirm that reproducible, commercial-scale production of the MC was possible. As such, the scientists involved did not have access to well-established, validated protocols. While safe and effective vaccine stabilates were produced, the process was not primarily intended to be a basis for registration, and as such there were several unique challenges to be met in the preparation of the registration dossier. Firstly, there were very few formal documents on which to base the dossier, particularly for the Quality (manufacturing) section. Secondly, the ILRI scientists had produced and evaluated the vaccine stabilate along scientific principles with less emphasis on regulatory processes and requirements. Thirdly, there were not the usual purpose-designed clinical studies for either Safety or Efficacy and hence the data were not as complete as would normally be found in a registration dossier. Also, those involved in the production were primarily research scientists with generally limited recognition and understanding of the regulatory systems in the agreed target countries of Kenya, Tanzania, Malawi and Uganda. So the task of registration began from a very low base in terms of what is normally required for registration. The following section documents the approach used to develop the dossier and how each of the challenges was addressed, and presents an outline version of the final registration dossier itself.

13.5.1 Structure and preparation of the ITM registration dossier

The dossier was structured as far as possible in line with the European Notice to Applicants (European Commission, 2007). The components of a typical European dossier are shown in Table 13.2. The preparation of the dossier is outlined below with emphasis on the critical features.

13.5.1.1 Part 1. The summary of product characteristics (SPC)

The SPC (formerly known as the 'Data Sheet') was drafted initially to ensure clarity and alignment on the exact specifications (sometimes referred to as the 'product profile') of the product and how it should be used. The SPC for the FAO MC vaccine stabilate is shown in Fig. 13.1 and was based purely on the data collected during development of the product.

Table 13.2. Description of the component parts and respective contents of the dossier.

Parts of dossier	Contents
Part 1	Introduction and summary of product characteristics
Part 2	Quality: manufacturing and control
Parts 3 and 4	Safety and efficacy
Part 5	Appendices Standard operating procedures Documentation on constituents, e.g. MSDS[a] Batch production record

[a]Material safety data sheets.

East Coast Fever ITM MC Vaccine.

Summary of Product Characteristics (SPC)

Composition. This is a live East Coast Fever (ECF) vaccine produced from 3 *Theileria parva* stocks: Muguga, Kiambu 5 and Serengeti-tranformed. They are suspended in Eagle's Minimum Essential Medium, containing 3.5% bovine serum albumin (Fraction V), 7.5% glycerol to protect the parasites during freezing and thawing, penicillin (150 units/ml) and streptomycin (150 µg/ml).

Presentation. The vaccine is presented as i) the concentrated vaccine stabilate (VS) in coloured 0.5ml straws sealed at one end and ii) the VS diluent in glass serum bottles containing the required volume for dilution of VS. The bottles are closed with grey butyl rubber stoppers and sealed with aluminium tear-off seals. On thawing the concentrated VS is an opaque dark brown finely particulate suspension. As a consequence upon thawing the VS should be carefully mixed, but without shaking, before addition to the VS diluent. Dilution of concentrated VS to provide the immunisation dose provides a light orange-brown solution, finely particulate.

Pharmacological Action. Immunisation allows the controlled establishment of the 3 component parasite stocks in cattle. Overt disease is prevented by simultaneous treatment with oxytetracycline. Immunised cattle develop full immunity within 4 weeks to the three stocks of *T. parva*.

Indications. The ECF vaccine is indicated in the following situations i) for *Bos indicus* calves over 1 month of age in ECF endemic areas, ii) for pure and cross-bred cattle susceptible to ECF in or moving into endemic areas and ii) other cattle not immune to ECF. The vaccine will not protect against theileriosis caused by *T. annulata* or *T. mutans*.

Contra-indications. Cattle should not be immunised if, they show evidence of incubating ECF, rather they should be treated with anti-theilerial drugs e.g. buparvaquone, calves less than 1 month of age, cattle in poor condition and / or suffering from other disease, cattle in the last 3 months of pregnancy, draught animals.

Storage and handling. The VS concentrate must be kept frozen in liquid nitrogen until use. The diluent must be kept frozen below -20C until required for use. In the field, the VS must be kept on ice, but not submerged.

Directions for use – Vaccine Stabilate dilution and immunisation procedure

(a) Vaccine Diluent: Thaw the vaccine diluent using warm water, as necessary, but below 40ºC, taking care to avoid immersing the bottle cap, since water may enter the bottle. Carefully mix the diluent bottle during thawing, but do not shake to avoid frothing. Check to ensure the diluent is completely thawed, dry the bottle and place immediately on ice. The temperature of the diluent during this process should not rise above about 10ºC. Once thawed, unused diluent should not be frozen and re-used.

(b) Vaccine Stabilate concentrate

1. Take out the number of straws required and the number of diluent bottles to be used (1 straw = 32 doses of current Vaccine Stabilate – minus handling losses). Thaw the straws by rolling them in between palms for 1-2 minutes. Normal safety precautions should be observed in handling liquid nitrogen.
2. Remove the contents of the straw into a pre-cooled sterile serum tube e.g. Nunc 2 ml tube. If 2 or more straws are to be used it is advisable to pool the straw contents.
3. Draw 0.4 ml of Vaccine Stabilate concentrate into a 1 ml syringe, and inject into one diluent bottle, but firstly drawing some diluent into this syringe, allowing for mixing of diluent and stabilate and injecting the mixture into the diluent bottle. This process should be repeated to ensure that the full volume of Vaccine Stabilate has been transferred. Keep diluent bottle inverted during this mixing to avoid air bubbles and frothing of the diluent bottle contents.Put prepared vaccine on ice in a suitable cool box, it can now last for 2 hours, with 4 hours maximum under optimal conditions. Do not allow cap of bottle to come into contact with or be immersed in ice-water.

1. Do not use prepared vaccine if colour is deep red or bright yellow. Normal colour should be in the range orange-red to orange-yellow.
2. Mix the prepared vaccine gently and avoid shaking the vaccine bottle as this will cause foam and loss of usable vaccine volume. Draw 1 ml of prepared vaccine in a suitable 1ml syringe from the diluent bottle and inoculate immediately as above. Return the vaccine bottle to storage on ice as quickly as possible. Do not fill the syringe unless the animal can be inoculated immediately, as keeping the filled syringe in the environment can result in deterioration of the vaccine.

Immunisation procedure

1. Tag the animal and record the number.
2. Weigh the animal and record the weight.
3. Injection of long acting oxtetracycline (OTC) 30% (1 ml/ 10 Kg), volumes of drug exceeding 15 ml should be injected in different sites, calves below 50 kg receive a standard 5 ml dose.
4. Inject 1 ml of prepared Vaccine Stabilate, diluted as below, subcutaneously close to the parotid gland (i.e. slightly below and in front of the base of the ear). Use this opportunity to check for possible gland swelling due to ECF and if detected do not immunise, but treat with anti-theilerial drugs e.g. Butalex.
5. Monitor the animals for 10-20 minutes after immunisation in order to observe possible allergic reaction (skin rash, lacrimation, salivation, swollen eyelids, rapid breathing). If severe allergic reactors are observed treat the animal with 2-4 ml of adrenaline (1:1000 dilution).
6. Monitor animals after immunisation in close collaboration with the livestock owner. Animals showing severe signs of ECF 2-3 weeks after immunisation must be treated with anti-theilerial drugs.

Safety (adverse reactions in cattle to immunisation)

The VS has been thoroughly tested in large numbers of cattle before release to provide a safe immunising dose. The use of 30mg/kg OTC has been shown to eliminate or minimise untoward reactions in cattle.

The vaccine supplier/immunising team will instruct livestock owners about monitoring of immunised cattle and on the action to take in the rare case of an adverse reaction to immunisation, as follows:

- Cattle should be monitored for 10-20 minutes after immunisation in order to observe possible allergic reactions
  - These could include: skin rash, lacrimation, salivation, swollen eyelids.
  - If severe allergic reactors are observed cattle should be treated with 2-4 ml of adrenaline (1:1000 dilution).
- Cattle should also be monitored for 2-3 weeks following immunisation in close collaboration with the livestock owner. Animals showing severe signs of ECF must be treated with anti-theilerial drugs e.g. Butalex ®

Efficacy

The trivalent live ECF vaccine will protect cattle against field challenge from a wide range of *Theileria parva* stocks, but the possibility of unknown and different immunogenic stocks breaking through this immunity cannot be excluded.

Additional precautions

The brand and concentration of OTC administered as treatment during immunisation can influence the response of cattle to immunisation and therefore the quality of the immune response. Only approved brands and drug concentrations should be used during immunisation.

- Standard safety precautions must be followed for the handling of liquid nitrogen.
- This vaccine may lose efficacy if the conditions for handling as described above are not followed precisely.

Fig. 13.1. SPC insert from the MC vaccine presentation.

13.5.1.2 Part 2. Quality (manufacture and quality control)

In outline, the Quality section includes the qualitative and quantitative composition of the product, a description of the manufacturing method, quality control of starting materials, control tests at both intermediate and final product stages, stability and further information on batch-to-batch consistency. These sections are shown in Table 13.3. The manufacturing procedure, including control tests, was described specifically for batch FAO 1 and some details included for FAO 2 where these differed significantly. A series of standard operating procedures was specifically written to inform the production process, and these were made available as part of the dossier. The manufacturing procedure is described in Chapter 12 of this volume and was published in detail for the ILRI 08 production by Patel *et al.* (2016).

13.5.1.3 Parts 3 and 4. Safety and efficacy

In a conventional European registration dossier, it is usual to present Safety and Efficacy as separate sections. However, for the ITM vaccine, the clinical evidence available to be used in the data package had evolved as a series of individual scientific studies without any specific regulatory pathway in mind, and many of the studies had been carried out to address both safety and efficacy simultaneously. Therefore, for the purposes of the dossier, it was decided that the two issues would be presented together in a single section by combining Parts 3 and 4 of the typical European dossier.

In regulatory terms, Safety can be defined as a lack of adverse local or systemic reactions following administration of the product. In statutory tests, this usually involves daily observations of vaccinated animals for a 14-day period post-vaccination. Vaccine Efficacy can be defined as a significant decrease in the severity of clinical signs, the level of infection or pathogen transmissibility exhibited by immunized individuals compared to unvaccinated controls following exposure to the pathogen, as evaluated in a series of different tests. The major subheadings for Safety and Efficacy in a European dossier are shown in Table 13.4.

The data supporting the Safety and Efficacy section were derived from the dose determination experiments for FAO 1 and 2 and ILRI 08. These data were supported by the results presented in multiple previous publications, which are summarized in Table 13.4. The data from these papers and reports were matched to the individual specific criteria shown in Table 13.5, as described in Peters *et al.* (2020).

The long-term stability of the vaccine had never been formally tested, although empirically it seemed to be stable for at least 10 years.

From the evidence presented in these studies, it was concluded that the MC vaccine is safe and efficacious when used per the directions in the SPC and that there is a significant positive benefit–risk relationship (the EU criterion for approval). This conclusion was strongly supported subsequently in a systematic review by Allan and Peters (2021).

Table 13.3. Part 2 of the dossier. Chemical, pharmaceutical and biological/microbiological information.

A	Qualitative and quantitative particulars of the constituents	Active ingredient details, excipients, usual terminology (PhEur, etc.), quantitative amounts of all actives and excipients
B	Description of the manufacturing method	Premises, methodology, validation
C	Control of starting materials	Provenance and QC tests on starting materials Packaging and closures TSE compliance
D	Control tests at intermediate stages	QC tests
E	Control tests on finished product	Specifications, compliance with specification. Safety tests, e.g. contaminants, endotoxins, etc.
F	Stability	Shelf life of active product, both in storage and in use
G	Further information	Batch-to-batch consistency

Table 13.4. The major safety and efficacy parameters to be addressed in vaccine registration.

Safety/efficacy parameter	Specific criteria
Safety	Single dose, repeated dose, overdose Live vaccines – reversion, shed and spread, dissemination Field safety Pregnancy and lactation Environmental safety User safety
Efficacy	Experimental challenge Immunogenicity[a] Dose determination Onset of immunity Duration of immunity Field efficacy
Other	Safety and efficacy of long-acting oxytetracycline Economic benefit/acceptance

[a]Immunogenicity is usually indicated by seroconversion. For ECF, although the serological response is not responsible for protection, it does reflect a response to inoculation of live parasites.

13.5.2 Dossier submission to national authorities

Due to its large file size, the dossier was prepared as a CD-Rom (now available from ILRI), and multiple copies were prepared for distribution to the agencies and individuals closely involved in the registration process. In the case of Kenya, this was submitted by an academic consultant on behalf of GALVmed. For Tanzania, a local technical representative (the VetAgro company owned by the late Drs Lieve Lynen and Guiseppe Di Giulio) was used in-country, and for Malawi, the dossier was submitted by the management of the CTTBD, Lilongwe. For Uganda an in-country technical representative was appointed to submit and negotiate approval of the dossier. The registrations were processed by the specific competent authorities in the respective countries, as shown in Table 13.6.

The vaccine was registered in Kenya, Tanzania and Malawi. Attempts at registration in Uganda have been singularly unsuccessful. The Ugandan National Drug Authority (NDA) in 2009 refused to approve the MC vaccine as it claimed that the Kiambu 5 strain persists in vaccinated cattle for several years, and furthermore declined to approve ILRI as a good manufacturing practice (GMP)-compliant manufacturing site. This was despite acceptance and support from farmers, researchers (Nsubuga-Mutaka *et al.*, 2000) and politicians, and approval by AU-PANVAC in 2008 of ILRI as a GMP manufacturer for ITM of MC (for the purpose of registering the ILRI 08 batch) following a GMP inspection. More recently (August 2024), the Uganda NDA certified that CTTBD is compliant with GMP for the manufacture of the ECF vaccine and diluent.

At the time of writing, it seems that all the registrations in Table 13.6 have been allowed to lapse. This does not signal an intention to abandon the vaccine, as it is still being used, including in Uganda, by special permission of the respective DVSs. It may reflect instead an insufficient incentive based on current market size for private distributors to maintain registration. Nevertheless, its use by special permission of the DVSs is a recognition by some stakeholders of the value of the vaccine.

13.6 Distribution and Uptake of the Muguga Cocktail Vaccine Stabilate

13.6.1 The establishment of distribution channels

At the same Task Force meeting in January 2009 referred to above (Section 13.3), applications for distribution in national markets were

Table 13.5. List of published papers and reports used in the Safety and Efficacy section.

Report number	Report title	Reference
SE1[a]	Determining a safe and protective immunizing dose for the FAO-1 *Theileria parva* composite stabilate for use in field vaccinations against East Coast fever.	(Mutugi *et al.*, 1997)
SE2	FAO-1 composite stabilate. Evaluation of efficacy at 1:80 and 1:100 dilutions and treatment with 30% oxytetracycline.	(Anon, 1998)
SE3	FAO-1–2 composite stabilate. Evaluation of efficacy at 1:80 direct dilution and treatment with 30% oxytetracycline.	(Anon, 1999a)
SE4	Titration of the FAO-1 stabilate.	(ILRI, 1996)
SE5	The persistence of component *Theileria parva* stocks in cattle immunized with the 'Muguga cocktail' live vaccine against east Coast fever in Uganda.	(Oura *et al.*, 2004)
SE6	*Theileria parva* live vaccination: parasite transmission, persistence and heterologous challenge in the field.	(Oura *et al.*, 2007)
SE7	An outbreak of East Coast fever on the Comoros: a consequence of the import of immunised cattle from Tanzania?	(De Deken *et al.*, 2007)
SE8	Infectivity/viability test of FAO-1 stabilate after 2.5 years storage, CTTBD, Lilongwe, Malawi.	(Anon, 1999b)
SE9	The potential of East Coast fever (ECF) vaccine on improved and indigenous cattle in Tanzania.	(Magwisha *et al.*, 2011)
SE10	Applying ITM immunisation in Tanzania using the FAO-1 vaccine batch (1998–2007).	(Anon, 2007)
SE11	Deployment of a live ECF vaccine in pastoral areas: lessons learned from Tanzania.	(Lynen *et al.*, 2005)
SE12	The use of a 30% formulation of oxytetracycline long-acting in East Coast Fever immunizations in Tanzania.	(Lynen *et al.*, 1999)
SE13	Use of two different dose rates of oxytetracycline in East Coast fever immunisation in Tanzania.	(Di Giulio *et al.*, 2000)
SE14	Technical meeting on the Infection and Treatment Method of East Coast Fever immunization and the way forward in Kenya.	(Turasha, 2005)
SE15	Molecular and immunological characterisation of *Theileria parva* stocks which are components of the 'Muguga cocktail' used for vaccination against East Coast fever in cattle.	(Bishop *et al.*, 2001)
SE16	The biological and practical significance of antigenic variability in protective T cell responses against *Theileria parva*.	(Morrison, 2007)
SE17	Current status of vaccine development against Theileria parasites.	(Morrison and McKeever, 2006)
SE18	East Coast fever: 1. Chemoprophylactic immunization of cattle against *Theileria parva* (Muguga) and five Theilerial strains. 2. Cross-immunity trials with a Kenya strain of *Theileria lawrencei*. 3. Chemoprophylactic immunization of cattle using oxytetracycline and a combination of theilerial strains.	(Radley *et al.*, 1975a) (Radley *et al.*, 1975b) (Radley *et al.*, 1975c)
SE19	Pharmacokinetics of two long-acting oxytetracycline products administered subcutaneously and intramuscularly.	(Clarke *et al.*, 1999)
SE20	Perception of cattle farmers of the efficacy of East Coast fever immunization in Southern Zambia.	(Fandamu *et al.*, 2006)

Continued

Table 13.5. Continued

Report number	Report title	Reference
SE21	Financial analysis of East Coast fever control strategies in traditionally managed Sanga cattle in central province of Zambia.	(Minjauw *et al.*, 1999)
SE22	Epidemiological aspects and economic impact of bovine theileriosis (East Coast fever) and its control: A preliminary assessment with special reference to Kibaha district, Tanzania.	(Kivaria *et al.*, 2007)

[a]The individual reports/publications were allocated a number SE for easy reference.

Table 13.6. Details of ECF ITM MC dossier submission and review by national regulatory authorities.

Country	Dossier submitted by	National regulatory 'competent authority'	Registration granted
Kenya	Academic consultant	Pharmacy and Poisons Board (now Veterinary Medicines Directorate)	2009
Tanzania	In-country technical representative	Tanzania Food and Drugs Agency	2009
Malawi	CTTBD management	National Drug Authority	2008
Uganda	In-country technical representative	Ugandan National Drug Authority	Not registered but certificate of compliance with GMP issued to CTTBD 2024

also considered. No tangible agreement was made for the Kenyan market, although two companies were suggested, but two companies were selected for support in the Tanzanian market. One of these was the Arusha-based company VetAgro Ltd, a husband and wife partnership of the late Drs Lieve Lynen and Beppe di Giulio. These two veterinarians merit special mention here due to their pioneering efforts to promote and deploy the use of ITM in northern Tanzania, southern Kenya and elsewhere for over 20 years (Lynen *et al.*, 2012). In doing so, they had not only demonstrated the benefits of vaccination, mostly to Maasai cattle pastoralists, and that distribution of the vaccine was commercially viable, but they had also collected large quantities of clinical data which were subsequently published in either the grey or peer-reviewed literature (Table 13.5, SE 11, 12, 13; Di Giulio *et al.*, 2009) and used extensively in the dossier as evidence of safety and efficacy. The second company appointed in Tanzania was Ronheam Ltd, based in Dar-es-Salaam.

In May 2010, GALVmed organized an ambitious launch event for the product in Arusha, Tanzania, which was attended by senior politicians from Tanzania and Uganda and about 60 other delegates, including interested scientists, government officials and cattle farmer representatives. The main output was a series of resolutions and recommendations which set the strategic direction for the future sustainability and adoption of the vaccine (GALVmed, 2010).

13.6.2 Uptake of the Muguga cocktail vaccine

The exact figures for the number of animals that have been vaccinated using the commercial batches of the MC stabilate are not available. The best estimate of this relies on the numbers of doses of the vaccine sold by ILRI and CTTBD. The correspondence between the number of animals vaccinated and doses sold will be affected by several factors, including the vaccine straws purchased but not used and vaccine 'wastage' from the contents of a diluted straw not being fully used in the field. Although being without doubt an overestimate of the actual number of animals that were correctly vaccinated, the figures do provide an indication of vaccine uptake by year and country (Tables 13.7 and 13.8).

The early batches (i.e. FAO 1 and 2) were mostly deployed in Tanzania and Kenya, due largely to the efforts of Drs Lynen and di Giulio. They were distributed from CTTBD and ILRI, respectively. The ILRI 08 batch was available from ILRI after depletion of the FAO 2 batch in 2009 until stocks were exhausted in 2013. Table 13.7 shows the sales figures available for FAO 2, although they are incomplete, and for ILRI 08. It can be seen that about 84% of the 1.1 m doses were sold in Tanzania, mostly by VetAgro Ltd.

Distribution of MCL01 from CTTBD started in 2015 after depletion of ILRI 08, and to date about 1.1 million doses have been sold (G. Chaka, CTTBD, 2025, personal communication).

As shown in Table 13.8, most of the CTTBD-produced vaccine was used in Tanzania, with Kenya and Uganda also taking up substantial quantities. More recently, other countries, such as Rwanda, Burundi and South Sudan, have imported the vaccine.

It can be seen from Tables 13.7 and 13.8 that about 2.2 million doses have been sold over the 16 years from 2007 to 2022, which corresponds to an average of about 138,000 doses per year. Overall, a disproportionate number (about 1.53 million doses, or 70%) were supplied to Tanzania. It is apparent that the number of doses produced (about 3.8 million; Table 13.1) is markedly greater than the number sold. The reasons for this include lack of data for the FAO 1 and 2 doses sold prior to 2007 and straws which have been used or retained for research purposes. Nevertheless, the figures do indicate that there is an adequate supply of the vaccine available for commercial uptake.

Based on these figures, it is fair to say that uptake of the ITM approach has not met expectations, and adoption rates have been disappointing for those advocating its use. The reasons for this have not been clearly established, and the authors are unaware of any substantive effort to characterize the whole distribution chain and to identify and address the constraints therein. Of particular concern is the apparent lack of awareness of the very existence of the vaccine, let alone knowledge of its cost-saving benefits, among a large proportion of livestock owners in affected regions. This may reflect the lack of a strong link between the manufacturer and the distributors/livestock owners. A further contributing factor may be the relatively low financial incentive perceived by vaccinators.

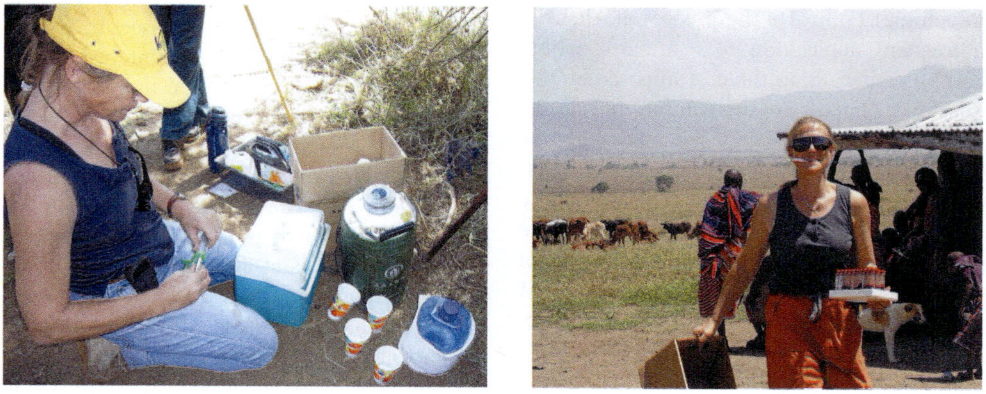

Fig. 13.2. Dr Lieve Lynen vaccinating Maasai cattle with the MC in northern Tanzania in 2008. (Photo credits: Andrew Peters (left) and Philip Toye (right).)

Table 13.7. Doses of the MC vaccine stabilate supplied by ILRI ([a]FAO 2 and [b]ILRI 08) between 2007 and 2013.

Country	2007[a]	2008[a]	2009[a&b]	2010[b]	2011[b]	2012[b]	2013[b]	Total
Kenya	990	1,500	1,200	16,000	15,000	31,000	5,600	71,290
Tanzania	63,000	75,000	47,800	100,000	140,000	125,000	378,000	928,800
Uganda	15,000	16,020				10,000	33,000	74,020
Malawi					16,000	12,000		28,000
Total	78,990	92,520	49,000	116,000	171,000	178,000	416,600	1,102,110

Table 13.8. Doses of the MC vaccine stabilate supplied by CTTBD.

Country	2016	2017	2018	2019	2020	2021	2022	Total
Kenya	210,000	3,200	10,000	10,000	5,000	22,000	15,000	275,200
Tanzania	186,360	34,222	100,000	46,080	66,000	129,120	38,000	599,782
Uganda	14,000		42,500		60,000	20,000		136,500
Malawi	6,960	3,880		2,040	520	520	200	14,120
Rwanda		6,000	15,920		5,880		34,299	62,099
Burundi					8,000			8,000
Sudan						2,080	7,160	9,240
Total	417,320	47,302	168,420	58,120	145,400	173,720	94,659	1,104,941

13.7 Where Are We? A Critical Appraisal of the Successes and Failures of the Commercialization of ITM to Date

There is no doubt that ECF is a very severe and economically important disease of cattle in eastern and southern Africa (see Chapter 2 of this volume). Control of the disease relies heavily on frequent application of acaricides, which contributes heavily to the cost imposed by this disease (see Chapter 2 of this volume) and carries a high risk of promoting the emergence of acaricide resistance among the tick population (see Chapter 15 of this volume). The availability of a safe, effective and readily available vaccine against ECF would greatly enhance control of the disease. As the MC delivered by the ITM fulfils these, the lack of its widespsread adoption has been both surprising and disappointing.

In analysing the reasons for this, it is useful to place the ITM in the context of the commercialization of veterinary vaccines in general. Some veterinary diseases and their medicines (pharmaceuticals and vaccines) are clearly private-sector issues, where an independent company can evaluate a market and can pursue a clear plan to produce and distribute to farmers at a profit, including a positive return on investment for the farmer. Examples here are pharmaceuticals for production diseases like nematode parasites or vaccines for bovine respiratory disease due to enzootic viruses. Others may be clearly public-sector issues, where there is a widely accepted interest for the greater good in controlling a specific disease and possibly where private industry will not invest due to perceived low market value. Diseases in this category would include rinderpest (now eradicated), peste des petits ruminants (currently the subject of publicly funded elimination campaigns), foot-and-mouth disease and other transboundary diseases where there is an advantage to the respective country's economy in controlling that disease. Another example is cysticercosis (*Taenia solium*) in the pig, where a very effective vaccine is available but which is not funded by the private sector because they do not see a viable market as there are few clinical signs in the pig. The vaccine is primarily intended to solve the human disease problem. Some diseases/products may fall between the two categories and so are amenable to a PPP approach. This is arguably how the ECF ITM project has been handled. In this case, the 'public' has been the production and registration of the vaccine (ILRI then CTTBD funded by donors) and market creation and awareness (initially and predominantly funded by donors), and the 'private' has predominantly been its distribution and delivery (distributors and vaccinators). What has been lost between the two is the promotion of awareness of the vaccine and its benefits by the private sector, the funding of studies to understand the economics of the distribution chain more fully and a strong, interdependent and mutually beneficial link between the 'public' and 'private' sectors. The underlying aim of the commercialization strategy, at least for the past 15 years, has been that the commercial enterprise involving ITM should be economically sustainable, that is, self-funding. The optimal way to do this is to establish a functional value chain where all participants in the chain benefit financially from it, and this is best achieved as a private-sector approach.

In the case of the MC, it is clear that the PPP has not worked very effectively in establishing a functional value chain. Several reasons can be put forward to explain this.

The first concerns the decision in 2009 to select CTTBD as the sole manufacturing site, a decision that divided opinion at the time for several reasons. It was felt that the manufacturing site should be more strategically located for the regions where there are greater numbers of exposed cattle and a higher demand for the product (e.g. Kenya or Tanzania), which would promote the development of a strong connection between the manufacturer and end-users. There were concerns that previous investments in CTTBD had not resulted in a long-term viable facility. This was compounded by the uncertainty around the ownership, and therefore management and financial accountability, of the centre (as outlined in Section 13.2.3). The facility also needed a substantial upgrade to meet the expected market demand, but there did not appear to be readily available resources to fund this. Thus, the final decision appears not to have been based solely on commercial or logistical grounds. It should also be noted that there was opinion that assistance should be given to a dedicated private enterprise start-up, with temporary technical and facility support from other institutions, such as ILRI, until it was self-sustaining. Thus, one of the main challenges that confronted GALVmed and partners in 2009 was to create and implement a sustainable business plan for the CTTBD facility. It was envisaged that the ultimate route to sustainability was to form a partnership with a commercial vaccine manufacturer who could invest in CTTBD to produce a portfolio of products at the site in addition to the MC. A number of companies have entered discussions, but to date none has taken the key step of active investment. The reasons for this are not clear, but it may be that the private sector needs to see broader evidence of a viable market for the unique product that is ITM, through actual sales beyond those achieved by VetAgro in northern Tanzania. The paradox is that a sufficient sales volume may only be reached with private-sector involvement to drive optimal uptake of the vaccine.

A second reason for the lack of widespread uptake of the vaccine is that there appears to be no meaningful connection between the production facility on the one hand and the livestock owners and end-suppliers of the vaccine on the other. The most severe outcome of this has been the considerable lack of awareness of the vaccine and of its financial benefits by the potential marketplace. In most commercial situations, the drive for creating awareness of a product and its benefits would be taken on by the manufacturer, although the business model most frequently found in Africa relies heavily on the distributor. For ITM, it appears that there was no specific entity responsible for coordinating and implementing a sustainable awareness campaign.

Thirdly, as mentioned above, there appears to have been a failure to understand fully the commercial landscape in which ITM is placed. With the benefit of retrospection, a glaringly obvious gap is the lack of real market research data for an ECF vaccine based on ITM and the clear identification of who in the PPP was best placed to generate these data. There have been efforts to seek the views of many stakeholders, including cattle farmers, notably by GALVmed, but to our knowledge there was no credible effort to understand the market in a rigorous and quantitative sense. Although several hundred farmers were consulted by GALVmed, it is not clear how representative the sample was for livestock owners in the *T. parva*-endemic region, nor how well informed they were of the financial benefits of ITM through reduced acaricide use. Most of the stakeholder opinion was really from officials in government, non-govenmental organizations (NGOs) and academics who argued that there was a big demand. However, they did not have any financial accountability for the success or otherwise of a commercial decision nor any real quantitative idea of the actual market size or demand. Importantly, there was never a clear quantitative understanding of the competition with the acaricide industry or indeed the use of therapeutics like parvaquone and buparvaquone. Again in retrospect, it became apparent that elements in the regional animal health industry have not been entirely supportive of ITM due to the perceived competition with and cannibalization of the existing acaricide and therapeutic markets.

In marketing the vaccine, it would appear to be essential to highlight the advantages of vaccination. These include especially the ability of only one inoculation to provide essentially lifelong immunity (see Chaper 12 of this volume) and less frequent application of expensive acaricides. With regard to the latter, Melewas *et al.* (1999) and Nsubuga-Mutaka (1999) recommended a 25–50% and a 50–60% reduction in dipping frequency in Tanzania and Uganda, respectively, based on experiences reported by livestock owners. Melewas *et al.* (1999, p. 21) further reported that the 'high cost of acaricides has been the most important reason for commercial farmers to take on ECF immunisation'. It is clear that a more comprehensive study is needed to provide strong evidence to support vaccine awareness efforts, although this does come with caveats (see item 5 in Section 13.9).

At the time of writing, GALVmed have ceased to invest in CTTBD, and its sustainable future is still uncertain. It is unclear why national governments or regional organizations have not supported the production of the vaccine, especially given the long history of public ownership of vaccine production facilities in Africa.

Despite the uptake of ITM to date being less than what was envisaged, it must be emphasized that the efforts of organizations like VetAgro in northern Tanzania have demonstrated that, with a sustained commitment to marketing and delivery, there is a strong and clear demand for the vaccine and that the distribution of the ITM vaccine is commercially viable. There is no obvious reason why this should not be replicated elswhere if linked to a dependable supply of the vaccine. What should not be lost in any analysis of the 'partial' success of the commercialization of the technology is that it is a very effective tool – a single inoculation provides effectively lifelong immunity with no substantiated reports of breakthrough in over 20 years of commercial deployment (Di Giulio *et al.*, 2009), apart from challenge from buffalo-derived parasites.

It must also be recognized that, unfortunately, there is as yet no alternative vaccine for ECF and no real prospects for one for at least a decade. Following the development of the ITM vaccine in the mid-1970s, doubts were expressed about the feasibility of its field application and, with rapid advances in immunology, the development of an alternative method of vaccination based on understanding the mechanisms of immunity to the parasite was set as a key deliverable for ILRAD. The development of such a vaccine for ECF was a priority for ILRAD and remains so for its successor, ILRI. However, it has proved to be a frustratingly elusive goal, despite some promising findings with subunit antigen preparations (see Chapter 11 of this volume). In addition, the conventional technical approaches of vaccines based on attenuated or inactivated parasites have been equally unproductive.

13.8 Improvements to the ITM Vaccination Technology to Enhance Commercial Uptake

In any effort directed at achieving sustained use of the vaccine, attention must be given to addressing the challenges associated with its production and distribution, which are outlined in Section 13.1. In an attempt to confirm and prioritize the importance of these challenges, a stakeholder workshop was organized by ILRI and GALVmed in 2014 (ILRI/ILRI/GALVmed, 2015). Participants represented a wide range of entities interested in the ITM vaccine and included distributors and vaccinators, government ministries responsible for animal health services in relevant countries, researchers, regulatory authorities and vaccine producers. The issues were discussed in detail and the list of desired improvements suggested at the meeting is reproduced in Fig. 13.3. This list was recorded without any filter for feasibility or expected impact, and it is recognized that some of these could be viewed as a wish list weakly tethered to a realistic outcome.

As discussed below, some of these points have since been addressed, to some extent at least.

13.8.1 Package size

As stated in the SPC (Fig. 13.1), the vaccine stabilate should be used within 4 h of thawing and diluting. The packaging of MC in quantities of 30–40 doses per straw is inconvenient where only a few animals are to be vaccinated and leads to vaccine wastage. An immediately apparent solution to this is to reduce the number of doses per straw by packaging a more dilute stabilate during production, and some of batch MCL03 and batch MCL04 at CTTBD were prepared as 10-dose straws. However, this approach relies on a reasonably accurate estimate of the stabilate potency prior to *in vivo* dose determination of the final product. It also requires an estimate of how much of the final stabilate should be diluted, and there are increased costs due to the greater number of straws and liquid nitrogen space required for storage.

An alternative approach is to thaw, dilute and refreeze already packaged vaccine of known potency, an approach which relies on minimal loss of sporozoite viability during the thaw–refreeze cycle. In addition to the advantages mentioned above, this method allows for the fewer-dose straws to be made according to demand. Mbao *et al.* (2006) recorded an average viability loss of 35% in sporozoite suspensions following thawing and refreezing. Guided by this, Patel *et al.* (2019) prepared 1:5 dilutions of the previously packaged ILRI 08 vaccine. The repackaged stabilate was tested at dilutions of 1:20 and 1:14 to provide a dosage equivalent to that recommended for the undiluted vaccine assuming no loss of sporozoite viability (1:20) or about a 35% loss of viability during repackaging (1:14). Both formulations were found to protect animals against an otherwise lethal challenge with the parental stabilate, which validated this approach for producing straws containing fewer doses from already packaged stabilate. Recently, CTTBD has thawed stabilates stored in packaged straws and in bulk in transfusion bags. The stabilates were thawed in iced water. When the potency of the repackaged stabilates was tested *in vivo* without dilution, they produced severe reactions similar to those observed in stabilate batches that did not undergo a thaw–freeze step (M. Chaka, CTTBD, 2025, personal communication).

13.8.2 Diluent modification

The vaccine diluent is a traditional cell culture medium, comprising Eagle's minimal essential medium, bovine serum albumin, glycerol as a cryoprotectant and antibiotics. A major drawback of this medium is that it must be kept at −20°C, which requires large freezer capacity. Given the short time between thawing and inoculation in which the sporozoites are suspended in the diluent, a simpler and more stable salt solution should be adequate. CTTBD has undertaken various in-house trials with PBS as diluent and sucrose as cryoprotectant with promising outcomes, but the results have not been published (M. Chaka, CTTBD, 2025, personal communication).

13.8.3 Liquid nitrogen storage

Traditionally, the vaccine stabilate has been stored in liquid nitrogen up until the point of dilution in the field. Liquid nitrogen cold chain facilities are not uncommon in Africa due to the use of artificial insemination, especially in dairy herds. Liquid nitrogen storage has the advantage of being more reliable than freezer storage in areas where electricity supply is frequently interrupted, if the supply of liquid nitrogen is not affected. Transport of vaccine stabilate from central depots to the field is also relatively straightforward with insulated flasks.

1. Improving the cold chain. There were several aspects to this:
    - Removing the need for liquid nitrogen to store the vaccine
    - Developing a simpler diluent which can be kept at room temperature
    - Improving the post-reconstitution viability to allow for a longer duration between administration and delivery – especially important in smallholder areas with straws of 40 doses or more.
    - Providing better storage equipment for transport of the vaccine
2. Removing the need for oxytetracycline
3. Removing the need for live animals during the production process
4. Developing ticks which can yield greater number of sporozoites
5. Eradicate the vector
6. Produce one vaccine which can be used in all countries
7. Provide the vaccine in a smaller dose packaging
8. Decrease the cost of the vaccine
9. Develop a sub unit vaccine
10. Develop an ECF vaccine which can be administered as an aerosol
11. Validate the use of other antibiotic formulations

Fig. 13.3. List of proposed improvements suggested by the ITM stakeholder workshop held at ILRI August 2014. (ILRI/GALVmed, 2015.)

Nevertheless, the requirement for liquid nitrogen storage and distribution is recognized as a severe limitation to the general availability of the vaccine, particularly in remote areas, and adds to the cost of vaccine distribution. To address this, there have been experiments to explore alternatives. Lyophilization of the vaccine stabilate was examined by Marcotty *et al.* (2003) using trehalose and sucrose as cryoprotectants. Although the authors estimated that less than 1% of the sporozoites survived lyophilization, the preparations kept at −5°C for 2 weeks and −20°C for up to 80 days were reported as being immunogenic and capable of inducing parasitosis and clinical signs, whereas no clinical reaction or parasitosis was observed in cattle inoculated with lyophilized parasites kept at room temperature for 7 days. Clearly, much longer storage times must be tested if this method is to be considered as an alternative to liquid nitrogen. There have also been reported studies showing minimal loss of infectivity if stabilates are kept for up to 6 weeks at −70°C (Mbassa *et al.*, 1998) or at −80°C for 30 days (Atuhaire *et al.*, 2020). The results suggest the possibility of temporary storage using dry ice (CO_2) for the 'last mile' of the distribution chain.

13.8.4 *In vitro* dose determination

The current method of determining a suitable dilution of any vaccine stabilate for field inoculation involves two to three rounds of immunization of cattle with titrated doses of the vaccine stabilate and observing the clinical outcome following a lethal challenge. This method is expensive, time-consuming and less than ideal from an animal welfare perspective.

There is currently no reliable *in vitro* method to estimate the potency of a sporozoite stabilate. Marcotty *et al.* (2004) attempted to use quantitative infection of bovine lymphocytes *in vitro* as an estimate of vaccine potency. They were able to discern a tenfold difference in the number of viable sporozoites between two vaccine stabilates. Corresponding differences were observed *in vivo* between the stabilates in the onset of fever and parasitosis, but not in the level of parasitosis or time to death. It must be noted that the numbers of animals used in these *in vivo* experiments were very small, and further work is required to incorporate this method in routine production of the vaccine stabilate.

Although less cumbersome than *in vivo* challenge experiments, cell culture methods are time-consuming and require well-trained operators. Alternative approaches have been considered. Estimates based on the number of infected acini in the ticks used for preparation of the stabilates do not take account of variation in the number or state of maturation of sporozoites in the acini, or loss of viability during the preparation and freezing of the stabilate. Direct counting of sporozites in the stabilate is thwarted by the tendency of the sporozoites to form clumps and does not take into account the viability of individual parasites. Methods based on DNA content alone will not distinguish between live and dead sporozoites, whereas estimates based on RNA content may circumvent this problem but have not yet been developed and validated.

13.9 Conclusions

The MC as an ITM vaccine has been shown to be a remarkably effective product in the field and amenable to commercially viable deployment, as evidenced by the efforts of pioneering distributors such as VetAgro in northern Tanzania. Several commercial-scale batches totalling over 2 million doses have been made and distributed from two different sites. The product has been successfully registered in three key countries and has been used by special consent of the respective animal health authority in a fourth. Although use of the vaccine has thus far been below expectations, it is imperative that efforts continue to build on this experience and base to achieve more widespread deployment. This is especially so given the low likelihood that a more attractive immunization alternative, such as a subunit vaccine, will appear in the next decade (see Chapter 10 of this volume). There is the alternative view that control should rely predominantly on tick control and treatment of clinical cases. Given the issues with increased use of acaricides (discussed in Chapter 15 of this volume), the cumulative cost of treating animals and need for close monitoring, and the possibility of widespread resistance to both acaricides and therapeutics, the authors believe this may be a dangerous approach. An additional approach, relying on the inherited resistance found in indicine cattle, is discussed in Chapter 7 of this volume.

The authors believe that, in order to achieve more effective deployment of ITM, several factors need to be addressed.

1. There must be a renewed effort to increase awareness of the benefits of the vaccine to livestock owners and their advisors. Central to this is to remedy the perceived disconnect between the production facility and the end-user, and to establish a clear, mutually beneficial and interdependent relationship between them.
2. Despite its pitfalls, a PPP is initially necessary in order to provide the resources to reinvigorate the project, but with the aim of its being a purely private enterprise once a sustainable market is achieved. This would involve renewed discussions with private-sector entities focused on identifying and removing the perceived barriers to their engagement in distributing and ultimately manufacturing the vaccine.
3. Further donor and public fund investment should be used initially to re-evaluate the size of the market for the vaccine, based on the experiences since 2009. This should incorporate an analysis of the optimal cost of vaccination and ensure that livestock owners whose opinions are sought are fully aware of the financial advantages that come with vaccination. Any assessment of the importance of the disease as perceived by livestock owners must acknowledge the

suppression of the disease due to current control methods using acaricides or therapeutics, and the use of resistant but less productive animals.

4. An assessment of the situation with respect to CTTBD, including ownership and suitability of location, must be undertaken, and an alternative site should be established if there is any doubt as to the future of CTTBD. If the reachable market is deemed large and potentially profitable enough, then a new commercial entity should be set up to produce and distribute the ITM product, in a location sufficiently close to existing scientific and production expertise and target markets (e.g. ILRI), which could be drawn down on an as-needed basis to keep down overhead costs. Such a facility would need to be built and operated to a GMP standard to allow full registration by key target countries that have now developed high-level regulatory standards (e.g. Uganda).
5. Despite the temptation to improve the product or the process, initial efforts must be focused on establishing a sustainable market. Although it seems obvious that an essential factor in this is a strong awareness campaign, what is not as clear is who is in the best position to undertake this. As mentioned above, most African business models rely on the distributors to promote the product. For ITM, where the distributorship is probably not as well developed, this role may have to fall to the manufacturer. If the sole manufacturer remains CTTBD, this underscores the importance of either resolving the issues around its ownership or partnering with a private-sector manufacturer.

   Any awareness campaign would benefit greatly from a rigorous study to determine the degree to which acaricide application can be reduced following vaccination and the consequent cost savings associated with this, and extensive publication of such data. The predominant reason to maintain acaricide application after vaccination is to reduce exposure to other tick-borne pathogens and to reduce direct damage caused by ticks *per se*. Any recommendation on the extent to which acaricide use may be safely reduced must allow for this and may be difficult due to variation in local factors such as the size of infected tick populations, cattle types, farming system and presence of wildlife.
6. Ultimately, profit should be large enough to include funding for an ongoing product improvement plan to address issues such as those outlined above.
7. It must be acknowledged that production of the ITM vaccine is a substantially more complicated production process than is needed for other vaccines. It requires people with a range of skills, knowledge and experience, which relatively few people possess. Similarly, the biological and infrastructural resources that are needed are not at all commonplace. A high priority must be placed on retaining these skills and resources.

Above all, a successful future for ITM will rely heavily on the full commitment of all parties, public and private, to ensure success.

Acknowledgements

Unlike other chapters in this volume, this chapter relies substantially on information not available in peer-reviewed literature. The authors are extremely grateful to Mihji Chaka and Nick Juleff for providing much valuable information and insight, and to Carolin Schumacher, Fiona Allan and Lois Muraguri for their comments on earlier versions of the chapter. Parts of this chapter first appeared in Peters *et al.* (2020) and are reproduced here with permission.

References

Allan, F.K. and Peters, A.R. (2021) Safety and efficacy of the East Coast fever Muguga cocktail vaccine: A systematic review. *Vaccines* 9(11), 1318. DOI: 10.3390/vaccines9111318.

Anon (1998) FAO-1 composite stabilate. Evaluation of efficacy at 1:80 and 1:100 dilutions and treatment with 30% oxytetracycline.

Anon (1999a) FAO-1-2 composite stabilate. Evaluation of efficacy at 1:80 direct dilution and treatment with 30% oxytetracycline.

Anon (1999b) *Infectivity/viability test of FAO-1 stabilate after 2.5 years storage*. CTTBD, Lilongwe.

Anon (2007) Applying ITM immunisation in Tanzania using the FAO-1 vaccine batch (1998-2007).

Atuhaire, D.K., Lieberman, D., Marcotty, T., Musoke, A.J. and Madan, D. (2020) An alternative cold chain for storing and transporting East Coast fever vaccine. *Veterinary Parasitology* 288, 109304. DOI: 10.1016/j.vetpar.2020.109304.

Berkvens, D.L., Geysen, D.M. and Brandt, J.R.A. (1998) Comments on the paper 'Sustainable tick and tickborne disease control in livestock improvement in developing countries'. *Veterinary Parasitology* 77(2–3), 211–215. DOI: 10.1016/s0304-4017(98)00096-x.

Bishop, R., Geysen, D., Spooner, P., Skilton, R., Nene, V. *et al.* (2001) Molecular and immunological characterisation of *Theileria parva* stocks which are components of the 'Muguga cocktail' used for vaccination against East Coast fever in cattle. *Veterinary Parasitology* 94(4), 227–237. DOI: 10.1016/s0304-4017(00)00404-0.

Clarke, C.R., Wang, Z., Cudd, L., Burrows, G.E., Kirkpatrick, J.G. *et al.* (1999) Pharmacokinetics of two long-acting oxytetracycline products administered subcutaneously and intramuscularly. *Journal of Veterinary Pharmacology and Therapeutics* 22(1), 65–67. DOI: 10.1046/j.1365-2885.1999.00181.x.

Cunningham, M.P., Brown, C.G.D., Burridge, M.J. and Purnell, R.E. (1973) Cryopreservation of infective particles of *Theileria parva*. *International Journal for Parasitology* 3(5), 583–587. DOI: 10.1016/0020-7519(73)90082-9.

De Castro, J.J. (1997) Sustainable tick and tickborne disease control in livestock improvement in developing countries. *Veterinary Parasitology* 71(2–3), 77–97. DOI: 10.1016/s0304-4017(97)00033-2.

De Castro, J.J. (1998) Reply to comments on the paper 'Sustainable tick and tickborne disease control in livestock in developing countries'. *Veterinary Parasitology* 71, 213–215.

De Deken, R., Martin, V., Saido, A., Madder, M., Brandt, J. *et al.* (2007) An outbreak of East Coast fever on the Comoros: A consequence of the import of immunised cattle from Tanzania? *Veterinary Parasitology* 143(3–4), 245–253. DOI: 10.1016/j.vetpar.2006.08.018.

Di Giulio, G., Lynen, G., Ulicky, E., Katende, J. and Morzaria, S. (2000) Use of two different dose rates of oxytetracycline in East Coast fever immunisation in Tanzania. In: *Tick and Tick-Borne Pathogens: Into the 21st Century. Proceedings of the 3rd International Conference, High Tatra Mountains, Slovakia*, pp. 121–123.

Di Giulio, G., Lynen, G., Morzaria, S., Oura, C. and Bishop, R. (2009) Live immunization against East Coast fever – current status. *Trends in Parasitology* 25(2), 85–92. DOI: 10.1016/j.pt.2008.11.007.

European Commission (2007) EudraLex - Volume 6 - Notice to Applicants and Regulatory Guidelines for Medicinal Products for Veterinary Use. Available at: https://ec.europa.eu/health/documents/eudralex/vol-6_en (accessed 3 April 2023).

Fandamu, P., Thys, E., Duchateau, L. and Berkvens, D. (2006) Perception of cattle farmers of the efficacy of East Coast fever immunization in Southern Zambia. *Tropical Animal Health and Production* 38(1), 9–16. DOI: 10.1007/s11250-006-4341-4.

GALVmed (2010) East Coast fever (ECF) Vaccine Launch. Available at: https://galvdox.galvmed.org/application/files/1216/6627/9208/8_ECF_Launch_0.pdf (accessed 3 April 2023).

ILRI (1996) *Titration of the FAO-1 stabilate*. Experiment K83K(4/2). Production Record for FAO Muguga Cocktail Vaccine Stabilate. ILRI internal document.

ILRI/GALVmed (2015) *Distribution, delivery and improvement of the Infection and treatment method vaccine for East Coast fever*. Report of a Workshop, Nairobi, Kenya, 19–20 August 2014. ILRI, Nairobi.

Kivaria, F.M., Ruheta, M.R., Mkonyi, P.A. and Malamsha, P.C. (2007) Epidemiological aspects and economic impact of bovine theileriosis (East Coast fever) and its control: A preliminary assessment with special reference to Kibaha district, Tanzania. *Veterinary Journal* 173(2), 384–390. DOI: 10.1016/j.tvjl.2005.08.013.

Latif, A.A. and Hove, T. (2011) History and critical review of *Theileria parva* (Boleni), the vaccine stock against Zimbabwean cattle theileriosis. *Ticks and Tick-Borne Diseases* 2(3), 163–167. DOI: 10.1016/j.ttbdis.2011.06.002.

Lynen, G., Melewas, J., Majaliwa, K., Bakuname, C. and Di Giulio, G. (1999) The use of a 30% formulation of oxytetracycline long-acting in East Coast fever immunizations in Tanzania. In: Mukaratirwa, S. and Obwolo, M.J. (eds) *Animal Health and Production for Development. Proceedings of IX International Conference of Associations of Institutions of Tropical Veterinary Medicine*, University of Utrecht Press, pp. 367–375 (Vol. 1).

Lynen, G., Di Giulio, G., Homewood, K., Reid, R. and Mwilawa, A. (2005) Deployment of a live ECF vaccine in pastoral areas: Lessons learned from Tanzania. In: *The Role of Biotechnology in Animal Agriculture to Address Poverty in Africa: Opportunities and Challenges. Proceedings of the 4th All African Conference on Animal Agriculture and the 31st Annual Meeting of the Tanzania Society for Animal Production*, pp. 193–201. Available at: https://www.cabidigitallibrary.org/doi/pdf/10.5555/20123160992

Lynen, G., Yrjö-Koskinen, A.E., Bakuname, C., Di Giulio, G., Mlinga, N. *et al.* (2012) East Coast fever immunisation field trial in crossbred dairy cattle in Hanang and Handeni districts in northern Tanzania. *Tropical Animal Health and Production* 44(3), 567–572. DOI: 10.1007/s11250-011-9936-8.

Magwisha, H.B., Ruheta, M.R., Mbwambo, H.A., Ranga, E.E. and Makungu, L.S. (2011) The potential of East Coast fever (ECF) vaccine on improved and indigenous cattle in Tanzania. *Journal of the Commonwealth Veterinary Association* 27, 87–92.

Mangani, M. (1999) ECF immunisation in Zambia. In: Morzaria, S. and Williamson, S. (eds) *Live Vaccines for Theileria parva: Deployment in Eastern, Central and Southern Africa. Proceedings of an FAO/ILRI/OAU-IBAR Workshop Held at ILRI (International Livestock Research Institute),* Nairobi, Kenya, March 10–12, 1997, pp. 30–33.

Marcotty, T., Berkvens, D., Besa, R.K., Losson, B., Dolan, T.T. *et al.* (2003) Lyophilisation and resuscitation of sporozoites of *Theileria parva*: Preliminary experiments. *Vaccine* 22(2), 213–216. DOI: 10.1016/s0264-410x(03)00564-4.

Marcotty, T., Speybroek, N., Berkvens, D., Chaka, G., Besa, R. *et al.* (2004) *In vitro* titration of *Theileria parva* tick derived stabilates. *Parasitology* 128, 131–137. DOI: 10.1017/S0031182003004323.

Mbao, V., Berkvens, D., Dolan, T., Speybroeck, N., Brandt, J. *et al.* (2006) Infectivity of *Theileria parva* sporozoites following cryopreservation in four suspension media and multiple refreezing: Evaluation by *in vitro* titration. *The Onderstepoort Journal of Veterinary Research* 73(3), 207–213. DOI: 10.4102/ojvr.v73i3.147.

Mbassa, G.K., Kweka, L.E. and Dulla, P.N. (1998) Immunization against East Coast fever in field cattle with low infectivity *Theileria parva* stabilate – preliminary assessment. *Veterinary Parasitology* 77(1), 41–48. DOI: 10.1016/s0304-4017(97)00138-6.

McKeever, D.J. (2007) Live immunisation against *Theileria parva*: Containing or spreading the disease? *Trends in Parasitology* 23, 565–568. DOI: 10.1016/j.pt.2007.09.002.

Melewas, J., Majaliwa, M. and Lynen, L. (1999) ECF immunisation in Tanzania. In: Morzaria, S. and Williamson, S. (eds) *Live Vaccines for Theileria parva: Deployment in Eastern, Central and Southern Africa. Proceedings of an FAO/ILRI/OAU-IBAR Workshop Held at ILRI (International Livestock Research Institute*), Nairobi, Kenya, March 10–12, 1997, p. 21.

Minjauw, B., Rushton, J., James, A.D. and Upton, M. (1999) Financial analysis of East Coast fever control strategies in traditionally managed Sanga cattle in Central Province of Zambia. *Preventive Veterinary Medicine* 38(1), 35–45. DOI: 10.1016/s0167-5877(98)00128-7.

Morrison, W.I. (2007) The biological and practical significance of antigenic variability in protective T cell responses against *Theileria parva*. *Veterinary Parasitology* 148(1), 21–30. DOI: 10.1016/j.vetpar.2007.05.007.

Morrison, W.I. and McKeever, D.J. (2006) Current status of vaccine development against Theileria parasites. *Parasitology* 133, S169–S187. DOI: 10.1017/S0031182006001867.

Morzaria, S., Spooner, P., Bishop, R. and Mwaura, S. (1999) The preparation of a composite stabilate for the immunization against East Coast fever. In: Morzaria, S. and Williamson, S. (eds) *Live Vaccines for Theileria parva: Deployment in Eastern, Central and Southern Africa. Proceedings of an FAO, OAU–IBAR and ILRI Workshop Held at ILRI (International Livestock Research Institute*), Nairobi, Kenya, March 10–12, 1997, pp. 56–61.

Mutugi, J., Njuguna, L., Musisi, F., Morzaria, S.P., Spooner, P.R. *et al.* (1997) Determining a Safe and Protective Immunizing Dose for the FAO-1 *Theileria parva* Composite Stabilate for Use in Field

Vaccinations against East Coast Fever. In: *FAO Technical Report AG:GCP/RAF/291/DEN & GCP/RAF/293/BEL, Report for Eastern, Central and Southern African Countries through the Organization of African Unity Inter-African Bureau for Animal Resources by Food and Agriculture Organization of the United Nations,* 1997, Rome.

Nsubuga-Mutaka, R. (1999) ECF immunisation in Uganda. In: Morzaria, S. and Williamson, S. (eds) *Live Vaccines for Theileria parva: Deployment in Eastern, Central and Southern Africa. Proceedings of an FAO/ILRI/OAU-IBAR Workshop Held at ILRI (International Livestock Research Institute*), Nairobi, Kenya, March 10–12, 1997, p. 28.

Nsubuga-Mutaka, R.C., Otim, C.P., Kakaire-Nyende, M., Erima, S. and Ongyera, S. (2000) Immunization against East Coast fever by Infection and Treatment Method in Uganda. *Uganda Journal of Agricultural Sciences* 5, 1–2.

Oura, C.A.L., Bishop, R., Wampande, E.M., Lubega, G.W. and Tait, A. (2004) The persistence of component *Theileria parva* stocks in cattle immunized with the 'Muguga cocktail' live vaccine against East Coast fever in Uganda. *Parasitology* 129(Pt 1), 27–42. DOI: 10.1017/s003118200400513x.

Oura, C.A.L., Bishop, R., Asiimwe, B.B., Spooner, P., Lubega, G.W. *et al.* (2007) *Theileria parva* live vaccination: Parasite transmission, persistence and heterologous challenge in the field. *Parasitology* 134(Pt 9), 1205–1213. DOI: 10.1017/S0031182007002557.

Patel, E., Mwaura, S., Kiara, H., Morzaria, S., Peters, A. *et al.* (2016) Production and dose determination of the Infection and Treatment Method (ITM) Muguga cocktail vaccine used to control East Coast fever in cattle. *Ticks and Tick-Borne Diseases* 7(2), 306–314. DOI: 10.1016/j.ttbdis.2015.11.006.

Patel, E., Mwaura, S., Giulio, G., Cook, E.A.J., Lynen, G. *et al.* (2019) Infection and Treatment Method (ITM) vaccine against East Coast fever: Reducing the number of doses per straw for use in smallholder dairy herds by thawing, diluting and refreezing already packaged vaccine. *BMC Veterinary Research* 15(1), 46. DOI: 10.1186/s12917-019-1787-y.

Payne, R. (1999) Preparation of stabilates for immunisation against East Coast fever at NVRC, Muguga, Kenya. In: Morzaria, S. and Williamson, S. (eds) *Live Vaccines for Theileria parva: Deployment in Eastern, Central and Southern Africa. Proceedings of an FAO/ILRI/OAU-IBAR, Workshop Held at ILRI (International Livestock Research Institute*), Nairobi, Kenya, March 10–12, 1997, pp. 62–65.

Perry, B.D. (2016) The control of East Coast fever of cattle by live parasite vaccination: A science-to-impact narrative. *One Health* 2, 103–114. DOI: 10.1016/j.onehlt.2016.07.002.

Peters, A.R., Toye, P., Spooner, P., Giulio, G. and Lynen, G. (2020) Registration of the East Coast fever Infection and Treatment Method vaccine (Muguga cocktail) in East Africa. *Gates Open Research* 4, 100. DOI: 10.21955/gatesopenres.1116653.1.

Radley, D.E., Brown, C.G.D., Burridge, M.J., Cunningham, M.P., Kirimi, I.M. *et al.* (1975a) East Coast fever: 1. Chemoprophylactic immunization of cattle against *Theileria parva* (Muguga) and five theilerial strains. *Veterinary Parasitology* 1(1), 35–41. DOI: 10.1016/0304-4017(75)90005-9.

Radley, D.E., Young, A.S., Brown, C.G.D., Burridge, M.J., Cunningham, M.P. *et al.* (1975b) East Coast fever: 2. Cross-immunity trials with a Kenya strain of *Theileria lawrencei*. *Veterinary Parasitology* 1(1), 43–50. DOI: 10.1016/0304-4017(75)90006-0.

Radley, D.E., Brown, C.G.D., Cunningham, M.P., Kimber, C.D., Musisi, F.L. *et al.* (1975c) East Coast fever: 3. Chemoprophylactic immunization of cattle using oxytetracycline and a combination of theilerial strains. *Veterinary Parasitology* 1(1), 51–60. DOI: 10.1016/0304-4017(75)90007-2.

Turasha, G. (2005) Technical meeting on the infection and treatment method of East Coast fever immunization and the way forward in Kenya. In: *A Meeting at Naivasha Country Club*, pp. 1–2. Available at: https://hdl.handle.net/10568/178611 (accessed 10 December 2025).

Ushewokunze-Obatolu, U. (1999) Immunisation against theileriosis in Zimbabwe. In: Morzaria, S. and Williamson, S. (eds) *Live Vaccines for Theileria parva: Deployment in Eastern, Central and Southern Africa. Proceedings of an FAO/ILRI/OAU-IBAR Workshop Held at ILRI (International Livestock Research Institute*), Nairobi, Kenya, pp. 34–36.

14 Treatment of Disease Caused by *Theileria parva*

Nick McHardy[†*]

14.1 Introduction

Until the introduction of Clexon™ in 1983, with the hydroxy-naphthoquinone compound parvaquone as its active ingredient, there was no effective treatment for East Coast fever (ECF) or any other theilerial disease of cattle. The search for a cure for ECF had begun soon after the massive outbreak of ECF in southern Africa, which began in 1901 and led to the identification of *Theileria parva* as the causal agent in 1904. The nascent pharmaceutical industry had little to offer, and none of the modest range of therapies available at the time to treat other diseases had any effect on ECF. Veterinarians relied on various dyes, such as acridine orange and methylene blue; these had some effect on the related tick-transmitted disease babesiosis, but their effect on ECF was at best 'modest'. Various other treatments were recommended, including fearsomely high doses of liquid paraffin given by mouth, but it is unlikely that these had any beneficial effect.

This chapter describes the search for a curative drug for ECF from the early work in the 1950s and the subsequent discovery of the anti-theilerial effects of the hydroxy-naphthoquinones and a few other compounds in the 1970s. Their development into effective anti-theilerial products and the most effective ways to use them are described here. The naphthoquinones were also shown to be effective in the treatment of the closely related disease caused by *Theileria annulata*. Unfortunately, resistance to the naphthoquinones has already been found in this parasite in several countries but, as yet, not in *T. parva*. The urgency of finding new treatments for all forms of theileriosis is recognized, and the early steps that have been taken in the search are also described.

14.2 Historical Perspective

Neitz (1957) reported that various 4- and 8-aminoquinolines affected the piroplasm stage of *T. parva* and that the 4-aminoquinoline chloroquine inhibited the schizont stage, but Barnett and Bailey (1957) and several others since were unable to confirm this. Oleandomycin and diethylcarbamazine were briefly touted as candidate anti-theilerials but their development was not pursued.

Neitz (1953, 1957) found that tetracycline compounds had a prophylactic action if administered orally or by injection daily during the incubation period of ECF, but only a minor and transitory beneficial action if they were given in the early clinical stages of the disease. This was confirmed by Brocklesby and Bailey (1962). Mugera *et al.* (1973) and Brown *et al.* (1977) also reported a modest therapeutic effect of tetracyclines, but only in the early stages of

*The editors were saddened by the sudden death of Dr Nick McHardy during the final stages of the preparation of this book.

 East Coast Fever: The Disease, its Impact and Control (eds W.I. Morrison and P. Toye)
DOI: 10.1079/9781800626324.0014

the disease. This essentially prophylactic method of control was used on some farms, particularly for valuable cattle at high risk of infection, but it was cumbersome and expensive and has been little used since the 1960s. Now, except in very specific risk situations, the use of tetracyclines in this way would be unacceptable for many reasons, among them environmental risk, cost and particularly in lactating cattle because of human safety concerns over drug residues in milk. Such 'blanket' use of tetracycline might also be expected to accelerate the development of resistance in bacteria, so it would be unattractive for this reason too. However, oxytetracycline is used very effectively as the 'blocking' drug in the Infection and Treatment Method (ITM) of immunization against ECF (see Chapters 12 and 13 of this volume).

A more focused approach to the search for an effective treatment for ECF began in the 1950s. The most extensive programme was that of Wilde and his team at the Wellcome Research Laboratory near Nairobi, established specifically for this purpose. There being no laboratory animal model of ECF, the programme used small groups of cattle infected by the attachment of ticks harvested from cattle suffering from clinical ECF. Over the subsequent 15 years, more than 100 compounds were tested, many of them novel, alone and in various combinations, as well as those compounds mentioned above which had been reported to have some anti-theilerial effect. Most of the novel compounds were made in Wellcome's own Synthetic Chemistry Laboratories as candidate treatments for a wide range of other purposes, including bacterial, viral, protozoal and helminth diseases. None of them were synthesized specifically for the treatment of ECF, because there was no 'active lead' chemical structure on which to base the search.

None of the compounds that Wilde tested had more than very minor effects on the course of ECF (Wilde, 1977). Pyrimethamine most consistently showed any evidence of activity, manifested by transient effects on macroschizonts and a modest extension of survival times, but out of 103 cattle treated with pyrimethamine, alone or in combination with various other compounds, only five recovered, which was similar to the survival rate in untreated cases.

14.3 Discovery and Development of Curative Drugs for ECF

The pharmaceutical industry in the 1970s apparently believed that the market for an ECF drug would be too small to justify the cost of the necessary research and development (R&D) programme. The failure rate of 'active leads' to become saleable products in the industry at the time was said to be around 99%, and there was not even an active lead for ECF. However, the Burroughs Wellcome company had the enlightened policy of allowing research scientists to spend 10% of their time on subjects of their own choosing, in the hope that this might lead to something 'useful' to Wellcome. The current author chose to investigate a potential cure for ECF, but using cultures of *T. parva* macroschizonts in bovine lymphoblasts, recently developed by Malmquist *et al.* (1970), rather than infected cattle, as the basis of the compound-screening system. The seed culture was kindly provided by the UNDP/ODA Project at the East African Veterinary Research Organization (EAVRO) near Nairobi. Almost 100% of the lymphoblasts in these cultures contained a theilerial macroschizont, and they could be maintained relatively easily as continuously growing cell lines.

The *in vitro* screening system, in microculture plates, had a capacity of 100 compounds per week. It was, therefore, possible to test most of the compounds that Wilde had tested very quickly. None of them, including pyrimethamine, had more than a minimal effect on the *T. parva* schizonts in the cultures. Importantly, this suggested that the *in vitro* screen was unlikely to show 'false positive' results, so it appeared to be an inexpensive and reliable tool for the search. However, with no active lead compound, the approach was to test a broad range of compounds with known activity against a selection of pathogens, including oxytetracycline and several other antibacterials (McColm and McHardy, 1984). None of them showed significant anti-theilerial activity. Oxytetracycline had no apparent effect on the macroschizonts or on their host lymphoblasts, even at 100 μg/ml (McHardy *et al.*, 1976; McHardy, 1978). It was concluded that the prophylactic effect of

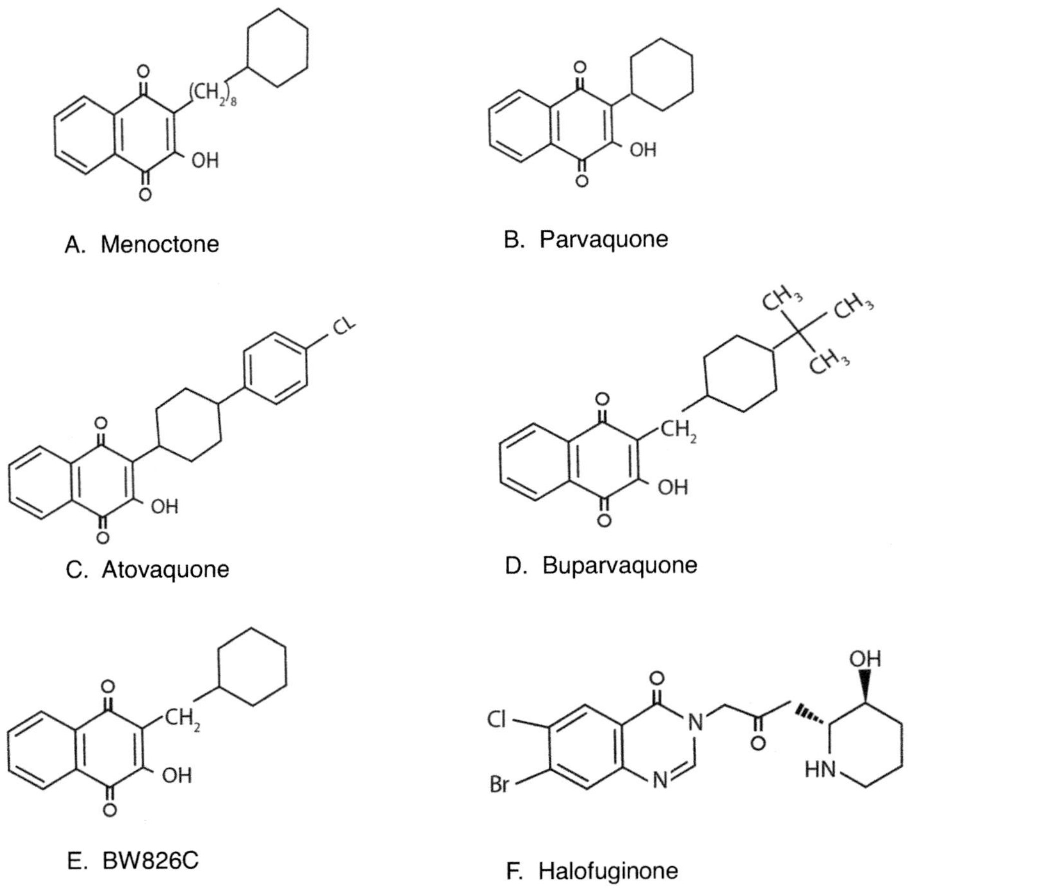

Fig. 14.1. The molecular structures of anti-theilerial therapeutic compounds.

tetracycline when administered to cattle immediately after infection was perhaps due to inhibition of the parasite's ability to transform its host lymphocytes into dividing lymphoblasts *in vivo*, or to an effect only on its pre-schizont stage immediately following infection. Subsequent studies by Spooner (1990) supported the former suggestion.

14.3.1 Menoctone – The first compound with anti-theilerial activity

The literature was searched for other compounds that had shown activity against a far wider range of diseases but which had not been developed as products for various reasons. Among these, several were active against malarial parasites, including the hydroxynaphthoquinone 'menoctone' (Fig. 14.1A; Fieser *et al.*, 1948).

After 48 h incubation with menoctone at concentrations of 1.0 and 0.1 μg/ml, only 23 and 27%, respectively, of the lymphoblasts contained a schizont, and most of the remaining schizonts were small with few nuclei. The schizont cytoplasm showed obvious signs of degeneration, and the lymphoblasts from which schizonts had been eliminated showed clear signs of reversion to normal lymphocyte appearance. Many had faintly stained remnants of schizonts where parasites had apparently been eliminated. As menoctone was the first compound ever to be shown to have significant lethal action on theilerial schizonts, a brief summary of further studies with it is provided here.

Titration of menoctone in *in vitro* cultures revealed EC50 values (the concentration that reduces parasitosis to 50% of that in untreated control cultures) against *T. parva* and *T. annulata* schizonts of 0.06 μg/ml and 0.08 μg/ml, respectively. None of the other 'failed' antimalarial compounds that were tested showed more than minimal anti-theilerial activity (McHardy, 1978). Following exposure of cultured cells to menoctone at 0.1 μg/ml, there was a small decrease in schizont numbers and in the number of nuclei in the schizonts within 6 h of exposure. The effect was maximal by around 48 h in the *T. annulata* cultures and after 72 h with *T. parva*.

Studies of the activity of menoctone in cattle infected experimentally by administering *T. parva* sporozoites were conducted in collaboration with the United Nations Development Programme (UNDP)/Overseas Development Administration (ODA) ECF Project in Kenya (see Chapter 1 of this volume). Intramuscular injection of 5 mg/kg menoctone on the day of infection followed by 1 mg/kg daily on the following 9 days suppressed the infection almost completely, and subsequently the animals were fully susceptible to challenge with the homologous parasite stabilate. In a further trial, animals received 5 mg/kg menoctone on the first day of fever with macroschizonts present in lymph node smears, then 1 mg/kg on each of the subsequent 5 days. The clinical course of the disease was rapidly halted and the animals were resistant to subsequent challenge. These findings and a small selection of *in vitro* screening results were published in Nature (McHardy *et al.*, 1976; correction in McHardy, 1978). This was the first demonstration that a well-established, potentially fatal ECF infection could be cured by drug treatment. Further trials (McHardy and Rae, 1981) showed that a single intramuscular injection of 10 mg/kg bodyweight of menoctone was curative in moderately severe ECF, and more severe infections could be cured, in most cases, by a further similar injection.

14.3.2 Parvaquone

Synthesis of menoctone involved a process of at least 16 stages, which would make it far too expensive for use as a veterinary drug. A small team of Wellcome's synthetic chemists, led by Dr Alan Hudson, was therefore enlisted to make analogues of menoctone in the hope of identifying a comparably active, but less expensive, naphthoquinone for development. Over a period of 4 years, several hundred of these compounds were synthesized. Testing them in the *T. parva in vitro* screen quickly revealed that the presence of a hydroxyl group in the -3 position on the naphthoquinone ring was 'mandatory' for significant anti-theilerial activity. Omission of the -OH or its replacement by anything else, such as a halogen, or anything more 'bulky', resulted in greatly reduced anti-theilerial action. Insertion of any grouping anywhere on the left of the two 6-carbon atom rings of the naphthoquinone 'core' also resulted in reduced activity, in some cases to near zero (Boehm *et al.*, 1981; Hudson *et al.*, 1985, 1986).

A number of compounds that were more closely analogous to menoctone were synthesized, and some of these showed activity equal to, or greater than, that of menoctone in the *in vitro* screen (Boehm *et al.*, 1981), but the manufacture of most of them would still be too expensive. However, among them was the simplest structure of them all, in which the cyclohexyl ring was attached directly in the 2-position on the naphthoquinone core, with no methylene groups between the core and the cyclohexyl ring (Fig. 14.1B). Surprisingly, it was almost exactly as effective against *T. parva* as menoctone, and it was relatively easy to synthesize. Like menoctone, it was slightly less active against *T. annulata* than against *T. parva*. Its serial number was 'BW993C', later given the pharmacopoeal name 'parvaquone'.

A series of trials with parvaquone was conducted in *T. parva*-infected cattle with more advanced clinical and parasitological signs of ECF than in the initial studies with menoctone, to compare the clinical efficacy of the two compounds. At the time of treatment, the animals had displayed schizonts in lymph node smears and a rectal temperature of at least 39.5°C for 3 consecutive days. Some had early signs of pulmonary oedema. Parvaquone cured all 14 cattle treated with a single intramuscular injection of 20 mg/kg, four of five treated with 10 mg/kg and three of five treated with 5 mg/kg (McHardy *et al.*, 1983). All five treated twice with 10 mg/kg parvaquone, with an interval of 3 days between treatments, were also cured. Menoctone cured seven of ten animals treated once with 5 mg/kg. All untreated control animals in this series of trials died of ECF.

Five other 3-hydroxy-naphthoquinones with various side-groups in the 2-position were also tested in infected cattle (McHardy *et al.*, 1983). One of them had only a side-chain of 12 methylene groups and a terminal methyl group, but no cyclohexyl ring. Three esters of naphthoquinones were also designed as 'pro-drugs', in the hope that they would be metabolized slowly into parvaquone to give a more extended period of schizonticidal action. However, they showed little activity in cattle, presumably because little or no metabolism to parvaquone occurred. These findings also appeared to confirm that a hydroxyl (and no other) group in the 3-position is mandatory for effective anti-theilerial activity.

The virulence of *T. parva* is known to vary across its geographical range, both between and within individual countries (see Chapter 6 of this volume). Dolan *et al.* (1984) examined the efficacy of two injections of 10 mg/kg of a simple formulation of parvaquone to treat clinical disease induced by stabilates of sporozoites of three geographically distinct isolates of *T. parva*, one each from Kenya, Tanzania and Uganda, and two from buffalo-derived isolates, which cause Corridor disease (CD) in cattle, known at that time as *Theileria parva lawrencei*, one from Kenya and one from Tanzania. Although the numbers of parasites in each stabilate inoculation were not determined, the time to first detection of macroschizonts in stained smears of lymph node aspirates was similar among the groups, indicating broadly similar infective doses. As expected, the pattern of disease varied between the groups, and in some cases the recovery period was prolonged. Cure rates in the groups infected with cattle-derived *T. parva* were, respectively, 3/7, 6/6 and 6/7. In those infected with buffalo-derived parasites, they were 5/7 and 6/7. These results suggested that there may be differences in susceptibility to parvaquone between these isolates, although the formulation of drug used in the study was not 'optimized' to give the most effective pharmacokinetic behaviour and the numbers of cattle were small.

A long-term follow-up study was made of the body weight changes in the animals in this study (Dolan, 1986a). Perhaps unsurprisingly, in view of the suboptimal treatment given to some of the animals, increases were less than impressive in some cases. Also, no treatments were given in either of these studies to control concurrent and intercurrent infections, nor were there any treatments of specific adverse clinical signs, including pulmonary oedema. Such treatments would be applied in the field in situations where veterinary care is available.

Field efficacy studies with parvaquone, in its optimized formulation as Clexon™, were conducted by various teams throughout eastern Africa in cattle naturally infected with *T. parva* (Musisi *et al.*, 1985, in Zambia; Chema *et al.*, 1986, in Kenya; Mbwambo *et al.*, 1987, in Tanzania). Each of these trials broadly confirmed laboratory findings that around 90% of early to moderately severe ECF cases could be cured with two injections of 10 mg/kg of parvaquone, with an interval of 2–3 days between them. In more advanced cases, some with clear signs of pulmonary oedema, additional injections were often necessary, but cure rates were still generally between 75% and 90%, depending largely on the severity of the pulmonary oedema and other clinical signs at the time of first treatment.

14.3.2.1 Pharmokinetics of parvaquone in bovine blood

The *in vitro* screen was adapted to determine concentrations of parvaquone (and other drugs) in the blood plasma of treated cattle (McHardy and Mercer, 1984). The results from this bioassay showed very similar values to those found later with a more sophisticated, HPLC-based, assay (Kinabo and Bogan, 1988). Parvaquone was detectable in plasma within 30 min after intramuscular injection. Its concentration peaked at around 180 × *in vitro* EC503 h after injection of 20 mg/kg parvaquone and around 90 × EC50 with 10 mg/kg. Concentrations then fell steadily to near zero 48 h after injection. When two injections of 10 mg/kg were given with an interval of 48 h, plasma concentrations after the first and second doses were almost identical, but the peak concentration was about half that following the 20 mg/kg dose. These findings were important in optimizing the formulation of parvaquone and in selecting the interval of 2 days between intramuscular injections of 10 mg/kg bodyweight as the recommended primary course of treatment of ECF with Clexon™.

14.3.2.2 Registration and launch of Clexon™

Parvaquone was registered as a product for sale as an anti-theilerial for use in food animals in 1982. Safety testing indicated that parvaquone caused no significant toxicity, apart from a modest inhibition of blood clotting at very high doses. This could be due to parvaquone's tenuous structural similarity to K vitamins. Withholding periods for milk and tissues of treated animals were established as 14 and 28 days, respectively, partly due to the persistence of small amounts of drug at injection sites in some animals. Clexon™ was launched by Burroughs Wellcome for the treatment of *T. parva* and *T. annulata* infections in 1983.

14.3.3 Buparvaquone and the antimalarial compound atovaquone

As a result of the findings on the efficacy of fairly simple hydroxy-naphthoquinones against *Theileria*, the coccidiosis and malaria teams at Wellcome became more interested in them, and the synthetic chemists focused their attention on these diseases rather than on theileriosis. However, testing of some of their output in the *T. parva in vitro* screen continued.

There was broad similarity between the results against *Theileria*, *Plasmodium* and *Eimeria* but no single compound was best against all three. The naphthoquinone compound most active against the poultry coccidian *Eimeria tenella*, serial number BW58C (Hudson *et al.*, 1985; Hudson *et al.*, 1986), was judged unlikely to be commercially viable as a product for livestock, and further work on it for coccidiosis was terminated, but attempts to optimize the activity of naphthoquinones as antimalarials continued. This culminated in 'atovaquone' (Fig. 14.1C), which was developed for the prophylaxis and treatment of malaria, and, in combination with the 'old' antimalarial compound proguanil, released as Malarone™. This is one of the few instances in which research on the treatment of a veterinary disease, theileriosis, instigated other studies which ultimately led to an important new human medicinal product.

While the many 'target' compounds that had been synthesized as potential antimalarials were tested in the *T. parva in vitro* screen, only a few of the many hundreds of 'intermediate' compounds produced on the often-complex routes in their synthesis had been tested 2 years later. One, BW720C, showed outstanding activity against *T. parva*. Its EC50 was 0.003 μg/ml – 20-fold less than that of parvaquone (0.06 μg/ml), and like parvaquone, it was only slightly less active against *T. annulata*. BW720C, later named buparvaquone, would be more expensive to manufacture than parvaquone, but the curative dose could also be expected to be considerably lower, perhaps making it an economic proposition as a veterinary drug.

It was also anticipated that generic copies of Clexon™ would be introduced in the foreseeable future, so it was decided to develop buparvaquone as a second-generation product to supersede Clexon™. Parvaquone's patent protection was relatively weak. It had been shown to have modest antimalarial activity in the original study of Fieser *et al.* (1948), and its action on *Theileria* was judged to be not particularly surprising as both organisms are apicomplexan parasites. In addition, a methodology for its synthesis was already 'known' from the Fieser publication. Buparvaquone, however, was not a 'known' compound, its structure was significantly different to that of menoctone, its enhanced anti-theilerial activity was not 'predictable' and its synthetic route was novel. The patent protection for buparvaquone, therefore, was relatively strong. It was named buparvaquone because it had a fairly bulky tertiary butyl group in the -4 position on the cyclohexyl ring of parvaquone (Fig. 14.1D). What made its outstanding anti-theilerial activity particularly surprising was that it also had a single methylene group between the cyclohexyl ring and the naphthoquinone 'core' of the molecule. This was entirely unexpected because insertion of a methylene group in this position in the parvaquone molecule (compound BW826C,

Fig. 14.1E) produced a tenfold reduction of anti-theilerial action *in vitro* (McHardy *et al.*, 1985).

A series of trials with buparvaquone in cattle infected with *T. parva* in Kenya, similar to the earlier ones with parvaquone, showed that a single injection of 2.5 mg/kg cured almost all animals with moderately severe ECF, and additional similar dose(s) cured many of the more advanced cases, compared with two or more injections of 10 mg/kg of parvaquone (McHardy *et al.*, 1985). So, a 20-fold increase in anti-schizont activity *in vitro* translated to an eightfold increase in therapeutic efficacy against clinical ECF, compared with parvaquone and menoctone. Importantly, BW720C was also more effective than parvaquone in the treatment of *T. annulata* infections.

Various publications on the results of field efficacy trials confirmed the activity of buparvaquone when used to treat cattle infected with *T. parva* or *T. annulata* (Dolan *et al.*, 1992; Wanjohi *et al.*, 1995; Muraguri *et al.*, 1999, 2006, against *T. parva*; Dhar *et al.*, 1987; Hashemi-Fesharki, 1991, against *T. annulata*).

The exhaustive series of safety studies necessary for its registration as a veterinary medicinal product showed that, like parvaquone, it was extremely safe. It had the additional advantage that it partitioned very weakly from blood to milk, so its milk withholding period was only 2 days compared with 14 days for the smaller parvaquone molecule in Clexon™. It was launched in 1993 with the tradename Butalex™. Butalex™ quickly became the preferred product for the treatment of both of the commonest forms of bovine theileriosis, largely because the primary course of treatment was a single injection. Pharmacokinetic studies showed that buparvaquone (as either Butalex™ or Buparvex™) was detected 15 min after inoculation into cattle and reached peak plasma concentration after 3 h. There was considerable variation in the peak plasma concentration in individual animals (32–589 ng/ml and 183–449 ng/ml for Butalex™ and Buparvex™, respectively), but there was no correlation between peak plasma concentration and the rapidity of clinical cure (Muraguri *et al.*, 2006). Generic buparvaquone products were also released, principally in markets in Asia, where European patents on buparvaquone and Butalex™ were not recognized.

Buparvaquone has been shown to be effective against *Theileria orientalis*/*T. buffeli*, some subtypes of which cause severe disease in Australasia (Minami *et al.*, 1985; Stewart *et al.*, 1990; referred to as *T. sergenti* in the former publication, before the nomenclature of this species was changed – see Chapter 1 of this volume). Zaugg and Lane (1989) reported that buparvaquone was effective in the treatment of *Babesia equi* (later re-named *Theileria equi*). A number of studies have also reported that buparvaquone has strong activity against *Leishmania donovani* (Croft *et al.*, 1992; Ortiz *et al.*, 2016), including when applied topically on infected mice (Garnier *et al.*, 2007).

14.3.4 Parvaquone and frusemide

Treatment of ECF with parvaquone and frusemide (furosemide), a sulphonamide 'loop' diuretic, was shown to be effective in the treatment of advanced cases of ECF with pulmonary oedema (Mbwambo *et al.*, 2002). (Two decades later, frusemide was found to be beneficial for treatment of oedema associated with human COVID-19 infections, although certain corticosteroids were even more effective in suppressing the oedema.) An injectable product containing parvaquone and frusemide was developed by the Irish veterinary company Bimeda. This product, Parvexon Plus™ (originally named Fruvexon™), cured around 75% of advanced field cases of ECF with obvious pulmonary oedema, compared with around 45% of those treated with parvaquone alone (Azuba Musoke *et al.*, 2004). Parvexon Plus™ quickly became the preferred product for the treatment of ECF in cases with pulmonary oedema.

14.3.5 Coccidiostats as anti-theilerials

Around the time that parvaquone was developed, another compound, halofuginone hydrobromide, was also shown to be active against *T. parva* (Schein and Voigt, 1979). Halofuginone hydrobromide and halofuginone lactate were both found to be active (Schein and Voigt, 1979; Dolan, 1986b). Halofuginone is a synthetic quinazolinone derivative of febrifugine, which was originally identified in the roots and leaves of a Chinese medicinal plant (*Dichroa febrifuga*; reviewed by McLaughlin *et al.*, 2014). Previous studies had shown that halofuginone was also active against several other apicomplexan parasites, including *Eimeria*, *Plasmodium*, *Toxoplasma* and *Cryptosporidia* species (Edgar and Flanagan, 1979; Silverlås *et al.*, 2009; reviewed by Gill and Sharma, 2022). Halofuginone hydrobromide had been registered as a poultry coccidiostat (Stenorol™), and the lactate salt of halofuginone was registered (Halocur™) for treatment of cryptosporidiosis. The structure of halofuginone is shown in Fig. 14.1F.

Initial experiments with halofuginone hydrobromide in cattle had shown that it caused significant tissue damage when administered by injection (Kinabo, 1989), so the oral route was used to examine its activity against *T. parva*. Oral treatment of *T. parva*-infected animals with only 1.2 mg/kg of halofuginone hydrobromide, repeated as clinically indicated, was curative in most cases (Schein and Voigt, 1979). Halofuginone's effect appeared to be principally on the macroschizont stage of the parasite, with very little, if any, effect on the subsequent piroplasm stage in the erythrocytes. Uilenberg *et al.* (1980) obtained essentially similar results with a dose of 1 or 2 mg/kg of halofuginone hydrobromide, repeated as clinically indicated. The 2 mg/kg dose caused diarrhoea in the cattle, and they reported that 4 mg/kg was fatal in mice, so this dosage was not tested in cattle. They also reported an effect on *T. parva* macroschizonts *in vitro*, down to 0.01 μg/ml.

Halofuginone hydrobromide was compared with parvaquone *in vitro* and in *T. parva* stabilate-infected cattle by Morgan and McHardy (1982). *In vitro* EC50 values were similar (0.03 and 0.06 μg/ml, respectively) but, oddly, while the *in vitro* dose–response curve of parvaquone was sigmoidal, that of halofuginone was bell-shaped (Fig. 14.2). Halofuginone's effect at 1.0 and 0.1 μg/ml appeared to be minimal in the *in vitro* system, but its activity increased to a peak at 0.015 μg/ml, then fell progressively, similarly to parvaquone's. The reason for higher concentrations of halofuginone apparently being less effective against *T. parva* schizonts *in vitro* than far lower concentrations has not been elucidated but might be explained by a non-lethal effect on

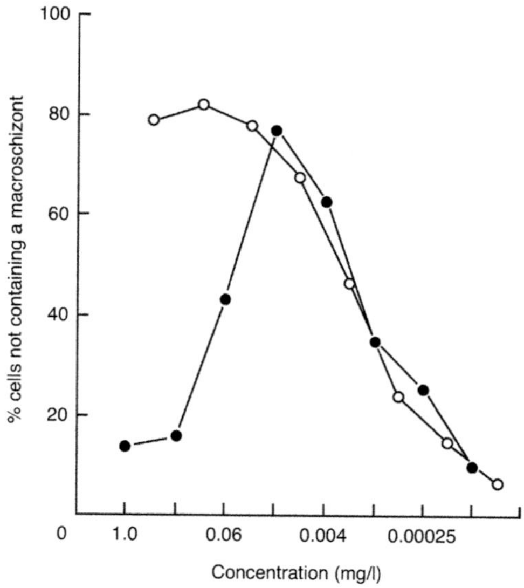

Fig. 14.2. Comparison of the effects of parvaquone (open circles) and halofuginone hydrobromide (filled circles) on *T. parva* macroschizonts *in vitro*, 48 h after addition of the compounds. In untreated cultures, about 98% of lymphoblasts contained a macroschizont. (From Morgan and McHardy, 1982.)

the host lymphoblasts that blocked the compound's access to the parasites. This is supported by results of experiments in which the schizonticidal action of parvaquone was abolished in cultures treated with a mixture of parvaquone and high concentrations of halofuginone (McHardy and Morgan, 1981).

Although it cured ECF, halofuginone hydrobromide given orally was also unacceptably irritant, causing gastric ulceration and bleeding, even at its minimum ECF curative dose. However, halofuginone lactate was similarly effective (Dolan, 1986b) and was shown to be less irritant. It was launched for the oral treatment of ECF (marketed by Hoechst as Terit™) at about the same time as Clexon™.

In field trials of the treatment of natural cases of ECF with Terit™ conducted by Njau *et al.* (1985) and Chema *et al.* (1987), cure rates were similar to those in the experimental studies. However, its lack of activity against the piroplasm stage rendered it unacceptable for the treatment of *T. annulata* infections, which produce higher levels of piroplasm parasitaemia and a much greater degree of anaemia compared to infections with *T. parva*. Most veterinary practitioners in East Africa showed a clear preference for Clexon™ over Terit™ for the treatment of ECF, and Terit™ was withdrawn from the market after only a few years, so parvaquone-based products remained the only effective treatment for ECF until Butalex™ was launched.

Two other anti-coccidial compounds, the ionophores monensin and lasalocid, were also found to be active against *T. parva* macroschizonts *in vitro* (McHardy and Rae, 1982). Their EC50 values were 0.02 and 0.25 µg/ml, respectively, making monensin about three times more active *in vitro* than parvaquone. Monensin is administered orally, in feed, for the prevention and treatment of coccidiosis. In a preliminary study in cattle treated with 5 mg/kg orally on 5 consecutive days, it showed no effect on ECF, presumably because it is not absorbed from the gut. In a second study, it was injected intravenously at 0.5 mg/kg for 5 consecutive days. While this had a clear anti-theilerial effect, it also caused unacceptable toxicity, and further development was not pursued. Lasalocid was not tested in cattle.

14.3.5.1 Mode of action of naphthoquinones and halofuginone

The mode of action of tetracyclines on ECF is discussed in Chapter 12 of this volume. The mode of action of hydroxynaphthoquinones against *T. parva* has not been studied directly. However, their likely activity could be inferred from knowledge of the antimalarial action of atovaquone, whose structure is broadly similar to that of buparvaquone. Atovaquone is a competitive inhibitor of ubiquinol, specifically inhibiting the mitochondrial electron transport chain at the bc1 complex, resulting in a loss of mitochondrial function (Nixon *et al.*, 2013). Like atovaquone, buparvaquone acts on all stages of the target parasite's life cycle and not on host cell mitochondrial or respiratory enzymes, which accounts for the extremely low toxicity of these compounds. This mode of activity is consistent with the finding of mutations in cytochrome b in buparvaquone-resistant isolates of *T. annulata* (discussed further in Section 14.4). In electron microscopic studies of *T. parva* exposed to buparvaquone (N. McHardy, 2024, personal communication) there was obvious disruption of organelles of the macroschizont and piroplasm stages of the parasite, beginning within an hour of exposure, but there was less damage to the boundary membrane or the nucleus of the parasites at this time. Twenty-four hours after exposure, disruption of the parasite's organelles was very obvious, reflecting light microscopic observations of Giemsa-stained lymphoid and blood smears from *Theileria*-infected cattle treated with buparvaquone. The host lymphoblastoid cells appeared to be completely unaffected by buparvaquone. The ladder-like membrane microstructure of their mitochondria, bearing their respiratory enzymes, was entirely normal throughout the study.

The main mode of action of halofuginone is inhibition of the activity of prolyl-tRNA synthetase (PRS), which catalyses the interaction of appropriate amino acids to the cognate tRNAs (reviewed by Gill and Sharma, 2022). Thus, it would be expected to affect a wide range of cellular activities that involve protein synthesis. Halofuginone has been shown to have a number of clinical activities in humans, including inhibition of fibrosis and slowing the progression of certain tumours (McLaughlin *et al.*, 2014). Halofuginone interacts with human glutamyl-prolyl-tRNA synthetase (EPRS), and the parasite and mammalian PRS proteins show a high level of sequence conservation (Keller *et al.*, 2012), which almost certainly accounts for at least some of the toxic side effects of the drug and its very low therapeutic index. It is strongly schizonticidal *in vitro* on *Theileria*-infected cells, even at low concentrations, but it does not appear to be active against the piroplasm stages, for reasons that are not understood.

Since halofuginone is no longer marketed as an anti-theilerial, its mode of action might be seen to be purely academic in this context, but Gill and Sharma (2022) have argued that knowledge of its activity on parasite PRS and the role of cross-reactivity with host PRS in the toxic side effects of the drug offers the possibility of developing a safer compound with the same mode of action but with greater selectivity for the parasite. This would be particularly relevant to *Theileria*, given the availability of only one class of therapeutic drug at present and in view of the emergence of resistance to naphthoquinones in *T. annulata* infections and the likelihood that resistance will, at some time, also occur in *T. parva*.

14.4 Drug Resistance

As yet (2025) there have been no reports of resistance to hydroxy-naphthoquinones in *T. parva*, but resistance in *T. annulata* has been reported in several countries, including Tunisia, Iran, Sudan, Pakistan, India and Turkey (Mhadhbi *et al.*, 2010; Sharifiyazdi *et al.*, 2012; Chatanga *et al.*, 2019; Ali *et al.*, 2022; Hacılarlıoglu *et al.*, 2023). Resistance to halofuginone in *T. parva* was not reported during the short period of availability of Terit™. The confirmed resistance to hydroxy-naphthoquinones in *T. annulata* is a cause for concern since these are the only drugs currently available for the treatment of clinical theileriosis, and it demonstrates the likely potential for similar resistance to develop in *T. parva*.

The genetic basis of resistance in *T. annulata* to buparvaquone has been investigated in a number of studies. Mutations in the cytochrome b gene in parasites from cattle exhibiting resistance to buparvaquone therapy have been reported in several countries (Mhadhbi *et al.*, 2010, 2015; Sharifiyazdi *et al.*, 2012; Chatanga *et al.*, 2019; Ali *et al.*, 2022; Hacılarlıoglu *et al.*, 2023). The mutations involved residues in the cytochrome b protein that lie within the putative buparvaquone binding site. Hacılarlıoglu *et al.* (2023) conducted a particularly thorough study in Turkey involving clonal analyses of parasites isolated from cattle in which intensive treatment with buparvaquone had failed to effect a cure. Two non-synonymous mutations in putative buparvaquone binding sites in the cytochrome b protein (residues 135 and 253) were identified in the resistant parasites. Comparison of parasite clones obtained prior to and following treatment provided convincing evidence of a strong association of these two mutations with drug resistance. The same authors detected these mutations at frequencies of 3.9 and 3.7%, respectively, in a large sample of field isolates of *T. annulata* and, significantly, there was an almost tenfold increase in the frequencies of the mutations in parasites collected between 2011 and 2012 compared to those collected between 1998 and 2007, indicating a marked increase in the incidence of drug-resistant parasites. Mutations in cytochrome b at position 253 were also detected in the resistant parasites in Pakistan (Ali *et al.*, 2022), and other mutations in or close to the putative buparvaquone binding site were detected in this study and in the studies of Tunisian and Sudanese resistant parasites (Mhadhbi *et al.*, 2015; Chatanga *et al.*, 2019).

T. annulata peptidyl-prolyl isomerase (TaPIN1) is secreted by the schizont into the host cell and has been shown to modulate oncogenic signalling pathways in the host cells (Marsolier *et al.*, 2015). These authors also reported that buparvaquone inhibits the activity of TaPIN1 *in vitro* and found a point mutation in TaPIN1 that reverses the ability of buparvaquone to inhibit its activity. This mutation has been detected in buparvaquone-resistant isolates of *T. annulata* from Tunisia and Sudan (Marsolier *et al.*, 2015). A study by Salim *et al.* (2019), which reported sequencing of TaPIN1 and cytochrome b genes in 67 Sudanese isolates of *T. annulata* from farms where drug resistance was reported, found 40 isolates with mutations in TaPIN1 and 18 with mutations in cytochrome b, including 11 with mutations in both genes. However, the cell lines in this study were uncloned and their drug resistance status was not rigorously demonstrated. Hence, a clear causal association of TaPIN1 with drug resistance has not yet been demonstrated. Moreover, the study reported by Hacılarlıoglu *et al.* (2023) failed to detect mutations in TaPIN1 in drug-resistant *T. annulata* isolates from Turkey.

14.5 Treatment of Disease Caused by *T. parva*

14.5.1 The acute and fatal nature of the disease

Once susceptible breeds of cattle become infected with *T. parva*, either the parasites that cause ECF or those transmitted from buffalo causing CD, clinical signs develop within 7–10 days, often resulting in death after a further 8–10 days (see Chapters 4 and 5 of this volume for further details). If left untreated, mortality approaches 100% in European (*Bos taurus*) breeds of cattle, and is only slightly lower in improved *B. indicus* breeds and their crosses with *B. taurus*. January disease, the milder form of disease caused by *T. parva* in Zimbabwe, usually results in less than 25% mortality. High levels of mortality also occur in cases of *T. annulata* infection.

The frequently acute and fatal nature of these diseases highlights the need for early and appropriate application of the therapeutic agents.

14.5.2 Response to therapy

Most early and moderately severe clinical cases respond rapidly to treatment with parvaquone or buparvaquone. Temperature rise is halted within 1 or 2 days, after which temperatures return to normal. In more advanced cases, particularly if pulmonary oedema is present, temperature may remain elevated, in which case a further dose of the drug is required. Macroschizonts are usually cleared from lymph node smears within a few days in relatively mild cases, but less quickly in more severe disease. In smears from heavily parasitized animals, microschizonts (i.e. parasites undergoing merogony) disappear rapidly and are likely to be difficult to find only 1 day after treatment. The effect on piroplasms in blood smears is usually dramatic; practically 100% of piroplasms are likely to be dead and pyknotic within 24 h of treatment, but erythrocytes containing pyknotic piroplasms may remain in the blood for more than a week following treatment. Blood leukocyte counts return rapidly to normal levels following successful treatment.

Cure rates of uncomplicated ECF, CD and January disease, treated correctly with the registered parvaquone or buparvaquone products, can approach 100%, but several key factors can influence the outcome of treatment, as described below.

14.5.3 Requirement for early diagnosis and treatment

As discussed in Chapters 4 and 11 of this volume, infection with *T. parva* causes disorganization and destruction of lymphoid tissues, which compromises the capacity to mount effective immune responses. Treatment of most infectious diseases benefits from an optimally functional immune system to aid the clearance of the infectious agent. Hence, identification of infection with *T. parva* in its early stages and prompt application of treatment provide the best chance of an effective cure. The main early clinical signs of the disease are enlargement of lymph nodes draining the site of tick attachment, particularly the parotid and prescapular nodes, coinciding with elevation of body temperature. A drop in milk yield may also be apparent in the early stages in dairy animals.

14.5.4 Detection and treatment of intercurrent infections

The effect on immune competence referred to above also renders animals more susceptible to infection with other pathogens, particularly in the later stages of the disease. These may be newly acquired infections or recrudescence of latent infections carried by affected animals. Cattle in areas infested with the tick vectors of *Babesia* and *Anaplasma* are likely to harbour carrier infections with these pathogens. In this regard, some early accounts of ECF describe anaemia and jaundice as clinical features of disease. However, these findings are likely to have been due to co-infection with other pathogens. *Anaplasma* parasitaemia in cases of ECF may be very much lower (i.e. less than 1%) than in primary uncomplicated infections, but still cause severe anaemia (McHardy and Kiara, 1996). Recognition of *Anaplasma* in stained blood smears from cases of ECF treated with naphthoquinones is difficult because dead *Theileria* piroplasms appear almost identical to healthy *Anaplasma* organisms, and are cleared slowly from the blood. Cases of ECF are also susceptible to infection with bacterial pathogens,

Table 14.1. Response to treatment with buparvaquone of cases of ECF with intercurrent infections with other pathogens.

Intercurrent infections	No. treated	No. cured	% cured
Bacterial, respiratory	29	26	89.5
Bacterial, enteric	12	11	91.5
Anaplasmosis (*A. marginale*)	10	10	100
Babesiosis (*B. bigemina*)	3	3	100
Bacterial + Anaplasmosis	6	5	83.5
Total with intercurrent infections	60	55	91.5
Total with no intercurrent infections	40	38	95.0

particularly those affecting the respiratory and alimentary tracts. In a study of 100 cases of ECF of various degrees of severity on farms in Kenya (Wanjohi *et al.*, 1995), 60 were found to be complicated by intercurrent conditions (Table 14.1). Prompt diagnosis and appropriate treatment produced a cure rate of 91.5% of these cases, compared with 95% of the 40 with uncomplicated ECF. For ethical reasons, a group with intercurrent infections from which specific treatment was withheld could not be included in this study.

14.5.5 Additional supportive therapy

In most fatal cases of ECF, the primary cause of death is pulmonary oedema, caused by a major inflammatory episode in the lungs. Effectively, the animal drowns in its own body fluids. Cases of ECF showing signs of pulmonary oedema should be treated with a diuretic along with parvaquone or buparvaquone.

Although corticosteroids are sometimes used together with theilericidal drugs to suppress inflammatory responses, there is no published evidence on their beneficial effect and they may be expected also to have an inhibitory effect on the immune response to theileriosis.

14.5.6 Appropriate use of curative drugs

At least ten so-called 'generic' parvaquone and ten buparvaquone products have reached the East African market since expiry of patents on the 'pioneer' products, Clexon™ and Butalex™, but few reports on their clinical efficacy and safety have been published. Unregistered products and products that may be genuinely generic, but without published evidence of efficacy, may contain less than (or even none of) the stated content of the active ingredient, or different oil and solvent vehicles compared to genuine generic and pioneer products. The 'correct' oil and solvent is particularly important in governing the pharmacokinetic behaviour and therefore the therapeutic performance of parvaquone and buparvaquone, because the hydroxy-naphthoquinones are almost completely insoluble in water. It took almost 2 years of trials to optimize the formulations of Clexon™ and Butalex™ and the selection of the best oil was a particularly difficult aspect of that programme. 'Policing' of 'pirate' and other unregistered products by regulatory authorities is difficult for many reasons, not least because of limited resources. However, products that contain no naphthoquinone may be identified by dropping a small volume into a glass of water. As the drop of product enters the water, parvaquone and buparvaquone come out of solution immediately and sink slowly as a pale yellow 'curtain'. This does not give a reliable indication of the concentration of active ingredient (if any is present), but with experience, an approximate estimation can be made by comparison with a product that is known to be genuine.

Misuse of curative drugs creates an increased risk of selecting drug-resistant strains of the parasite. Given that treatment with suboptimal doses is a frequent cause of drug resistance in many diseases, the use of sub-standard theilericidal drug products would be expected to increase the risk of resistance developing in *Theileria* parasites. Sustained prophylactic use of any of these products may also be a risk and is also contraindicated, except in carefully supervised circumstances.

14.6 The Search for New Anti-theilerial Drugs

At the time of writing (2025), products containing parvaquone or buparvaquone are the only ones available specifically for the treatment of ECF (and other theilerioses). It is now 50 years since the activity of menoctone was demonstrated and almost 40 years since the first naphthoquinone product was launched. Given the lack of investment in new therapeutics for the disease, it is unlikely that any new products will reach the market in the immediate future. Typically, the 'lead time' from first demonstration of activity in a novel candidate compound until it reaches the market as a finished and registered product is about 10 years. The minimum cost of development, including the extensive package of efficacy and formulation optimization, and studies of safety for treatment of animals and for human consumption of tissues and milk from treated animals, necessary for its registration by regulatory bodies, is unlikely to be much less than US$100 million. However, a drug that is already registered for another indication might be 'repurposed' for the treatment of theileriosis, in which case the lead time and cost of development could be substantially lower. The quinazolinone halofuginone (in Terit™) was repurposed from being an anti-coccidial drug in far less time, and at much lower cost, than it took to discover and develop the naphthoquinone compounds. For these reasons, the search for new anti-theilerial drugs has focused on 'open source' compounds, mostly from banks of antimalarial compounds.

The concept of open source boxes to investigate therapeutics was developed to provide open access to panels of compounds with known biological activity that could potentially provide therapeutic activity against a pathogen or group of pathogens. Two such boxes are the Medicines for Malaria Venture Malaria Box and the Medicines for Malaria Venture Pathogen Box (Van Voorhis *et al.*, 2016).

Four studies using these open boxes in theileriosis have been reported. Nyagwange *et al.* (2019) screened about 800 compounds from both the malaria and the pathogen boxes against cultures of bovine lymphoblastoid cells infected with *T. parva*. They monitored inhibition of the uptake of tritiated thymidine by infected cells rather than microscopic examination as an indicator of anti-theilerial effect, using buparvaquone as their positive control compound. The Nyagwange study identified nine 'malaria box' and eight 'pathogen box' compounds with anti-theilerial activity, but most of them were also relatively toxic for the host lymphoblast cells. However, two had 'promising' specific anti-theilerial activity with IC50 values of $0.78 \pm 0.61\,\mu M$. They also found that the anti-leukaemia drug 'dasatinib' had an EC50 of 5.0 nM. Dasatinib's toxicity for the host bovine lymphoblastoid cells, > 10 µM, seems surprisingly low for a drug used for the treatment of lymphoid leukaemia, but its identification is encouraging, although there is no mention of investigating it, or related compounds, further as potential treatments for theileriosis.

Hostettler *et al.* (2016) examined about 400 malaria box compounds by testing them against cultures of cells infected with *T. annulata*. They assayed activity using a quantitative real-time PCR, focusing on the *T. annulata* surface protein (TaSP) gene. They found five active compounds, two of them with EC50 values of 0.5 and 0.2 µM, respectively, broadly similar to that of buparvaquone. These compounds were moderately toxic to the host macrophage cells, but electron microscopic examination of treated cultures showed clear preferential toxicity for the *Theileria* macroschizonts.

A third study, by Villares *et al.* (2022), with the malaria box compounds, using an automated microscopy assay, detected nine compounds that reduced the viability of the infected cells to < 25% after 48 h. Only two of these reduced the number of parasites per host cell. By far the most active was that containing trifloxystrobin, an anti-fungal compound used for crop protection. Trifloxystrobin kills the host cells of *T. parva* and *T. annulata*, and hence also their schizonts, with an EC50 value similar to that of buparvaquone. Loss of its anti-fungal activity has been linked to mutations in the fungal cytochrome b gene (Miao *et al.*, 2020). However, Villares *et al.* (2022) reported that it was active against buparvaquone-resistant *T. annulata* parasites harbouring mutations in cytochrome b, suggesting that trifloxystrobin has a different mode of action to buparvaquone. These findings are promising for producing an effective alternative treatment for ECF, but further studies to evaluate the feasibility of using the drug *in vivo* will be required to determine whether it is a viable candidate.

Perhaps there should be some unease about the cytotoxic effects of some of these new 'lead' compounds on bovine lymphoblasts. For example, halofuginone was withdrawn from the market partly because of its cytotoxic side effects.

Repurposing a human medical drug for use in veterinary medicine could be problematical for several reasons, particularly if its therapeutic index is low, and because of patenting and differential pricing restrictions. There is also the possibility, if not the likelihood, that the veterinary product would be misused in human medicine, particularly if its price was significantly lower than for its human use. While the new anti-theilerial leads discussed above are encouraging, they are only the first step on the path to a new theilericide. Nevertheless, given the current availability of only two effective compounds, both of which are at risk of development of drug resistance, it is important that the search for new anti-theilerials is pursued vigorously.

14.7 Concluding Remarks

Reliance on ECF drugs with a single mode of action to which, presumably, resistance in ECF will appear at some time, as it has in *T. annulata*, is very worrying, but the search for new or 'repurposable' drugs with different modes of action has begun. In a marketplace dominated by generic naphthoquinone products at prices that are only a small fraction of those of the pioneer products when they were launched, the cost of new product development is a formidable financial disincentive. However, for cattle owners in affected countries, ECF (and other tick-transmitted diseases) will continue to be extremely costly problems for which effective remedies are essential.

Meanwhile, although resistance to buparvaquone has been identified in *T. annulata* in several countries, it is not yet a serious and widespread problem everywhere, and resistance has not been found at all in *T. parva*. The aim, therefore, must be to continue to use all three of the available tools for the management of ECF – tick control, immunization and curative drugs – in the best combination to suit each farming system, and to encourage the use of curative drugs (and acaricides) in ways that will minimize the rate at which resistance to them develops.

The pioneer naphthoquinone-based products were only developed by Wellcome for the treatment of theileriosis because of the enlightened view of Dr Paul Capstick, the company's veterinary R&D Director at the time of their discovery. When asked to approve the progress of parvaquone from the discovery phase into development as a product, he said, 'Yes - because Sir Henry would have wanted us to.' 'Sir Henry' was Sir Henry Wellcome, co-founder of the Burroughs Wellcome company. He was a keen amateur parasitologist and the founder of the Wellcome Museum of the History of Medicine. Surely, Sir Henry would also have been pleased that the Wellcome Trust is now the key funder of the 'open box' initiative for tropical diseases – the basis of the current search for new drugs to treat theileriosis.

References

Ali, Q., Zahid, O., Mhadhbi, M., Jones, B., Darghouth, M.A. *et al.* (2022) Genetic characterisation of the *Theileria annulata* cytochrome b locus and its impact on buparvaquone resistance in bovine. *International Journal for Parasitology: Drugs and Drug Resistance* 20, 65–75. DOI: 10.1016/j.ijpddr.2022.08.004.

Azuba Musoke, R., Tweyongyere, R., Bizimenyera, E., Waiswa, C., Mugisha, A. *et al.* (2004) Treatment of East Coast fever of cattle with a combination of parvaquone and frusemide. *Tropical Animal Health and Production* 36(3), 233–245. DOI: 10.1023/B:TROP.0000016832.69136.68.

Barnett, S.F. and Bailey, K.P. (1957) *Chemotherapy of East Coast fever*. Annual Report. East African Veterinary Research Organization 1956-1957. EAVRO, Nairobi.

Boehm, P., Cooper, K., Hudson, A.T., Elphick, J.P. and McHardy, N. (1981) *In vitro* activity of 2-alkyl-3-hydroxy-1,4-naphthoquinones against *Theileria parva*. *Journal of Medicinal Chemistry* 24(3), 295–299. DOI: 10.1021/jm00135a011.

Brocklesby, D.W. and Bailey, K.P. (1962) Oxytetracycline hydrochloride in East Coast fever (*Theileria parva* infection). *British Veterinary Journal* 118(3), 81–85. DOI: 10.1016/S0007-1935(17)43151-4.

Brown, C.G.D., Radley, D.E., Burridge, M.J. and Cunningham, M.P. (1977) The use of tetracyclines in the chemotherapy of East Coast fever (*Theileria parva* infection of cattle). *Tropenmedizin und Parasitologie* 28, 513–520.

Chatanga, E., Mosssad, E., Abdo Abubaker, H., Amin Alnour, S., Katakura, K. *et al.* (2019) Evidence of multiple point mutations in *Theileria annulata* cytochrome b gene incriminated in buparvaquone treatment failure. *Acta Tropica* 191, 128–132. DOI: 10.1016/j.actatropica.2018.12.041.

Chema, S., Waghela, S., James, A.D., Dolan, T.T., Young, A.S. *et al.* (1986) Clinical trial of parvaquone for the treatment of East Coast fever in Kenya. *The Veterinary Record* 118(21), 588–589. DOI: 10.1136/vr.118.21.588-a.

Chema, S., Chumo, R.S., Dolan, T.T., Gathuma, J.M., Irvin, A.D. *et al.* (1987) Clinical trial of halofuginone lactate for the treatment of East Coast fever in Kenya. *The Veterinary Record* 120(24), 575–577. DOI: 10.1136/vr.120.24.575.

Croft, S.L., Hogg, J., Gutteridge, W.E., Hudson, A.T. and Randall, A.W. (1992) The activity of hydroxy-naphthoquinones against *Leishmania donovani*. *The Journal of Antimicrobial Chemotherapy* 30(6), 827–832. DOI: 10.1093/jac/30.6.827.

Dhar, S., Malhotra, D.V., Bushan, C. and Gautam, O.P. (1987) Treatment of clinical cases of bovine tropical theileriosis with buparvaquone (BW720C). *Indian Veterinary Journal* 64, 331–334.

Dolan, T.T. (1986a) Chemotherapy of East Coast fever: The long term weight changes, carrier state and disease manifestations of parvaquone treated cattle. *Journal of Comparative Pathology* 96(2), 137–146. DOI: 10.1016/0021-9975(86)90004-6.

Dolan, T.T. (1986b) Chemotherapy of East Coast fever. *Acta Tropica* 43, 1765–1773.

Dolan, T.T., Young, A.S., Leitch, B.L. and Stagg, D.A. (1984) Chemotherapy of East Coast fever: Parvaquone treatment of clinical disease induced by isolates of *Theileria parva*. *Veterinary Parasitology* 15(2), 103–116. DOI: 10.1016/0304-4017(84)90026-8.

Dolan, T.T., Injairu, R., Gisemba, F., Maina, J.N., Mbadi, G. *et al.* (1992) A clinical trial of buparvaquone in the treatment of East Coast fever. *The Veterinary Record* 130(24), 536–538. DOI: 10.1136/vr.130.24.536.

Edgar, S.A. and Flanagan, C. (1979) Efficacy of Stenorol® (halofuginone) for the control of coccidiosis in turkeys. *Poultry Science* 58(6), 1483–1489. DOI: 10.3382/ps.0581483.

Fieser, L.F., Heymann, H. and Seligman, A.M. (1948) Naphthoquinone antimalarials, XVIII. Metabolic oxidation products. *The Journal of Pharmacology and Experimental Therapeutics* 94(2), 112–124. DOI: 10.1016/S0022-3565(25)03481-0.

Garnier, T., Mantyla, A., Jarvinen, T., Lawrence, J., Brown, M. *et al.* (2007) *In vivo* studies on the antileishmanial activity of buparvaquone and its pro-drugs. *Journal of Antimicrobial Chemotherapy* 60(4), 802–810. DOI: 10.1093/jac/dkm303.

Gill, J. and Sharma, A. (2022) Prospects of halofuginone as an antiprotozoal drug scaffold. *Drug Discovery Today* 27(9), 2586–2592. DOI: 10.1016/j.drudis.2022.05.020.

Hacılarlıoglu, S., Bilgic, H.B., Bakırcı, S., Tait, A., Weir, W. *et al.* (2023) Selection of genotypes harbouring mutations in the cytochrome b gene of *Theileria annulata* is associated with resistance to buparvaquone. *PloS ONE* 18(1), e0279925. DOI: 10.1371/journal.pone.0279925.

Hashemi-Fesharki, R. (1991) Chemotherapeutic value of parvaquone and buparvaquone against *Theileria annulata* infection of cattle. *Research in Veterinary Science* 50(2), 204–207. DOI: 10.1016/0034-5288(91)90107-y.

Hostettler, I., Müller, J. and Hemphill, A. (2016) *In vitro* screening of the open-source Medicines for Malaria Venture Malaria Box reveals novel compounds with profound activities against *Theileria annulata* schizonts. *Antimicrobial Agents and Chemotherapy* 60(6), 3301–3308. DOI: 10.1128/AAC.02801-15.

Hudson, A.T., Randall, A.W., Fry, M., Ginger, C.D., Hill, B. *et al.* (1985) Novel anti-malarial hydroxynaphthoquinones with potent broad spectrum anti-protozoal activity. *Parasitology* 90(Pt 1), 45–55. DOI: 10.1017/s0031182000049003.

Hudson, A.T., Pether, M.J., Randall, A.W., Fry, M., Latter, V.S. *et al.* (1986) ChemInform abstract: *In vitro* activity of 2-cycloalkyl-3-hydroxy-1,4-naphthoquinones against *Theileria*, *Eimeria* and *Plasmodium* species. *Chemischer Informationsdienst* 17(52), 271–275. DOI: 10.1002/chin.198652144.

Keller, T.L., Zocco, D., Sundrud, M.S., Hendrick, M., Edenius, M. *et al.* (2012) Halofuginone and other febrifugine derivatives inhibit prolyl-tRNA synthetase. *Nature Chemical Biology* 8(3), 311–317. DOI: 10.1038/nchembio.790.

Kinabo, L.D.B. (1989) Pharmacology of the new antitheilerial drugs: Parvaquone, buparvaquone and halofuginone. *Veterinary Bulletin* 59, 961–968.

Kinabo, L.D.B. and Bogan, J.A. (1988) Parvaquone and buparvaquone: HPLC analysis and comparative pharmacokinetics in cattle. *Acta Tropica* 45, 87–94.

Malmquist, W.A., Nyindo, M.B.A. and Brown, C.G.D. (1970) East Coast fever: Cultivation *in vitro* of bovine spleen cell lines infected and transformed by *Theileria parva*. *Tropical Animal Health and Production* 2(3), 139–145. DOI: 10.1007/BF02359680.

Marsolier, J., Perichon, M., DeBarry, J.D., Villoutreix, B.O., Chluba, J. *et al.* (2015) *Theileria* parasites secrete a prolyl isomerase to maintain host leukocyte transformation. *Nature* 520(7547), 378–382. DOI: 10.1038/nature14044.

Mbwambo, H.A., Mkonyi, P.A. and Chua, R.B. (1987) Field evaluation of parvaquone against naturally occurring East Coast fever. *Veterinary Parasitology* 23(3–4), 161–168. DOI: 10.1016/0304-4017(87)90001-x.

Mbwambo, H.A., Sudi, F.F., Mkonyi, P.A., Mfinanga, J.M., Mella, E.S. *et al.* (2002) Comparative studies of the efficacy of parvaquone and parvaquone-plus-frusemide in the treatment of *Theileria parva* infection (East Coast fever) in cattle. *Veterinary Parasitology* 108(3), 195–205. DOI: 10.1016/s0304-4017(02)00195-4.

McColm, A.A. and McHardy, N. (1984) Evaluation of a range of antimicrobial agents against the parasitic protozoa, *Plasmodium falciparum*, *Babesia rodhaini* and *Theileria parva in vitro*. *Annals of Tropical Medicine and Parasitology* 78(4), 345–354. DOI: 10.1080/00034983.1984.11811831.

McHardy, N. (1978) *In vitro* studies on the action of menoctone and other compounds on *Theileria parva* and *T. annulata*. *Annals of Tropical Medicine and Parasitology* 72(6), 501–511. DOI: 10.1080/00034983.1978.11719354.

McHardy, N. and Rae, D.G. (1981) Treatment of stabilate-induced East Coast fever with menoctone. *Tropical Animal Health and Production* 13(4), 227–239. DOI: 10.1007/BF02237932.

McHardy, N. and Rae, D.G. (1982) Antitheilerial activity of the coccidiostat monensin. *Tropical Animal Health and Production* 14(1), 13–14. DOI: 10.1007/BF02281094.

McHardy, N. and Kiara, H.K. (1996) Super-infection with *Theileria parva* in calves previously infected with *Babesia bigemina* or *Anaplasma marginale*. In: *Proceedings of a Scientific Conference, National Veterinary Research Centre, Muguga, Kenya*, pp. 49–54.

McHardy, N. and Mercer, J.P. (1984) Bioassay of parvaquone in the serum of cattle infected with *Theileria parva* and treated with Clexon. *Kenya Veterinarian* 8, 9–14.

McHardy, N., Haigh, A.J.B. and Dolan, T.T. (1976) Chemotherapy of *Theileria parva* infection. *Nature* 261(5562), 698–699. DOI: 10.1038/261698a0.

McHardy, N. and Morgan, D.W.T. (1981) Studies *in vivo* and *in vitro* with 993C and halofuginone. In: Irvin, A.D., Cunningham, M.P. and Young, A.S. (eds) *Advances in the Control of Theileriosis*. Martinus Nijhoff Publishers, The Hague, The Netherlands, pp. 209–211.

McHardy, N., Hudson, A.T., Morgan, D.W.T., Rae, D.G. and Dolan, T.T. (1983) Activity of 10 naphthoquinones, including parvaquone (993C) and menoctone, in cattle artificially infected with *Theileria parva*. *Research in Veterinary Science* 35(3), 347–352.

McHardy, N., Wekbsa, L.S., Hudson, A.T. and Randall, A.W. (1985) Antitheilerial activity of BW720C (buparvaquone): A comparison with parvaquone. *Research in Veterinary Science* 39(1), 29–33. DOI: 10.1016/S0034-5288(18)31765-X.

McLaughlin, N.P., Evans, P. and Pines, M. (2014) The chemistry and biology of febrifugine and halofuginone. *Bioorganic & Medicinal Chemistry* 22(7), 1993–2004. DOI: 10.1016/j.bmc.2014.02.040.

Mhadhbi, M., Naouach, A., Boumiza, A., Chaabani, M.F., BenAbderazzak, S. *et al.* (2010) *In vivo* evidence for the resistance of *Theileria annulata* to buparvaquone. *Veterinary Parasitology* 169(3–4), 241–247. DOI: 10.1016/j.vetpar.2010.01.013.

Mhadhbi, M., Chaouch, M., Ajroud, K., Darghouth, M.A. and BenAbderrazak, S. (2015) Sequence polymorphism of cytochrome b gene in *Theileria annulata* Tunisian isolates and its association with buparvaquone treatment failure. *PLoS ONE* 10(6), e0129678. DOI: 10.1371/journal.pone.0129678.

Miao, J., Zhao, G., Wang, B., Du, Y., Li, Z. *et al.* (2020) Three point-mutations in cytochrome b confer resistance to trifloxystrobin in *Magnaporthe oryzae*. *Pest Management Science* 76(12), 4258–4267. DOI: 10.1002/ps.5990.

Minami, T., Nakano, T., Shimizu, S., Shimura, K., Fujinaga, T. *et al.* (1985) Efficacy of naphthoquinones and imidocarb dipropionate on *Theileria sergenti* infections in splenectomized calves. *The Japanese Journal of Veterinary Science* 47(2), 297–300. DOI: 10.1292/jvms1939.47.297.

Morgan, D.W.T. and McHardy, N. (1982) Comparison of the antitheilerial effect of wellcome 993C and halofuginone. *Research in Veterinary Science* 32(1), 84–88. DOI: 10.1016/S0034-5288(18)32443-3.

Mugera, G.M., Mworia, G.M. and Munyua, W.K. (1973) Treatment of East Coast fever with aureomycin. *Bulletin of Epizootic Diseases of Africa* 21(4), 501–505.

Muraguri, G.R., Kiara, H.K. and McHardy, N. (1999) Treatment of East Coast fever: A comparison of parvaquone and buparvaquone. *Veterinary Parasitology* 87(1), 25–37. DOI: 10.1016/s0304-4017(99)00154-5.

Muraguri, G.R., Ngumi, P.N., Wesonga, D., Ndungu, S.G., Wanjohi, K. *et al.* (2006) Clinical efficacy and plasma concentrations of two formulations of buparvaquone in cattle infected with East Coast fever (*Theileria parva* infection). *Research in Veterinary Science* 81, 119–126. DOI: 10.1016/j.rvsc.2005.09.012.

Musisi, F.L., Morgan, D.W.T. and Schels, H.F. (1985) Treatment of theileriosis with parvaquone in Zambia. *Veterinary Record* 117(13), 338–339. DOI: 10.1136/vr.117.13.338.

Neitz, W.O. (1953) Aureomycin in *Thieileria parva* infection. *Nature* 171(4340), 34–35. DOI: 10.1038/171034a0.

Neitz, W.O. (1957) Theileriosis, gonderioses and cytoxoonoses: A review. *Onderstepoort Journal of Veterinary Medicine* 27, 275–430.

Nixon, G.L., Moss, D.M., Shone, A.E., Lalloo, D.G., Fisher, N. *et al.* (2013) Antimalarial pharmacology and therapeutics of atovaquone. *The Journal of Antimicrobial Chemotherapy* 68(5), 977–985. DOI: 10.1093/jac/dks504.

Njau, B.C., Mkonyi, P.A., Mleche, W.C.H., Kitaly, J.I. and Maiseli, N.C. (1985) Treatment of field cases of East Coast fever with halofuginone lactate. *Tropical Animal Health and Production* 17(4), 193–200. DOI: 10.1007/BF02356976.

Nyagwange, J., Awino, E., Tijhaar, E., Svitek, N., Pelle, R. *et al.* (2019) Leveraging the Medicines for Malaria Venture malaria and pathogen boxes to discover chemical inhibitors of East Coast fever. *International Journal for Parasitology* 9, 80–86. DOI: 10.1016/j.ijpddr.2019.01.002.

Ortiz, D., Forquer, I., Boitz, J., Soysa, R., Filwiler, A. *et al.* (2016) Targeting the cytochrome bc1 complex of *Leishmania* parasites for discovery of novel drugs. *Antimicrobial Druga Chemotherapy* 60, 4972–4982. DOI: 10.1128/AAC.00850-16.

Salim, B., Chatanga, E., Jannot, G., Mossaad, E., Nakao, R. *et al.* (2019) Mutations in the TaPIN1 peptidyl prolyl isomerase gene in *Theileria annulata* parasites isolated in Sudan. *International Journal for Parasitology: Drugs and Drug Resistance* 11, 101–105. DOI: 10.1016/j.ijpddr.2019.11.001.

Schein, E. and Voigt, W.P. (1979) Chemotherapy of bovine theileriosis with halofuginone: Short communication. *Acta Tropica* 36(4), 391–394.

Sharifiyazdi, H., Namazi, F., Oryan, A., Shahriari, R. and Razavi, M. (2012) Point mutations in the *Theileria annulata* cytochrome b gene is associated with buparvaquone treatment failure. *Veterinary Parasitology* 187(3–4), 431–435. DOI: 10.1016/j.vetpar.2012.01.016.

Silverlås, C., Björkman, C. and Egenvall, A. (2009) Systematic review and meta-analyses of the effects of halofuginone against calf cryptosporidiosis. *Preventive Veterinary Medicine* 91(2–4), 73–84. DOI: 10.1016/j.prevetmed.2009.05.003.

Spooner, P.R. (1990) Oxytetracycline inhibition of mitochondrial protein synthesis in bovine lymphocytes infected with *Theileria parva* or stimulated by mitogen. *Parasitology* 101(3), 387–393. DOI: 10.1017/S0031182000060583.

Stewart, N.P., Vos, A.J., McHardy, N. and Standfast, N.F. (1990) Elimination of *Theileria buffeli* infections from cattle by concurrent treatment with buparvaquone and primaquine phosphate. *Tropical Animal Health and Production* 22(2), 116–122. DOI: 10.1007/BF02239836.

Uilenberg, G., Jongejan, F., Perie, N.M. and Franssen, F.F.J. (1980) Chimiotherapie des theilerioses bovines par un anticoccidien, l'halofuginone. *Revue d'elevage et de Medicine Veterinaire Pays Tropicaux* 33, 33–43.

Van Voorhis, W.C., Adams, J.H., Adelfio, R., Ahyong, V., Akabas, M.H. *et al.* (2016) Open source drug discovery with the Malaria Box compound collection for neglected diseases and beyond. *PLoS Pathogens* 12(7), e1005763. DOI: 10.1371/journal.ppat.1005763.

Villares, M., Lourenço, N., Berthelet, J., Lamotte, S., Regad, L. *et al.* (2022) Trifloxystrobin blocks the growth of *Theileria parasites* and is a promising drug to treat buparvaquone resistance. *Communications Biology* 5(1), 1253. DOI: 10.1038/s42003-022-03981-x.

Wanjohi, J.M., Muraguri, G.R., Rumberia, R.M., Kariuki, D.P. and McHardy, N. (1995) Chemotherapy of East Coast fever: Buparvaquone treatment of field cases occurring in Kikuyu and Limuru divisions of Kiambu district, Kenya. *East African Agricultural and Forestry Journal* 60(3), 131–135. DOI: 10.1080/00128325.1995.11663233.

Wilde, J.K.H. (1977) The control of *Theileriosis*. In: *Theileriosis. Report of a Workshop Held in Nairobi, Kenya*. ILRI (aka ILCA and ILRAD), Nairobi, Kenya, pp. 76–85.

Zaugg, J.L. and Lane, V.M. (1989) Evaluations of buparvaquone as a treatment for equine babesiosis (*Babesia equi*). *American Journal of Veterinary Research* 50(5), 782–785.

15 Biological Properties and Control of the Tick Vectors of *Theileria parva*

Maxime Madder*
Clinglobal, Tamarin, Mauritius

15.1 Introduction

The geographic distribution of East Coast fever (ECF), the disease caused by *Theileria parva*, is dictated by the distribution of the tick vectors, which in turn depends on climatic conditions and other factors that sustain their survival and reproduction. As discussed in Chapter 4 of this volume, the acute and fatal nature of ECF presents a significant challenge to efforts to control the disease. The commonly used approaches to prevent or control other infectious diseases, such as vaccination or therapeutics, have met with limited application for ECF (discussed in Chapters 12, 13 and 14 of this volume). Therefore, control of infestation by the tick vector remains the most widely used method for controlling ECF.

Effective tick control not only prevents the transmission of ECF but also helps in reducing other tick-borne diseases, promoting overall cattle health and safeguarding the economic well-being of farmers. Tackling the tick problem is therefore not just a matter of disease control; it is an issue of food security, economic stability and sustainable agriculture in some of the most vulnerable regions of the world.

This chapter briefly summarizes available information on the tick vector species and development of *T. parva* in the tick, and discusses the methods currently used to control ECF by prevention of tick infestation. Discussion of the use of acaricides includes consideration of the emerging problem of acaricide resistance.

15.2 The Tick Vector

15.2.1 General

The transmission of the protozoan parasite *T. parva* is intricately linked to the life cycle and feeding behaviour of the tick vector. Understanding the capacity of ticks to act as vectors for *T. parva* is critical in unravelling the complexities of ECF transmission and in developing effective control strategies. This capacity is not merely a consequence of the tick's susceptibility to infection by the parasite, but is also heavily influenced by the tick's feeding behaviour and developmental stages.

T. parva is transmitted trans-stadially, that is, infections acquired by feeding tick larvae and nymphs are transmitted to a new host, following moulting, by the nymphal and adult stages, respectively. The different stages of the tick vector, therefore, need to feed on different individuals of the same species to achieve transmission of the parasite.

*Corresponding author: Maxime.Madder@clinglobal.com

 East Coast Fever: The Disease, its Impact and Control (eds W.I. Morrison and P. Toye)
DOI: 10.1079/9781800626324.0015

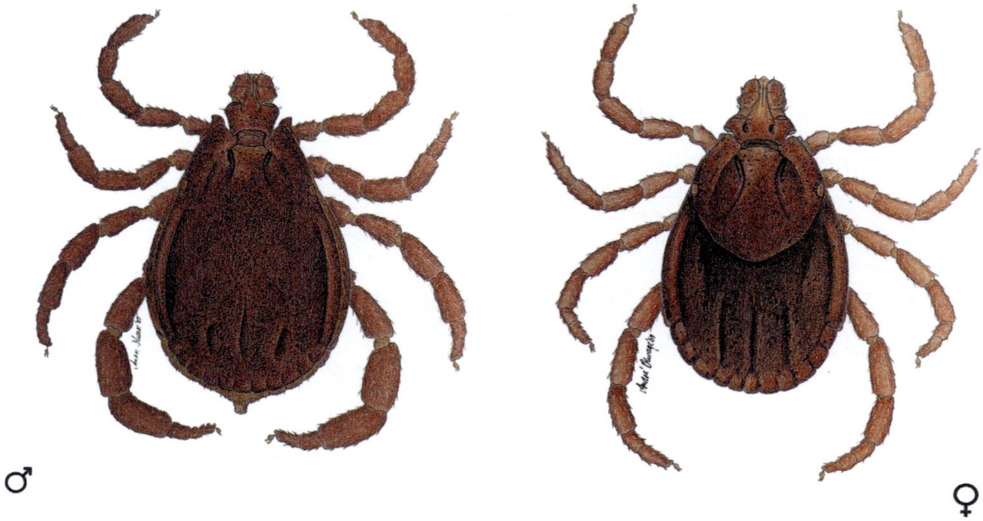

Fig. 15.1. *Rhipicephalus appendiculatus* ticks. (Reproduced with permission from Norval, 1994.)

15.2.2 Tick vector species

The principal vector of *T. parva*, *Rhipicephalus appendiculatus* (Fig. 15.1), is a three-host tick (i.e. the larvae, nymphs and adults all have a free-living phase and quest for a host) found throughout a large part of eastern and southern sub-Saharan Africa (Fig. 15.2).

A closely related tick species, *Rhipicephalus zambeziensis*, which is largely confined to southern Africa (see Chapter 6, Fig. 6.1, this volume), has also been shown experimentally to be a competent vector. Although there is evidence that it transmits the parasite in the field, its importance as a vector of disease is unclear. According to some authors, *R. zambeziensis* is implicated more in the transmission of Corridor disease, caused by buffalo-derived *T. parva*, rather than classical ECF. However, it is also associated with transmission of *Theileria taurotragi* and the bacterium *Ehrlichia bovis*, which cause benign bovine theileriosis and bovine ehrlichiosis, respectively (Walker *et al.*, 2003). Several other species of ticks can be infected with *T. parva* experimentally, but do not act as vectors of the parasite because the larval and nymphal stages feed on non-bovine hosts in the field.

Both *R. appendiculatus* and *R. zambeziensis* have a wide host range, feeding on several species of large and medium-sized ungulates, including buffalo. Among domestic species, cattle are the preferred hosts. The adult stages attach in large numbers to the ears (resulting in the tick frequently being referred to as the 'brown ear tick'), but are also found on other parts of the body. Larvae and nymphs show less of a preference for the ears but rather attach on the feet and legs (Walker *et al.*, 2003).

The geographic distribution of these tick species is influenced by climatic conditions, principally ambient temperature and humidity, and availability of suitable hosts. *R. zambeziensis* is found in hotter, drier areas in southern Africa, where there is limited overlap of its distribution with that of *R. appendiculatus*. Studies of the presence of the two *Rhipicephalus* species in Zimbabwe found that *R. appendiculatus* was present in areas with an annual rainfall of 500–2000 mm and a mean annual temperature of less than 22.5°C, whereas the areas populated by *R. zambeziensis* had annual rainfalls of 500–700 mm and a mean annual temperature that exceeded 20°C (Norval *et al.*, 1982). Experimental studies of survival of the two species of ticks under conditions of different temperature and humidity have provided further confirmation of differences in optimal conditions for survival of the tick species (Madder *et al.*, 2005).

Populations of *R. appendiculatus* in tropical regions and more southern temperate areas display different behavioural characteristics. In tropical regions, a long rainy season favours

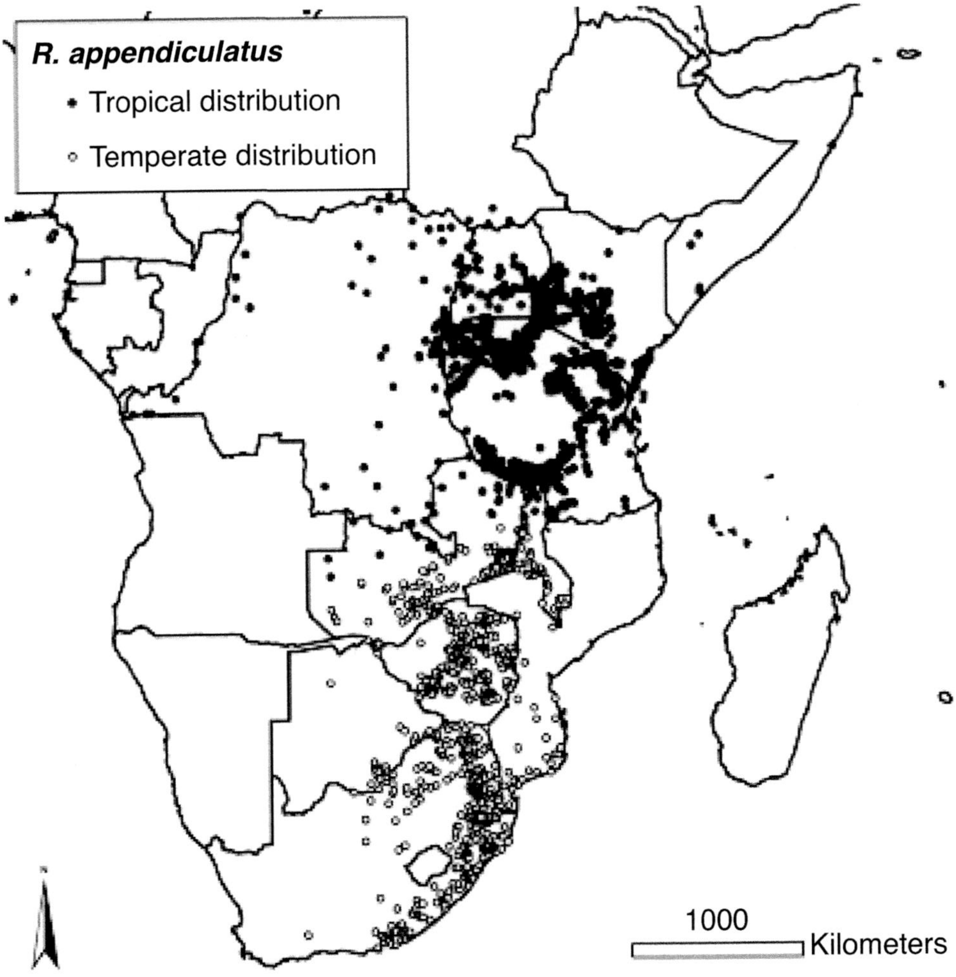

Fig. 15.2. The recorded distribution of *R. appendiculatus* in sub-Saharan Africa. (Reproduced with permission from Leta *et al.*, 2013.)

survival and reproduction throughout the year, whereas in southern temperate areas, ticks must survive long periods of unfavourable conditions necessitating dormancy expressed as behavioural diapause in the unfed adult stage (Madder *et al.*, 2002).

Mathematical modelling, using ecological and climatic parameters that influence the suitability of habitat to support *R. appendiculatus*, has been employed to develop an ecoclimatic index to predict the distribution of this tick species in Africa (Lessard *et al.*, 1990; Perry *et al.*, 1990). These studies demonstrated a close correlation between the ecoclimatic index and the recorded distribution of *R. appendiculatus* in much of eastern and southern Africa, albeit including some areas where the tick was not present. However, the model also predicted suitable habitat in a large coastal strip of West Africa extending from Cameroon to northern Angola, where there is no evidence that the tick has ever been present. The low density of cattle and wild ungulate species in this area may have rendered it unsuitable to sustain the tick.

High-resolution predictive mapping for *R. appendiculatus* has also been performed

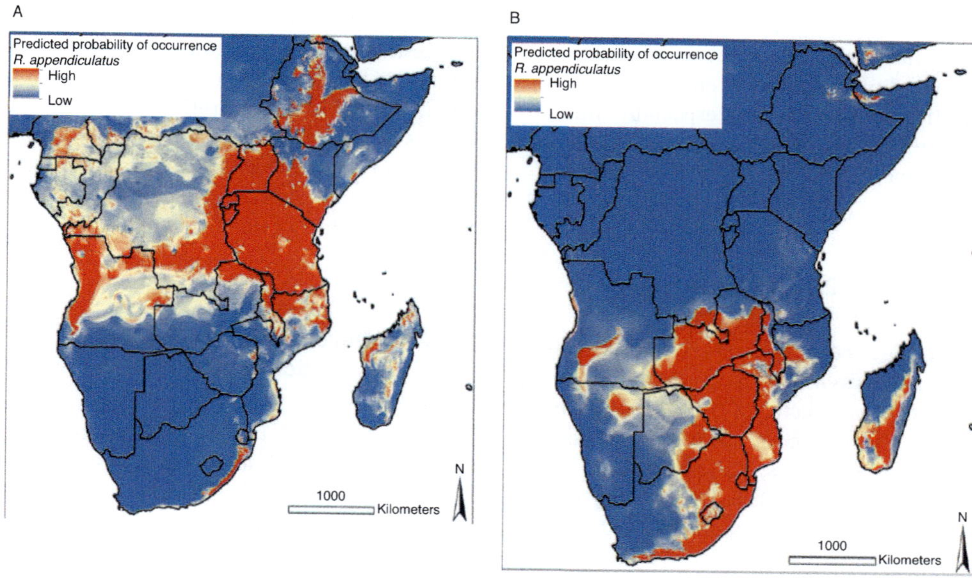

Fig. 15.3. Predicted habitat suitability *for R. appendiculatus* in the Horn of Africa based on tropical (A) and temperate (B) occurrence records. (Reproduced with permission from Leta *et al*., 2013.)

for regions in the Horn of Africa (Leta *et al.*, 2013). The predicted habitat suitability for *R. appendiculatus*, calculated based on its tropical distribution in sub-Saharan Africa, showed that highly suitable habitat is found in the highlands of Ethiopia and some areas in southern Eritrea (Fig. 15.3A). In contrast, the use of data from the temperate populations showed very few areas of suitable habitat, apart from small areas in north-eastern Ethiopia and north-western Somalia (Fig. 15.3B). The difference between the model based on temperate and that based on tropical distribution might be related to the population characteristics and specifically to the difference in diapausing phenology, as discussed above.

The absence of *R. appendiculatus* in areas where its suitability was predicted highlights the importance of active monitoring, especially in those areas where introduction is possible by human migration, cattle trade movement or importation by road or air. Leta *et al.* (2013) proposed that spread of the tick into Ethiopia has been prevented by the large area of unsuitable habitat between Ethiopia and the endemic areas of South Sudan and Kenya. Any introduction of the tick and parasite into Ethiopia would be 'catastrophic', given the exceptionally high numbers of cattle there (see Chapter 2 of this volume). In 2003 and 2004, ECF decimated a large proportion of the cattle population on the Grand Comore island, off the east coast of Africa, because of live cattle importations from Tanzania without adequate quarantine (De Deken *et al.*, 2007). Multilocus genotyping revealed that the *T. parva* parasites isolated in the Comoros were similar to those in the Muguga cocktail vaccine used in Tanzania to immunize cattle. The findings indicated but did not establish unequivocally that ECF reached the Comoros through imported livestock that had been infected in Tanzania, suggested by the authors as resulting from exposure to ticks that had fed on cattle vaccinated with the Muguga cocktail. Another striking example of the introduction of ticks as a result of cattle importation without proper quarantine has been described in West Africa, where *Rhipicephalus microplus* was introduced on live cattle originating from Brazil in the beginning of the 21st century and has now colonized most of the West African countries (Madder *et al.*, 2007, 2012; Adakal *et al.*, 2013; Lontsi-Demano *et al.*, 2020). It can be concluded that the geographic distribution of ticks is influenced by a combination of host mobility, variations in environmental and climatic conditions, and especially human-mediated factors, resulting in ongoing shifts in their range.

15.2.3 Tick feeding

The feeding behaviour of ixodid ticks is a complex process that facilitates both its survival and its role as a vector of pathogens. *R. appendiculatus* attaches to its hosts and feeds over a period of several days. The attachment period for *R. appendiculatus* feeding on cattle ranges from 6 to 12 days for adult females, 4 to 7 days for nymphs and 3 to 6 days for larvae. Unlike these stages, which feed continuously and engorge over several days, adult males exhibit intermittent feeding. They attach to the host for shorter periods to consume blood and then detach, while remaining on the host, to search for mates. This behaviour can span the entire time they remain on the host, which may last up to 2 months (Sonenshine and Roe, 2014).

The feeding process begins when the tick locates a suitable host, guided by sensory cues detected through Haller's organ. These cues include heat, carbon dioxide and host odours. Once on the host, the tick selects an attachment site. Ticks become firmly attached to host skin by secreting substances that harden to form a 'cement' around the embedded mouthparts of the tick. Saliva secreted into the feeding site contains anticoagulants, immunomodulators and enzymes that suppress the host's immune response, prevent clotting and create an environment conducive to prolonged feeding. The composition of *R. appendiculatus* saliva has not been examined in any detail. However, studies of saliva of related tick species (reviewed in Binnington and Kemp, 1980; Šimo *et al.*, 2017) have identified a wide range of activities, including molecules that inhibit vasoconstriction, platelet adherence and blood clotting, as well as components that inhibit host inflammation and immune responses and ablate pain and itching at the tick feeding site. These salivary components are also crucial for the transmission of pathogens like *T. parva*. There is an initial period of slow feeding followed, in the last few days, by ingestion of larger volumes of blood, which result in up to a 200-fold increase in the starting weight of the tick. Concentration of the ingested blood is achieved by excretion of water from digestion of ingested blood into the saliva of the tick. Secretion of ions also ensures retention of osmolarity of the tick haemolymph.

15.2.4 Development of *T. parva* in the tick vectors

The development of *T. parva* in its mammalian and arthropod hosts is discussed in Chapter 3 of this volume and will only be briefly summarized here. Piroplasms ingested by feeding ticks are released following lysis of infected erythrocytes in the tick gut and differentiate within a few days to form distinct morphological forms considered to represent micro- and macro-gametes. Fusion of pairs of gametes results in formation of zygotes, which, following invasion of the gut epithelium, undergo meiosis to generate (haploid) kinetes (Mehlhorn *et al.*, 1978; Fawcett *et al.*, 1982; Mehlhorn and Shein, 1984). The motile kinetes enter the haemolymph and migrate to the salivary glands, where they invade salivary gland epithelial cells. In nymphal ticks, kinete production occurs just after they moult to the adult stage, usually about 3 weeks after detachment. The parasites undergo sporogony in the salivary gland cells (Fawcett *et al.*, 1982). However, development of sporogony is usually suspended until the ticks commence feeding on a new host. Tick feeding provokes rapid nuclear division of the parasites within a complex multinucleate labyrinthine syncytium, which after 3–5 days undergoes fission to generate the uninucleate sporozoites that are released into the saliva. Thus, there is a delay of several days between tick attachment and release of sporozoites into the bovine host (Purnell and Joyner, 1968; Shaw and Young, 1995). Although there is experimental evidence that sporogony can occur in ticks incubated at high temperatures (28°C or 37°C; Young *et al.*, 1984) or placed on pasture where maximal monthly temperatures are 27–32°C (Young *et al.*, 1987), it is unclear whether this is of relevance in naturally infected ticks in the field.

The *T. parva* genome is haploid throughout its life cycle in the mammalian host but undergoes diploid and tetraploid stages in the tick (Gauer *et al.*, 1995), during which sexual recombination can occur between genotypically different strains of the parasite. The occurrence of sexual recombination during development of the tick has been confirmed experimentally by demonstrating frequent recombination events in parasites obtained from ticks fed on animals co-infected with two genotypically distinct parasite isolates (Katzer *et al.*, 2011; Henson *et al.*, 2012).

The correlation between the level of piroplasm parasitaemia in the calf at times of nymphal detachment and the subsequent prevalence and abundance of infection (i.e. the proportion of ticks infected and the number of infected salivary gland acini, respectively) in adult ticks is non-linear, as tick mortality seems to increase with increasing levels of infection in the ticks (Watt and Walker, 2000). This non-linear relationship of piroplasm levels and tick infectivity suggests that factors beyond the initial parasite load influence the development of infection within the tick's salivary glands. Moreover, the finding of increased mortality in ticks with higher levels of infectivity indicates that heavy parasite burdens impose a cost on tick survival. This complex interplay between parasite load, infection development and tick survival emphasizes the importance of considering these dynamics in understanding the transmission of *T. parva*.

Climatic conditions influence the duration of the life cycle. Studies of infected ticks in an experimental paddock in Kenya showed that the minimum time required for transmission of infection acquired by nymphal ticks was 30 days during the warm season but 62 days during the cold season, where the mean temperature differed by 4°C (Young *et al.*, 1981). In southern Africa, adult *R. appendiculatus* ticks have a seasonal diapausing behaviour, that is, ticks overwinter in a low metabolic state of suspended development (Randolph, 1997). Eastern African *R. appendiculatus* ticks do not exhibit diapause when exposed to a South African environment (Madder *et al.*, 2002). During diapause, adult ticks delay host-seeking and feeding.

Several authors also report vectorial competence of *R. appendiculatus* and *R. zambeziensis* ticks for different *T. parva* strains (Tempia, 1997; Ochanda *et al.*, 1998; Odongo *et al.*, 2009). It was found that southern African *R. appendiculatus* showed a lower infection rate compared to eastern African ticks when fed at the same time on cattle infected with eastern or southern African strains of *T. parva*. In addition, at least some southern African *T. parva* strains are significantly less virulent compared to eastern African strains. In Zimbabwe, where virulent *T. parva* causing ECF was eliminated in the mid-20th century, the remaining parasites were less virulent (Uilenberg, 1999), which allowed immunization of cattle with live sporozoites, using the Boleni isolate, without the need for tetracyclines (Kanhai *et al.*, 1997). A study that compared the virulence of a Zambian isolate (Chitongo) with the eastern African Muguga strain demonstrated that the former was significantly less virulent both *in vivo* (longer pre-patent phase, lower parasitosis and less mortality) and *in vitro* (4-day longer pre-infection time). To eliminate any bias by dose-dependent reactions, an *in vitro* standardized dose was used in these experiments to initiate infection (Tindih *et al.*, 2010). However, further studies are required to determine whether or not this is a general feature of Zambian *T. parva*.

The difference in vector competence among the geographically distinct *R. appendiculatus* populations and the virulence of the *T. parva* strains most likely evolved as a result of the environmental characteristics in the different geographies. In eastern Africa, *R. appendiculatus* shows a low degree of diapause, high tick numbers on cattle and several generations of ticks throughout the year, with all stages feeding simultaneously. The disease is transmitted by both nymphs and adults. The high tick numbers throughout the year facilitate the survival of the parasite in the ticks because the parasite in animals with clinically apparent infection will most probably be picked up by several larvae and nymphs before the animal becomes a carrier or dies. The relative resistance of local indigenous cattle breeds (zebu-type) to *T. parva* infections allows many animals to survive infections with virulent stocks and become carriers. In this situation, ECF can be present throughout the year. In southern Africa with diapausing tick populations, tick instars have well-defined feeding periods with minimal overlap in feeding. In this region, almost no transmission of infection acquired by larvae occurs because larvae appear to be very poor at picking up the parasite from carrier animals (Norval *et al.*, 1992; Tempia, 1997), which are the main source of infection. The occurrence of the disease is therefore seasonal and normally coincides with the rainy season, when adult ticks feed. Survival of the parasite in the ticks over the diapause period is rather doubtful because (i) the abundance of the parasite in adults that had fed as nymphs on carrier animals is quite low, and (ii) because of the long period of diapause of the adults, the survival of the parasites in the ticks is likely to decline. Survival of the parasite in the host occurs mainly in the form of a carrier status in cattle (mainly sanga-type), which favours the selection of less virulent *T. parva* stocks as sanga-type cattle are more susceptible to *T. parva* infection compared to zebu-type.

15.2.5 Survival of *R. appendiculatus* and *T. parva* in the field

Ticks can survive on pasture and retain infection without feeding for prolonged periods of time. As early as 1911, Theiler reported that in South Africa ticks harbouring infection with *T. parva* could survive for over a year (Theiler, 1911). Two studies conducted in Kenya involving introduction of *R. appendiculatus* ticks into double-fenced paddocks previously free of ticks provided detailed information on the survival of the tick and infection with *T. parva* under field conditions (Young *et al.*, 1983; Newson *et al.*, 1984). Newson and colleagues (1984) examined survival of different stages of the tick. Most larvae were found to survive for 6–7 months but showed a rapid decline in numbers over the subsequent 4 months; maximal numbers of nymphs were maintained for about 1 year, with a decline in the population over the subsequent 6 months; maximal numbers of adults were maintained for about 18 months but declined over the next 6 months. In the study by Young *et al.* (1983), similar results were obtained for survival of adult ticks. In addition, by feeding ticks collected at different times from the paddock on susceptible cattle, they demonstrated consistent transmission of lethal infection by ticks that had fed up to 1 year previously, but thereafter transmission was detected only intermittently and resulted in mild infections. The study by Young *et al.* (1983) was conducted in climatic conditions that were considered near optimal for *R. appendiculatus*. In a subsequent study, the same researchers (Young *et al.*, 1987) examined ticks infected experimentally with *T. parva* and then placed in nylon mesh containers on pasture in the Trans-Mara Division of Kenya, where the mean maximal monthly temperature ranged from 28 to 33°C. Over 80% of the ticks survived up to 10 months, after which their viability gradually declined. High levels of infection with *T. parva* were retained for 7 months and subsequently declined. However, ticks that had fed for 294–439 days all produced lethal infections when fed on susceptible cattle.

While the studies discussed above provide valuable information on the longevity of infections with *T. parva* in the tick, it is important to bear in mind that they were conducted with experimentally infected ticks, which have a high incidence and level of infection. The incidence of infection in naturally infected ticks in endemically infected areas is usually less than 3%, and many of the infected ticks contain only one or two infected salivary gland acini. Therefore, the duration of survival of the parasite in the field is likely to be significantly shorter. In any event, very few of the ticks in areas stocked by cattle or other host species are likely to remain unfed for the prolonged periods of time tested in these experimental studies.

Advancing knowledge about the survival strategies of *T. parva* in its tick vector provides critical leverage points for controlling ECF. By focusing on the parasite's dependence on the tick for its life-cycle progression, researchers can devise novel, sustainable and targeted approaches to curb this economically devastating disease.

15.2.6 Susceptibility of hosts to tick infestation

The burdens of ticks feeding on buffalo are much lower than those found on cattle (Khan *et al.*, 2013) due to several key biological, behavioural and ecological factors. Buffalo have evolved stronger innate resistance to ticks compared to domestic cattle (Akhtar *et al.*, 2011). Their immune system reacts more aggressively to tick infestations, leading to rapid inflammatory responses that impair tick feeding. Studies have shown that buffalo develop localized skin reactions that cause ticks to detach before completing their feeding cycle, reducing overall tick burden (Benitez *et al.*, 2012).

Bos indicus cattle generally show greater resistance to tick infestation than *B. taurus* animals (Roberts, 1968), and infestation in cross-bred cattle decreases proportionately with the fraction of *B. taurus* genetic composition of the animal (Perotto *et al.*, 2025). This difference between *B. taurus* and *B. indicus*, which has been studied most thoroughly with the one-host tick *R. microplus*, is genetically determined and is due predominantly to superior acquired resistance in *B. indicus* animals, as the levels of tick infestation are initially similar in naïve animals of each type (Wagland, 1978; Piper *et al.*, 2009). The relative resistance manifests as a decrease in the proportion of ticks that can complete feeding due to acquisition of partial immunity following initial tick exposure (Roberts, 1968). *Bos indicus* cattle carry 10–20% of the numbers of ticks carried by *B. taurus* (Jonsson *et al.*, 2014) and show superior resistance to the tick-borne diseases babesiosis and anaplasmosis (Bock *et al.*, 1997). However, given that severe ECF can be caused by a single infected tick (see Chapter 7 of this volume), the degree of resistance to ticks shown by *B. indicus* cattle does not prevent infection with *T. parva* and therefore does not obviate the need for disease control measures.

15.3 Control of Tick Infestation

15.3.1 General

The tick, *R. appendiculatus*, plays a central role in the epidemiology of ECF, as it serves as the exclusive vector of *T. parva* allowing transmission between cattle. Managing the tick population is therefore a cornerstone of ECF control. Tick-control strategies aim to reduce the level of infestation of cattle with *R. appendiculatus*, thereby minimizing the transmission of *T. parva*. These strategies encompass a range of interventions, including chemical acaricides, biological control, breeding for tick-resistant cattle and environmental management to disrupt tick habitats.

15.3.2 Chemical control

Since the early 20th century, the control of disease caused by *T. parva* has relied predominantly on prevention of infestation of cattle by the tick vector by application of acaricides. The first acaricide used to control *R. appendiculatus* in southern Africa was an arsenic compound introduced from Australia, where it was used to control *Boophilus microplus* ticks (referred to as 'blue ticks' and now reclassified as *R. microplus*), which transmit babesiosis (Dolan, 1999). Although it was successful for these one-host ticks, arsenic compounds were too toxic to be applied at the short intervals required to control three-host ticks like *R. appendiculatus* in southern Africa (Norval *et al.*, 1992).

In the following decades, a variety of chemical compounds were developed, including organochlorines (1945), organophosphates (1955), amitraz (1975), synthetic pyrethroids (1978), macrocyclic lactones (1981), fluazuron (1994) and fipronil (1995) (Gallina *et al.*, 2024; FAO, 2025). Most recently, isoxazolines have been developed and brought to the market for the control of cattle ticks in South America and Australia, especially to control *R. microplus/australis* (Coopers, 2025; MSD, 2025). Although very effective against one-host ticks, this new class of acaricides has not reached the market to control ticks on cattle in low- and middle-income countries (LMIC) in Africa because of its long withdrawal period in meat-producing animals (about 3 months) and restriction of use in female cattle which are producing or may in the future produce milk or milk products for human consumption. In the absence of established withdrawal periods and residue limits for dairy products, off-label use of acaricides carries a significant public health risk.

The development of new acaricides is a cornerstone of modern efforts to control tick populations and mitigate the diseases they transmit, particularly to address the increasing prevalence of acaricide resistance. However, the process of bringing a novel acaricide to market is fraught with economic and scientific challenges, primarily stemming from high costs of research and development, and market limitations. These factors collectively shape the trajectory of innovation in the field, underscoring the need for strategic investments and interdisciplinary approaches to overcome these obstacles.

15.3.3 The classes of acaricides and methods of application

The principal chemical groups used to control ticks on cattle include organophosphates, synthetic pyrethroids, amidines, macrocyclic lactones, insect growth regulators, phenylpyrazoles and the newer isoxazoline compounds (Table 15.1).

15.3.3.1 Organophosphates (OPs)

The OPs, such as chlorpyrifos and coumaphos, were among the first acaricides introduced for tick control. These compounds act by inhibiting acetylcholinesterase, leading to the accumulation of acetylcholine in synapses and sustained nerve

Table 15.1. Classes of acaricides commonly used to control tick infestation of cattle.

Acaricide class	Common application methods	Mode of action	API[a] used for tick control in cattle
Organophosphates	Dip, spray, pour-on, ear-tags	Inhibit acetylcholinesterase → accumulation of acetylcholine → neuromuscular paralysis	chlorfenvinphos chlorpyrifos coumaphos
Synthetic pyrethroids	Dip, spray, pour-on	Modify sodium channel gating → repetitive nerve firing → paralysis	cyfluthrin cypermethrin (=alphacypermethrin) deltamethrin flumethrin permethrin
Formamidines	Dip, spray	Octopamine receptor agonist → nervous system disruption and death	amitraz cymiazole
Phenylpyrazoles	Pour-on	Block GABA (Gamma-aminobutyric acid)-gated chloride channels → uncontrolled neuronal activity	fipronil
Insect growth regulators (IGRs)	Pour-on, feed additive	Disrupt tick development by mimicking/inhibiting hormones (e.g. juvenile hormone analogues)	fluazuron
Macrocyclic lactones	Injection, pour-on	Bind glutamate-gated chloride channels → paralysis and death	abamectin doramectin eprinomectin ivermectin moxidectin
Isoxazolines	Pour-on	Block GABA- and glutamate-gated chloride channels → hyperexcitation → death	fluralaner

[a]Active pharmaceutical ingredient.

stimulation. OPs are typically applied through dip tanks, spray races or hand sprays. Despite their initial effectiveness, resistance is now observed, and concerns remain regarding their environmental impact and operator safety.

15.3.3.2 Synthetic pyrethroids (SPs)

SPs, including cypermethrin and flumethrin, target voltage-gated sodium channels, causing prolonged depolarization and paralysis of the tick. These compounds are most commonly administered via pour-on formulations, hand spraying or dipping. Although they were initially highly effective and relatively safe, resistance has become common, often due to metabolic cross-resistance with OPs.

15.3.3.3 Amidines

Amidines, with amitraz being the principal representative, function as octopamine receptor agonists, disrupting the tick's nervous system and leading to detachment and death. These are applied similarly to OPs and SPs, often as pour-on or hand sprays. While amitraz has a different mode of action than other acaricides, resistance has increasingly been reported, often associated with behavioural changes in ticks. These changes include repellency, disorientation or hyperactivity as the compounds act primarily on octopamine receptors in the nervous system of ticks.

15.3.3.4 Macrocyclic lactones (MLs)

MLs, such as ivermectin and doramectin, act systemically by enhancing the permeability of glutamate-gated chloride channels, resulting in flaccid paralysis. These compounds are typically administered as injectables, oral drenches or pour-ons. MLs are also active against internal parasites, which has led to their frequent use and, consequently, the development of resistance, especially in *R. microplus* populations but to a lesser extent in *R. appendiculatus* populations (Evans *et al.*, 2024).

15.3.3.5 Insect growth regulators (IGRs)

IGRs, particularly fluazuron, exert their effect by inhibiting chitin synthesis, disrupting the development and moulting of immature tick stages. These compounds are applied topically, most commonly in pour-on formulations. While IGRs are not effective against adult ticks, their role in reducing larval populations makes them valuable in integrated tick management strategies.

15.3.3.6 Phenylpyrazoles

Phenylpyrazoles, such as fipronil, function as antagonists of GABA-gated chloride channels, resulting in uncontrolled neural excitation and death. Although widely used in companion animals, their use in livestock is limited due to residue concerns and regulatory restrictions. However, they represent an alternative class with a distinct mode of action.

15.3.3.7 Isoxazilines

The most recent addition to tick-control arsenals is the isoxazoline class, including compounds such as fluralaner and afoxolaner. These molecules inhibit both GABA- and glutamate-gated chloride channels, producing strong acaricidal effects with high specificity for arthropods. Currently used in companion animals via oral administration, isoxazolines are under evaluation for use in livestock in Africa. As mentioned above, they have been registered in Australia and Brazil for cattle but with a long withdrawal period in meat-producing animals and prohibited use in dairy animals. Notably, there is no reported cross-resistance between isoxazolines and older acaricide classes.

In conclusion, the successful management of *R. appendiculatus* requires a deep understanding of the pharmacological properties and application methods of available acaricide classes. Given the pervasive issue of resistance, integrated tick management strategies, including acaricide rotation, targeted application and non-chemical approaches, are essential to preserve efficacy and support sustainable cattle production.

15.4 Acaricide Resistance

15.4.1 General

The emergence of resistance to several acaricide classes presents a serious challenge to

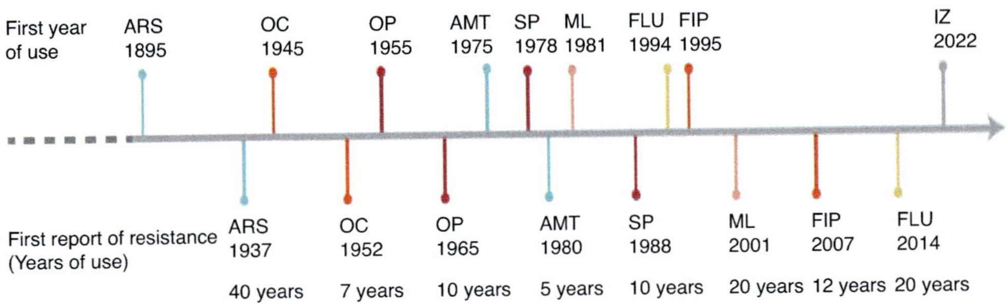

Note: AMT: amitraz, ARS: arsenicals, FLU: fluazuron, FIP: fipronil; IZ: Isoxazolines, ML: Macrocyclic lactones, OC: organochlorines, OP: organophosphates, SP: synthetic pyrethroids.

Fig. 15.4. History of the initial reports of resistant ticks following commercialization of chemical acaricide class or its representative. Compiled from data in George *et al.*, 2004; Rodriguez-Vivas *et al.*, 2012; Agwunobi *et al.*, 2021; Obaid *et al.*, 2022.

sustainable control of ticks and the diseases they transmit. Acaricide resistance has emerged as one of the most significant driving forces behind the demand for new tick-control solutions. As depicted in Fig. 15.4, over decades of intensive use, resistance to widely utilized acaricide classes such as organophosphates, pyrethroids, and amidines has become a pervasive problem (FAO, 2025).

Ticks have evolved complex resistance mechanisms, including target site insensitivity, enhanced detoxification pathways and behavioural adaptations that reduce exposure to chemicals. This resistance undermines the efficacy of existing products, forcing livestock owners to use higher doses or more frequent applications, which exacerbates environmental impacts and increases production costs. The global agricultural sector, particularly in LMIC where livestock production is central to livelihoods, is the most heavily affected by these challenges. Resistance not only reduces productivity by allowing higher tick burdens but also elevates the risk of tick-borne disease outbreaks, compounding economic losses.

Despite the pressing need for alternatives, the high costs and protracted timelines of acaricide development remain formidable barriers. Bringing a new acaricide to market requires significant investment in discovery, formulation, testing and regulatory compliance. Initial stages involve extensive screening of chemical libraries or natural products to identify candidates with acaricidal activity, followed by validation of efficacy across different tick species and life stages. Advances in genomics and molecular biology have expanded the pool of potential targets, but this has also increased the complexity and costs associated with target validation and compound optimization. Moreover, the development process must account for environmental safety, non-target effects and compatibility with integrated pest management systems, adding further layers of scrutiny.

Regulatory requirements represent another major economic hurdle. In most jurisdictions, acaricides are classified as pesticides, subjecting them to rigorous safety and environmental assessments before approval. These evaluations are designed to ensure that products pose minimal risks to human health, animal welfare and ecosystems. The regulatory landscape often demands lengthy and resource-intensive studies, which can discourage investment from companies, especially smaller firms with limited financial resources. The relatively small market for acaricides compared to pharmaceuticals for human use further compounds the challenge. Most demand for acaricides arises from regions with limited purchasing power, such as sub-Saharan Africa and parts of Asia and Latin America, where the livestock industry forms the backbone of rural economies. For manufacturers, this translates into a lower return on investment, reducing the incentive to develop innovative products.

Examination of available resistance data for *R. appendiculatus*, determined mainly from use of *in vitro* bioassays such as the Larval Packet Test (LPT), reveals that resistance has been identified for several acaricide classes, although, in comparison to the one-host tick *R. microplus*, it appears to be more limited. Studies performed by Evans and colleagues (Evans *et al.*, 2024) demonstrated medium to high levels of resistance to chlorfenvinphos and amitraz in stocks of *R. appendiculatus* from Tanzania and Uganda, and, in the latter stocks, medium levels of resistance to ivermectin were also detected. Most strains of *R. appendiculatus* were susceptible to alpha-cypermethrin. Overall, based on the bioassays, no resistance was detected for fipronil and a very low degree of resistance to ivermectin. The long withdrawal period of fipronil and the high cost of fipronil-based pour-ons might limit its use and therefore development of resistance. Also for macrocyclic lactones like ivermectin, the higher cost compared to acaricide sprays might have affected the frequency of use. Previous reports from western Uganda (Vudriko *et al.*, 2016; Miyama *et al.*, 2020), Benin (Adehan *et al.*, 2016) and Tanzania (Nagagi *et al.*, 2020) confirm these findings related to acaricide resistance and frequency of use.

In vivo studies strategically designed to consider the ticks' predilection sites and tick attachment cues enabled a comprehensive assessment of acaricidal efficacy at different sites of acaricide application at multiple time points following treatment or tick challenge (Evans *et al.*, 2024). The authors showed that the route of administration and dosage, particularly for pour-on formulations, emerged as critical factors influencing efficacy. Direct application of acaricides to the ears produced more rapid tick knock-down for *R. appendiculatus*, whereas applying the product as a dorsal stripe enhanced residual activity. Although substantially more resource-intensive and time-consuming than *in vitro* assays, *in vivo* evaluations offer significantly deeper insights into product performance under realistic biological and behavioural conditions.

Up-to-date, isoxazoline-based formulations for control of ticks in large production animals in Africa have not been registered, except for the control of poultry mites in South Africa by fluralaner-based products. Isoxazolines have been tested *in vivo* against *R. appendiculatus*. Recently isolated field tick strains from eastern Africa showed a moderately higher level of tolerance to fluralaner compared to the fully susceptible reference isolate. As no selection pressure could have caused this finding, it is an important factor to consider in future acaricide control options (Evans *et al.*, 2024).

The availability of compounds with distinct modes of action for use in rotation is critical to effective resistance management. However, the high financial burden associated with developing compounds with novel modes of action, coupled with increasingly stringent regulatory frameworks driven by environmental concerns, and the frequent withdrawal of existing acaricides, continues to narrow the range of currently accessible and future tick-control options (De Rouck *et al.*, 2023).

15.4.2 Bioassays used to detect resistance

Acaricide resistance is a growing global concern, with significant implications for the control of tick populations and the management of tick-borne diseases in livestock and humans. Accurate and reliable detection of resistance is critical for guiding control strategies, monitoring resistance trends and informing the development of new acaricides. Bioassays, which directly assess the susceptibility of ticks to acaricidal compounds, remain the gold standard for detecting and quantifying resistance. Bioassays are experimental methods that measure the biological response of ticks to varying concentrations of an acaricide, the phenotypic resistance. They provide a quantitative means to assess the susceptibility or resistance of tick populations, typically expressed as lethal concentrations (LC50 or LC90) or the percentage of mortality at a given concentration. Resistance is identified when mortality rates are significantly lower than those observed in a susceptible reference population. In contrast, genotypic resistance to acaricides is measured by detecting genetic mutations or markers that are known to confer resistance to specific classes of acaricides. The phenotypic and genotypic assays can provide different types of information which, when combined, can give a better view of the observed and potential resistance of the ticks or future threats if mutations are already observed genetically but not expressed in the phenotype, especially when dealing with recessive mutations. In addition, resistance of tick populations of neighbouring farms might be completely different and most likely are guided by the use of acaricides on that farm. Sampling strategies are key but not always easy to determine.

The FAO has recently published updated *Guidelines for Sustainable Tick Control and Acaricide Resistance Management in Livestock*, summarizing different bioassays (FAO, 2025). Although mainly related to the one-host tick *R. microplus*, these bioassays also offer opportunities to evaluate resistance in two- and three-host tick species. In addition, protocols for tick sampling and available bioassays suitable for detecting acaricide resistance in livestock ticks are described in detail in this technical documentation ('Diagnosis and monitoring of acaricide resistance', FAO, 2025, pp.1–44).

There are several bioassays commonly used to detect and measure acaricide resistance in ticks, each with specific applications, depending on the tick life-cycle stage and the type of acaricide.

15.4.2.1 The larval packet test (LPT)

The LPT, established by Stone and Haydock (1962), is one of the most widely adopted methods and is considered the gold standard by the FAO. In this assay, tick larvae are placed inside packets made of filter paper that has been treated with various concentrations of an acaricide. After 24 hours of exposure, mortality is assessed, providing a clear picture of resistance levels based on dose-response. The complete process typically requires approximately 6 weeks. LPT protocols are available for all major acaricide classes, except insect growth regulators (IGRs) such as fluazuron, which disrupt the moulting process, a biological event not assessed within the LPT framework.

15.4.2.2 The larval immersion test (LIT)

The LIT, initially developed by Shaw (1966) and later refined by Sabatini *et al.* (2001), involves immersing tick larvae in acaricide solutions within microcentrifuge tubes (m-LIT). This method demonstrates enhanced sensitivity for detecting resistance to MLs when compared to the LPT (Klafke *et al.*, 2006; Klafke *et al.*, 2012). It is similar to the LPT in that the assay duration spans approximately 6 weeks, from tick collection to mortality assessment, and it is also unsuitable for evaluating resistance to moulting inhibitors such as fluazuron.

15.4.2.3 The adult immersion test (AIT)

The AIT, described by Drummond *et al.* (1973), is applied to engorged adult female ticks to evaluate *in vitro* acaricidal efficacy. The assay focuses on measuring reproductive parameters, particularly reductions in oviposition and egg viability, following exposure to acaricides. Results are typically obtained within 2 weeks post-treatment. AIT can be conducted using either dose-response protocols or discriminating concentrations. Although more demanding in terms of sample size, AIT remains the only validated method for diagnosing resistance to certain IGRs, notably fluazuron, due to its impact on reproductive physiology rather than larval mortality.

15.4.2.4 The larval tarsal test (LTT)

The LTT is a more time-efficient and sensitive bioassay for screening multiple acaricide compounds and concentration ranges. Larvae are exposed to treated surfaces (e.g. multi-well plates), allowing evaluation of contact toxicity through tarsal (leg) absorption. Studies by Lovis *et al.* (2011, 2013) demonstrated that LTT can produce resistance ratios comparable to those observed in the LPT, despite using significantly lower lethal concentrations, sometimes up to 150-fold lower. This method simplifies handling by eliminating the need for direct manipulation of mobile larvae, thereby improving throughput and consistency.

15.4.2.5 The syringe immersion test (SIT)

The SIT is a practical adaptation of the m-LIT, wherein tick larvae are exposed to acaricide-treated environments within modified syringes lined with mesh or cloth. Eggs are allowed to hatch directly within the syringe chamber, minimizing the handling of live larvae. Initially introduced by Souza *et al.* (2008) for acaricide screening, SIT was later adapted for testing natural products, including plant extracts, against *R. (Boophilus) microplus* (Sindhu *et al.*, 2012). Comparative studies between SIT, m-LIT and LPT indicate that, at least for amitraz, LPT offers superior reliability for resistance diagnostics (Santos *et al.*, 2013). Nonetheless, recent assessments (Robaina *et al.*, 2023) suggest that SIT is equally effective as m-LIT in determining ML toxicity in *R. microplus* populations in Brazil. Together, these bioassays provide complementary insights into resistance patterns and help guide effective tick-control strategies.

15.4.3 Molecular assays used to detect resistance

Specific single nucleotide polymorphisms (SNPs) associated with acaricide resistance in *R. appendiculatus* have not been conclusively identified. While resistance mechanisms have been studied, detailed molecular characterizations, particularly SNPs linked to resistance, remain limited. In contrast, extensive research on *R. microplus* has identified several SNPs associated with resistance to various acaricide classes (Rodriguez-Vivas *et al.*, 2018; FAO, 2025). The correlation between the frequency of resistance-conferring alleles (as determined by molecular assay) in a specific tick population and their phenotypic resistance (as measured by bioassay or *in vivo* testing) is not always strong or consistent. The inconsistency raises concerns about the reliability of molecular assays alone for accurately predicting phenotypic resistance, and this limits their standalone utility in guiding treatment decisions for farmers.

On the other hand, specific SNPs associated with acaricide resistance can occur in either a homozygous or heterozygous state, and this distinction plays a crucial role in understanding the dynamics of resistance within tick populations. In a study performed in *R. microplus* from Brazil and South Africa, ticks homozygous for the kdr (knock-down resistance)-type allele were less susceptible to the acaricide, particularly at higher concentrations (Heylen *et al.*, 2024). These homozygous ticks are often able to survive standard acaricide treatments and can pass the resistance trait to all offspring if they mate with another homozygous resistant individual, leading to a rapid spread of resistance through the population. In contrast, ticks that are heterozygous for the resistance allele exhibit partial resistance or reduced sensitivity to the acaricide, indicating the mutation is considered a recessive mutation, as previously reported by other authors (Li *et al.*, 2014). In some cases, these ticks might still be killed by treatment, but if the resistance trait is dominant or co-dominant, they may survive and continue to propagate the allele.

Monitoring the frequency of homozygous and heterozygous individuals in a population provides essential insights into the stage and severity of resistance development. A high proportion of heterozygotes may indicate the early emergence of resistance in a tick population, serving as an early warning for resistance management interventions. Conversely, a high number of individuals homozygous for the resistance allele signals that the resistance is well established, and the acaricide in question may no longer be effective. This genetic information is therefore vital for guiding the selection of acaricides, implementing rotational strategies and developing sustainable tick-control programmes.

If only presence/absence of a resistance allele is required, fast and reliable PCR-based field tests for acaricide resistance offer a significant advantage over traditional bioassays by providing rapid, precise and mechanism-specific detection of resistance. Unlike bioassays, which often require weeks to complete due to the need for tick collection, rearing and exposure to acaricides, molecular tests can yield results within hours to a few days. These assays, such as quenching of unincorporated amplification signal reporters (QUASR)-PCR (Meiring and Labuschagne, 2024), allow for the direct identification of resistance-associated mutations (e.g. kdr mutation) without the need for live tick handling or *in vivo* testing. Their high sensitivity enables early detection of resistance alleles in field populations, supporting timely and targeted intervention strategies. As such, molecular tools, if available, represent a powerful complement to conventional methods, particularly in integrated resistance management programmes. As mentioned in the recently published FAO guidelines (FAO, 2025), development of an integrated surveillance system for ticks, tick-borne diseases and acaricide resistance is a long-term goal for the risk assessment and adaptation of control strategies. The fragmented data available from different geographies indicate the importance of monitoring capabilities at the regional/country level.

15.5 Vaccines

The vast majority of studies of immunity to ticks and vaccine development in cattle have focused on the one-host tick *R. microplus* because of its economic importance in cattle production throughout large parts of Australasia, Central and South America and Africa. In addition to acting as a vector for babesiosis and anaplasmosis, heavy infestations with the tick cause reduced productivity and sometimes death of the host. Herein, approaches to vaccine development against *R. microplus* will be outlined and their applicability to *R. appendiculatus* briefly discussed.

15.5.1 Naturally acquired resistance

As discussed above (in Section 15.2.2), cattle acquire a degree of resistance to tick infestation following initial exposure to tick challenge. *Bos indicus* cattle develop much higher levels of resistance compared to *B. taurus*, resulting in tick burdens that are 10–20% of those observed in *B. taurus*. In the case of cattle with acquired resistance to *R. microplus*, loss of ticks following tick challenge occurs mainly in the first 24 hours following larval attachment. Ticks find resistant animals unsuitable for feeding in that some fail to feed and those that do so make more frequent and shorter attachments and, on completion of feeding, have lower body weights than ticks fed on naïve animals (Kemp *et al.*, 1986). Attachment of ticks to hosts with acquired resistance provokes a marked immediate type hypersensitivity reaction. Since this response is stronger in the more resistant *B. indicus* animals compared to *B. taurus*, it is considered to be important in mediating resistance (Willadsen *et al.*, 1978). It is characterized by cellular infiltrates into the tick attachment sites, containing numerous polymorphonuclear leukocytes, eosinophils and mast cells, many of which are degranulating, accompanied by serous exudation that contains elevated levels of histamine (Schleger *et al.*, 1976; Robbertse *et al.*, 2018). Increased numbers of B and T lymphocytes are also present in the bite site. The hypersensitivity reactions cause irritation at the tick feeding sites, which results in increased grooming in animals with acquired resistance, contributing to loss of ticks (Snowball, 1956).

15.5.2 Immunization against tick infestation

Cattle with acquired resistance to *R. microplus* produce antibodies reactive with proteins in tick saliva. Some these proteins have been isolated and shown to provoke cutaneous immediate type hypersensitivity reactions when inoculated intradermally into resistant cattle (Willadsen *et al.*, 1978). Attempts to immunize cattle with these and other salivary proteins have resulted in a degree of immunity, but the levels of immunity have been no better than, and often inferior to, that achieved following natural exposure to the tick (Willadsen, 1980).

Tick saliva contains immunomodulatory proteins that suppress host immune responses to saliva, which, along with other activities in saliva, facilitates prolonged feeding (Wikel, 1999). Such modulation is likely to limit the efficacy of vaccine-induced responses to salivary antigens following tick challenge. Therefore, subsequent efforts to induce immunity have pursued an alternative strategy based on immunization with tick antigens that are not normally exposed to the host immune system (so-called 'concealed antigens') (Willadsen, 2004; De la Fuente *et al.*, 2007). Earlier studies by Allen and Humphreys (1979) had shown that immunization of guinea pigs with antigens prepared from the internal organs of *Dermacenter andersoni* ticks resulted in significant levels of protection against tick challenge. A series of studies of *R. microplus* in Australia demonstrated that immunization of cattle with homogenates and subsequently with tick gut fractions resulted in highly significant reduction in the tick burden following tick challenge (Kemp *et al.*, 1986). Fractionation of the tick guts led to the identification of a protective antigen (Bm86) (Willadsen *et al.*, 1989), which, when used to immunize cattle, resulted in approximately 80% reduction in tick burdens and a marked reduction in egg output from the surviving ticks. Anti-Bm86 antibodies caused death of feeding ticks as a result of direct damage to the tick gut epithelium and leakage of blood from the gut, the damaged ticks taking on a translucent red appearance (Agbede and Kemp, 1986; Kemp *et al.*, 1989). A recombinant version of Bm86 was used in a commercial vaccine that has been marketed in Australia and in South America (Willadsen *et al.*, 1995). The use of Bm86 as an immunomodulator has also been registered as a Conditionally Licensed product in the USA for the control of *R. microplus* and *R. annulatus* ticks in the Rio Grande Valley of Texas and Mexico border. Although the vaccine has proved to be effective in many areas, the immunity is not boosted by natural challenge and therefore frequent re-vaccination is required.

The success of Bm86 stimulated an upsurge of interest in anti-tick vaccines. Earlier studies of ticks and insects had shown that mammalian immunoglobulins in ingested blood cross the gut epithelium, allowing entry into the haemolymph. They retain their antigen-binding specificities (Schlein *et al.*, 1976), thus providing opportunities to target a variety of internal tick organs by vaccination. Recent advances in tick genome sequencing and transcriptomics have led to the identification of a plethora of antigens predicted to be potential targets for vaccination. These are discussed in a number of recent reviews (van Oosterwijk and Wikel, 2021; Abbas *et al.*, 2023). Recent research has provided evidence that combinations of two or more antigens that target different tick organ systems can provide enhanced immunity (reviewed by Ndawula and Tabor, 2020). Although promising results have been obtained with some of these antigens, no further commercial vaccines have been produced to date.

15.5.3 Applicability of vaccination to *R. appendiculatus*

There have been very few studies to investigate vaccination against *R. appendiculatus*. The antigens tested, including an orthologue of Bm86 (Ra86), have generally performed very poorly compared to the protection achieved with Bm86 against the one-host tick *R. microplus* (Imamura *et al.*, 2008; Olds *et al.*, 2012; Sabadin *et al.*, 2017). It should be noted that a subsequent study, which examined the sequences of Ra86 in field isolates of *R. appendiculatus* ticks, detected extensive sequence polymorphism, raising doubt about its value as a vaccine target antigen (Kamau *et al.*, 2016).

Based on current evidence that an anti-tick vaccine is unlikely to provide complete protection against tick infestation, it is unlikely to be of value as a primary tool for controlling ECF. However, use of an effective anti-tick vaccine might be of value alongside a vaccine for *T. parva* to reduce tick damage and further reduce the use of acaricides, but development of such a vaccine would require substantial financial investment.

15.5.4 Transmission-blocking vaccines

In recent years, there has been increasing interest in the possibility of vaccinating animal or human hosts to inhibit transmission of pathogens to arthropod vectors, as a means of reducing the reservoir of infection in the field. In the case of tick vectors, the concept is to generate antibodies to pathogen antigens that are involved in development in the tick, thus preventing establishment of infection. This approach has not been investigated for *T. parva*, but development of such an immunization protocol should be possible and one potential target antigen has been identified based on studies in mice (Havlíková *et al.*, 2009). However, it is doubtful whether a vaccine of this type would make a significant impact on the disease caused by *T. parva* in most field situations. A high level of transmission-blocking 'immunity' would be required, and all of the cattle in a given location would need to be vaccinated to have an impact on the parasite population. Since *T. parva* establishes a carrier state in cattle, animals already immune to *T. parva* would need to be vaccinated. Moreover, the presence of (unvaccinated) buffalo could undermine the effect of cattle vaccination.

15.6 Other Potential Control Measures

15.6.1 Pasture burning

Maintaining pastures and grazing areas through practices such as mowing, controlled burning and removing leaf litter can reduce tick habitats and population density. Implementing rotational grazing, where pastures are rested and rotated, can help break the tick life cycle and reduce the buildup of tick populations (George *et al.*, 2004). Field burning, particularly prescribed burning, has been shown to significantly reduce the density of *R. appendiculatus* ticks. A study conducted in Zambia compared tick burdens across areas with early burning, late burning and no burning. The results indicated that areas without burning had the highest tick burdens, with up to 200 ticks per transect, while both early and late burning regimes resulted in substantially lower tick densities. Although no significant differences were observed between early and late burning, both were effective in reducing tick populations compared to areas with no burning (Bhagoos *et al.*, 2023). On the other hand, previous studies performed in the Kruger National Park in South Africa revealed a temporary reduction of tick populations of *R. appendiculatus* after burning, which indicated limited practical use as control option. In particular, subsequent host influx when the vegetation recovers might substantially negate the overall benefit of burning, and without the exclusion of major tick hosts in the burned area, burning would not be recommended as a tick-control option (Spickett *et al.*, 1992).

In most African countries, rotational grazing or field burning is limited, especially as grazing land is shared among community members and regulated by traditional authorities rather than individual legal ownership.

15.6.2 Biological control

Conventional methods of tick control, primarily relying on synthetic acaricides, have been widely employed to reduce tick populations and mitigate disease transmission in many parts of the world, especially in LMIC where livestock production is challenged by ticks and the pathogens they transmit. However, prolonged and indiscriminate use of acaricides has led to the emergence of resistance in multiple tick species, environmental contamination and residues in animal products, necessitating the exploration of sustainable alternatives (Abbas *et al.*, 2014; Rodriguez-Vivas *et al.*, 2018; Evans *et al.*, 2024). Biological control offers a promising alternative by leveraging natural enemies of ticks and environmentally friendly agents to suppress tick populations. As discussed below, this approach includes the use of entomopathogenic fungi, nematodes, predators, parasitoids and microbial pathogens, as well as plant-based compounds with acaricidal properties.

15.6.2.1 Entomopathogenic fungi

Among the most studied biological agents for tick control are entomopathogenic fungi, particularly *Metarhizium anisopliae* (now often referred to as *M. brunneum*) and *Beauveria bassiana*. These fungi infect ticks through direct contact, with conidia adhering to the tick's cuticle, germinating and penetrating the exoskeleton. Subsequent fungal proliferation within the host leads to its death. These fungi have demonstrated effectiveness against multiple tick species in controlled settings, but environmental factors like humidity and temperature significantly influence their efficacy (Fernandes and Bittencourt, 2008; Samish *et al.*, 2014; Kaaya and Hassan, 2000).

The use of *Metarhizium* spores to reduce tick loads by environmental spraying when applied in suburban settings is unlikely to cause meaningful reductions in the abundance of non-target arthropods, resulting in limited impact on biodiversity (Fischhoff *et al.*, 2017).

15.6.2.2 Natural predators

Predation represents a key ecological mechanism in regulating arthropod populations and may contribute to the suppression of tick densities when incorporated into Integrated Tick Management programmes.

Oxpeckers (*Buphagus erythrorhynchus* and *B. africanus*) are obligate ectoparasite feeders native to the savannahs and open grasslands of sub-Saharan Africa. These birds frequently associate with large wild and domestic ungulates and are known to feed on engorged adult ticks. Observational studies suggest that oxpeckers can reduce tick burdens by mechanically removing ticks during grooming, although the efficacy varies depending on host accessibility and oxpecker population density (Weeks, 2000). Given the preference of oxpeckers for feeding on blood at wounds or the feeding site of a previously removed tick, and the inability of cows to prevent oxpeckers from doing so, they may not be beneficial in the end (Weeks, 1999).

Guinea fowl (*Numida meleagris*), a domesticated bird species commonly kept in rural and peri-urban African settings, are ground foragers that consume various arthropods, including ticks. Although empirical evidence on their predatory efficiency against ticks is limited, reports and small-scale trials have suggested that guinea fowl can significantly reduce tick populations in grazing areas (Massawe, 2019). Their effectiveness, however, may be influenced by seasonal availability of ticks and competing food sources. Additionally, guinea fowl are hosts of the immature stage of different tick species.

However, in addition to avian wildlife species, keeping domestic chicken with cattle may serve as an easy alternative as they can ingest several species of ticks and up to 81 ticks per chicken per hour (Dreyer *et al.*, 1997).

15.6.2.3 Entomopathogenic nematodes (EPNs)

EPNs, particularly those from the Steinernematidae and Heterorhabditidae families, have garnered attention as potential biological control agents against ticks, including species prevalent in Africa. EPNs infect ticks by entering through natural openings, releasing symbiotic bacteria that proliferate within the host, leading to its death. Unlike their interaction with insect hosts, EPNs do not reproduce within tick cadavers, which may influence their long-term efficacy in tick population control (Samish *et al.*, 2000). Innovative delivery methods, such as using infected insect cadavers, have been explored to enhance EPN efficacy. This approach has shown promise in semi-field conditions, particularly against *R. microplus* (Filgueiras *et al.*, 2023).

15.6.2.4 Entomoparasitic wasps

Entomoparasitic wasps, particularly *Ixodiphagus hookeri*, have been studied for their potential in biologically controlling tick populations, including species prevalent in Africa. *Ixodiphagus hookeri* is a minute encyrtid wasp (approximately 0.8–0.9 mm in length) that parasitizes ticks by laying its eggs inside them. The wasp's larvae develop within the tick, ultimately leading to the host's death. The presence of the symbiotic bacterium *Wolbachia pipientis* in *I. hookeri* may aid in suppressing the tick's immune response, facilitating successful parasitism. In Africa, *I. hookeri* has been observed parasitizing tick species such as *Amblyomma variegatum* and *R. appendiculatus*. A field study in Kenya involved releasing approximately 150,000 *I. hookeri* wasps over a year on a 4 ha pasture with ten zebu cattle. The study reported a 95% reduction in *A. variegatum* populations on the cattle, while no significant effect was observed on *R. appendiculatus* (Mwangi *et al.*, 1997; Demas *et al.*, 2002).

15.6.2.5 Botanical substances

Botanical extracts and essential oils are gaining recognition as alternative acaricides in the management of ixodid ticks, with active compounds derived from various plant parts, including leaves, stems, bark, roots, seeds and flowers. These plant-based substances act through multiple mechanisms, disrupting nerve transmission, respiration and membrane permeability, and often show both lethal and sub-lethal effects, such as repellency, feeding deterrence, growth inhibition and reduced reproductive potential.

Three broad categories are distinguished: (i) plants *in situ*, (ii) plant extracts and (iii) essential oils. *In situ* control involves using intact plants with anti-tick properties. For instance, *Melinus minutiflora* and *Andropogon gayanus* reduce *R. microplus* larval activity in pasture, while *M. minutiflora* repels *R. appendiculatus* instars (Mwangi *et al.*, 1995). However, effects tend to be modest and slow to manifest (Showler and Saelao, 2022). Despite advantages such as organic status, multi-modal activity and resistance suppression, challenges remain: inconsistent efficacy due to plant variability, short residual action, non-target effects and scalability constraints. Nevertheless, botanical acaricides offer promising tools in integrated tick management, especially in regions where conventional chemicals face resistance or regulatory barriers.

15.7 Integrated Control Strategies

In many ECF-endemic areas, control of the disease is heavily reliant on use of acaricides to reduce tick infestation and prevent challenge with *T. parva*. However, the use of acaricides alone is labour-intensive and costly, and their intensive use runs the risk of selecting acaricide resistance in the tick population. The latter can be alleviated by rotational use of different classes of acaricides. However, the integrated use of acaricides with other disease control measures, by reducing the amounts and frequency of application of acaricide required, would provide cheaper and more sustainable means of controlling ECF. Use of the Infection and Treatment Method (ITM) ECF vaccine (and any other vaccines that become available in the future) is an obvious option. In circumstance where calves can be closely monitored for early clinical signs of ECF, as described by Nanteza *et al.* (2023), early chemotherapy of affected animals, in conjunction with reduced acaricide use, could be employed. Reduced acaricide use is also possible in indigenous breeds of cattle, which exhibit a degree of resistance to ECF.

Integrated ECF control programmes should be locally tailored, cost-effective and community-supported. Combining vaccination, smart tick control, resistant cattle and improved grazing practices offers the best long-term solution, especially for small-scale farmers in LMICs.

15.8 Concluding Remarks

Controlling *R. appendiculatus* in Africa with the aim of limiting clinical cases of ECF and increasing productivity will continue to rely heavily on the use of chemical acaricides, although their use has some disadvantages. Resistance to acaracides has been detected in *R. appendiculatus*, although it is not clear how quickly or broadly it will spread, nor whether it will extend to all classes of acaricides. There are also realistic concerns about environmental contamination and the health impacts of acaricides. Despite these, and the monetary and labour-associated costs involved, farmers will continue to rely on chemical control as the most effective and affordable option to control ticks. As discussed elsewhere in this volume, other means of control of the tick vector or the disease caused by *T. parva* are promising but will not supplant acaricide use in the immediate future. They may play an increasing role in integrated management of the disease and delay the emergence of resistance to acaricides.

In summary, locally adapted, farmer-led integrated control programmes based around decreasing the use of acaricides offer the best path towards sustainable management of tick-borne diseases across diverse African landscapes. Alternative approaches have limitations and require further research and development before they can be implemented in the field. The focus, therefore, should still be on minimizing acaricide resistance.

References

Abbas, M.N., Jmel, M.A., Mekki, I., Dijkgraaf, I. and Kotsyfakis, M. (2023) Recent advances in tick antigen discovery and anti-tick vaccine development. *International Journal of Molecular Sciences* 24(5), 4969. DOI: 10.3390/ijms24054969.

Abbas, R.Z., Zaman, M.A., Colwell, D.D., Gilleard, J. and Iqbal, Z. (2014) Acaricide resistance in cattle ticks and approaches to its management: The state of play. *Veterinary Parasitology* 203(1–2), 6–20. DOI: 10.1016/j.vetpar.2014.03.006.

Adakal, H., Biguezoton, A., Zoungrana, S., Courtin, F., De Clercq, E.M. *et al.* (2013) Alarming spread of the Asian cattle tick *Rhipicephalus microplus* in West Africa – another three countries are affected: Burkina Faso, Mali and Togo. *Experimental & Applied Acarology* 61(3), 383–386. DOI: 10.1007/s10493-013-9706-6.

Adehan, S.B., Biguezoton, A., Adakal, H., Assogba, M.N., Zoungrana, S. *et al.* (2016) Acaricide resistance of *Rhipicephalus microplus* ticks in Benin. *African Journal of Agricultural Research* 11(14), 1199–1208. DOI: 10.5897/AJAR2015.10619.

Agbede, R.I.S. and Kemp, D.H. (1986) Immunization of cattle against *Boophilus microplus* using extracts derived from adult female ticks: Histopathology of ticks feeding on vaccinated cattle. *International Journal for Parasitology* 16(1), 35–41. DOI: 10.1016/0020-7519(86)90062-7.

Agwunobi, D.O., Yu, Z. and Liu, J. (2021) A retrospective review on ixodid tick resistance against synthetic acaricides: Implications and perspectives for future resistance prevention and mitigation. *Pesticide Biochemistry and Physiology* 173, 104776. DOI: 10.1016/j.pestbp.2021.104776.

Akhtar, M., Muhammad, F., Lodhi, L.A., Hussain, I. and Anwar, M.I. (2011) Immunity against ticks – a review. *Pakistan Veterinary Journal* 31, 529–536.

Allen, J.R. and Humphreys, S.J. (1979) Immunization of guinea-pigs and cattle against ticks. *Nature* 280, 491–493. DOI: 10.1038/280491a0.

Benitez, D., Cetra, B. and Florin-Christensen, M. (2012) *Rhipicephalus (Boophilus) microplus* ticks can complete their life cycle on the water buffalo (*Bubalus bubalis*). *Journal of Buffalo Science* 1(2), 193–197. DOI: 10.6000/1927-520X.2012.01.02.11.

Bhagoos, M., Siame, T., Munyeme, M. and Mwase, E.T. (2023) Comparative analysis of tick burden, diversity, and distribution in intensively managed wildlife estates with and without prescribed burning. *GSC Advanced Research and Reviews* 17(3), 169–180. DOI: 10.30574/gscarr.2023.17.3.0483.

Binnington, K.C. and Kemp, D.H. (1980) Role of tick salivary glands in feeding and disease transmission. *Advances in Parasitology* 18, 315–339. DOI: 10.1016/S0065-308X(08)60403-0.

Bock, R.E., de Vos, A.J., Kingston, T.G. and McLellan, D.J. (1997) Effect of breed of cattle on innate resistance to infection with *Babesia bovis*, *B bigemina* and *Anaplasma marginale*. *Australian Veterinary Journal* 75(5), 337–340. DOI: 10.1111/j.1751-0813.1997.tb15706.x.

Coopers (2025). Available at: https://www.coopersanimalhealth.com.au (accessed 25 June 2025).

De Deken, R., Martin, V., Saido, A., Madder, M., Brandt, J. *et al.* (2007) An outbreak of East Coast fever on the Comoros: A consequence of the import of immunised cattle from Tanzania? *Veterinary Parasitology* 143(3–4), 245–253. DOI: 10.1016/j.vetpar.2006.08.018.

De la Fuente, J., Almazán, C., Canales, M., Pérez de la Lastra, J.M., Kocan, K.M. *et al.* (2007) A ten-year review of commercial vaccine performance for control of tick infestations on cattle. *Animal Health Research Reviews* 8(1), 23–28. DOI: 10.1017/S1466252307001193.

De Rouck, S., İnak, E., Dermauw, W. and Van Leeuwen, T. (2023) A review of the molecular mechanisms of acaricide resistance in mites and ticks. *Insect Biochemistry and Molecular Biology* 159, 103981. DOI: 10.1016/j.ibmb.2023.103981.

Demas, F.A., Mwangi, E.N., Hassanali, A., Kunjeku, E.C. and Mabveni, A.R. (2002) Visual evaluation and recognition of hosts by the tick parasitoid, *Ixodiphagus hookeri* (Hymenoptera: Encyrtidae). *Journal of Insect Behavior* 15(4), 477–494. DOI: 10.1023/A:1016377132585.

Dolan, T.T. (1999) Dogmas and misunderstandings in East Coast fever. *Tropical Medicine & International Health* 4(9). DOI: 10.1046/j.1365-3156.1999.00445.x.

Dreyer, K.A.R.I.N., Fourie, L.J. and Kok, D.J. (1997) Predation of livestock ticks by chickens as a tick-control method in a resource-poor urban environment. *Onderstepoort Journal of Veterinary Research* 64, 273–276.

Drummond, R.O., Ernst, S.E., Trevino, J.L., Gladney, W.J. and Graham, O.H. (1973) *Boophilus annulatus* and *B. microplus*: Laboratory tests of insecticides. *Journal of Economic Entomology* 66(1), 130–133. DOI: 10.1093/jee/66.1.130.

Evans, A., Madder, M., Fourie, J., Halos, L., Kumsa, B. *et al.* (2024) Acaricide resistance status of livestock ticks from East and West Africa and *in vivo* efficacy of acaricides to control them. *International Journal for Parasitology: Drugs and Drug Resistance* 25, 100541. DOI: 10.1016/j.ijpddr.2024.100541.

FAO (2025) *Guidelines for Sustainable Tick Control and Acaricide Resistance Management in Livestock*. FAO, Rome. Available at: https://openknowledge.fao.org/server/api/core/bitstreams/5ebf63fd-6ca5-470c-a652-f58d9ed929a5/content (accessed 25 June 2025).

Fawcett, D.W., Büscher, G. and Doxsey, S. (1982) Salivary gland of the tick vector of East Coast fever. III. The ultrastructure of sporogony in *Theileria parva*. *Tissue and Cell* 14(1), 183–206. DOI: 10.1016/0040-8166(82)90017-9.

Fernandes, É.K.K. and Bittencourt, V.R.E.P. (2008) Entomopathogenic fungi against South American tick species. *Experimental and Applied Acarology* 46(1–4), 71–93. DOI: 10.1007/s10493-008-9161-y.

Filgueiras, M.D.G., Matos, R.S., Barreto, L.P., Mascarin, G.M., Rizzo, P.V. *et al.* (2023) From the laboratory to the field: Efficacy of entomopathogenic nematodes to control the cattle tick. *Pest Management Science* 79(1), 216–225. DOI: 10.1002/ps.7190.

Fischhoff, I.R., Keesing, F. and Ostfeld, R.S. (2017) The tick biocontrol agent *Metarhizium brunneum* (= *M. anisopliae*) (strain F52) does not reduce non-target arthropods. *PLoS ONE* 12(11), e0187675. DOI: 10.1371/journal.pone.0187675.

Gallina, T., dos Santos Lagranha, C., Bilo, G., Malavolta, C., Ferreira, L.L. *et al.* (2024) Control of *Rhipicephalus microplus* on taurine cattle with fluralaner in a subtropical region. *Parasites & Vectors* 17(1), 101. DOI: 10.1186/s13071-024-06200-0.

Gauer, M., Mackenstedt, U., Mehlhorn, H., Schein, E., Zapf, F. *et al.* (1995) DNA measurements and ploidy determination of developmental stages in the life cycles of *Theileria annulata* and *T. parva*. *Parasitology Research* 81(7), 565–574. DOI: 10.1007/BF00932023.

George, J.E., Pound, J.M. and Davey, R.B. (2004) Chemical control of ticks on cattle and the resistance of these parasites to acaricides. *Parasitology* 129(Suppl. S1), S353–S366. DOI: 10.1017/s0031182003004682.

Havlíková, S., Roller, L., Koci, J., Trimnell, A.R., Kazimírová, M. *et al.* (2009) Functional role of 64P, the candidate transmission-blocking vaccine antigen from the tick, *Rhipicephalus appendiculatus*. *International Journal for Parasitology* 39(13), 1485–1494. DOI: 10.1016/j.ijpara.2009.05.005.

Henson, S., Bishop, R.P., Morzaria, S., Spooner, P.R., Pelle, R. *et al.* (2012) High-resolution genotyping and mapping of recombination and gene conversion in the protozoan *Theileria parva* using whole genome sequencing. *BMC Genomics* 13, 503. DOI: 10.1186/1471-2164-13-503.

Heylen, D.J.A., Labuschagne, M., Meiring, C., van der Mescht, L., Klafke, G. *et al.* (2024) Phenotypic and genotypic characterization of acaricide resistance in *Rhipicephalus microplus* field isolates from South Africa and Brazil. *International Journal for Parasitology: Drugs and Drug Resistance* 24, 100519. DOI: 10.1016/j.ijpddr.2023.100519.

Imamura, S., Konnai, S., Vaz, I. da S.J., Yamada, S., Nakajima, C. *et al.* (2008) Effects of anti-tick cocktail vaccine against *Rhipicephalus appendiculatus*. *The Japanese Journal of Veterinary Research* 56(2), 85–98.

Jonsson, N.N., Piper, E.K. and Constantinoiu, C.C. (2014) Host resistance in cattle to infestation with the cattle tick *Rhipicephalus microplus*. *Parasite Immunology* 36(11), 553–559. DOI: 10.1111/pim.12140.

Kaaya, G.P. and Hassan, S. (2000) Entomogenous fungi as promising biopesticides for tick control. *Experimental & Applied Acarology* 24(12), 913–926. DOI: 10.1023/A:1010722914299.

Kamau, L.M., Skilton, R.A., Githaka, N., Kiara, H., Kabiru, E. *et al.* (2016) Extensive polymorphism of RA86 genes in field populations of *Rhipicephalus appendiculatus* from Kenya. *Ticks and Tick-Borne Diseases* 7(5), 772–781. DOI: 10.1016/j.ttbdis.2016.03.011.

Kanhai, G.K., Pegram, R.G., Hargreaves, S.K., Hove, T. and Dolan, T.T. (1997) Immunisation of cattle in Zimbabwe using *Theileria parva* (Boleni) without concurrent tetracycline therapy. *Tropical Animal Health and Production* 29(2), 92–98. DOI: 10.1007/BF02632324.

Katzer, F., Lizundia, R., Ngugi, D., Blake, D. and McKeever, D. (2011) Construction of a genetic map for *Theileria parva*: Identification of hotspots of recombination. *International Journal for Parasitology* 41(6), 669–675. DOI: 10.1016/j.ijpara.2011.01.001.

Kemp, D.H., Agbede, R.I.S., Johnston, L.A.Y. and Gough, J.M. (1986) Immunization of cattle against *Boophilus microplus* using extracts derived from adult female ticks: Feeding and survival of the parasite on vaccinated cattle. *International Journal for Parasitology* 16(2), 115–120. DOI: 10.1016/0020-7519(86)90096-2.

Kemp, D.H., Pearson, R.D., Gough, J.M. and Willadsen, P. (1989) Vaccination against *Boophilus microplus*: Localization of antigens on tick gut cells and their interaction with the host immune system. *Experimental & Applied Acarology* 7(1), 43–58. DOI: 10.1007/BF01200452.

Khan, A., Mushtaq, M.H., Ahmad, M., Tipu, Y., Khan, A. *et al.* (2013) Tick infestation rate in cattle and buffalo in different areas of Khyber Pakhtunkhwa, Pakistan. *Journal of Veterinary and Animal Sciences (Lahore)* 3, 31–35.

Klafke, G.M., Sabatini, G.A., de Albuquerque, T.A., Martins, J.R., Kemp, D.H. *et al.* (2006) Larval immersion tests with ivermectin in populations of the cattle tick *Rhipicephalus (boophilus) microplus* (Acari: Ixodidae) from state of Sao Paulo, Brazil. *Veterinary Parasitology* 142(3–4), 386–390. DOI: 10.1016/j.vetpar.2006.07.001.

Klafke, G.M., Castro-Janer, E., Mendes, M.C., Namindome, A. and Schumaker, T.T.S. (2012) Applicability of bioassays for the diagnosis of ivermectin resistance in *Rhipicephalus microplus* (Acari: Ixodidae). *Veterinary Parasitology* 184(2–4), 212–220. DOI: 10.1016/j.vetpar.2011.09.018.

Lessard, P.L., L'Eplatterier, R., Norval, R.A.I., Kundert, K., Dolan, T.T. *et al.* (1990) Geographic information systems for studying the epidemiology of cattle diseases caused by *Theileria parva*. *Veterinary Record* 126, 255–262.

Leta, S., Clercq, E.M. and Madder, M. (2013) High-resolution predictive mapping for *Rhipicephalus appendiculatus* (Acari: Ixodidae) in the horn of Africa. *Experimental and Applied Acarology* 60, 531–542. DOI: 10.1007/s10493-013-9670-1.

Li, A.Y., Davey, R.B., Miller, R.J., Guerrero, F.D. and George, J.E. (2014) Genetics and mechanisms of permethrin resistance in the Santa Luiza strain of *Boophilus microplus* (Acari: Ixodidae). *Journal of Medical Entomology* 45, 427–438.

Lontsi-Demano, M., Ngnindji-Youdje, Y., Laroche, M., Bamou, R., Talom, A.D. *et al.* (2020) Cattle trading favors the introduction and establishment of the invasive tick *Rhipicephalus (boophilus) microplus* in Menoua division, west region of Cameroon. *Journal of Entomology and Zoology Studies* 8, 207–214.

Lovis, L., Perret, J.-L., Bouvier, J., Fellay, J.-M., Kaminsky, R. *et al.* (2011) A new *in vitro* test to evaluate the resistance level against acaricides of the cattle tick, *Rhipicephalus (boophilus) microplus*. *Veterinary Parasitology* 182(2–4), 269–280. DOI: 10.1016/j.vetpar.2011.06.004.

Lovis, L., Mendes, M.C., Perret, J.-L., Martins, J.R., Bouvier, J. *et al.* (2013) Use of the larval tarsal test to determine acaricide resistance in *Rhipicephalus (boophilus) microplus* Brazilian field populations. *Veterinary Parasitology* 191(3–4), 323–331. DOI: 10.1016/j.vetpar.2012.09.011.

Madder, M., Speybroeck, N., Brandt, J., Tirry, L., Hodek, I. *et al.* (2002) Geographic variation in diapause response of adult *Rhipicephalus appendiculatus* ticks. *Experimental & Applied Acarology* 27(3), 209–221. DOI: 10.1023/a:1021694207456.

Madder, M., Speybroeck, N., Bilounga, A., Helleputte, D. and Berkvens, D. (2005) Survival of unfed *Rhipicephalus appendiculatus* and *Rhipicephalus zambeziensis* adults. *Medical and Veterinary Entomology* 19(3), 245–250. DOI: 10.1111/j.1365-2915.2005.00566.x.

Madder, M., Thys, E., Geysen, D., Baudoux, C. and Horak, I. (2007) *Boophilus microplus* ticks found in West Africa. *Experimental and Applied Acarology* 43(3), 233–234. DOI: 10.1007/s10493-007-9110-1.

Madder, M., Adehan, S., De Deken, R., Adehan, R. and Lokossou, R. (2012) New foci of *Rhipicephalus microplus* in West Africa. *Experimental and Applied Acarology* 56(4), 385–390. DOI: 10.1007/s10493-012-9522-4.

Massawe, U.E. (2019) Effectiveness of guinea fowl as biological control method for ticks in protected areas: A case of Saanane Island National Park, Mwanza region Tanzania. Doctoral dissertation, The Open University of Tanzania.

Mehlhorn, H. and Shein, E. (1984) The piroplasms: Life cycle and sexual stages. *Advances in Parasitology* 23, 37–103. DOI: 10.1016/s0065-308x(08)60285-7.

Mehlhorn, H., Schein, E. and Warnecke, M. (1978) Electron microscopic studies on the development of kinetes of *Theileria parva* Theiler 1904 in the gut of the vector ticks *Rhipicephalus appendiculatus*. *Revue Scientifique et Technique, Office International Des Epizooties* 34, 599–611.

Meiring, C. and Labuschagne, M. (2024) Using QUASR-PCR as a field-based genotyping assay for a tick acaricide resistance marker. *Scientific Reports* 14(1), 13584. DOI: 10.1038/s41598-024-64401-0.

Miyama, T., Byaruhanga, J., Okamura, I., Uchida, L., Muramatsu, Y. *et al.* (2020) Effect of chemical tick control practices on tick infestation and *Theileria parva* infection in an intensive dairy production region of Uganda. *Ticks and Tick-Borne Diseases* 11(4), 101438. DOI: 10.1016/j.ttbdis.2020.101438.

MSD (2025). Available at: https://www.exzolt.com.br (accessed 25 June 2025).

Mwangi, E.N., Essuman, S., Kaaya, G.P., Nyandat, E., Munyinyi, D. *et al.* (1995) Repellence of the tick *Rhipicephalus appendiculatus* by the grass *Melinis minutiflora*. *Tropical Animal Health and Production* 27(4), 211–216. DOI: 10.1007/BF02250692.

Mwangi, E.N., Hassan, S.M., Kaaya, G.P. and Essuman, S. (1997) The impact of *Ixodiphagus hookeri*, a tick parasitoid, on *Amblyomma variegatum* (Acari: Ixodidae) in a field trial in Kenya. *Experimental & Applied Acarology* 21(2), 117–126. DOI: 10.1023/b:appa.0000031790.30821.57.

Nagagi, Y.P., Kimaro, E.G. and Temba, V. (2020) Practical application and the possible emergence of tick resistance to commonly used acaricides in various districts of Tanzania. *Livestock Research for Rural Development* 32(8), 127.

Nanteza, A., Nsadha, Z., Nsubuga, J., Oligo, S., Kazibwe, A. *et al.* (2023) Assessment of the impact of early diagnosis and early treatment in the integrated control of East Coast fever (ECF) involving acquired immunity induced by natural infection in Ankole cattle. *Pathogens* 12(1), 115. DOI: 10.3390/pathogens12010115.

Ndawula, C. and Tabor, A.E. (2020) Cocktail anti-tick vaccines: The unforeseen constraints and approaches toward enhanced efficacies. *Vaccines* 8(3), 457. DOI: 10.3390/vaccines8030457.

Newson, R.M., Chiera, J.W., Young, A.S., Dolan, T.T., Cunningham, M.P. *et al.* (1984) Survival of *Rhipicephalus appendiculatus* (Acarina: Ixodidae) and persistence of *Theileria parva* (Apicomplexa: Theileriidae) in the field. *International Journal for Parasitology* 14(5), 483–489. DOI: 10.1016/0020-7519(84)90029-8.

Norval, R.A.I., Walker, J.R. and Colborne, J. (1982) The ecology of *Rhipicephalus zambeziensis* and *Rhipicephalus appendiculatus* (Acarina: Ixodae) with particular reference to Zimbabwe. *Ondersteport Journal of Veterinary Research* 49, 181–190.

Norval, R.A.I., Perry, B.D. and Young, A.S. (1992) *The Epidemiology of Theileriosis in Africa*. Academic Press, London.

Norval, R.A.I. (1994) Vectors: Ticks. In: Coetzer, J.A.W., Thomson, G.R. and Tustin, R.C. (eds) *Infectious Diseases of Livestock Diseases, with Special Reference to Southern Africa*. Oxford University Press, Cape Town, pp. 3–24.

Obaid, M.K., Islam, N., Alouffi, A., Khan, A.Z., da Silva Vaz Jr, I. *et al.* (2022) Acaricides resistance in ticks: Selection, diagnosis, mechanisms, and mitigation. *Frontiers in Cellular and Infection Microbiology* 12, 941831. DOI: 10.3389/fcimb.2022.941831.

Ochanda, H., Young, A.S., Medley, G.F. and Perry, B.D. (1998) Vector competence of 7 *Rhipicephalid tick* stocks in transmitting 2 *Theileria parva* parasite stocks from Kenya and Zimbabwe. *Parasitology* 116(Pt 6), 539–545. DOI: 10.1017/s0031182098002613.

Odongo, D.O., Ueti, M.W., Mwaura, S.N., Knowles, D.P., Bishop, R.P. *et al.* (2009) Quantification of *Theileria parva* in *Rhipicephalus appendiculatus* (Acari: Ixodidae) confirms differences in infection between selected tick strains. *Journal of Medical Entomology* 46(4), 888–894. DOI: 10.1603/033.046.0422.

Olds, C., Mwaura, S., Crowder, D., Odongo, D., van Oers, M. *et al.* (2012) Immunization of cattle with Ra86 impedes *Rhipicephalus appendiculatus* nymphal-to-adult molting. *Ticks and Tick-Borne Diseases* 3(3), 170–178. DOI: 10.1016/j.ttbdis.2012.03.003.

Perotto, D., Silva, N.L. da, Leite, M.C. de P., Souza, C.F. de and Souza, J.C. de (2025) Populational model of *Rhipicephalus microplus* in beef cattle in the southern region of Paraná, Brazil. *Veterinary Sciences* 12(3), 206. DOI: 10.3390/vetsci12030206.

Perry, B.D., Lessard, P., Norval, R.A., Kundert, K. and Kruska, R. (1990) Climate, vegetation and the distribution of *Rhipicephalus appendiculatus* in Africa. *Parasitology Today* 6(4), 100–104. DOI: 10.1016/0169-4758(90)90224-r.

Piper, E.K., Jonsson, N.N., Gondro, C., Lew-Tabor, A.E., Moolhuijzen, P. *et al.* (2009) Immunological profiles of *Bos taurus* and *Bos indicus* cattle infested with the cattle tick, *Rhipicephalus (boophilus) microplus*. *Clinical and Vaccine Immunology* 16(7), 1074–1086. DOI: 10.1128/CVI.00157-09.

Purnell, R.E. and Joyner, L.P. (1968) The development of *Theileria parva* in the salivary glands of the tick, *Rhipicephalus appendiculatus*. *Parasitology* 58(3), 725–732. DOI: 10.1017/s0031182000029036.

Randolph, S.E. (1997) Abiotic and biotic determinants of the seasonal dynamics of the tick *Rhipicephalus appendiculatus* in South Africa. *Medical and Veterinary Entomology* 11(1), 25–37. DOI: 10.1111/j.1365-2915.1997.tb00286.x.

Robaina, D., Caballero, J. and Suárez, G. (2023) Syringe immersion test as *in vitro* bioassay against *Rhipicephalus microplus*: Macrocyclic lactones dose-response relationship. *Open Veterinary Journal* 13(10), 1259–1267. DOI: 10.5455/OVJ.2023.v13.i10.4.

Robbertse, L., Richards, S.A., Clift, S.J., Barnard, A.-C., Leisewitz, A. *et al.* (2018) Comparison of the differential regulation of T and B-lymphocyte subsets in the skin and lymph nodes amongst three cattle breeds as potential mediators of immune-resistance to *Rhipicephalus microplus*. *Ticks and Tick-Borne Diseases* 9(4), 976–987. DOI: 10.1016/j.ttbdis.2018.03.034.

Roberts, J.A. (1968) Acquisition by the host of resistance to the cattle tick, *Boophilus microplus* (Canestrini). *The Journal of Parasitology* 54(4), 657. DOI: 10.2307/3277013.

Rodriguez-Vivas, R.I., Hodgkinson, J., Rosasdo-Aguilar, J.A., Villegas-Perez, S.L. and Trees, A.J. (2012) The prevalence of pyrethroid resistance phenotype and genotype in *Rhipicephalus (Boophilus) microplus* in Yucatan, Mexico. *Veterinary Parasitology* 184(2–4), 221–229. DOI: 10.1016/j.vetpar.2011.09.017.

Rodriguez-Vivas, R.I., Jonsson, N.N. and Bhushan, C. (2018) Strategies for the control of *Rhipicephalus microplus* ticks in a world of conventional acaricide and macrocyclic lactone resistance. *Parasitology Research* 117(1), 3–29. DOI: 10.1007/s00436-017-5677-6.

Sabadin, G.A., Parizi, L.F., Kiio, I., Xavier, M.A., da Silva Matos, R. *et al.* (2017) Effect of recombinant glutathione s-transferase as vaccine antigen against *Rhipicephalus appendiculatus* and *Rhipicephalus sanguineus* infestation. *Vaccine* 35(48), 6649–6656. DOI: 10.1016/j.vaccine.2017.10.026.

Sabatini, G.A., Kemp, D.H., Hughes, S., Nari, A. and Hansen, J. (2001) Tests to determine LC50 and discriminating doses for macrocyclic lactones against the cattle tick, *Boophilus microplus*. *Veterinary Parasitology* 95(1), 53–62. DOI: 10.1016/S0304-4017(00)00406-4.

Samish, M., Alekseev, E. and Glazer, I. (2000) Biocontrol of ticks by entomopathogenic nematodes: Research update. *Annals of the New York Academy of Sciences* 916(1), 589–594. DOI: 10.1111/j.1749-6632.2000.tb05341.x.

Samish, M., Rot, A., Ment, D., Barel, S., Glazer, I. *et al.* (2014) Efficacy of the entomopathogenic fungus *Metarhizium brunneum* in controlling the tick *Rhipicephalus annulatus* under field conditions. *Veterinary Parasitology* 206(3–4), 258–266. DOI: 10.1016/j.vetpar.2014.10.019.

Santos, T.R.B., Klafke, G.M., Pappen, F.G., Nizoli, L.Q., Biegelmeyer, P. *et al.* (2013) Comparison of three larval bioassays to evaluate susceptibility of *Rhipicephalus (boophilus) microplus* to amitraz. *Revista Brasileira de Parasitologia Veterinária* 22(4), 495–501. DOI: 10.1590/S1984-29612013000400008.

Schleger, A.V., Lincoln, D.T., McKenna, R.V., Kemp, D.H. and Roberts, J.A. (1976) *Boophilus microplus*: Cellular responses to larval attachment and their relationship to host resistance. *Australian Journal of Biological Sciences* 29(6), 499–512. DOI: 10.1071/BI9760499.

Schlein, Y., Spira, D.T. and Jacobson, R.L. (1976) The passage of serum immunoglobulins through the gut of *Sarcophaga falculata*. *Annals of Tropical Medicine & Parasitology* 70(2), 227–230. DOI: 10.1080/00034983.1976.11687116.

Shaw, R.D. (1966) Culture of an organophosphorus-resistant strain of *Boophilus microplus* (Can.) and an assessment of its resistance spectrum. *Bulletin of Entomological Research* 56(3), 389–405. DOI: 10.1017/s0007485300056480.

Shaw, M.K. and Young, A.S. (1995) Differential development and emission of *Theileria parva* sporozoites from the salivary gland of *Rhipicephalus appendiculatus*. *Parasitology* 111(2), 153–160. DOI: 10.1017/S0031182000064891.

Showler, A.T. and Saelao, P. (2022) Integrative alternative tactics for ixodid control. *Insects* 13(3), 302. DOI: 10.3390/insects13030302.

Šimo, L., Kazimirova, M., Richardson, J. and Bonnet, S.I. (2017) The essential role of tick salivary glands and saliva in tick feeding and pathogen transmission. *Frontiers in Cellular and Infection Microbiology* 7, 281. DOI: 10.3389/fcimb.2017.00281.

Sindhu, Z., Jonsson, N.N. and Iqbal, Z. (2012) Syringe test (modified larval immersion test): A new bioassay for testing acaricidal activity of plant extracts against *Rhipicephalus microplus*. *Veterinary Parasitology* 188(3–4), 362–367. DOI: 10.1016/j.vetpar.2012.03.021.

Snowball, G.J. (1956) The effect of self-licking of cattle on infestation of cattle tick *Boophilus microplus*. *Australian Journal of Agricultural Research* 7, 227–237. DOI: 10.1071/AR9560227.

Sonenshine, D.E. and Roe, R.M. (eds) (2014) *Biology of Ticks*, Vol. 2. Oxford University Press, New York.

Souza, A.P. de, Veiga, L.P.H.N., Bellato, V., Sartor, A.A., Cardoso, C.P. *et al.* (2008) Proposta para teste carrapaticida por imersão de larvas de *Rhipicephalus (boophilus) microplus*: avaliação em cipermetrina e amitraz. *Revista Brasileira de Parasitologia Veterinária* 17(4), 242–245. DOI: 10.1590/S1984-29612008000400014.

Spickett, A.M., Horak, I.G., Van Niekerk, A. and Braack, L.E. (1992) The effect of veld-burning on the seasonal abundance of free-living ixodid ticks as determined by drag-sampling. *The Onderstepoort Journal of Veterinary Research* 59(4), 285–292.

Stone, B.F. and Haydock, K.P. (1962) A method for measuring the acaricide-susceptibility of the cattle tick *Boophilus microplus* (Can.). *Bulletin of Entomological Research* 53(3), 563–578. DOI: 10.1017/S000748530004832X.

Tempia, S. (1997) Comparison of the vectorial capacity of *R. appendiculatus* (Acari: Ixodidae) nymphs and adults originating from Eastern and Southern provinces of Zambia infected by *Theileria parva* Katete stock. MSc thesis, Institute for Tropical Medicine, Antwerp, Belgium.

Theiler, A. (1911) The artificial transmission of East Coast fever. [Report of the Government Veterinary Bacteriologist]. Pretoria: Government Printer and Stationery Office, pp. 7–55.

Tindih, H.S., Marcotty, T., Naessens, J., Goddeeris, B.M. and Geysen, D. (2010) Demonstration of differences in virulence between two *Theileria parva* isolates. *Veterinary Parasitology* 168(3–4), 223–230. DOI: 10.1016/j.vetpar.2009.11.006.

Uilenberg, G. (1999) Immunization against diseases caused by *Theileria parva*: A review. *Tropical Medicine & International Health* 4(9), A12–A20. DOI: 10.1046/j.1365-3156.1999.00446.x.

van Oosterwijk, J.G. and Wikel, S.K. (2021) Resistance to ticks and the path to anti-tick and transmission blocking vaccines. *Vaccines* 9(7), 725. DOI: 10.3390/vaccines9070725.

Vudriko, P., Okwee-Acai, J., Tayebwa, D.S., Byaruhanga, J., Kakooza, S. *et al.* (2016) Emergence of multi-acaricide resistant *Rhipicephalus ticks* and its implication on chemical tick control in Uganda. *Parasites & Vectors* 9(1), 4. DOI: 10.1186/s13071-015-1278-3.

Wagland, B.M. (1978) Host resistance to cattle tick (*Boophilus microplus*) in Brahman (*Bos indicus*) cattle. II.* The dynamics of resistance in previously unexposed and exposed cattle. *Australian Journal of Agricultural Research* 29(2), 395–400. DOI: 10.1071/AR9780395.

Walker, A.R., Bouattour, A., Camicas, J.L., Estrada-Peña, A., Horak, I.G. *et al.* (2003) *Ticks of Domestic Animals in Africa: A Guide to Identification of Species*. Biosciences Reports, Edinburgh, UK.

Watt, D.M. and Walker, A.R. (2000) Pathological effects and reduced survival in *Rhipicephalus appendiculatus* ticks infected with *Theileria parva* protozoa. *Parasitology Research* 86(3), 207–214. DOI: 10.1007/s004360050033.

Weeks, P. (1999) Interactions between red-billed oxpeckers, *Buphagus erythrorhynchus*, and domestic cattle, *Bos taurus*, in Zimbabwe. *Animal Behaviour* 58(6), 1253–1259. DOI: 10.1006/anbe.1999.1265.

Weeks, P. (2000) Red-billed oxpeckers: Vampires or tickbirds? *Behavioral Ecology* 11(2), 154–160. DOI: 10.1093/beheco/11.2.154.

Wikel, S.K. (1999) Tick modulation of host immunity: An important factor in pathogen transmission. *International Journal for Parasitology* 29(6), 851–859. DOI: 10.1016/s0020-7519(99)00042-9.

Willadsen, P. (1980) Immunity to ticks. *Advances in Parasitology* 18, 293–311. DOI: 10.1016/s0065-308x(08)60402-9.

Willadsen, P. (2004) Anti-tick vaccines. *Parasitology* 129(Suppl. 1), S367–S387. DOI: 10.1017/s0031182003004657.

Willadsen, P., Williams, P.G., Roberts, J.A. and Kerr, J.D. (1978) Responses of cattle to allergens from *Boophilus microplus*. *International Journal for Parasitology* 8(2), 89–95. DOI: 10.1016/0020-7519(78)90003-6.

Willadsen, P., Riding, G., McKenna, R., Kemp, D., Tellam, R. *et al.* (1989) Identification of a protective antigen from *Boophilus microplus*. *Journal of Immunology* 143, 1346–1351. DOI: 10.4049/jimmunol.143.4.1346.

Willadsen, P., Bird, P., Cobon, G.S. and Hungerford, J. (1995) Commercialisation of a recombinant vaccine against *Boophilus microplus*. *Parasitology* 110(Suppl), S43–S50. DOI: 10.1017/s0031182000001487.

Young, A.S., Leitch, B.L. and Newson, R.M. (1981) The occurrence of a *Theileria parva* carrier state in cattle from an East Coast fever endemic area of Kenya. In: Irvin, A.D., Cunningham, M.P. and Young, A.S. (eds) *Advances in the Control of Theileriosis. Current Topics in Veterinary Medicine and Animal Science*. Springer, Dordrecht, The Netherlands, pp. 60–62.

Young, A.S., Leitch, B.L., Dolan, T.T., Newson, R.M., Ngumi, P.N. *et al.* (1983) Transmission of *Theileria parva* by a population of *Rhipicephalus appendiculatus* under simulated natural conditions. *Parasitology* 86(2), 255–267. DOI: 10.1017/S0031182000050423.

Young, A.S., Leitch, B.L. and Mutugi, J.J. (1984) Some factors controlling the stimulation of sporogony of *Theileria parva* in its tick vector *Rhipicephalus appendiculatus*. *International Journal for Parasitology* 14(1), 97–102. DOI: 10.1016/0020-7519(84)90018-3.

Young, A.S., Leitch, B.L., Morzaria, S.P., Irvin, A.D., Omwoyo, P.L. *et al.* (1987) Development and survival of *Theileria parva* in *Rhipicephalus appendiculatus* exposed in the Trans-Mara, Kenya. *Parasitology* 94(3), 433–441. DOI: 10.1017/S0031182000055785.

16 Future Research Priorities and Opportunities

W. Ivan Morrison[1]* and Philip Toye[2]
[1]*Roslin Institute, University of Edinburgh, Edinburgh, UK;* [2]*International Livestock Research Institute, Nairobi, Kenya*

16.1 Introduction

The assembly in this book of current knowledge on the diseases caused by *Theileria parva* and the measures used for their control has provided an opportunity to consider gaps in our understanding that constrain efforts to develop improved methods of control. Herein, we provide a brief outline of the areas we believe require further research. A convincing case can be made for investment in research on all or most of the topics discussed in this book, and specific research areas are covered in the individual chapters. However, some areas are of higher strategic importance with respect to developing novel and improved methods to control East Coast fever (ECF), and these are discussed in more depth in this chapter.

Section 16.2 presents two areas of research which, if successful, would transform the ECF landscape and possibly have application outside this disease. Both take advantage of the natural immunobiological features of the cattle hosts and the parasite. Section 16.3 includes other areas of research that would improve or safeguard current control measures, whilst Section 16.4 addresses issues of significant biological interest that may have a longer-term effect on disease control.

16.2 Research to Develop Novel Methods of Control

16.2.1 Vaccination

Ever since the first formal recognition of ECF and identification of *T. parva* as the causal agent, it has been recognized that animals that survive an initial infection develop robust immunity that prevents further episodes of the disease. It is obvious that vaccination to reproduce this artificially would be the most effective and sustainable method for controlling the disease. However, development of a widely acceptable method of vaccination has proved frustratingly difficult. The use of live parasites in the Infection and Treatment Method (ITM) of vaccination, developed in the 1970s, has been shown to provide robust, long-lasting immunity following a single inoculation. Although commercialization of the ITM vaccine was eventually achieved, the complexity of the production process and, more significantly, deficiencies in the distribution and marketing of the vaccine have limited its uptake. These shortcomings need to be addressed if the vaccine is to survive as a commercial entity. In any event, there is a need to establish a realistic strategy for development of more practical methods of vaccination against *T. parva*. Over the past three

*Corresponding author: Ivan.Morrison@ed.ac.uk

(eds W.I. Morrison and P. Toye)
DOI: 10.1079/9781800626324.0016

decades, research to develop such a vaccine has largely focused on testing candidate antigens, with little emphasis placed on addressing aspects of the host–parasite relationship that are barriers to vaccine development (so-called 'discovery research'). The 'quick-fix' approach of attempting to develop a vaccine within the 3–4 year lifespan of a research project is unrealistic and, unsurprisingly, has not been successful.

Investigation of approaches to vaccination must therefore be underpinned by studies to resolve biological and technical issues that are critical to achieving successful outcomes. A particularly glaring technical deficiency is the lack of methods for genetic manipulation of the parasite. The past decade has seen rapid advances in techniques that allow genetic modification of apicomplexan parasites. These techniques are now being used extensively in studies of malaria parasites to study the function of gene products and to ablate or modify gene expression. Yet, there have been no sustained attempts to establish these procedures for *T. parva*. As discussed below (Section 16.2.1.1), the availability of methods to genetically manipulate *T. parva* is required to fully explore development of a cell line-based vaccine. The need for these methods has also been highlighted in Chapter 10 of this volume as a major impediment to understanding the cell biology of the parasite and how it causes disease.

Attempts to immunize with sporozoite antigens, despite inducing high titres of neutralizing antibodies, have been unsuccessful, and achieving sustained levels of protective antibodies against this stage of the parasite seems unlikely. Given the overwhelming evidence that naturally acquired immunity against *T. parva* is mediated by T cell responses against schizont-infected cells, future research needs to focus on inducing immunity against this stage of the parasite.

16.2.1.1 Immunization with infected cells

Cultured *Theileria*-infected cell lines have been used successfully for many years to vaccinate cattle against *Theileria annulata*. However, the same approach has proved impractical for *T. parva* because of the much greater numbers of cells that are required to reproducibly induce immunity (~10^8 compared to ~10^6 for *T. annulata*). Induction of immunity against *T. annulata* and *T. parva* using infected cells depends on transfer of the parasite into the cells of recipient animals, which recent evidence indicates occurs as a result of spontaneous cell fusion between some of the infected cells and cells of recipient animals. Such fusion occurs much more frequently with cells infected with *T. annulata* than with *T. parva*. Hence, devising a means of increasing the efficiency of parasite transfer from *T. parva*-infected cells would allow immunization with smaller numbers of infected cells, which could be exploited to produce a commercially viable vaccine. This would entail genetically manipulating the infected cells to enhance their ability to fuse with cells of recipient animals. Appropriate modifications may become evident through identification of the host proteins that mediate cell fusion in *T. annulata* and that are not expressed as strongly in *T. parva*-infected cells. One such molecule under current investigation is Sirp A, which is involved in mediating fusion of human macrophages infected with *Mycobacterium tuberculosis* and is expressed on *T. annulata*-infected cells.

While use of parasite-infected cells for immunization would still have some of the disadvantages of a live vaccine, it would overcome many of the shortcomings of ITM. It would involve an entirely *in vitro* production process with greatly simplified standardization and quality control procedures, which would be more suitable for commercial development. Moreover, buffalo-derived strains of the parasite could be included, which is not possible with ITM. Although such a vaccine would still require cold storage, it could be distributed in a refrigerated form to end-users, similar to processes used for the *T. annulata* cell vaccines.

One of the disadvantages of using any live Theileria vaccine is the perceived risk of introducing the parasite genotypes in the vaccine into field tick populations. In the case of *T. annulata*, this has prohibited the use of a universal vaccine and has resulted in each country producing its own vaccine. For *T. parva*, it should be borne in mind that the parasite populations have been quite fluid due to the movement of hosts with carrier infections and opportunities for sexual recombination during tick transmission. The availability of methods to genetically manipulate the parasite should allow interference with the ability of parasites in cell line vaccines to infect erythrocytes, thus negating tick transmissibility.

Again, this would not be possible with parasites used in ITM, as the production process is dependent on tick transmission.

16.2.1.2 Development of an anti-schizont subunit vaccine

The evidence that parasite-specific CD8 T cell responses play a vital role in immunity has prompted research aimed at developing a vaccine using parasite antigens targeted by the protective CD8 response. Although several CD8 T cell target antigens have been identified, attempts to immunize cattle with some of these antigens delivered in viral vectors have provided protection in only a small proportion of animals. Continuation of this research is required, albeit with a renewed and tighter focus. Rather than 'blindly' testing different vaccine formulations, research needs initially to focus on areas that are critical in deciding which antigen delivery systems/formulations are appropriate for vaccine testing by (i) more clearly defining the characteristics of the protective T cell response and (ii) assessing which parasite antigens are most suitable for vaccination.

16.2.1.2.1 THE NATURE OF THE PROTECTIVE T CELL RESPONSE. Attempted immunization procedures using viral vectors resulted in CD8 T cell responses whose functional activity differed from that of CD8 T cells from animals immunized with live parasites, as evidenced by lack of cytotoxic activity. As argued in Chapter 11 of this volume, the functional defect of the CD8 T cell response may relate to the nature of the CD4 T cell response that regulates differentiation of the CD8 T cell response. Elucidating the functional characteristics of the T cell responses that mediate immunity will guide the choice of antigen delivery systems that are most likely to induce an appropriate immune response.

The induction of functionally defective T cell responses is also a feature of responses to primary infections with *T. parva*. As discussed in Chapters 4 and 11 of this volume, there is evidence that primary infection of naïve animals results in modulation of the host's T cell response, undermining its ability to recover and develop immunity. Unlike other parasites that also inhibit or avoid the host immune response, *T. parva* generates an early vigorous T cell response, but in contrast to the response generated in immune animals, the response in naïve animals lacks any effector activity against the parasite. This is believed to have evolved to delay clearance of the parasite and development of immunity. Furthermore, there is evidence that the immunomodulatory activity of the parasite is associated with infected T cells, as infections initiated with infected T cells result in lethal infections, whereas those initiated with infected B cells develop mild self-limiting infections.

These different systems provide powerful experimental models to interrogate the features of protective immune responses to *T. parva*, by conducting the following comparisons:

- the non-protective responses induced by immunization with viral vectors compared to the responses of immune animals;
- the non-protective response induced by infection of naïve animals compared to responses of immune animals; and
- the responses induced by infected T cells compared to responses induced by infected B cells.

16.2.1.2.2 THE CHOICE OF ANTIGENS FOR INCLUSION IN A SUBUNIT VACCINE. Experimental and field studies have revealed that the immunity against *T. parva* induced with live parasites can be parasite strain-restricted, reflecting polymorphism of the target antigens. However, several observations indicate that strain specificity of the immune response may not be as great an obstacle as might be envisaged (discussed in Chapter 11 of this volume), including the finding that only some of the target antigens identified to date exhibit substantial sequence polymorphism. The strain restriction of CD8 T cell responses to *T. parva* has been shown to be due to a profound immunodominance, resulting in individual animals responding to only one or a few of the CD8 T cell epitopes against which they are capable of responding. Further work is required to expand the list of known CD8 T cell antigens and to determine their degree of polymorphism. The aim of vaccine studies would be to focus on those antigens that show limited sequence polymorphism and to undertake experiments to identify antigens capable of inducing responses in animals of different MHC types.

16.2.2 Understanding and exploiting inherited resistance

Several long-standing studies clearly demonstrated the existence of resistance to ECF in indigenous cattle residing in endemic areas. In contrast to susceptible breeds of cattle, which suffer very high levels of mortality, a small percentage of the indigenous stock succumb upon initial exposure as calves, but most survive and develop immunity. Early researchers recognized the potential of this genetic pool, but attempts to exploit it through traditional breeding programmes were hindered by the low productivity of the indigenous cattle. The advent of powerful genomic technologies, by enabling identification of the genetic basis of the resistance, may now provide an avenue to redress that situation.

Recent progress has been made through a series of studies involving identification of a lineage of (usually susceptible) Boran cattle that survived infection with *T. parva* when introduced into a site where there is a high level of challenge from infected buffalo. Analyses of the inheritance in these animals identified a region in the genome that is strongly linked to the resistance phenotype. Further studies are required to identify precisely the causal allele, which would provide a more reliable marker for selection of resistance and may provide an indication of the mechanism of the resistance. In this regard, *in vitro* studies of cells from resistant animals have yielded initial evidence that resistance is associated with decreased multiplication of infected cells, results which were supported by earlier *in vivo* observations. Further studies are required to determine whether this is due to a direct effect on the infected cell, such as interference with the parasite's ability to induce proliferation, or is a result of another cell type that acts on the infected cells. Refinement of *in vitro* methods to reflect the resistance phenotype could facilitate development of an *in vitro* biological assay for predicting resistance status.

In order to explore the feasibility of commercial exploitation of this resistance genotype, available data need to be analysed to estimate the financial benefit to livestock owners of using resistant cattle, through reduced mortality and morbidity and decreased use of acaricides.

Based on the findings of the earlier studies, it is clear that other genes are also involved in determining resistance in indigenous breeds of cattle. In the longer term, with further advances in genetics, analyses of the resistance in these animals should be pursued to identify additional markers of resistance.

16.3 Research to Support Current Control Measures

16.3.1 Up-to-date information on the impact of the disease

While there is little doubt that *T. parva* remains one of the most important pathogens of cattle in Africa and causes enormous economic losses, precise information on the current economic burden of the disease is fragmentary and of variable quality. Such information is required not only to inform policy makers and research funders but also to provide a baseline against which new interventions to control the parasite can be evaluated. In Chapter 2 of this volume, a standardized framework for collecting field data is proposed, which can be used to obtain more accurate figures on the cost of the disease by collecting data from representative livestock production systems in different countries. This would also allow meaningful comparisons of the impact of the disease in different regions and different cattle management systems. Whilst it is acknowledged that obtaining the raw data to populate the framework is a non-trivial exercise, the refined methodology and some of the population data would extend to other livestock diseases. Indeed, full justification of the funding to undertake this exercise would necessitate its encompassing several important diseases in addition to ECF. Without this approach, the true impact of ECF and the effectiveness of any control measure will be difficult to assess accurately.

16.3.2 Surveillance for resistance to current acaricides

Prevention of tick infestation by subjecting cattle to regular application of acaricides has remained the principal means of controlling ECF for most of the past century. The acute and fatal nature of the disease requires intensive use of acaricides in many areas to achieve effective control. It is not uncommon for cattle to be treated with acaricide every 5 days. In addition to the costs of materials and labour and the attendant environmental contamination, such intensive use of acaricides poses a significant threat of selecting for acaricide resistance in the tick populations. More extensive surveillance for acaricide resistance in tick populations is required to ensure that resistance can be detected at an early stage, allowing modifications in tick-control practices to minimize the impact of resistance. This should include all pathogen-transmitting tick species and not just *Rhipicephalus appendiculatus*.

16.3.3 Development of novel acaricides and therapeutics

In Chapters 14 and 15 of this volume, a strong case is made for the development of novel acaricides and therapeutics. For the former, these are required to combat the anticipated increase in resistance, and for the latter, another low-cost therapeutic with a different mode of action than buparvaquone would be very valuable to counteract the likelihood of emergence of resistance to buparvaquone. Given the scope and methodology required to develop these compounds, this area of research lies much more in the realm of established commercial entities.

16.4 Other Aspects of the Biology of the Parasite

16.4.1 Tick transmissibility of *T. parva*

Infections of cattle with parasites transmitted from buffalo rarely develop to the piroplasm stage, which is necessary for further transmission of the parasite. The more restricted genetic diversity of cattle-maintained *T. parva* compared to that of parasites found in buffalo is thought to be due to a subset of buffalo parasites that adapted to tick transmission in cattle. The continued divergence of the two parasite populations indicates that such adaptation to cattle does not occur, or occurs very infrequently, in current parasite populations. However, as discussed in Chapter 5 of this volume, three experimental studies have reported that repeated passage of buffalo parasites in cattle using large numbers of ticks resulted in the emergence of readily transmissible parasites similar to those found in naturally infected cattle. That this 'behavioural transformation' rarely occurs in the field is probably because the conditions of these experiments (i.e. serial passage of the same parasite population with large numbers of ticks) are unlikely to be replicated under field conditions.

Recent rapid advances in genetic tools to study *T. parva* now provide an opportunity to investigate the genetic basis of tick transmissibility of these parasites. Although this topic of research might be viewed as of lower strategic relevance than the topics discussed above, it could yield insight into the genes involved in differentiation of the parasite during merogony, and provide genetic markers to predict the likely tick transmissibility of buffalo parasites. These markers could be used to select appropriate parasite types for use in live vaccines in response to concerns about 'vaccine' genotypes entering field circulation.

16.4.2 Host cell invasion and cell tropism

Studies conducted in the 1980s with East African isolates of *T. parva* demonstrated that sporozoites are able to infect T and B lymphocytes, including CD4, CD8 and gamma/delta T cell subsets. Sporozoites also bound to and entered monocytes and dendritic cells but were unable to establish infection in these cell types. More recently, a Zambian isolate of *T. parva* (Chitongo), which is of lower virulence than East African strains, was shown to infect only CD8 T cells. It is unclear whether this is a frequently occurring phenotype, and its precise role in affecting virulence of the parasite is not understood. As discussed in Chapter 3 of this volume, invasion of bovine lymphocytes by sporozoites involves a complex series of events, implying that multiple molecular interactions are likely to be involved. Studies of immune responses to the sporozoite stage of the parasite in the 1980s identified a sporozoite surface protein (p67) that is involved in initial binding to target lymphocytes and induces antibody responses capable of neutralizing the infectivity of sporozoites *in vitro*. The sequence of the p67 gene in the Chitongo strain is identical to that of East African strains, indicating that other proteins must be involved in determining the different tropism. Since the mid-1990s, studies of sporozoite invasion of bovine lymphocytes have largely been abandoned, and there has been little effort to identify other parasite proteins involved in the cell invasion process, although a recent study has identified another two sporozoite proteins that stimulate strong neutralizing antibody responses. Correspondingly, the host cell proteins involved in binding and entry of sporozoites have not been identified. Given the crucial importance of the sporozoite–lymphocyte interaction in infection, there is a need to renew efforts in this area to identify the proteins involved in cell invasion and the molecular basis of differences in tropism.

Index

Note:– Page numbers in **bold** type refer to figures; page numbers in *italic* type refer to tables.

Printed and bound by CPI Group (UK) Ltd, Croydon, CR0 4YY
13/09/2026
14961113-0004